CLINICAL TRANSESOPHAGEAL ECHOCARDIOGRAPHY

A PROBLEM-ORIENTED APPROACH

SECOND EDITION

CLINICAL TRANSESOPHAGEAL ECHOCARDIOGRAPHY

A PROBLEM-ORIENTED APPROACH

SECOND EDITION

Editors

STEVEN N. KONSTADT, M.D.

Professor
Department of Anesthesiology
Co-Director
Division of Cardiothoracic Anesthesia
The Mount Sinai Medical Center
New York, New York

STANTON K. SHERNAN, M.D.

Assistant Professor
Department of Anesthesiology
Perioperative and Pain Medicine
Brigham & Women's Hospital
Boston, Massachusetts

YASU OKA, M.D.

Professor Emeritus
Department of Anesthesiology
Albert Einstein College of Medicine
Bronx, New York
Professorial Lecturer
Department of Anesthesiology
Mount Sinai Medical Center
New York, New York

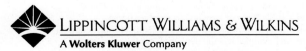

LIPPINCOTT WILLIAMS & WILKINS
A **Wolters Kluwer** Company

Philadelphia • Baltimore • New York • London
Buenos Aires • Hong Kong • Sydney • Tokyo

Acquisitions Editor: R. Craig Percy
Developmental Editor: Jenny Kim
Production Editor: Jennifer Vogt
Manufacturing Manager: Benjamin Rivera
Cover Designer: Karen Quigley
Compositor: TechBooks

© 2003 by LIPPINCOTT WILLIAMS & WILKINS
530 Walnut Street
Philadelphia, PA 19106 USA
LWW.com

Printed in China

Library of Congress Cataloging-in-Publication Data

Clinical transesophageal echocardiography : a problem-oriented approach / [edited by]
Steven N. Konstadt, Stanton K. Shernan, Yasu Oka.— 2nd ed.
    p. ; cm.
   Includes bibliographical references and index.
   ISBN 0-7817-3938-1
   1. Transesophageal echocardiography.   I. Konstadt, Steven N.   II. Shernan, Stanton K.
III. Oka, Yasu.
   [DNLM: 1. Echocardiography, Transesophageal.   WG 141.5.E2 C6415 2003]
RD52.T73C55   2003
616.1′207543—dc21

                                                    2003040088

Care has been taken to confirm the accuracy of the information presented and to describe generally accepted practices. However, the authors, editors, and publisher are not responsible for errors or omissions or for any consequences from application of the information in this book and make no warranty, expressed or implied, with respect to the currency, completeness, or accuracy of the contents of the publication. Application of this information in a particular situation remains the professional responsibility of the practitioner.

The authors, editors, and publisher have exerted every effort to ensure that drug selection and dosage set forth in this text are in accordance with current recommendations and practice at the time of publication. However, in view of ongoing research, changes in government regulations, and the constant flow of information relating to drug therapy and drug reactions, the reader is urged to check the package insert for each drug for any change in indications and dosage and for added warnings and precautions. This is particularly important when the recommended agent is a new or infrequently employed drug.

Some drugs and medical devices presented in this publication have Food and Drug Administration (FDA) clearance for limited use in restricted research settings. It is the responsibility of the health care provider to ascertain the FDA status of each drug or device planned for use in their clinical practice.

10 9 8 7 6 5 4 3 2 1

Dedicated to my family for their boundless support and inspiration
S.N.K.

CONTENTS

CONTRIBUTING AUTHORS

Solomon Aronson, M.D. Chicago, Illinois

Alexander N. Chapochnikov, M.D., Ph.D. Rockford Anesthesiologists Associated; Swedish-American Hospital; and OSF St. Anthony Medical Center, Rockford, Illinois

Albert T. Cheung, M.D. Associate Professor, Department of Anesthesiology, University of Pennsylvania; and Division of Cardiothoracic Anesthesia and Critical Care, Hospital of the University of Pennsylvania, Philadelphia, Pennsylvania

Randall Correia, M.D. Department of Anesthesiology, Cleveland Clinic Foundation, Cleveland, Ohio

Lori Bray Croft, M.D. Assistant Professor and Attending Physician, Department of Cardiology, The Mount Sinai Medical Center, New York, New York

A. Jackson Crumbley III, M.D. Associate Professor, Department of Surgery; and Chief, Thoracic Organ Transplantation Service, Medical University of South Carolina, Charleston, South Carolina

Ellise Delphin, M.D., M.P.H. Professor and Chair, Department of Anesthesiology, UMDNJ–New Jersey Medical School; and Chief of Service, Department of Anesthesiology, UMDNJ–University Hospital, Newark, New Jersey

James A. DiNardo, M.D. Associate Professor, Department of Anesthesia, Boston Children's Hospital, Harvard Medical School, Boston, Massachusetts

Edward A. Fisher, M.D. Associate Clinical Professor and Associate Attending, Department of Medicine, Mount Sinai Hospital, New York, New York

Martin E. Goldman, M.D. Dr. Arthur and Hilda Mester Professor of Medicine, Department of Medicine/Cardiology, Mount Sinai Medical School; and Director of Echocardiography, Department of Cardiology, Mount Sinai Hospital, New York, New York

Katherine P. Grichnik, M.D. Associate Professor, Department of Anesthesiology, Duke University Medical Center, Durham, North Carolina

Gregg S. Hartman, M.D. Associate Professor of Anesthesiology, Director of Cardiac Anesthesia, Department of Anesthesiology, Dartmouth Medical School, Hanover, New Hampshire; and Department of Anesthesiology, Dartmouth-Hitchcock Medical Center, Lebanon, New Hampshire

Kristine J. Hirsch, M.D. Assistant Professor, Department of Anesthesia, Halifax Infirmary, Queen Elizabeth II Health Sciences Center, Halifax, Nova Scotia, Canada

David Jayakar, M.D. Assistant Professor and Attending Physician, Department of Cardiac Surgery, University of Chicago, Chicago, Illinois

Ronald A. Kahn, M.D. Associate Professor of Anesthesiology and Surgery, Divisional Director of Vascular Anesthesia, Department of Anesthesiology, The Mount Sinai Medical Center, New York, New York

Marc Kanchuger, M.D. Assistant Professor and Co-Director of Cardiothoracic Anesthesiology, Department of Anesthesiology, New York University School of Medicine, New York, New York

Steven N. Konstadt, M.D. Professor, Department of Anesthesiology, Co-Director, Division of Cardiothoracic Anesthesia, The Mount Sinai Medical Center, New York, New York

A. Stephane Lambert, M.D. Assistant Professor, Department of Anesthesia, St. Michael's Hospital, University of Toronto, Toronto, Ontario, Canada

Martin J. London, M.D. Professor of Clinical Anesthesia, Department of Anesthesia and Perioperative Care, University of California, San Francisco; and Attending Anesthesiologist, Anesthesia Service, Veterans Affairs Medical Center, San Francisco, California

Eric K. Louie, M.D. Professor, Department of Medicine, Division of Cardiology, Stritch School of Medicine, Loyola University, Maywood, Illinois; and Manager, Medicine and Neurology Service Line, Edward Hines, Jr. Veterans Affairs Hospital, Hines, Illinois

Jonathan B. Mark, M.D. Professor and Vice Chairman, Department of Anesthesiology, Duke University Medical Center; and Chief, Department of Anesthesiology Service, Veterans Affairs Medical Center, Durham, North Carolina

Andrew Maslow, M.D. Department of Anesthesiology, Rhode Island Hospital; and Assistant Professor, Department of Anesthesiology, Brown University Medical School, Providence, Rhode Island

Bonnie Milas, M.D. Assistant Professor, Department of Anesthesiology, University of Pennsylvania, Hospital of the University of Pennsylvania, Philadelphia, Pennsylvania

Yasu Oka, M.D. Professor Emeritus, Department of Anesthesiology, Albert Einstein College of Medicine, Bronx, New York; and Professorial Lecturer, Department of Anesthesiology, Mount Sinai Medical Center, New York, New York

Kazumasa Orihashi, M.D. Assistant Professor, Department of Surgery, Programs for Applied Medicine, Graduate School of Biomedical Sciences, Hiroshima University; and Chief, Division of Thoracic and Cardiovascular Surgery, Hiroshima University Hospital, Hiroshima, Japan

Enrique J. Pantin, M.D. Assistant Professor, Department of Anesthesiology, University of Medicine and Dentistry of New Jersey; and Assistant Professor, Department of Anesthesiology, Robert Wood Johnson University Hospital, New Brunswick, New Jersey

Scott T. Reeves, M.D. Associate Professor, Department of Anesthesia and Perioperative Medicine, Medical University of South Carolina, Charleston, South Carolina

David L. Reich, M.D. Professor, Department of Anesthesiology, The Mount Sinai Medical Center, New York, New York

Sandra I. Reynertson, M.D. Associate Professor, Department of Medicine, Stritch School of Medicine, Loyola University, Maywood, Illinois; and Medical Director, Coronary Care Unit, Department of Medicine, Edward Hines, Jr. Veterans Affairs Hospital, Hines, Illinois

Adam B. Rosenbluth, M.D. Fellow, Department of Cardiology, Mount Sinai Hospital, New York, New York

Ivan S. Salgo, M.D. Corporate Technical Staff, Philips Medical Systems, Andover, Massachusetts

Robert M. Savage, M.D. Staff, Department of Anesthesiology, Cleveland Clinic Foundation, Cleveland, Ohio

Joseph S. Savino, M.D. Associate Professor, Department of Anesthesia, University of Pennsylvania School of Medicine; and Section Chief, Cardiovascular Thoracic Anesthesia and Intensive Care Unit, Department of Anesthesia, Hospital of the University of Pennsylvania, Philadelphia, Pennsylvania

Rebecca A. Schroeder, M.D. Associate Professor, Department of Anesthesiology, Duke University Medical Center, Durham, North Carolina

Jack S. Shanewise, M.D. Associate Professor and Director of Cardiothoracic Service, Department of Anesthesia, Emory University, Atlanta, Georgia

Stanton K. Shernan, M.D. Assistant Professor, Department of Anesthesiology, Perioperative, and Pain Medicine, Brigham & Women's Hospital, Harvard Medical School, Boston, Massachusetts

Linda Shore-Lesserson, M.D. Associate Professor, Department of Anesthesiology, Mount Sinai School of Medicine; and Attending Anesthesiologist, Department of Anesthesiology, Mount Sinai New York University Medical Center, New York, New York

Alann Solina, M.D. Associate Professor, Vice Chairman, and Division Chief of Cardiac Anesthesiology, UMDNJ-Robert Wood Johnson Medical School, New Brunswick, New Jersey

Marc E. Stone, M.D. Assistant Professor, Department of Anesthesiology, The Mount Sinai Medical Center, New York, New York

Scott C. Streckenbach, M.D. Instructor, Department of Anesthesia, Harvard Medical School; and Assistant Anesthetist, Department of Anesthesia and Critical Care, Massachusetts General Hospital, Boston, Massachusetts

Christopher A. Troianos, M.D. Chair and Program Director, Department of Anesthesiology, Mercy Hospital of Pittsburgh, Pittsburgh, Pennsylvania

PREFACE

Since its introduction into clinical practice in the 1980s, the utility of perioperative transesophageal echocardiography (TEE) has become increasingly more evident as anesthesiologists, cardiologists, and surgeons continue to appreciate its potential applications. Initially TEE was used only to examine left ventricular function, then to diagnose a broad range of hemodynamic problems. Now it is recognized as a tool to make complex diagnostic decisions and to guide and evaluate pharmacological and surgical interventions.

A recent survey of 155 United States academic institutions reported that 91% of these institutions routinely use perioperative TEE (1). TEE provides real time, noninvasive imaging of the heart and great vessels while simultaneously permitting quantification of blood flow and overall cardiac performance without interrupting the surgical procedure. The popularity of perioperative TEE is based on the fact that it may significantly impact perioperative cardiac surgical decision-making by providing pertinent information regarding hemodynamic management, cardiac valvular function, and the diagnosis of congenital heart lesions and great vessel pathology (2,3). Consequently, the information provided by a comprehensive echocardiographic examination can significantly contribute to the perioperative management of cardiac surgical patients.

Recent publications describing the indications for performing perioperative TEE and the technique for acquiring a comprehensive TEE examination have facilitated the growth of this important diagnostic tool (4,5). In addition, the introduction of guidelines for credentialing and certification, including the development of examinations sponsored by the National Board of Echocardiography (6), have all supported an increasing demand for interdisciplinary education and training in the optimal utilization of perioperative TEE. Another advance in the field of perioperative TEE is the Standardized Perioperative Report form created by a joint task force of the Society of Cardiovascular Anesthesiologists and the American Society of Echocardiography. With all of these developments in perioperative TEE, the echocardiographer has to meet higher standards.

Rapid advances in technology and application of perioperative TEE have provided the incentive to produce the second edition of *Clinical Transesophageal Echocardiography: A Problem-Oriented Approach.* The key improvements of this new edition are briefly summarized here:

- This edition combines the elements of our two earlier books (*Oka & Goldiner* and *Clinical Transesophageal Echocardiography: A Problem Oriented Approach,* First Edition) with both didactic basic and advanced chapters as well as case-based discussions.
- To enhance learning, there is a new format with bulleted summary points and suggested readings indicated in bold.
- New surgical procedures such as minimally invasive aortic repair are covered.
- Multiplane imaging has almost entirely replaced biplane imaging.

In more detail throughout the text multiple diagrams, graphic illustrations, and superior quality two-dimensional, M-mode, and Doppler TEE images are used to emphasize the importance of visual imagery in interpreting echocardiographic data. Section I of this text provides a concise foundation of practical information pertaining to the basic principles of ultrasound image acquisition, optimization, and artifacts as well as the interpretation and orientation of echocardiographic anatomical views. In addition, guidelines for education and safety along with perioperative service-related topics in perioperative TEE are reviewed. Section II of the text focuses on specific clinical applications of perioperative TEE including detailed evaluations of ventricular function and hemodynamics, as well as valvular, aortic, pericardial, and great vessel pathology. This section also reviews the utility of echocardiography for evaluating endocarditis, masses, defects, and surgical devices. Section III of this text is unique in its format of using problem-oriented case discussions to emphasize the relevance and utility of perioperative TEE. Commonly encountered clinical scenarios including mitral valve disease, congestive heart failure, myocardial ischemia and infarction, aortic pathology, trauma, lung transplantation, and the echocardiographic evaluation of perioperative hypotension are reviewed.

It is our sincere hope that this text will serve as a classic resource of practical information by providing an interdisciplinary foundation of clinically relevant knowledge for both novice and experienced practitioners of perioperative TEE.

Steven N. Konstadt, M.D.
Stanton K. Shernan, M.D.
Yasu Oka, M.D.

References

1. Poterack KA. Who uses transesophageal echocardiography in the operating room? *Anesth Analg* 1995;80:454–458.
2. Savage RM, Lytle BW, Aronson S, et al. Intraoperative echocardiography is indicated in high-risk coronary artery bypass grafting. *Annals of Thoracic Surgery* 1997;64:368–373.
3. Mishra M, Chauhan R, Sharma KK, et al. Real-time intraoperative transesophageal echocardiography—how useful? Experience of 5,016 cases. *J Cardiothorac Vasc Anesth* 1998;12:625–632.
4. Shanewise JS, Cheung AT, Aronson S, et al. ASE/SCA Guidelines for performing a comprehensive intraoperative multiplane transesophageal echocardiography examination: recommendations of the American Society of Echocardiography Council for Intraoperative Echocardiography and the Society of Cardiovascular Anesthesiologists task force for certification in perioperative transesophageal echocardiography. *Anesth Analg* 1999;89:870–874.
5. Cahalan MK, Abel M, Goldman M, et al. American Society of Echocardiography and Society of Cardiovascular Anesthesiologists task force guidelines for training in perioperative echocardiography. *Anesth Analg* 2002;94:1384–1388.
6. Aronson S, Thys D. Training and certification in perioperative transesophageal echocardiography: a historical perspective. *Anesth Analg* 2001;93:1422–1427.

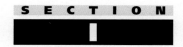

BASIC PRINCIPLES

PRINCIPLES OF ULTRASOUND

RONALD A. KAHN
IVAN S. SALGO

ULTRASOUND WAVE PROPERTIES

Sound waves are mechanical vibrations that may be transmitted through a given media. These sound waves may be described by several characteristics: frequency, wavelength, and amplitude. Frequency is defined as the number of oscillations per unit time. The usual unit of frequency is hertz (Hz), which is defined as cycles per second. While the range of frequencies that may be heard by the human ear is 20 to 20,000 Hz, ultrasound frequencies begin above 20 kHz. Medical echocardiographic imaging usually uses frequencies from 3 to 10 MHz.

Wavelength is defined as the distance between each individual cycle of ultrasound, usually expressed in millimeters. The relationship between frequency and wavelength is:

$$c = \gamma \bullet f$$

where c is the propagation speed of the ultrasound signal in a given medium, γ is the wavelength, and f is the frequency. If the propagation speed is constant, frequency and wavelength are inversely related. Since the propagation velocity of ultrasound in the soft tissue is 1,540 m/s, wavelength and frequency may be deduced by the following relationship:

$$1.54 = \gamma(\text{mm}) \bullet f(\text{Mhz})$$

The resolution of a particular ultrasound signal is limited by its wavelength: the shorter the wavelength (e.g., the higher the ultrasound frequency), the higher the resolution. Although fine resolution is desired during diagnostic evaluation, these high-frequency ultrasound signals are rapidly attenuated during propagation, resulting in poor ultrasound penetration. Lower-frequency ultrasound is attenuated less during propagation, resulting in deeper penetration of the ultrasound signal. The fine resolution associated with high frequencies must be balanced against the ability to image deeper structures with lower frequencies.

R. A. Kahn: Department of Anesthesiology, The Mount Sinai Medical Center, New York, New York.
I. S. Salgo: Philips Medical System, Andover, Massachusetts.

The height of an ultrasound wave is described as its amplitude. The usual unit of amplitude is decibel (dB), which is the logarithmic ratio of the signal to a given reference signal. This logarithmic expression of scale allows compression of many orders of magnitude into a compact range. This conversion simplifies the process of signal amplification and attenuation; signal amplitudes may be added or subtracted, respectively, thus avoiding the more complex computations associated with multiplication and division.

ULTRASOUND INTERACTIONS

Acoustic impedance is defined as the velocity that an ultrasound signal traverses a particular media multiplied by the media's density. Normally an ultrasound wave travels along a straight line though a medium of a homogeneous acoustical impedance. When an ultrasound wave reaches an interface of differing impedances, it will either be reflected or refracted. The basis of ultrasound imaging depends on the reflection of the ultrasound waves from a given tissue interface or boundary to the ultrasound transducer; the greater the difference in tissue impedance, the greater the reflection of the ultrasound wave. Bone has a very high acoustical impedance (high density and high propagation velocity), whereas gas has a low acoustical impedance (low density and low propagation velocity). Because of these extreme differences in acoustical impedances compared with soft tissue, ultrasound waves are predominately reflected from any air or bone interfaces, thus limiting deeper ultrasound penetration and imaging.

When large smooth objects (with respect to the ultrasound wavelength) are encountered by the ultrasound, they reflect ultrasound waves smoothly and at predictable angles like a mirror; this reflection is known as a specular reflection. These specular reflections are produced when the width of the reflecting object is larger than one fourth of the wavelength of the ultrasound, explaining the dependency of axial resolution on frequency. The display of specular echos is highly dependent on angle. Specular echos will return to the transducer only if the ultrasound is perpendicular to the reflected interface; if this interface is not perpendicular, the ultrasound may be reflected away from the transducer. This phenomenon explains the lower resolution associated with structures parallel to the ultrasound beams such as the lateral and septal myocardial boarders. In contrast to specular reflection, ultrasound may be scattered by tissue interfaces significantly smaller than the ultrasound wavelength. This scatter results in the random deflection of ultrasound signals throughout tissue, significantly decreasing the return of ultrasound signals to the transducer. These scattered echos are important both in the visualization of either homogeneous or small objects as well as the visualization of structures that are parallel to the ultrasound waves. Finally, the direction of the ultrasound wave may be changed, which is known as refraction. Refraction may result in the misregistration of a structure in an ultrasound image.

Attenuation refers to the loss of ultrasound power as it traverses tissue. Tissue attenuation is dependent on ultrasound reflection, scattering, and absorption. The absorption occurs as a result of the conversion of ultrasound energy into heat. The greater the ultrasound reflection and scattering, the less ultrasound energy is available for penetration and resolution of deeper structures; this effect is especially important during scanning with higher frequencies. While water, blood, and muscle have low tissue impedance with resultant low ultrasound attenuation, air and bone have very high tissue ultrasound impedance, limiting the ability of ultrasound to traverse these structures.

IMAGE FORMATION

Transducers

Piezoelectric crystals convert ultrasound and electrical signals. When presented with a high-frequency electrical signal, these crystals produce ultrasound energy, which is directed toward the areas to be imaged. Commonly, a short ultrasound signal is emitted from the piezoelectric crystal. After ultrasound wave formation, the crystal "listens" for the returning echoes for a given period of time and then pauses prior to repeating this cycle. This cycle length is known as the pulse repetition frequency (PRF). This cycle length must be long enough to provide enough time for a signal to travel to and return from a given object of interest. Typically, PRF varies from 1 to 10 kHz, which results in 0.1 to 1 msec between pulses. When reflected, ultrasound waves return to these piezoelectric crystals, and they are converted into electrical signals, which may be appropriately processed and displayed. Electronic circuits measure the time delay between the emitted and received echo. Since the speed of ultrasound through tissue is a constant, this time delay may be converted into the precise distance between the transducer and tissue.

The three-dimensional shape of the ultrasound beam is dependent on both the physical aspects of the ultrasound signal as well as the design of the transducer. An unfocused ultrasound beam may be thought of as an inverted funnel, where the initial straight columnar area is known as the "near

field" (also known as the Fresnel zone) followed by conical divergent area known as the "far field" (also known as the Fraunhofer zone). The length of the near field is directly proportional to the square of the transducer diameter and inversely proportional to the wavelength, specifically,

$$F_n = D^2/4\lambda$$

where F_n is the near field length, D is the diameter of the transducer, and λ is the ultrasound wavelength. Increasing the frequency of the ultrasound increases the length of the near field. The angle of the far field convergence (θ) is directly proportional to the wavelength and inversely proportional to the diameter of the transducer and is expressed by the equation:

$$\sin \theta = 1.22\lambda/D$$

Further geometric shaping of the beam may be adjusted using acoustical lenses or the shaping of the piezoelectric crystal. Ideally, imaging should be performed within the near field or focused aspect of the ultrasound beam, since the ultrasound beam is most parallel and the tissue interfaces are most perpendicular to these ultrasound beams.

Resolution

An ultrasound image may be described by its axial, lateral, or elevational resolution. Resolution defines the ability to define two point targets as distinct. *Axial resolution* is the minimum separation between two interfaces located in a direction parallel to the beam so that they can be imaged as two different interfaces. The most precise image resolution is along this axial plane. The higher the frequency of the ultrasound signal, the greater the axial resolution, since ultrasound waves of shorter wavelengths may be used. The shorter the burst of the emitted ultrasound wave (e.g., the shorter the pulse length), the greater the axial resolution, because of the increased ability to differential adjacent interfaces. Pulse duration should be no greater than two or three cycles. The range of frequencies contained within a given ultrasound transmission is referred to as the frequency bandwidth. Generally the shorter the pulse of the ultrasound produced, the greater the frequency bandwidth. Because of the relationship between short pulse lengths and high bandwidths, high bandwidths are associated with better axial resolution. High transducer bandwidths also allows for better resolution of deeper structures.

Lateral resolution is the minimum separation of two interfaces aligned along a direction perpendicular to the ultrasound beam. The most important determinant of lateral resolution is the ultrasound beam width or ultrasound beam focusing; the narrower the beam, the better the lateral resolution. If a small object appears within the near field, it can be resolved laterally accurately; if it appears within the far field, however, the size of this small object will appear to increase with the increased width of the ultrasound beam.

This increase in size with far field imaging results in blurring of deeper structures. *Elevational resolution* refers to the ability to determine differences in the thickness of the imaging plane. The thickness of the ultrasound beam is a major determinant of elevational resolution. Some probes can focus in the elevation direction as well, keeping the focus on target.

Instrumentation

Ultrasound machines allow for standard image controls. Preprocessing describes the modifications performed on the analog and digital signal prior to storage in the computer memory, whereas postprocessing refers to image manipulation after its entry into memory. The output power of the ultrasound beam is the amplitude of the power of the ultrasound signal delivered by the transducer. As previously discussed, a given ultrasound signal decreases in strength with deeper penetration, because of reflection and scatter. Without adjustment, the closer structure would appear to be brighter because of stronger specular echo, whereas deeper structures would appear darker because of this diminution of ultrasound power. Time gain compensation (TGC) controls allow for the separate adjustment of gain based on the depth of a particular structure. The TGC controls are usually adjusted such that near structures are set for lower gains with gradually increasing gains of deeper structures. The depth control adjusts the PRF, allowing for less or greater image penetration. If interrogation of deeper structures is required, the PRF must be decreased, which results in decreases in temporal resolution, since lower frame rates must be used.

The gain and attenuation controls of a scanner increase and decrease the intensity of all signals proportionally, changing the number of detected echo signals by bringing them above or below the rejection threshold of the dynamic range (DR). The receiver gain adjusts the scale that reflected ultrasound signals are displayed. This adjustment has parallels with the volume control of audio equipment, which increase or decrease the volume of a given signal. To deal with the potential loss of image quality caused by the display of the larger number of insignificant echoes obtained at high settings, a "damping" adjustment exists. Damping does not modify the received signal directly, but it decreases the strength of the emitted ultrasound beam by limiting the duration of the pulses that form the beam. Because less power is sent toward the target, fewer noise signals are generated. Damping also enhances the image because it improves resolution by decreasing the number of cycles in each ultrasound pulse.

The intensity of echo signals spans a wide range from very weak to very strong. Very strong signals falling beyond the saturation level and very weak signals below the sensitivity of the instrument are automatically eliminated. The DR of the instrument is defined by the limits at which extremely strong or weak signals are eliminated. This DR may be expressed as the ratio of the highest to the lowest amplitude signal in decibels. In this manner, signals of low intensity that contain little useful information, and mostly noise, can be selectively rejected.

A wide DR is needed for high resolution, whereas a narrow range facilitates the discrimination between true image signals and noise. In clinical echocardiography, strong signals that arise from dense tissues (e.g., cardiac valves) and weaker signals arising from soft tissues (e.g., myocardium) are of interest. To give the weaker signals a greater representation in the DR, an amplifier converts the linear signal intensity scale into a logarithmic scale. Although this increases the number of weaker signals detected, it also amplifies noise. Compression may be used to selectively amplify weaker signals, and postprocessing of signals may be used to map signals of different amplitudes into a specific display brightness, further influencing displayed image brightness and contrast.

TWO-DIMENSIONAL IMAGING

As suggested above, sound waves create areas of compression and refraction that can be generated by piezoelectric crystal vibrations. These vibrations are produced by applying an electric current whose voltage is proportional to the amplitude of the produced sound waves. The inverse happens as well: as sound waves strike the face of piezoelectric crystals, mechanical vibrations are converted into electrical energy. This voltage can be plotted over time (e.g., voltage V vs. time t). This plot is referred to as radiofrequency (RF) data. Because time is distance in ultrasound, plotting V versus t is parallel to plotting V versus depth (13.0 μs$\rightarrow$ 1 cm, not 6.5 μs, it's round trip). This voltage measurement is directly proportional to amplitude, so amplitude versus depth plots may be created. If one converts amplitude to a number of gray levels (such as 256), then pixel brightness over depth will yield an M-mode plot. Finally, sweeping M-mode plots across a sector yields the familiar two-dimensional brightness (B)-mode image. Logarithmic compression is used to express a large DR into a smaller gray scale plot of amplitudes (8-bit gray, 2^8). Factors that increase the time of flight for an echo, such as larger sector width or deeper depth, reduce frame rate and hence temporal resolution.

DOPPLER TECHNIQUES

Most modern echo scanners combine Doppler capabilities with their two-dimensional imaging capabilities. After the desired view of the heart has been obtained by two-dimensional echocardiography, the Doppler beam, represented by a cursor, is superimposed on the two-dimensional image. The operator positions the cursor as parallel as possible to the assumed direction of blood flow and then empirically adjusts the direction of the beam to optimize the audio and visual representations of the reflected Doppler signal. At the present time, Doppler technology can be used in at least four different ways to measure blood velocities:

pulsed, high-repetition frequency, continuous-wave (CW), and color flow.

The Doppler Effect

The Doppler effect was described by an Austrian physicist in the 1800s. When an object is moving toward a fixed reference point, the frequency of an emitted signal increases; conversely, if an object is moving away from a fixed reference point, the emitted signal frequency decreases. Information on blood flow dynamics can be obtained by applying Doppler frequency shift analysis to echoes reflected by the moving red blood cells. Blood flow velocity, direction, and acceleration can be instantaneously determined. The Doppler principle states that the frequency of ultrasound reflected by a moving target (such as red blood cells) will be different from the frequency of the transmitted ultrasound. The magnitude and direction of the frequency shift is related to the velocity and direction of the moving target.

This blood velocity may be calculated by the following equation:

$$v_{\mathrm{BLOOD}} = \frac{c(f_T - f_R)}{2\,f_T \cos\theta}$$

where c is the speed of sound, v_{BLOOD} is the speed of the object, f_T is the transmitted frequency, f_R is the received frequency, $(f_T - f_R)$ is thus the observed frequency shift, and θ is the angle of incidence (the angle between the direction of moving target and the ultrasound signal). Flow velocity may be underestimated if the angle of incidence is large. Angles of less than 20 degrees are clinically acceptable; these measurements would result in a 6% error (cosine 20 degrees = 0.94). If the blood moves more than half the wavelength, the signal will "alias," so it is preferable to use longer wavelengths (lower frequencies) for Doppler measurements.

Based on the Doppler shift principle, blood flow velocity can be used to determine pressure gradients. The modified Bernoulli equation describes the relationship between pressure gradients (P_1 and P_2) and blood flow velocities. When flow acceleration and viscous friction variables of blood are ignored and flow velocity proximal to a fixed obstruction (V_1) is significantly less than flow velocity after the obstruction (V_2), then the following formula can be used to calculate the pressure gradient across a fixed orifice:

$$P_1 - P_2 = 4(V_2)^2$$

Pulsed-Wave Doppler

In pulsed-wave (PW) Doppler, blood flow parameters can be determined at precise locations by emitting repetitive short bursts of ultrasound at a specific frequency (PRF) and analyzing the frequency shift of the reflected echoes (Figure 1.1). A time delay between the emission of the ultrasound signal burst and the sampling of the reflected signal determines the depth at which the velocities are sampled. The delay is proportional to the distance between the transducer and the location of the velocity measurements. To sample at a given depth (D), sufficient time must be allowed for the signal to travel a distance of $2D$ (from the transducer to the sample volume and back).

The depth of sampling can be adjusted by varying the time delay between the emission of the ultrasonic signal and the sampling of the reflected wave. In practice, the sampling location or *sample volume* is represented by a small marker, which can be positioned at any point along the Doppler beam by moving it up or down the Doppler cursor.

If the PRF exceeds the minimum for a particular depth sample volume, range ambiguity will occur. This ambiguity occurs because the system must wait for the earlier pulse to return before it sends out the next. Range ambiguity worsens for larger sector sizes and volumes that are farther away from the transducer, because the pulses must wait a longer time before being fired again. (Phase changes and hence velocities inside the gate of the RF wave are used to find the frequency shift by a process known as quadrature phase demodulation. The frequency shift is "demodulated" or pulled apart from the original RF wave.

The trade-off for the ability to measure flow at precise locations is that ambiguous information is obtained when flow velocity is very high. A simple reference to Western movies will clearly illustrate this point. When a stagecoach gets underway, its wheel spokes are observed as rotating in the correct direction. As soon as a certain speed is attained, however, rotation in the reverse direction is noted because the camera frame rate is too slow to correctly observe the motion of the wheel spokes. The Nyquist sampling theorem may be explained using the analogy of a moving stagecoach in an old Western film. If the wheels move too quickly for the shutter speed, the wheels appear to go backwards even though the coach can be seen to move forward, because the movie frame rate is not high enough to capture accurately the spinning motion of the wheel. This is known as undersampling of the shutter rate and results in aliasing. The Nyquist sampling theorem in signal processing states that a wave must be sampled with at least twice the sampling frequency of the original phenomenon frequency in order to avoid ambiguity in the determination of direction of flow. This artifact can be avoided by increasing the sampling frequency, but this limits the range. Alternatively, the Doppler shift may be decreased by minimizing the frequency of the emitted ultrasound signal.

High Pulse Repetition Frequency Doppler

On some instruments, PW Doppler can be modified to a high-PRF mode. Whereas in conventional PW Doppler only a single burst of ultrasound is considered to be in the body at any given time, in high-PRF Doppler two to five sample volumes are simultaneously present in the tissues. Information coming back to the transducer may be coming back from

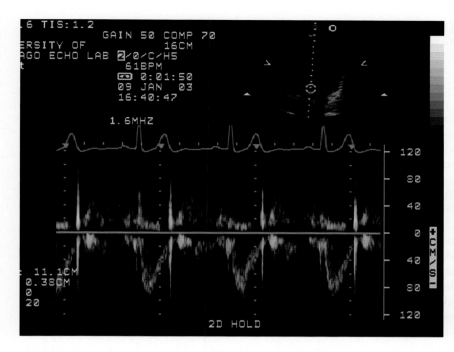

FIGURE 1.1. Pulsed Doppler image of a transthoracic echo. The apex of the left ventricle is at the apex of the 2D image at the upper right. The spectral trace is shown below. Note the value "cm/s." Flow away from the probe goes below the baseline, in this case flow related to left ventricular outflow. There is flow above the baseline after the T wave of the electrocardiogram (ECG), which shows the presence of aortic insufficiency. The sample gate shown along the 2D image is placed in the left ventricular outflow. The flow below the baseline shows peak flow approximately 80 cm/s.

depths of two, three, or four times the initial sample volume depth. The returning signals can be a mix of signals that have previously been emitted and have traveled to distant gates, and other signals that were just sent and returned from the first range gate.

The high-PRF mode allows increasing the sampling frequency since the scanner does not wait for the return of the information from distant gates. It nonetheless receives that information back within the specified time gate period. Higher velocities can be measured with this method than with PW Doppler; however, the depth from which spe-

cific gate the velocity signals are reflected is unknown (range ambiguity).

Continuous-Wave Doppler

If ultrasound signals are continuously emitted and sampled, higher velocities may be determined accurately, since the PRF is infinitely small. Although this technique allows accurate detection of a greater range of blood velocities without aliasing, spatial specificity is sacrificed (Figure 1.2). Continuous-wave Doppler only defines blood velocity along

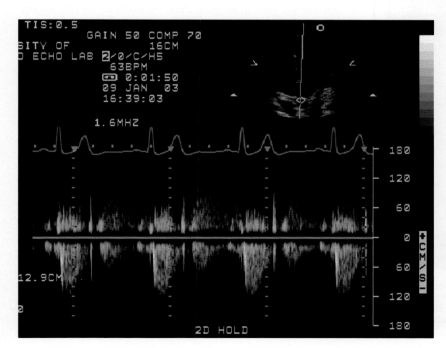

FIGURE 1.2. Continuous Wave (CW) Doppler image of a transthoracic echo. The apex of the left ventricle is at the apex of the 2D image at the upper right. Since flow is not range gated, the velocity shown in the spectral image cannot be localized along the line. Hence CW does not point over a particular structure. Note how the left ventricle (LV) outflow trace here shows many components.

a line instead of at a point in space like PW Doppler. Thus, one must be careful in attributing a velocity to a specific structure.

Color-Flow Mapping

Color flow Doppler is based on the use of many PW gates, and the results of the Doppler interrogation are superimposed on a simultaneously obtained two-dimensional image. In addition to showing the location, direction, and velocity of cardiac blood flow, the images produced by these devices allow estimation of flow acceleration and differentiation of laminar and turbulent blood flow. Blood flow velocities are calculated within a given echocardiographic sector. At each point, these blood flow velocities are represented in real time by an arbitrary color map, where flow toward the probe is usually represented by red and flow away from the probe is usually represented by blue. The faster the velocity, the greater the color intensity that is depicted. "Aliasing" is represented by a change in color between blue and red. A variance map may be added by addition of the color green if the blood acceleration is greater than a preset amount. In other words, the brightness of the red or blue colors at any location and time is usually proportional to the corresponding flow velocity, while the hue is proportional to the temporal rate of change of the velocity (Figure 1.3).

Image Storage

Videotape has been the classical method to store echo images. It still represents an extremely dense form of compression.

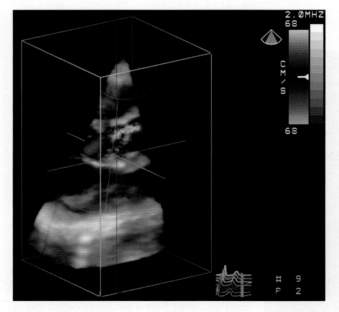

FIGURE 1.3. 3D Color Flow Doppler. The parasternal transthoracic image shows the anterior mitral valve leaflet near the red axis. The left ventricular outflow is just above. A 3D jet of aortic insufficiency is shown going through the aortic valve.

Typically, echo images are stored in super-video home system (VHS) format, which has a slightly higher resolution (more raster lines) than conventional videocassette recorders (VCRs). Because these are stored as magnetic fields within a tape, an analog form of communication, there is loss of information and it may appear slightly different each time it is played. Nonetheless, videotape is a clinically accepted form of storage.

Digital sampling refers to the quantization of a signal. The sampling rate refers to how much temporal information is saved from the original signal. For example, a photograph may be sampled to 256 (8 bits or 2^8) shades of gray. Humans are not able to perceive much more than 7 or 8 bits of gray; however, they are quite good at distinguishing colors. The ultrasound system converts the analog ultrasound signal to the digital domain and creates an image. Storing to a VCR tape requires an additional step of digital to analog conversion with an associated loss of information. An alternative method is digital storage. Since the image is kept in its initial form, it will appear identically each time it is shown. It can be compressed using lossless compression, so repeated pixels can be compressed without losing any information. There are mathematical techniques to compress images even further; this is known as lossy compression. Images can be averaged over areas of space within one frame using blocks as a discrete cosine transform as in Joint Photographic Expert Group (JPEG) compression formats. At compression rates higher than 20:1, the image can appear "blocky." Moving pictures can be averaged over time as well. Motion Picture Experts Group (MPEG) format represents an extremely efficient form of compression, which may provide compression rates of 100:1 to 200:1.

The medical standard Digital Imaging and Communication in Medicine (DICOM) defines a vendor-independent format for storing medical data. As listed on its official site (*medical.nema.org*), "The DICOM Standards Committee exists to create and maintain international standards for communication of biomedical diagnostic and therapeutic information in disciplines that use digital images and associated data." The American Society of Echocardiography maintains its collaboration with the DICOM working group as well as representatives of the major ultrasound vendors in order to define common standards. The standards define not only image data but also other information such as patient data.

Transesophageal Echocardiography Transducers

Transesophageal echocardiography (TEE) transducers are mechanically precise devices that must be watertight at the insertion tube level, electrically isolated from patients, and resist agents used to perform high-level disinfection. Multiplane systems contain a piezoelectric assembly that rotates on a mechanical assembly or turntable from 0 to 180 degrees. This crystal can be rotated either mechanically or by an electric stepper motor. Most manufacturers do not use latex components on their gastroscope assembly, so TEE probes are safe to use in patients with latex allergies. Some manufacturers add shielding to their probes or use isolated amplifiers in order to suppress electrocautery noise. Newer TEE probes include harmonic imaging capabilities. It is important to use bite guards in order to prevent trauma to the probe itself.

KEY POINTS

- The basis of ultrasound imaging depends on the reflection of the ultrasound waves from a given tissue interface or boundary to the ultrasound transducer.

- The resolution of a particular ultrasound signal is limited by its wavelength: the higher the ultrasound frequency, the higher the resolution.
- Piezoelectric crystals in the transducers convert ultrasound and electrical signals.
- The resulting voltage can be plotted over time and is referred to as radiofrequency data.
- This voltage measurement is directly proportional to amplitude, which is converted to a gray scale to create the image.
- The Doppler principle states that the frequency of ultrasound reflected by a moving target will be different from the frequency of the transmitted ultrasound. The magnitude and direction of the frequency shift is related to the velocity and direction of the moving target

Clinical Transesophageal Echocardiography: A Problem-Oriented Approach, Second Edition. Edited by S. N. Konstadt et al. Lippincott Williams & Wilkins © 2003.

2

EMERGING TECHNOLOGIES IN ECHOCARDIOGRAPHY

IVAN S. SALGO

Echocardiography has undergone sweeping changes over the past three decades. As we enter the 21st century, two-dimensional (2D) B-mode, color Doppler, spectral analysis, and M-mode represent the mainstay of cardiac examination. New entrants such as contrast and three-dimensional (3D) echocardiography have been undergoing constant evolution in processing technology and pharmaceutical development, and ascertaining appropriate clinical usage in scanning sessions remains the key question for these developing technologies. This chapter provides an overview of two emerging technologies: contrast and 3D echocardiography.

CONTRAST ECHOCARDIOGRAPHY

The Physics of Bubble Detection

A contrast agent is a substance that attenuates, absorbs, scatters, reflects, modulates, distorts, or interacts in some way with the interrogating energy used to image patients. Numerous constraints are placed on these families of agents, the most important of which is that the substance be nontoxic. This requirement is not completely met by some agents in use today, namely certain iodinated agents used by x-ray techniques such as fluoroscopy and computed tomography. These agents are accommodated clinically because they are judged to meet an "acceptable" risk-benefit ratio in making diagnoses.

Ultrasound contrast agents are tiny microbubbles designed to pass through capillaries and increase the signal strength of returning echoes. Generally they have a "safer" risk profile than many x-ray imaging agents. By "vibrating" in a nonlinear way, ultrasound agents simply increase the radiofrequency signal returned to the transducer. The signals produced by these agents are much stronger than classic echoes returned by scatterers such as blood and become more easily detectable within the dynamic range of the system.

Two general types of acoustic interactions occur in microbubbles: *nonlinear oscillations* and *destruction*. Because

I. S. Salgo: Philips Medical Systems, Andover, Massachusetts.

bubbles expand more easily than they can be compressed, they exhibit a physical nonlinearity that can be detected using signal-processing techniques (Fig. 2.1). Microbubble compressibility is the most important factor in determining how well they can be "seen." Other variable factors are statistical distribution of size within the injection, stability, bloodstream concentration, shell composition, and core composition. The properties of a "good" echo contrast agent include:

Nontoxicity: particle size
Nontoxicity: metabolic
Finite transit life: not too long, not too short
Detection: good backscatter of ultrasound
Physiology: "advantageous" constituent interactions

Mean capillary diameter is approximately 6 μm, so the first nontoxicity requirement is that, in order to avoid creating tissue infarcts, the particles not be larger than 6 μm. The next nontoxicity requirement is that the agent's shell be easily metabolized. Sonicated 5% albumin has been a popular choice because it is essentially a natural substance. Other shell agents include sugars and lipids. The approval of these agents has varied across the globe, with different agents having approval in different countries. Moreover, this evolution changes so quickly that tables in printed texts become quickly outdated. Sonicated albumin contains air (21% O_2 and 79% N_2) with other trace gases. Unfortunately, the intrinsic diffusivity of oxygen and nitrogen means that the gas escapes from the core. Because the scattering cross section is proportionate to its radius, the bubble soon becomes undetectable (1).

The next logical approach is to use gases of lower diffusiveness such as halogenated gases: fluorocarbons or sulfur hexafluoride. These agents have a longer life in the bloodstream and survive transpulmonary passage more easily. There are also agents known as "phase-shift" agents that convert from liquid at room temperature to gas at 37°C, but these agents are not as widely used. Median bubble sizes for all of these agents are 2 to 4 μm.

From this discussion it should be obvious that the technique of contrast administration can affect the success of the

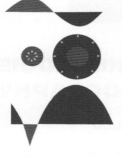

Incident RF acoustic field

A bubble can get only so small, but it can expand to a large size

Resulting asymmetrical vibrations produce harmonics

FIGURE 2.1. Depiction of contrast agent interaction with ultrasonography. Echocardiography contrast harmonic microbubble vibrations expand more easily than contract. This unevenness creates nonlinear vibrations and generates harmonic signals. *RF,* radiofrequency.

examination. For example, destruction of bubbles can be caused prematurely by pressure effects in the tubing. Moreover, use of agents can be more difficult in the operating room since patients are mechanically ventilated, frequently on 100% inspired O_2 and are cooled to 32°C or below. The blood and agents are cooled to this temperature. This represents a more aggressive environment for the microbubble, making its destruction more likely, and potentially increasing patient risk by alteration of the microbubble's physical properties.

The first publication that reported use of an echo contrast agent was in 1969. At that time agitated saline or indocyanine green was used. In fact, the most commonly used agent today remains agitated saline. This application and those that followed to the present day were intended to produce cavity opacification. The most evident use was in detecting atrial and ventricular septal defects. These applications are used as accepted clinical practice today. However, the use of venous injections of saline limited the clinical possibilities because of the statistical distribution of particle size—the bubbles are simply too big to survive transpulmonary passage. This limitation is caused by the extremely important phenomenon of venous (micro) embolus elimination by the lungs. In fact, use of contrast is safe if the dose and particle size are small enough and the amount of intracardiac right-to-left passage is limited or nonexistent.

Today many centers still use intravenous injections of saline or blood/saline agitated with air. Although a long-standing practice, this method does not incorporate quality control of bubble size and can certainly produce bubbles capable of capillary lodgment. Administration of an agent by an infusion reduces the peak concentration of agent compared with bolus injection, making bioeffects less probable.

Harmonic and Nonlinear Imaging Techniques

When a system sends out a fundamental pulse centered at 2 megahertz (MHz) and receives mainly at 2 MHz, fundamental imaging is said to occur. Physics demonstrates

that waves of higher and lower frequencies may be generated as this fundamental signal passes through a medium. These waves occur at many frequencies, but are quite strong at integer multiples, for example, at 4 MHz for a 2-MHz pulse. Receiving at twice the emitted frequency is known as second-harmonic imaging (not to be confused with musical terminology in which 4 MHz would be the first overtone.) The nonlinear behavior of bubbles creates strong second-harmonic signals and makes it easier for the ultrasound system to "see" the contrast agent.

This physical fact led to the development of harmonic imaging for echocardiography. Because sound represents compression and expansion of material created by acoustic waves, the alterations in pressure returning to the acoustic elements are transduced into an electrical signal (sometimes noted as a radiofrequency or RF signal). Mathematical manipulation of the transmitted signal can be used to distinguish between blood and tissue, as in Doppler echo, for example. The acoustic compressibility of tissue is different from that of bubbles. It is often said that "bubbles have much more nonlinear behavior" than tissue. With this in mind, developers set out to adapt imaging systems so that they could more easily detect signals generated from microbubbles and blood laden with contrast agent. Contrast signal acquisition techniques developed for this purpose can be classified as using low or high mechanical index (MI), fundamental or harmonic frequency, phase cancellation or no phase cancellation, and gated or nongated acquisition (Fig. 2.2).

One significant factor that affects microbubble interaction is the MI to which the microbubbles are exposed. Mechanical index is indicative of the peak negative pressure of an ultrasound pulse. For example, bubbles may oscillate at lower transmit energies but be destroyed at high ones. Doppler techniques send multiple pulses (collectively known as a packet). These are useful as a contrast physical change detector. For example, if the bubble is destroyed by the third

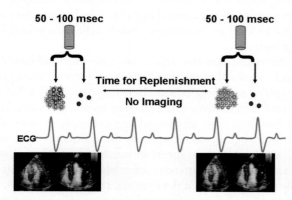

FIGURE 2.2. Gated contrast echocardiography techniques. Multiple frame triggering (*MFT*) images of echocardiography contrast can be obtained intermittently. Because ultrasound can destroy contrast agent, the first image shows perfusion while the next image is devoid of agent since it has been destroyed. Several heartbeats later, the agent has reperfused into the myocardium.

pulse in a five-pulse Doppler packet, this difference is demodulated by the system and bubbles can be recognized in the image. The pulse can be manipulated by other methods as well.

Pulse inversion is one of the first phase-cancellation techniques used to find nonlinear scatterers such as bubbles. If two pulses are sent and one is the mirror image of the other, the mostly linear interaction of tissue can be canceled out. However, bubbles respond quite differently, so their effect can be detected over and above the tissue signal. Another example of phase cancellation is amplitude (or power) modulation in which the first signal is twice as strong as the second. In tissue imaging, this signal can be subtracted out by using a correction factor of two and subtracting the waves. Microbubbles do not behave linearly, so this subtraction technique does not work with contrast.

However, a second-harmonic phenomenon allows tissue to be more easily detected with second-harmonic techniques even without ultrasound contrast. During early contrast research, it was noted that the speed of sound is different for compressed waves (in which sound travels faster) than for expanded waves. This unexpected finding means that second harmonic imaging can be used to improve imaging when contrast agents are not used. However, structures such as valve leaflets may appear thicker, so this newer modality must be considered in context against fundamental modes.

When imaging systems were first used to detect bubbles, it was found that the ultrasound beam destroyed the agent. When bolus techniques were used only to image the left ventricular (LV) cavity, this was not a problem, since the concentration of agent was quite high. However, to image the myocardium itself, the concentrations needed to be lowered, since the chamber blood pool filled with contrast would obscure the myocardium. For this reason, it was felt that the myocardium need only be seen during one phase of systole, so electrocardiogram (ECG)-triggered techniques were used. With the system applying intermittent imaging, a bolus was injected.

Applications: Cardiac Chamber Opacification

There are two major clinical applications for ultrasound contrast imaging: chamber opacification and myocardial perfusion imaging. Opportunities for using agents in the operating room include (2–5):

- Detection of cavity defects
- Analysis of global and regional ventricular function
- Assessment myocardial perfusion before bypass surgery
- Assessment of cardioplegia adequacy during bypass surgery
- Assessment of myocardial perfusion after bypass surgery
- Augmentation of Doppler echocardiography (better signal)

- Assessment of the presence of atrial appendage thrombus
- Assessment of renal perfusion

Most chamber opacification is performed within the left ventricle, and thus the acronym LVO (left ventricle opacification) is frequently used. Chamber opacification is used to detect anomalous structures, intracardiac shunts and improve analysis of segmental wall motion abnormalities. For example, a useful maneuver in detecting the presence of a persistent left superior vena cava (LSVC) is to give a bolus injection of echo contrast in the left antecubital vein. If present, the persistent LSVC will be identified by contrast entering the right atrium through a dilated coronary sinus before being seen at the normal entrance of the superior vena cava. Moreover, contrast agents can be used to detect the presence of shunting such as an atrial or ventricular septal defect. If the presence of a defect is known *a priori,* prudence dictates not using echo contrast agents, either commercial agents or those generated on site, unless specifically labeled. The pulmonary circulation provides an excellent safeguard for the peripheral venous circulation against large particulates from reaching the left-sided cardiac circulation. Particulates in the arterial circulation can create infarcts of critical organs such as the brain.

Probably the most widely used application in transthoracic echocardiographic clinical practice for ultrasound contrast agents are in improving images in the difficult-to-image patient. This application received first approval several years ago from regulatory agencies. Elucidating regional wall motion for stress echocardiography examinations represents one application. Chest wall echo is encumbered by a transducer aperture that must fit between rib spaces. Smaller apertures degrade lateral resolution. Furthermore, the fascial layers of the chest wall create a phenomenon known as clutter. Clutter is created by aberrations in the waves of ultrasound as they pass through inhomogeneous material. Clutter appears as structures typically within the blood pool. Naturally, TEE has much lower levels of clutter since there are less aberrations between the transducer and myocardium. For this reason, contrast agents are used much less frequently for LVO executed by TEE. Nonetheless, there are patients in whom identifying segmental wall motion abnormalities is difficult even by TEE. Hence, the blood–tissue interface is delineated more clearly with contrast agent.

Applications: Detection of Myocardial Perfusion

Use of echo contrast agents has received intense research focus over the past decade on another application: assessment of myocardial perfusion (6–8). Classically, regional wall motion abnormalities have been used to infer adequacy of coronary flow. Exercise stress and pharmacologic techniques are commonly used to find a biphasic response consistent with viable but (abnormally) perfusion-limited myocardium: increased wall motion at mild stress but wall

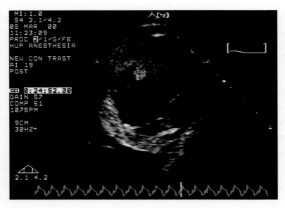

FIGURE 2.3. Aortic root injection of sonicated 5% albumin into an ovine test subject. The darker risk zone is on the lower right and was created by ligating a coronary artery.

motion abnormalities at peak stress recoverable after rest. In fact, the phenomenon of border zone myocardium exhibits an area of myocardial tissue that is normally perfused but hypocontractile due to tethering. Eventually, the penumbra of decreasing flow over time can recruit this viable myocardium into the infarct, worsening abnormal remodeling. The bottom line is that wall motion alone does not reveal all the physiologic variables necessary to evaluate acute or chronic ischemia or infarction.

There are generally two approaches to perfusion imaging: finding the "all-or-none" risk area and actually quantifying flow. The risk area is that of the myocardium "at risk of infarcting" during an acute obstruction to coronary flow, typically due, for example, to a ruptured plaque. There are only hours available to salvage myocardium at risk of necrosis. Essentially, there is no blood flow to this area, and blood perfusing the myocardium with the appropriate agent will "light up" normal myocardium but the risk zone will appear dark (Figs. 2.3 and 2.4). Bolus techniques with intermit-

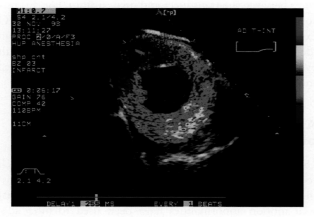

FIGURE 2.4. "Pseudo-colorization" of contrast images. It is easier to perceive changes in hue rather than gray level so areas of higher video intensity (and hence perfusion in this case) can be shaded.

tent still images of the myocardium at systole can be used, provided the echo contrast agent survives transpulmonary passage. The general trend in recent years, however, is to use lower MI, nontriggered techniques in which a live image of the moving myocardium is seen perfusing with contrast. In the latter, wall motion can be compared with the myocardial darkening, allowing two physiologic variables to be assessed while theoretically improving diagnostic confidence. Gated techniques are still in use when motion imaging is not necessary. Perfusion techniques can be used to assess the transmurality of an infarct (9).

Myocardial perfusion detected by contrast agent generally represents capillary flow and is essentially the myocardial blood volume. This is because a major portion of arterial and venous blood volume resides in the epicardium (10,11). Note that X-ray angiographic techniques image down to approximately 150 μm. The "no-reflow" phenomenon whereby angiographic flow is seen after percutaneous transluminal coronary angioplasty (PTCA) despite persistent wall motion abnormalities can nonetheless be elucidated by perfusion imaging. Disrupted plaque may embolize distally after balloon inflation, and while the lesion appears corrected by x-ray techniques, a risk zone of infarction still appears by perfusion echo.

Recent techniques have advanced the state of the art further. In fact, perfusion echo can be used to quantify the replenishment of blood in the myocardial bed. The principle is relatively simple. A steady-state concentration of agent is set up in the bloodstream by using an intravenous infusion rather than a bolus. A high-energy ultrasound frame can be fired to destroy an agent within the myocardial capillaries. Triggering after this flash can be altered: 1:1, 1:2, 1:4, 1:8, and so forth. "1:8" means that after the flash, imaging for the presence of contrast was done eight beats later with no other echoes fired in the interim. Intuition reveals that high coronary flow rates will replenish early and be seen at 1:3, for example, whereas impeded flow might only first be seen late since it took seven or eight beats to replenish ischemic myocardium. This represents a wash-in curve. These curves can be created by putting a region of interest cursor (perhaps a circle with a 0.5-cm diameter) over different perfusion segments. Blood flow in this instance is actually being quantified by echocardiography.

Contrast perfusion echo techniques have not been adopted for mainstream application due to several reasons. Many factors affect the accuracy of the examination: echo-transmit power, RF signal-processing techniques, image-processing techniques, agent used, infusion technique, inhomogeneous destruction of agent by the beam, and so forth. These factors have contributed to restricting the realm of perfusion echo imaging for research applications in general. Clinicians still need expertise in image processing, physics, and contrast pharmacology to be able to discern artifacts. Moreover, the operating room environment is much more dynamic. The patient's physiologic state changes quickly (e.g., cardiac output, temperature, inspired gas content, etc.), so it is more difficult to create a state favorable for agent kinetics. Direct aortic root injections of contrast agent imply that the "safety net" of the pulmonary circulation is not in play, so particle size distribution must be even more tightly controlled.

Contrast agents can be engineered to carry antibodies to fibrin, inflammatory targets or other receptors of choice, drugs, and even genes (12–15). These applications will move echocardiography from being a purely diagnostic modality to one that embraces therapeutics as well. This will be catalyzed by real-time 3D echocardiographic techniques.

THREE DIMENSIONAL ECHOCARDIOGRAPHY

Three-dimensional echocardiography involves the acquisition, processing, and display of the three spatial dimensions scanned during ultrasound imaging (16). Unlike two-dimensional echocardiography, this facilitates the complete visualization and analysis of cardiac structures as they move through space and time. As with 2D echocardiography, information can be used for either *visualization* or *quantification.*

The concept of using ultrasonic scanning in 3D is not new, but technologic advances have facilitated the development of 3D echocardiography. Over the past two decades, limitations in acquisition (i.e., a 3D probe and beam former) and in computer processing have posed significant obstacles to the technologic advancement of 3D echocardiographic imaging (17–23). The advent of fast desktop computers has sped up development of visualization techniques. The problem that remains for 3D is acquisition.

Three Dimensional Echo Acquisition

There are two general methods for gathering ultrasound information in three dimensions: ECG triggered (gated)

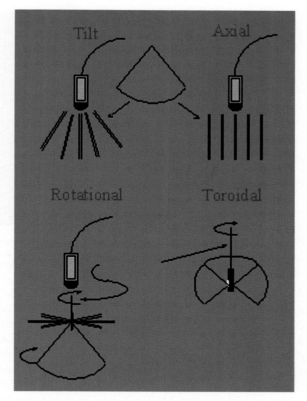

FIGURE 2.5. Three-dimensional acquisition by two-dimensional scanning. A conventional transducer can be swept through space. This can be tilted, moved in parallel, twisted, or rotated. Multiplane transducers naturally fall into the rotation category.

acquisition or real-time scanning. Triggered acquisition is commonly used in other applications such as contrast echocardiography. A sequence of 2D loops gathered over one cardiac cycle is stored digitally. These sequences can be collected freehand, in parallel ("axially breadloafed"), by twisting ("toroid/lighthouse"), by tilting, or by rotating (Figs. 2.5 and 2.6). Because multiplane transesophageal probes are becoming the standard of care (especially for complex

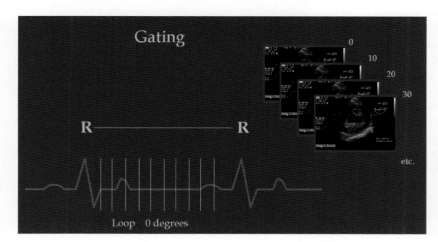

FIGURE 2.6. Gated acquisition for three-dimensional (3D) echo. Loops over one heartbeat are collected for each multiplane angle (0, 10, and 20 degrees, etc.). Then the loops can be recollated for angle sets rather than the heart cycle (electrocardiogram/time). Collectively, all the images at one temporal point in the R-R cycle represent a 3D set of data.

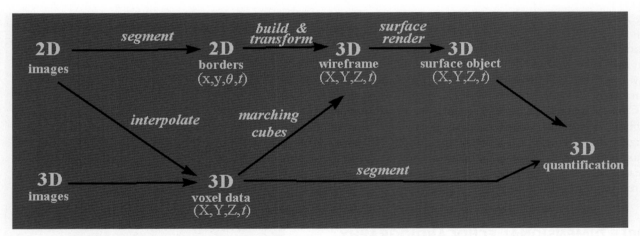

FIGURE 2.7. Pathway for three-dimensional (3D) image processing. Data can be acquired in conventional two-dimensional or newer 3D acquisition transducers. The data can then be volume rendered for visualization or surface rendered for quantification.

congenital and valvular surgical procedures), rotational acquisition is most commonly practiced. When the cardiac rhythm is regular, the loops acquired over different multiplane angles have good temporal correlation. One of the long-standing advantages of this technique is that conventional transducer technology can be used and the 2D images are of high quality. Unfortunately, triggered acquisition has several disadvantages as well: parts of the heart not scanned have to be "filled in" or interpolated, sequences can be difficult or impossible to obtain in patients with arrhythmias such as atrial fibrillation, patient or probe movement introduces significant spatial artifacts, and the acquisition of one virtual cardiac cycle takes several minutes (Fig. 2.7).

Another method of acquiring ultrasound information is to scan a 3D volume in space. A conventional phased-array probe scans in a 2D plane (it uses a one-dimensional series of piezoelectric elements to do this). Conversely, one can use a 2D matrix array of elements to fire a beam into 3D space by firing in the depth dimension laterally (as before) as well as in the elevation dimension (Fig. 2.8). Although this seems the logical approach, real-time scanning has several challenges. First, unlike magnetic resonance imaging (MRI) and X-ray computed tomography (CT), which use electromagnetic radiation traveling at the speed of light, echo uses sound that travels much more slowly. When the interrogating depth is deep within the body and the 3D field of view is large, the transmit–wait duty cycle over the whole set takes an inordinate amount of time to acquire. In order to overcome this limitation of physics, *parallelism* was introduced in receiving acoustic information. That is, for one transmit event, there are 2, 4, 8, 16, 32, etc. receive events going on at the matrix array. This can speed up acquisition so that scanning can occur at clinically feasible depths and sizes. (Naturally, if the scanning depth was kept to 2 cm and the sector widths were quite small, very high frame rates could be achieved.)

However, despite the ever-increasing ability in computing technology, due to acoustic signal limitations, parallelism cannot be increased indefinitely because image degradation occurs after a certain point.

Visualization

Once the ultrasound data are acquired, they must be reassembled for display and analysis. A matrix array can be used to

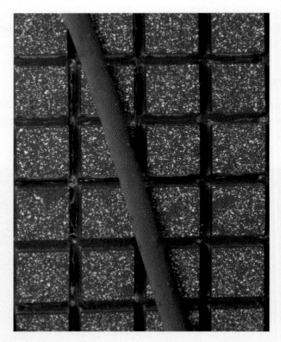

FIGURE 2.8. Scanning electron micrograph of matrix array elements. This matrix array can steer an ultrasound beam in three-dimensional space. Also visible is a human hair. (Courtesy of Philips Medical Systems.)

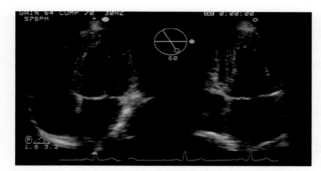

FIGURE 2.9. Instantaneous biplane imaging. Matrix array transducers allow the acquisition of more than one two-dimensional slice at a time. The clinical benefit is allowing visualization of anatomic structures from different perspectives simultaneously, such as wall or valvular motion.

show simultaneous 2D images (Fig. 2.9). For 3D visualization, there are two general methods: surface versus volume rendering. Each has benefits and drawbacks (Fig. 2.10 and 2.11).

Volume rendering can be understood as follows. Understanding that 2D echocardiograms have 2D gray level blocks known as pixels, volume rendering requires 3D gray level blocks known as voxels. Gated techniques use the 2D images to interpolate or fill in the blocks, whereas volume scanning fills in the voxels directly using a 3D scan converter. Naturally, since one cannot "see inside" a solid set of gray level voxels, special processing known as "volume rendering" must be used to create a 3D image of the heart onto a 2D screen. This is done using a computer that passes "rays" through the voxel cube onto a "photographic" plate. The concept is similar to creating a chest radiograph but it is done mathematically and with more 3D effect. The final plate is what

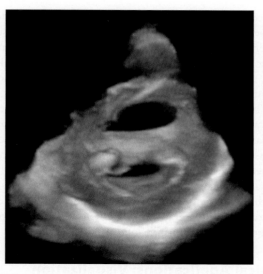

FIGURE 2.11. Three-dimensional transthoracic image obtained using a fully sampled matrix array. The mitral valve is shown during ventricular diastole. The anterior leaflet is shown from the viewpoint of the cardiac apex. The tip of the posteromedial papillary muscles can be seen in the foreground just above the anterior leaflet.

is shown on a 2D screen. The appearance can be adjusted by making low-level echoes (e.g., blood) transparent to the ray-casting algorithm and by adjusting the translucency of the tissue voxels.

Surface rendering is the 3D equivalent to tracing an outline, such as of the LV cavity. Surface rendering has been commonly used for gated acquisition data because many traces can be put together to form the endocardial surface of the left ventricle. Surface rendering is commonly used to show

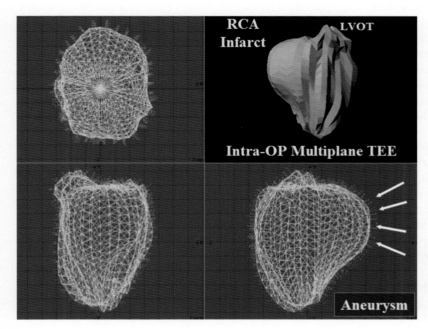

FIGURE 2.10. Surface rendering. A wire frame representation of the left ventricle in a patient with a right coronary infarct that progressed to a basal aneurysm is shown. This representation is useful for quantifying volumes, for example, but it is not useful for visualizing tissue detail.

the borders of cardiac chambers. The margins of a leaflet can be traced in 2D, however, so it is possible to perform surface rendering of tissue, but because this is rarely performed in 2D echocardiography, it likewise is rarely done in 3D. Finally, surface rendering contains no information inside the boundary.

When is each technique used? Classically, surface rendering was use in gated acquisition because it naturally extends to quantifying the blood volume within it. Volume rendering was used to visualize tissue structure but not quantification. (Generally the endocardial cavity is traced on a 2D echocardiogram before its area is known. The blood pool is said to have been segmented from the surrounding tissue.) Because the voxels are only gray levels but not classified as blood or tissue voxels, no quantification can be made.

Clinical Applications: Visualization

One of the common pitfalls in technologic development is to assume that the ingenuity of a device is all that is necessary for acceptance. One of the problems that have affected contrast and 3D echocardiography has been the lack of clinical applicability combined with ease of use. Is there any more diagnostic information? If so, is it justified by the extra time needed for gated scanning? These questions have remained unanswered for 3D echocardiography. As scanning time is reduced or becomes real time, will there be applications that can benefit?

One of the most straightforward applications involves imaging complex congenital heart defects. The benefit, even for simple defects, is to allow visualization of the defect as it is in space, which is what surgeons are accustomed to viewing. Even simple defects such as atrial and ventricular septal defects can be seen in juxtaposition to their surrounding anatomy, giving a vivid representation of the defect itself. More complicated defects require the expertise of those accustomed to imaging congenital heart disease. Experienced echocardiographers become proficient at reassembling 2D images, but they must communicate what they see in their mind's eye to other physicians. Therefore, 3D volume rendering has the potential to become useful as a communication tool for those just learning echocardiography and for referring physicians.

The above discussion makes apparent that volume rendering is useful for perioperative planning, and this is true in adult cardiac surgery as well. Over a decade ago, it was shown that the mitral annulus is not planar but rather conforms to a saddle shape. Moreover, understanding the spatial position of the leaflet with respect to coaptation leads to an understanding of the spatial orientation of regurgitant jets and helps the surgeon visualize and plan repair before going on to cardiopulmonary bypass.

Potentially new applications for volume rendering may appear as frame rates get faster and resolution gets finer.

Subtle motions in leaflet motion may become apparent in 3D. A more profound application may include visualizing wall motion defects in 3D. Problems with twisting and through-plane motion impede the ability to define regional wall motion abnormalities. Visualization of wall motion in 3D has the potential to improve the sensitivity and specificity of analyzing hypokinesis qualitatively.

Clinical Applications: Quantification

Quantification of cardiac function is essential in gauging the efficacy of therapy or the progression of disease. Although significant changes can be seen visually (e.g., dilated cardiomyopathy), subtle changes that can have a bearing on therapy are much more difficult to appreciate. Moreover, problems of inter- and intraobserver variability amplify the need for uniform measurement and communication. Because the heart is an intrinsically 3D structure, quantification of 2D slices naturally has limitations. For example, single and even biplane methods of LV volume computation can be inaccurate in aneurysmal ventricles. Through-plane motion can lead to inaccuracies in defining regional wall motion abnormalities. Recall that the act of tracing performs segmentation (24). Therefore, surface rendering has been generally associated with quantification. Note that this not the only way. Volume rendering can be used to quantify the blood pool as well. If the voxels associated with blood are added up, then the whole blood volume can be computed.

The most common application of quantification for 3D echocardiography has been the assessment of LV volume. It has been shown that three intersecting planes ("a poor person's 3D echocardiogram") are sufficient for obtaining accurate volumes. In fact, the biplane Simpson rule is remarkably accurate for symmetric ventricles. The key to these last two applications is that the images must be acquired at the same time or the measurement is subject to error. The images must not be foreshortened nor the probe moved during acquisition. Three-dimensional echocardiograms acquired in one heartbeat overcome these limitations by acquiring the whole volume so that even if only two orthogonal 2D images are acquired, it is known that they are exactly 90 degrees to each other. Volume calculation requires less spatial resolution than regional wall motion analysis because volume is a more forgiving metric than area or distance. Imaging endo- and epicardial shells allows quantification of endocardial volume, myocardial mass, and ventricular shape. Understanding the nature of shape is key in following ventricular remodeling.

More cutting edge applications involve quantifying regional wall motion and leaflet function (20,25). Because 3D cardiac (magnetic resonance) MR, CT, or echocardiographic methods have not been standards of care, clinicians have not appreciated the 3D nature of regional excursion and thickening. Current techniques to quantify local motion include creating regional subvolumes or calculating local changes

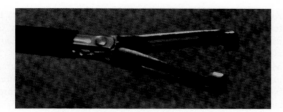

FIGURE 2.12. Surgical grasping device.

in endocardial surface area. Coupling material analysis with 3D shapes allows elucidation of the structural stresses that occur within leaflets, which can cause chordal rupture, for example.

Three-dimensional color Doppler allows visualization of the jet orientation, which is commonly used to judge mitral leaflet coaptation. Other 3D techniques could potentially allow fully automated measurement of regurgitant volume. Finding 3D power velocity integrals using matrix arrays are one such example of technologic evolution.

Clinical Applications: Catheter Guidance

Real-time imaging allows visualization of catheters and instruments as they move within vessels and cardiac chambers (Figs. 2.12 and 2.13). Catheter-based techniques are becoming increasingly popular for closing atrial septal defects, thereby avoiding sternotomy and cardiopulmonary bypass. Other applications include catheter placement used in ablation for electrophysiologic procedures. A significant aspect of this approach is that instruments create significant artifacts, including shadowing, multipath reflections, reverberations, and side lobes. Nonetheless, pressures to reduce morbidity, length of hospital stays, and health-care cost will continue to drive minimally invasive techniques.

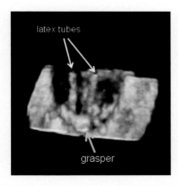

FIGURE 2.13. Three-dimensional (3D) echocardiography of grasping surgical grasping device. This figure demonstrates a 3D echo of a grasping device pinching two latex tubes together. This *in vitro* experiment was performed blinded to the surgical operator. (Courtesy of Jeremy Cannon, M.D., Cardiothoracic Surgery, Boston Children's Hospital.)

KEY POINTS

- Contrast agents increase the signal strength of returning echoes and should be nontoxic.
- Contrast echocardiography is commonly used for chamber opacification. When performed in the left ventricle, this is abbreviated as LVO.
- Contrast echocardiography can be used for detection and quantification of myocardial perfusion. This technique is currently applied less frequently than LVO.
- Future applications of contrast agents include adding ligands with biologic activity such as antifibrin antibodies for thrombus detection and gene delivery.
- Older techniques of 3D echocardiographic acquisition entail gating sequences of 2D images over several heart cycles. This is susceptible to artifacts from probe movement and patient arrhythmias.
- Newer acquisition methods for 3D echocardiography include use of matrix array probes to perform 3D scanning.
- 3D echocardiography can be used to visualize congenital heart defects, valvular morphology for perioperative planning and intraoperative assessment, and wall motion.
- Quantification of LV global and regional function using 3D echocardiography has been shown to be more accurate than conventional 2D methods.
- Future applications of 3D echocardiography include guiding instruments within the beating heart.

REFERENCES

1. Wei K, Skyba DM, Firschke C, et al. Interactions between microbubbles and ultrasound: *in vitro* and *in vivo* observations. *J Am Coll Cardiol* 1997;29:1081–1088.
2. **Aronson S, Savage R, Toledano A, et al. Identifying the cause of left ventricular systolic dysfunction after coronary artery bypass surgery: the role of myocardial contrast echocardiography. *J Cardiothorac Vasc Anesth* 1998;12:512–518.**
3. Aronson S, Lee BK, Wiencek JG, et al. Assessment of myocardial perfusion during CABG surgery with two-dimensional transesophageal contrast echocardiography. *Anesthesiology* 1991; 75:433–440.
4. Aronson S, Lee BK, Liddicoat JR, et al. Assessment of retrograde cardioplegia distribution using contrast echocardiography. *Ann Thorac Surg* 1991;52:810–814.
5. Voci P, Heidenreich P, Aronson S, et al. Quantitation of renal blood flow by contrast ultrasonography: preliminary results. *Cardiologia* 1989;34:1001–1006.
6. **Kaul S. Myocardial contrast echocardiography: 15 years of research and development. [Review] [81 refs]. *Circulation* 1997;96:3745–3760.**
7. Kaul S, Senior R, Dittrich H, et al. Detection of coronary artery disease with myocardial contrast echocardiography: comparison with 99mTc-sestamibi single-photon emission computed tomography. *Circulation* 1997;96:785–792.
8. Kaul S, Jayaweera AR. Coronary and myocardial blood volumes: noninvasive tools to assess the coronary microcirculation? [Letter; comment]. [Review] [45 refs]. *Circulation* 1997;96:719–724.

9. Price RJ, Skyba DM, Kaul S, et al. Delivery of colloidal particles and red blood cells to tissue through microvessel ruptures created by targeted microbubble destruction with ultrasound. *Circulation* 1998;98:1264–1267.

10. **Wei K, Le E, Jayaweera AR, et al. Detection of noncritical coronary stenosis at rest without recourse to exercise or pharmacological stress. *Circulation* 2002;105:218–223.**

11. Bowen FW, Hattori T, Narula N, et al. Reappearance of myocytes in ovine infarcts produced by six hours of complete ischemia followed by reperfusion. *Ann Thorac Surg* 2001;71:1845–1855.

12. Christiansen JP, Leong-Poi H, Klibanov AL, et al. Noninvasive imaging of myocardial reperfusion injury using leukocyte-targeted contrast echocardiography. *Circulation* 2002;105:1764–1767.

13. Mayer S, Grayburn PA. Myocardial contrast agents: recent advances and future directions [Review] [71 refs]. *Prog Cardiovasc Dis* 2001;44:33–44.

14. Laskar R, Grayburn PA. Assessment of myocardial perfusion with contrast echocardiography at rest and with stress: an emerging technology [Review] [81 refs]. *Prog Cardiovasc Dis* 2000;43:245–258.

15. **Shohet RV, Chen S, Zhou YT, et al. Echocardiographic destruction of albumin microbubbles directs gene delivery to the myocardium. *Circulation* 2000;101:2554–2556.**

16. **Salgo IS. Three-dimensional echocardiography [Review] [78 refs]. *J Cardiothorac Vasc Anesth* 1997;11:506–516.**

17. Camarano G, Jones M, Freidlin RZ, et al. Quantitative assessment of left ventricular perfusion defects using real-time three-dimensional myocardial contrast echocardiography. *J Am Soc Echocardiogr* 2002;15:206–213.

18. King DL, El Khoury CL, Maurer MS. Myocardial contraction fraction: a volumetric index of myocardial shortening by free-hand three-dimensional echocardiography. *J Am Coll Cardiol* 2002;40:325–329.

19. Marx GR, Sherwood MC. Three-dimensional echocardiography in congenital heart disease: a continuum of unfulfilled promises? No. A presently clinically applicable technology with an important future? Yes [Review] [122 refs]. *Pediatr Cardiol* 2002;23:266–285.

20. Salgo IS, Gorman JH III, Gorman RC, et al. Effect of annular shape on leaflet curvature in reducing mitral leaflet stress. *Circulation* 2002;106:711–717.

21. Angelini ED, Laine AF, Takuma S, et al. LV volume quantification via spatiotemporal analysis of real-time 3-D echocardiography. *IEEE Trans Med Imaging* 2001;20:457–469.

22. Belohlavek M, Tanabe K, Jakrapanichakul D, et al. Rapid three-dimensional echocardiography: clinically feasible alternative for precise and accurate measurement of left ventricular volumes. *Circulation* 2001;103:2882–2884.

23. Chuang ML, Hibberd MG, Beaudin RA, et al. Patient motion compensation during transthoracic 3-D echocardiography. *Ultrasound Med Biol* 2001;27:203–209.

24. Mele D, Fehske W, Maehle J, et al. A simplified, practical echocardiographic approach for 3-dimensional surfacing and quantitation of the left ventricle: clinical application in patients with abnormally shaped hearts. *J Am Soc Echocardiogr* 1998;11:1001–1012.

25. He S, Weston MW, Lemmon J, et al. Geometric distribution of chordae tendineae: an important anatomic feature in mitral valve function. *J Heart Valve Dis* 2000;9:495–501.

3

TRANSESOPHAGEAL ECHOCARDIOGRAPHIC TRAINING AND PERFORMANCE STANDARDS

STEVEN N. KONSTADT

TRAINING

We have entered an era in medicine in which the observance of guidelines for training, credentialing, certifying, and recertifying medical professionals has become increasingly common. Although there have been warnings (1) and objections (2) to anesthesiologists making diagnoses and aiding in surgical decision making, there is no inherent reason that an anesthesiologist cannot provide this valuable service to the patient. The key factors are proper training, extensive experience with intraoperative echocardiography (IOE), and available backup by a recognized echocardiographer. Transesophageal echocardiographic (TEE) training should begin with a dedicated training period. This is most easily accomplished during cardiac anesthesia fellowship, but can be pursued by postgraduate physicians as well. The subject can be approached through a combination of tutorials, scientific review courses, self-instruction with teaching tapes, interactive learning programs, and participation in echo reading sessions (3,4). Frequently, a symbiotic relationship with the cardiology division can be established in which anesthesiologists can teach the fundamentals of airway management, operating room physiology, and the use of local anesthetics while learning the principles of echocardiography from the cardiologists. To accelerate learning in the perioperative setting, it is important to perform a complete examination whenever possible, discuss the actual pathologic findings with the surgeon, and to bring diagrams and heart models into the operating room to enhance the examination.

In cardiovascular medicine, formal policy standards for performing diagnostic and therapeutic techniques have been recommended by a number of societies. In 1990, a task force from the American College of Physicians, the American College of Cardiology (ACC), and the American Heart Associa-

tion (AHA) created initial general guidelines for echocardiography (5). The American Society of Echocardiography also provided recommendations for general training in echocardiography and has introduced a self-assessment test for measuring proficiency. These organizations recommended the establishment of three levels of performance with a minimum number of cases for each level: level 1, introduction and an understanding of the indications [120 two-dimensional (2D) and 60 Doppler cases]; level 2, independent performance and interpretation (240 2D and 180 Doppler cases); and level 3, laboratory direction and training (590 2D and 530 Doppler cases) (2,6). However, these guidelines are limited because they are not based on objective data or achievement. Furthermore, because different individuals learn at different rates, meeting these guidelines does not ensure competence. Nor does failure to meet these guidelines preclude competence. In addition, these guidelines do not focus on intraoperative applications of echocardiography. In 1997, a revision of these same guidelines by the ACC and AHA also did not include specific recommendations for intraoperative applications (7). The American Society of Echocardiography and the Society of Cardiovascular Anesthesiologists (SCA) has created a task force to establish guidelines for training in perioperative echocardiography. These guidelines are available on the SCA website: *www.scahq.org/sca3/tee_guidelines.pdf*. This report proposed the creation of two levels of training: basic and advanced. Basic training requires the understanding of the principles of ultrasonography, the indications for perioperative echocardiography, mastery of the complete examination, the ability to make hemodynamic assessments, and the assessment of native valve lesions. To achieve this level of training the trainee must personally perform at least 50 complete examinations and study at least 150 examinations. The advanced level of training includes all of the basic components: detailed knowledge of native and prosthetic valve function, congenital heart disease, disease of the great vessels, and advanced

S. N. Konstadt: Department of Anesthesiology, Division of Cardiothoracic Anesthesia, The Mount Sinai Medical Center, New York, New York.

quantitative assessment. This level requires the personal performance of 150 examinations and the study of a total of 300 examinations. The basic examinations count toward the advanced requirements. The guidelines also recognize that individuals may have obtained training in practice. The guidelines recommend that these individuals should have at least 20 hours of CME in echocardiography for basic and 50 hours of CME in echocardiography for advanced training.

Previous work has shown that an examination focused on intraoperative procedures can serve as a test of TEE competence (8). In addition to training guidelines, the American Society of Echocardiography and SCA have worked to create a test of competence in perioperative echocardiography. The mission of the SCA's Task Force on Certification for Perioperative TEE was to develop a process that would acknowledge basic competence and offer the opportunity to demonstrate advanced competence as outlined by the SCA/American Society of Anesthesiology (ASA) practice parameters. The American Society of Echocardiography joined the effort, and this process led to the creation of an examination. The perioperative TEE is now administered by the National Board of Echocardiography and is given annually. The test is in a multiple-choice format and includes still and video image analysis. Key topics on the examination include the following:

- Fundamentals of Ultrasonic Imaging
- Cardiac Anatomy and Imaging planes
- Ventricular Function
- Valvular Abnormalities
- Intracardiac Masses
- Thoracic Aorta

Successful completion of the examination results in the title of "Testamur."

The combination of the TEE training guidelines and the TEE test may serve to create the basis for certification in perioperative TEE. Certification usually is granted by a national organization and is standardized. Credentialing is a process undertaken in each institution, and the criteria are unique to each institution. Credentialing defines who can perform a technique, when they can perform it, and where they can perform it. In our institution we have a credentialing process that mirrors the basic and advanced training requirements. Additionally, we have an expert level that allows the use of TEE outside of the perioperative arena. The three levels are defined in Table 3.1.

Performance Standards

The use of perioperative echocardiography places additional responsibilities on the anesthesiologist. For example all examinations should be recorded and stored, a report must be placed in the chart and kept on file, a log of all patients studied must be kept, and there must be a quality control system. To help the anesthesiologist deal with these challenges, several of the component societies have created task forces to create guidelines. The ASA and SCA recently worked together to create a document on practice parameters for perioperative TEE (9). These parameters outlined the recognized indications for perioperative echocardiography and divided these indications into categories based on the level of scientific evidence for the indication. The SCA and American Society of Echocardiography also created a task force to formulate a standardized perioperative report form. The goals of the report are listed below.

- Promote quality by defining the basic core of measurements and diagnostic statements required in a report.
- Facilitate the comparison of serial echocardiograms performed in patients at the same site or different sites.
- Improve communication by expediting development of structured report form software.
- Facilitate multicenter research and analyses of cost effectiveness.
- Facilitate billing compliance and collections.

This report can be downloaded from the SCA website at the following address: *www.scahq.org/sca3/teereport.shtml.*

Quality control is an area in which there are few specific guidelines for TEE performance. Rafferty et al. proposed one model for quality assurance (10). At the very least, each echocardiogram should be recorded in a standardized fashion and accompanied by a written report for inclusion in the patient's chart. Images may also be copied and included in the chart. Careful records of any complications should be maintained. To ensure that the proper images are being obtained and that the interpretations are correct, the studies should be periodically reviewed. This is another area in which the relationship between cardiology and anesthesiology can be productive.

It is important to recognize that practice guidelines are systematically developed *recommendations* that assist the practitioner and patient in making decisions about health care. These recommendations may be adopted, modified, or

TABLE 3.1. CONTINUING MEDICAL EDUCATION

	Basic	Advanced	Expert
Training	150 TEE exams	1 year of training	5 years of experience
Diagnostic range	Ventricular function	Full diagnostic range	Full diagnostic range
Location		OR, PACU	OR, PACU, ER, (ICU)
Annual performance		50 exams/year	50 exams/year
TEE testing status		TEE Testamur	TEE Testamur

rejected according to clinical needs and constraints. Practice guidelines are not intended as standards or absolute requirements and their use cannot guarantee any specific outcome. Practice guidelines are subject to revisions from time to time as medical knowledge, technology, and technique evolve. Guidelines are supported by analysis of the current literature and by synthesis of expert opinion, open forum commentary, and clinical feasibility data.

REFERENCES

1. Kaplan JA. Monitoring technology: advances and restraints. *J Cardiothorac Anesth* 1989;3:257.
2. Pearlman AS, Gardin JM, Martin RP, et al. Guidelines for optimal physician training in echocardiography. Recommendations of the American Society of Echocardiography Committee for Physician Training in Echocardiography. *Am J Cardiol* 1987;60:158–163.
3. Calahan MK, Foster E. Training in transesophageal echocardiography: in the lab or on the job? *Anesth Analg* 1995;81:217–218.
4. Savage RM, et al. Educational program for intraoperative transesophageal echocardiography. *Anesth Analg* 1995;81:399–403.
5. Popp RL, Williams SV, et al. ACP/ACC/AHA Task Force on Clinical Privileges in Cardiology: clinical competence in adult echocardiography. *J Am Coll Cardiol* 1990;15:1465–1468.
6. Pearlman AS, Gardin JM, Martin RP, et al. Guidelines for physician training in transesophageal echocardiography: recommendations of the American Society of Echocardiography Committee for Physician Training in Echocardiography. *J Am Soc Echocardiogr* 1992;5:187–194.
7. Cheitlin MD, Ritchie JL, et al. Committee on Clinical Application of Echocardiography: ACC/AHA Guidelines for the clinical application of echocardiography: executive summary. *J Am Coll Cardiol* 1997;29:862–879.
8. Konstadt SN, Reich DL, Rafferty T. Validation of a test of competence in transesophageal echocardiography. *J Cardiothorac Vasc Anesth* 1996;10:311–313.
9. Thys DT, Abel M, Bolen B, et al. Practice parameters for intraoperative echocardiography. *Anesthesiology* 1996;84:986–1006.
10. Rafferty T, LaMantia KR, Davis E, et al. Quality assurance for intraoperative transesophageal echocardiography monitoring: a report of 836 procedures. *Anesth Analg* 1993;76:228–232.

SAFETY OF INTRAOPERATIVE TRANSESOPHAGEAL ECHOCARDIOGRAPHY

STANTON K. SHERNAN

Transesophageal echocardiography (TEE) is an invaluable, intraoperative diagnostic monitor for the management of cardiac surgical patients. A recent survey of 155 U.S. academic institutions reported that 91% routinely use intraoperative TEE (1). The popularity of TEE is based on the fact that it may significantly impact intraoperative cardiac surgical decision making by providing pertinent information regarding hemodynamic management, cardiac valvular function, and the diagnosis of congenital heart lesions and great vessel pathology (2,3).

Compared with other hemodynamic monitoring and diagnostic modalities, TEE is considered to be relatively safe and noninvasive (4–6). The incidence of serious TEE-associated complications has been reported to be in the range of 0 to 0.5% (3,7–9). Morbidity and mortality rates of TEE are comparable with those of upper gastrointestinal (GI) endoscopy, which has a complication rate of 0.08% to 0.13% and a mortality rate of 0.004% (7,10,11). In a multicenter survey of 10,419 predominantly conscious, adult patients undergoing TEE, a complication rate of 0.18%, including one death, was reported (7). An incidence of 2.4% adverse events associated with TEE was noted in a study of 1,650 pediatric cardiac surgical patients (12). Furthermore, in a series of 7,200 adult, cardiac surgical patients, intraoperative TEE was associated with comparable morbidity (0.2%) and mortality (0%) (13) (Table 4.1). The purpose of this chapter is to review the safety of TEE, identify specific complications, and propose a set of relative and absolute contraindications to probe placement.

MECHANISM OF GASTROINTESTINAL INJURY ASSOCIATE WITH TRANSESOPHAGEAL ECHOCARDIOGRAPHY

Insertion and manipulation of the TEE probe has most commonly been associated with oropharyngeal, esophageal, and gastric trauma, occurring in approximately 0.2% of cardiac surgical patients (13). Direct trauma of the GI tract (i.e., dental injury, or esophageal laceration, perforation, or abrasion) may be associated with "blind" insertion and advancement of the probe, the large size of the probe tip relative to the normal esophagus, the wide range of probe tip flexion and manipulation required to obtain certain images, and the presence of unknown esophageal and gastric pathology. Indirect GI trauma (e.g., mucosal erythema, odynophagia, or dysphagia) may be related to excessive or prolonged, continuous pressure at the TEE probe–mucosal interface resulting in tissue ischemia and necrosis (14). Urbanowicz et al., however, demonstrated the absence of significant esophageal wall pressure (<17 mm Hg) and mucosal injury even with maximum TEE probe tip flexion in an animal model (15). Furthermore, a maximum TEE probe tip–esophageal wall contact pressure of 60 mm Hg in humans was not associated with adverse sequelae (15). Alternatively, GI injury may occur secondary to thermal injury produced by piezoelectric crystal vibration at the TEE probe tip or from ultrasound energy absorption by the adjacent tissue (15,16). Although esophageal thermal injury has been reported in patients with severe atherosclerotic cardiovascular disease in whom the esophageal circulation was presumed to be compromised (16), experimental studies in animals have failed to demonstrate any gross anatomic or microscopic evidence of injury directly related to ultrasound energy transmission (17). Esophageal mucosal injury may be limited by using minimal gain and acoustic power settings when obtaining images, and turning off the TEE unit during cardiopulmonary bypass (CPB). Furthermore, most TEE probes have a thermocouple to monitor transducer tip temperature and an automatic shutdown mechanism when a

S. K. Shernan: Department of Anesthesiology, Perioperative, and Pain Medicine, Brigham & Women's Hospital, Harvard Medical School, Boston, Massachusetts.

TABLE 4.1. INTRAOPERATIVE TRANSESOPHAGEAL ECHOCARDIOGRAPHY–ASSOCIATED COMPLICATIONS IN A CASE SERIES OF 7,200 CARDIAC SURGICAL PATIENTS

Complications	No. of Patients	% of All Cases (N = 7,200)	% of All Complications (N = 14)
Odynophagia	7	0.10%	50%
Swallowing abnormality	1	0.01%	7%
Esophageal abrasions	4	0.06%	29%
No associated pathology	2	0.03%	14%
Upper gastrointestinal hemorrhage	2	0.03%	14%
Esophageal perforation	1	0.01%	8%
Dental injury	2	0.03%	14%
Endotracheal tube malposition	2	0.03%	14%
Total	14	0.20%	100%

Reprinted from Kallmeyer I, Collard C, John A, et al. The safety of intraoperative transesophageal echocardiography: a case series of 7200 cardiac surgical patients. *Anesth Analg* 2001;92:1126–1130, with permission.

critical, preset temperature threshold (42°–44°C) is reached (18).

COMPLICATIONS ASSOCIATED WITH INTRAOPERATIVE TRANSESOPHAGEAL ECHOCARDIOGRAPHY

Pharyngeal and Esophageal Perforation

Pharyngeal and esophageal perforations are relatively rare yet serious TEE-associated complications (16), which most likely represent a more severe form of injury that is initiated by a mechanism similar to that, which produces gastroesophageal lacerations. The incidence of esophageal perforations secondary to TEE in the emergency room and critical care environment has been reported to be in the range of 0.02% to 0.03% (19). To date, at least 12 cases of perioperative TEE-associated pharyngeal or esophageal perforations have been reported in neonates and adult surgical patients (13,16,20–27). The vast majority of these cases have involved patients undergoing cardiac surgical procedures (13,20–25).

The exact location of esophageal injury associated with TEE probe insertion and manipulation is variable. It has been previously demonstrated that in obtaining the "transgastric" left ventricular short axis view, in 73% of patients the tip of the TEE probe was located in the stomach, in 14% at the gastroesophageal junction, and in 13% in the esophagus (28). Obtaining this particular view usually requires significant anteflexion, thus subjecting the gastroesophageal junction to injury while acting as a hinge for the TEE probe (15,29). The cricopharyngeal region also may be an area prone to TEE-related injury because the posterior esophageal mucosa at the Lannier triangle is only covered by fascia (21,30). One fatal case actually involved an esophago-

tracheal perforation (25). In reality the hypopharynx (22), along with the entire length of the esophagus, including the upper (level of cricopharyngeus) (21,23,27), middle (24,25), and lower (13,16,20,24,26) regions, are all at risk for injury.

Severe pharyngeal or esophageal injury is more likely to occur when TEE probe insertion is difficult or in patients with preexisting GI pathology (e.g., esophageal strictures, varices, tumors, diverticula, recent surgery, achalasia, Boerhaave syndrome). Several additional potential risk factors for TEE-associated gastroesophageal injury also have been proposed (Table 4.2). Children may be specifically prone to injury. In one series of 50 children in whom TEE was performed after congenital heart surgery, esophageal abnormalities including erythema (54%), edema (24%), hematoma (22%), mucosal erosion (14.1%), and petechiae (4.1%) were identified endoscopically in 64% of the patients, especially those weighing less than 9 kg (31). In contrast, esophageal injury was not observed in a study involving postmortem examination of infants following congenital heart surgery (32), or in an investigation involving animals weighing 5 kg (17). Nonetheless, the correlation between small body size or low weight and risk of TEE-related esophageal injury has been recognized by some manufacturers who recommend that even pediatric biplane TEE probes with distal tip dimensions of 9.1 × 8.8 mm (Philips Medical Systems, Andover, MA, U.S.A.), should only be used in patients weighing at least 3 kg (15,21,33,34).

The identification of those at increased risk for TEE-associated pharyngeal or esophageal perforation may be difficult because in some patients in whom esophageal perforation occurred there were no previous signs, symptoms (e.g., dysphagia, odynophagia, hematemesis, severe gastroesophageal reflux), or reported knowledge of esophageal pathology (13). Some reports have identified difficulty in inserting or advancing the TEE probe (15,22,23) and

TABLE 4.2. RISK FACTORS FOR TRANSESOPHAGEAL ECHOCARDIOGRAPHY–ASSOCIATED GASTROESOPHAGEAL INJURY

Risk Factor	Reference
Gastroesophageal pathology	13,35,42
Difficulty with TEE probe insertion	15,22,23
Advanced age	24
Infants/children	12,31,32
Small body habitus	21,25
Cardiomegaly	20
Preoperative steroids	24
History of thoracic radiation	24,27,42
Chronic vasculopathy	16
Cervical arthritis	27,42
Cricopharyngeal sphincter hypertrophy	22,27
Prolonged surgical duration/TEE probe insertion time	25

unusually poor image quality, whereas others have specifically indicated that TEE probe manipulation and image acquisition were uneventful (13,16,20,24–26). In addition, traumatic perforation of the cervical esophagus following endotracheal intubation (30) and esophageal injury associated with nasogastric tube placement (29) also have been implicated as potential causes of injury aside from TEE probe placement. The relatively low incidence of this important complication has made it difficult to attribute a direct correlation with intraoperative TEE. However, the significant morbidity and 10% to 25% mortality rate associated with pharyngeal or esophageal perforation demand that caution

and vigilance be observed during TEE examination (35,36). Consequently, in an attempt to improve safety and reduce morbidity associated with intraoperative TEE, the following precautions should be considered (29):

1. Preinsertion probe inspection for structural integrity
2. Gentle introduction and positioning of a well-lubricated probe
3. Avoiding forceful probe advancement or excessive manipulation in a flexed position
4. Avoiding leaving the TEE probe tip flexed for a prolonged period of time

The initial presentation of severe esophageal or pharyngeal trauma may include excessive hemorrhage (14), subcutaneous emphysema (23), or even the appearance of the probe in the surgical field (21,22) (Fig. 4.1). However, patients who are intubated postoperatively and are not immediately fed may remain asymptomatic for several hours to days until they present with dyspnea while eating or drinking (13,21,24,26) (Fig. 4.2). The Meckler triad of vomiting, pain, and subcutaneous emphysema relating to spontaneous esophageal perforation is often absent (20), and 33% of initial chest radiographs are normal (37). In considering the etiology of a pneumothorax or pleural effusion diagnosed in the immediate postoperative period, the potential for esophageal rupture associated with TEE probe manipulation should not be ignored. A definitive diagnosis may require chest radiography demonstrating a widened mediastinum

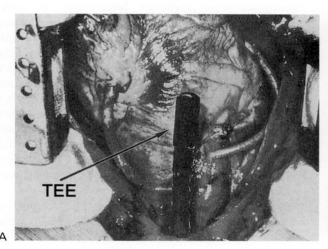
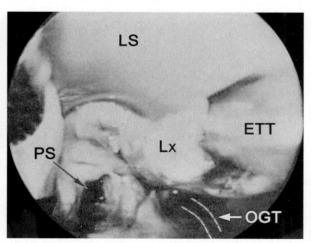

FIGURE 4.1. Esophageal perforation following difficult transesophageal echocardiographic (TEE) probe insertion in a 75-year-old woman undergoing emergent coronary artery bypass graft surgery. **A:** The probe tip (*TEE*) was found protruding from the upper mediastinum into the operating field and onto the anterior surface of the heart and was immediately removed. **B:** Rigid hypopharyngoscopy performed immediately postoperatively revealed a perforation (*PS*) on the left side of the hypopharynx, 2.2 cm proximal to a massively hypertrophied cricopharyngeal muscle obscuring a highly stenotic esophageal entrance. The defect was surgically repaired and the patient was discharged on the 49th postoperative day. *LS,* laryngoscope; *Lx,* larynx; *ETT,* endotracheal tube; *OGT,* orogastric tube. (Reproduced from Spahn DR, Schmid S, Carrel T, et al. Hypopharynx perforation by a transesophageal echocardiography probe. *Anesthesiology* 1995;82:581–583, with permission.)

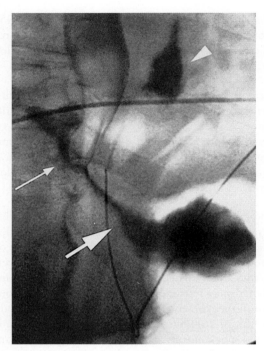

FIGURE 4.2. Distal esophageal perforation not diagnosed until 8 days following intraoperative transesophageal echocardiography performed in a 72-year-old man with an acute myocardial infarction undergoing emergency surgery for a perforated duodenal ulcer. Perforation of the distal esophagus was confirmed during an upper gastrointestinal series revealing contrast extravasation (*thin arrow*). The patient fully recovered following conservative management and was eventually discharged from rehabilitation 4½ months postoperatively. *Arrowhead*, extraluminal contrast in the dorsal mediastinum; *large arrow,* cardiac region of the stomach. (Reproduced from Zalunardo MP, Bimmler D, Grob UC, et al. Late oesophageal perforation after intraoperative transoesophageal echocardiography. *Br J Anaesth* 2002;88(4):595–597, with permission.)

or infiltrates, computed tomography scanning, Gastrografin (Bracco Diagnostics, Inc., Princeton, N.J., U.S.A.) esophagography swallow, or esophagogastroduodenoscopy (EGD). Early diagnosis and management of these injuries can prevent significant morbidity and mortality (35,36,38–40).

Gastrointestinal Bleeding

Gastrointestinal trauma associated with the use of intraoperative TEE may initially present as an upper GI hemorrhage. In two reported cases, acute upper GI hemorrhage was first noted in the operating room at the end of surgery and subsequently confirmed by EGD (13). Both patients were elderly women who had undergone valve replacements (one aortic, one mitral). Only one of these patients had a history of significant esophageal or gastric pathology (i.e., a surgically corrected and asymptomatic Zenker diverticulum). After uneventful TEE probe insertion and manipulation followed by benign intraoperative courses, orogastric aspirates revealed a significant amount of fresh blood and "coffee grounds" (>600 mL) in each patient. Both patients

required blood transfusions in the postoperative period and underwent EGD. In one patient the EGD examination revealed several linear esophageal erosions and a large contusion with a mucosal tear at the gastroesophageal junction that was consistent with a Mallory-Weiss tear most likely related to the TEE probe. In the second patient, EGD revealed erythema and diffuse oozing at the gastroesophageal junction without any other discrete lesions. Although an association with the TEE probe was considered, this patient was also severely coagulopathic. Gastric hemorrhage resolved in both patients with conservative nonsurgical management.

Significant upper GI hemorrhage associated with intraoperative TEE often presents as copious bright red blood or "coffee grounds" (from 500 to 9,000 mL) during orogastric suctioning in the immediate postoperative period (13,29, 41–44). The patient who experienced the 9-L hemorrhage actually died on the 90th postoperative day due to multisystem organ failure (respiratory distress syndrome, low cardiac output, and renal failure) following massive transfusion (29). Frequently, there is no evidence of difficulty in the TEE probe placement or the manipulation of imaging. Some reports also have speculated that the cause of the hemorrhage may be related to difficulty with nasogastric tube placement (29).

Diagnostic endoscopy has shown that most lacerations associated with TEE probe placement are Mallory-Weiss tears located in the vicinity of the gastroesophageal junction or in the gastric cardia (41,42) (Fig. 4.3). As previously mentioned, the lower gastroesophageal junction is prone to injury due to its relative narrowing and location as a common site for obtaining the left ventricular short axis view, which often requires significant anteflexion. Interestingly, two cases of TEE-associated splenic hilar injury also have been reported (43,44). Advancing the TEE probe laterally into the gastric cardia places the tip in a position adjacent to the spleen. Subsequent probe tip manipulation may put tension on the splenic hilum indirectly through the gastrosplenic ligament, which contains the short gastric vessels, thus subjecting the patient to potential splenic hemorrhagic injury (44). Significant hemorrhage associated with a parapharyngeal injury extending from the right soft palate to the right pyriform sinus has been reported following a difficult TEE probe insertion in a patient undergoing mitral valve replacement who eventually died from sepsis (14).

Occult GI bleeding associated with TEE also has been studied. Hulyalkar et al. determined that the 2% risk of upper GI hemorrhage in cardiac surgical patients was independent of the use of intraoperative TEE (45). In this particular report, the incidence of occult blood in the postoperative nasogastric aspirate of those patients in whom TEE was performed was actually lower than in those in whom TEE was not performed (48% vs. 54%, respectively).

Although direct GI trauma following TEE probe insertion and manipulation may contribute to the incidence of postoperative upper GI bleeding, one must consider that the overall incidence of GI complications following cardiac surgery is reported to be in the range of 0.7% to 2%

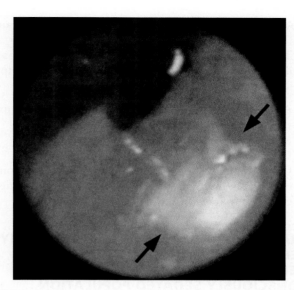

FIGURE 4.3. Endoscopic view of a 5-cm linear laceration in the cardiac region of the stomach (*arrows*) following intraoperative transesophageal echocardiography (TEE) in a 65-year-old man who had undergone elective aortic valve replacement. Immediately after TEE probe removal at the end of the procedure, 150 mL of blood was initially suctioned from the stomach followed by an additional 500 mL after admission to the intensive care unit. The patient was transfused with 3 units of packed red blood cells for a hematocrit of 26%, and subsequently made a full recovery. (Reproduced from Latham P, Hodgins L. A gastric laceration after transesophageal echocardiography in a patient undergoing aortic valve replacement. *Anesth Analg* 1995;81(3):641–642, with permission.)

(46,47). In a retrospective review, postoperative GI complications were diagnosed in 86 (1.9%) of 4,463 consecutive cardiac surgical patients. By logistic multivariate analysis, the following eight parameters were identified as predictors of postoperative GI complications: age greater than 70 years, CPB duration, need for blood transfusions, reoperation, triple-vessel coronary artery disease, New York Heart Association functional class IV, peripheral vascular disease, and congestive heart failure (48). Anticoagulant administration and perioperative visceral hypoperfusion also may exacerbate perioperative GI complications. Thus, factors other than TEE-associated trauma must be considered as potential risk factors for postoperative GI complications following cardiac surgery.

Dysphagia and Odynophagia

An independent correlation between intraoperative TEE and postoperative dysphagia or odynophagia has not been consistently demonstrated (15,45,49,50). The reported incidence of swallowing dysfunction in adult patients following cardiac surgery is in the range of 2% to 4% and is associated with advanced age, duration of tracheal intubation, the presence of an orogastric tube, cerebral vascular accident, and recurrent laryngeal nerve injury (49,51,52). In a study of 57 patients prospectively randomized to undergo cardiac surgery with or without TEE, no differences between the two groups were

noted for minor complaints of odynophagia or nausea, nor was evidence of oral injury (i.e., pharyngeal reddening, lip injury) on pharyngeal inspection. In another review investigating 1,245 cardiac surgical patients, 20 patients (1.6%) were identified as having postoperative dysphagia (51). There were no differences in the incidence of dysphagia between the 4 of 217 patients (1.8%) who had undergone TEE and the 16 of 1,028 (1.6%) who had not. In contrast, other studies have implicated a correlation between intraoperative TEE and painful swallowing or dysmotility. In a nonrandomized study of 7,200 cardiac surgical patients, 7 patients (0.1%) complained of severe odynophagia warranting further investigation by EGD or Gastrografin swallow (13). Dysphagia or evidence of esophageal injury was demonstrated in 5 (0.07%) of these patients. In another study of 838 consecutive cardiac surgical patients undergoing TEE, after controlling for other significant factors (stroke, left ventricular ejection fraction, intubation time, duration of operation), multiple logistic regression analysis showed that the odds of dysphagia for TEE patients was 7.8 times greater than for non-TEE patients (50). Finally, in a study of 869 cardiac surgical patients, swallowing dysfunction was diagnosed in 34 patients (4%) and was associated with documented pulmonary aspiration in 90% of the patients, increased frequency of pneumonia, need for tracheostomy, length of stay in the intensive care unit, and duration of postoperative hospitalization (49). Independent predictors of postoperative dysphagia determined by multivariate logistic regression included age ($p < 0.001$), length of postoperative tracheal intubation ($p = 0.001$), and intraoperative TEE ($p = 0.003$, odds ratio = 4.68, 95% confidence interval 1.76–12.43). However, the researchers stated that these results suggested only an "association" and not necessarily a causal relationship, and that the "benefits of TEE during cardiac operations may still dictate the use of this device" (49). Although a direct correlation between intraoperative TEE and dysphagia following cardiac surgery has yet to be proven, the likelihood for the occurrence of this potential complication must be taken into consideration when deciding whether or not to use intraoperative TEE.

Airway Obstruction

Airway obstruction has been reported in 1% to 2% of all pediatric patients undergoing TEE (12). Stevenson et al. studied pediatric patients in whom the majority of TEE-associated complications were related to the airway (obstruction/compression, right mainstem advancement of the endotracheal tube, inadvertent tracheal extubation) or vascular compression by the probe (12). Compared with adults, pediatric surgical patients may be more predisposed to these complications due to the presence of anatomic variants and the proportionally smaller size of the oropharynx and mediastinum relative to the TEE probe. Increases in peak inspiratory pressure during positive pressure ventilation, increases in end-tidal CO_2, decreases in exhaled tidal volume, and impaired lung deflation have been observed in some infants following TEE probe advancement from the hypopharynx into the esophagus (53,54). In one case describing a infant with a double aortic arch, passage of a pediatric biplane probe (tip dimensions of 9.1 × 8.8 mm; Philips Medical Systems, Andover, MA) from the esophagus into the stomach produced a cyclic gurgling sound coincident with respirations. The TEE probe was removed with subsequent normalization of ventilation. Further inspection of the magnetic resonance image revealed a 10 mm diameter vascular ring compressing the trachea and esophagus (55). Airway obstruction also has been reported in an adult patient with a dissecting aneurysm of the ascending aorta and arch (56). Complete removal of the TEE probe, or at least withdrawing the probe into the hypopharynx when not in continuous use, have both been recommended when the presence of partial airway obstruction is detected (53,57).

An airway-obstructing hematoma developed in a 73-year-old anticoagulated patient with a history of transient ischemic attacks, who was referred for TEE under conscious sedation (58). Several hours following the TEE examination, the patient complained of dysphagia. The next day, shortly after the barium swallow was performed (Fig. 4.4), the patient developed stridor and experienced a respiratory arrest. Bedside cricothyroidotomy relieved the hypoxia. Direct laryngoscopy revealed a massive hematoma across the posterior pharyngeal walls, meeting at the midline at the level of the larynx accompanied by anterior swelling obscuring the epiglottis and arytenoids. The tracheostomy was re-

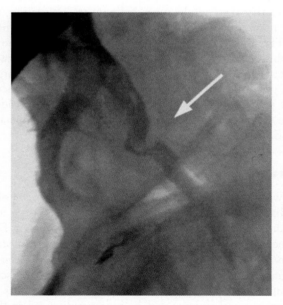

FIGURE 4.4. Roentgenogram (lateral view) of a barium swallow demonstrating an abnormal indentation (*arrow*) in the cricopharyngeal region of the esophagus. (Reproduced from Saphir JR, Cooper JA, Kerbavez RJ, et al. Upper airway obstruction after transesophageal echocardiography. *J Am Soc Echocardiogr* 1997;10(9):977–978, with permission.)

moved 10 days later and the patient was subsequently treated conservatively.

The researchers of this case report recommended observation of the following safety measures to avoid this complication:

1. Administer adequate sedation to facilitate TEE probe passage and prevent hemodynamic volatility.
2. Minimize the procedure time.
3. Consider using a small, pediatric probe.
4. Consider attenuating or discontinuing anticoagulation if difficulty in probe insertion is encountered or the patient complains of persistent dysphagia.

TRANSESOPHAGEAL ECHOCARDIOGRAPHY PERFORMANCE IN PATIENTS UNDER GENERAL ANESTHESIA VERSUS THE CONSCIOUSLY SEDATED POPULATION

The vast majority of intraoperative TEE examinations are performed by experienced ultrasonographers in cardiac surgical patients only after induction of general anesthesia, endotracheal intubation, and administration of neuromuscular relaxants. However, many diagnostic TEE examinations are performed in sedated, nonendotracheally intubated patients. The patients in the case series of Daniels et al. were mostly conscious yet sedated, and experienced a greater incidence of pulmonary (bronchospasm, hypoxia) and cardiac complications (transient dysrhythmias, angina pectoris) although proportionally fewer GI-related adverse events (7) compared with those in other large series of intubated cardiac surgical patients (13).

The presence of a secured airway in an anesthetized patient may afford a degree of safety from airway and reflexive hemodynamic complications that are more likely to be experienced by sedated, nonintubated patients. However, accidental placement of a TEE probe into the trachea has been described in sedated, nonendotracheally intubated patients (59,60). Signs of tracheal probe placement include resistance to probe advancement beyond 30 cm, airway obstruction/hypoventilation, and poor image quality. Interestingly, unique long-axis views of the aortic arch similar to those obtained from a suprasternal transthoracic transducer position may be diagnostic (Fig. 4.5). Although general anesthesia and airway protection may facilitate TEE probe placement, endotracheal intubation does not prevent the inadvertent placement of a TEE probe into the trachea (61). Furthermore, anesthetized patients may be predisposed to a relatively increased risk of esophageal injury due to the impediment of the endotracheal tube in the oropharynx, the relaxation of the esophagus with subsequent predominance of tissue folds, and the inability to provide verbal feedback regarding discomfort from probe malposition (14). Endotracheal tubes may be malpositioned during TEE probe manipulation, thereby causing hypoxemia (13). Thus, ultrasonographers

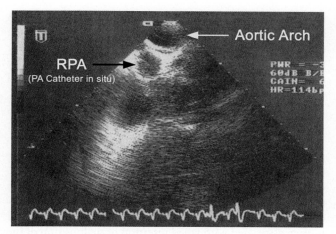

FIGURE 4.5. Accidental transtracheal imaging with a transesophageal echocardiographic (TEE) probe in a 79-year-old man during TEE examination under conscious sedation. Transverse imaging at 26 cm from the incisors revealed the aortic arch appearing as a fluid-filled chamber in the long-axis view adjacent to the transducer. The right pulmonary artery (*RPA*) and *in situ* pulmonary artery (*PA*) catheter appeared as a second fluid filled-chamber in the short-axis view, immediately distal to the aortic arch. Tracheal placement of the TEE probe was suspected when the patient coughed upon encountering resistance at 32 cm. The TEE probe was removed and reinserted in the upper esophagus under direct vision via direct laryngoscopy. (Reproduced from Sutton DC. Accidental transtracheal imaging with a transesophageal echocardiography probe. *Anesth Analg* 1997;85:760–762, with permission.)

must be vigilant in maintaining awareness for potential complications while inserting or manipulating a TEE probe in patients even after endotracheal intubation and general anesthesia induction.

MISCELLANEOUS COMPLICATIONS

Although the vast majority of morbidity attributed with TEE has involved gastroesophageal injury and airway complications, a variety of miscellaneous complications also have been reported (Table 4.3).

Contraindications to Transesophageal Echocardiography Probe Placement

Contraindications to the insertion of a TEE probe generally include either signs or symptoms of gastroesophageal disease (severe dysphagia, odynophagia, reflux, hematemesis) or a known history of pathology. In a series of 7,200 cardiac surgical patients (13), insertion of the TEE probe was contraindicated in 35 patients (0.5%) for reasons similar to those cited elsewhere (6,7,74,75) (Table 4.4). Patients with hiatal hernias usually tolerate TEE examination without complications, although imaging may be compromised. TEE, however, may be contraindicated when patients with hiatal hernias are severely symptomatic. TEE probe insertion also may be contraindicated in some patients with tho-

TABLE 4.3. MISCELLANEOUS COMPLICATIONS ATTRIBUTED TO TRANSESOPHAGEAL ECHOCARDIOGRAPHY

Complication	Reference (Number)
Fatal pulmonary embolism	Cavero et al. (62)
Aortic dissection rupture	Silvey et al. (69)
Bradycardia	Suriani et al. (63)
Transient recurrent laryngeal nerve injury	Zwetsch et al. (64)
Bacteremia	MacGowan et al. (65)
	Korsten et al. (66)
	Nikutta et al. (67)
Dental injury	Kallmeyer et al. (13)
Esophageal stethoscope displacement	Yasick et al. (68)
Vascular compression	Janelle et al. (70)
	Frommelt et al. (71)
	Bensky et al. (72)
	Lunn et al. (73)

racic aortic aneurysms. TEE probe manipulation within the esophagus has been directly associated with adjacent aortic injury (69). In addition, esophageal compression by a thoracic aortic aneurysm may cause significant dysphagia (13). If there is concern for the presence of esophageal pathology when the use of TEE is warranted, an intraoperative endoscopic examination should be performed to confirm the absence of significant disease (76).

There is controversy in the literature regarding the relative risk of TEE in patients with mild dysphagia in the absence of known esophageal pathology. Routine barium swallow or EGD prior to TEE probe insertion for all of these patients might be useful, although not necessarily cost effective. Proceeding with caution and maintaining a low threshold to abandon the procedure if resistance is encountered during insertion or advancement of the probe may be an acceptable

TABLE 4.4. CONTRAINDICATIONS TO TRANSESOPHAGEAL ECHOCARDIOGRAPHY PROBE INSERTION

Absolute
  Esophageal pathology
    Stricture
    Diverticula
    Varices
    Achalasia
    Esophagitis
    Mallory-Weiss tear
    Tumor
    Esophageal compression by thoracic aortic aneurysm
    Recent esophageal surgery
  Gastric pathology
    Recent upper gastrointestinal hemorrhage
    Recent gastric surgery

Relative
  Dysphagia/odynophagia
  Gastroesophageal reflux
  Hiatal hernia

approach, because the majority of these patients tolerate the procedure without complications (75). The use of intraoperative epicardial and epiaortic probes is also a reasonable alternative when TEE is contraindicated.

Failure to Place a Transesophageal Echocardiography Probe

Failure to successfully insert or advance the TEE probe occurs in 0.7% to 1.9% of awake, sedated patients (7,75) and in 0.8% of anesthetized pediatric patients (31). In Kallmeyer's series of anesthetized and endotracheal intubated adults, the incidence of failed probe insertion was considerably lower (0.18%) (13). In one of the patients in this case series, an 89-year-old man who presented for emergency coronary artery bypass grafting, resistance was encountered while attempting to advance the TEE probe into the proximal esophagus. Insertion of the TEE probe was immediately abandoned. The

patient's perioperative course was unremarkable, although he developed recurrent aspiration pneumonia after discharge from the hospital. EGD revealed the presence of a previously unknown Zenker diverticulum. The patient subsequently underwent a Zenker diverticulopexy and cricopharyngeal myotomy.

Explanations for failed TEE probe insertion in conscious adults include patient intolerance, operator inexperience, and limiting anatomic variants (double aortic arch, interrupted aortic arch, tracheal rings) in the pediatric population. Buckling of the TEE probe tip occurred during 2.8% of TEE probe insertions in one study of anesthetized patients and can contribute to difficult or failed placements (28). Because injury to the oropharynx or dysphagia following TEE is often associated with failed insertion or malposition of the probe, the procedure should be abandoned if difficulty or resistance is encountered with probe insertion or advancement (14) (Fig. 4.6).

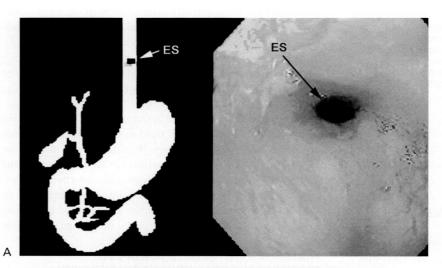

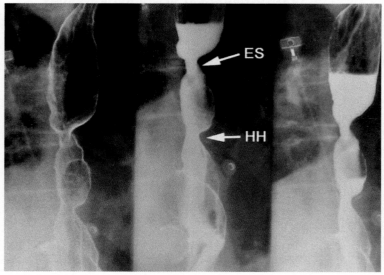

FIGURE 4.6. Endoscopic and radiographic evidence of an esophageal stricture in a 68-year-old man scheduled for coronary artery bypass grafting. Intraoperative transesophageal echocardiographic probe insertion was abandoned after resistance to advancement was encountered at a depth of 30 cm from the incisors. **A:** Upper gastrointestinal endoscopy performed intraoperatively revealed an esophageal stricture (*ES*) with a 10 mm diameter distal lumen, and a 1-cm linear ulcer approximately 30 cm from the incisors. **B:** Modified barium swallow performed 3 days after the operation revealed a midesophageal stricture (*ES*) and a hiatal hernia (*HH*). (Reproduced from Paiste J, Williams JP. Unsuccessful placement of transesophageal echocardiography probe because of esophageal pathology. *Anesth Analg* 2001;92:870–871, with permission.)

Biologic Safety

Ultrasound waves can be produced that contain sufficient mechanical energy to damage or destroy biologic tissue (77). However, low-intensity ultrasonography used in clinical medicine is generally well tolerated and not associated with serious side effects. The biologic effects of ultrasonography depend on the total energy flux across a particular area, the spatial distribution of energy within the sound beam, the duration and pattern over which a biologic system is exposed to the sound energy, the frequencies contained within the sound wave, and the sensitivity of the exposed tissue system (78).

Ultrasonography may produce heat locally, especially when sound energy is concentrated by scattering and reflection (78). More dense tissues such as muscle tend to heat more rapidly than less dense tissues such as fat (79). However, the loss of generated heat by local blood flow (convection) and direct diffusion (conduction) may ultimately limit deleterious effects. In addition, inserted heat-sensing devices are also used to shut off the transducer if a certain temperature is reached (18). High-intensity ultrasonography exposure also can cause *cavitation,* which refers to the creation or vibration of small gas-filled bubbles. Although cavitation is unlikely to occur in blood or soft tissue because of the relatively high viscosity, the resultant vibration of contrast agent microbubbles may cause them to absorb energy, which may subsequently be released as heat (80,81).

The American Institute of Ultrasound in Medicine has proposed the following guidelines for limiting diagnostic ultrasonographic exposure (82,83):

1. A diagnostic exposure that produces a temperature elevation of 1°C or less above normal
2. An exposure intensity of less than 1 W/cm^2 for focused ultrasound beams

Current diagnostic ultrasound systems have outputs ranging from 10 mW/cm^2 for imaging to as high as 430 mW/cm^2 for pulse wave Doppler ultrasonography (82). Although hazardous biologic effects associated with ultrasonography are possible, all evidence thus far indicates that echocardiography is a safe medical imaging tool.

SUMMARY

Many studies may underestimate the true incidence of TEE-associated complications due to conservative definitions of clinically significant adverse events, limitations in standardizing the evaluation of patients' subjective complaints, and ascribing truly related complications to other causes. In addition, it is difficult to assess consequences associated with the "distraction factor" of intraoperative multitasking and patient care while performing TEE (84). Morbidity associated with intraoperative TEE may be minimized by avoiding its use in patients with obvious contraindications to gastroesophageal manipulation, adhering to conservative judgment in abandoning probe insertion when significant resistance is encountered, and maintaining strict vigilance while continuing to observe and care for patients during the examination. The relatively low reported incidence of morbidity suggests that intraoperative TEE is a relatively safe diagnostic monitor that continues to serve as an invaluable tool in the perioperative management of cardiac surgical patients.

KEY POINTS

- The morbidity and mortality of TEE is comparable with that of upper gastrointestinal endoscopy, which has a complication rate of 0.08% to 0.13% and a mortality rate of 0.004%.
- Trauma to the GI tract may be associated with "blind" insertion and advancement of the TEE probe, the large size of the probe tip relative to the normal esophagus, the wide range of probe tip flexion and manipulation required to obtain certain images, excessive or prolonged continuous pressure at the TEE probe–mucosal interface, and the presence of unknown esophageal and gastric pathology.
- Severe pharyngeal or esophageal injury is more likely to occur when TEE probe insertion is difficult or in patients with preexisting GI pathology. However, the identification of those patients at increased risk for TEE-associated pharyngeal or esophageal perforation may be difficult because there may not be any previous signs, symptoms, or reported knowledge of esophageal pathology in some patients in whom esophageal perforation occurs.
- In patients who are intubated postoperatively and are not immediately fed, the initial presentation of severe esophageal or pharyngeal trauma may be delayed for several hours to days.
- While direct GI trauma following TEE probe insertion and manipulation may contribute to the incidence of postoperative upper GI bleeding, factors other than TEE-associated trauma also must be considered as potential risk factors for postoperative GI complications following cardiac surgery.
- Although a direct correlation between intraoperative TEE and dysphagia following cardiac surgery has yet to be proven, the likelihood for the occurrence of this potential complication must be taken into consideration when determining the risk/benefit ratio of intraoperative TEE.
- Airway obstruction has been reported in 1% to 2% of all pediatric patients undergoing TEE.
- Contraindications to the insertion of a TEE probe generally include either signs and symptoms of gastroesophageal disease (severe dysphagia, odynophagia, reflux, hematemesis) or a known history of pathology.
- Failure to successfully insert or advance the TEE probe has been reported to occur in 0.7% to 1.9% of sedated

patients that are awake, 0.8% of anesthetized pediatric patients, and 0.18% of anesthetized and endotracheally intubated adults.

■ Although hazardous biologic effects associated with ultrasonography are possible, all evidence thus far indicates that echocardiography is a safe medical imaging tool.

REFERENCES

1. Poterack KA. Who uses transesophageal echocardiography in the operating room. *Anesth Analg* 1995;80:454–458.
2. Savage RM, Lytle BW, Aronson S, et al. Intraoperative echocardiography is indicated in high-risk coronary artery bypass grafting. *Ann Thorac Surg* 1997;64:368–373.
3. Mishra M, Chauhan R, Sharma KK, et al. Real-time intraoperative transesophageal echocardiography—-how useful? Experience of 5,016 cases. *J Cardiothorac Vasc Anesth* 1998;12:625–632.
4. Shah KB, Rao TLK, Laughlin S, et al. A review of pulmonary artery catheterization in 6,245 patients. *Anesthesiology* 1984;61:271.
5. Davies MJ, Cronin KD, Domaingue CM. Pulmonary artery catheterization. An assessment of risks and benefits in 220 surgical patients. *Anaesth Intens Care* 1982;10:9.
6. Sise MJ, Hollingsworth P, Brimm JE, et al. Complications of the flow-directed pulmonary artery catheter: a prospective analysis in 219 patients. *Crit Care Med* 1981;9:315.
7. **Daniel WG, Erbel R, Kasper W, et al. Safety of transesophageal echocardiography. A multicenter survey of 10,419 examinations. *Circulation* 1991;83:817–821.**
8. **Seward JB, Khandheria BK, Oh JK, et al. Critical appraisal of transesophageal echocardiography: limitations, pitfalls, and complications. *J Am Soc Echocardiogr* 1992;5:288–305.**
9. Khandheria BK. The transesophageal echocardiographic examination: is it safe? [Editorial]. *Echocardiography* 1994;11:55–63.
10. Silvis SE, Nebel O, Rogers G, et al. Endoscopic complications. Results of the 1974 American Society for Gastrointestinal Endoscopy Survey. *JAMA* 1976;235:928–930.
11. Miller G. Komplikationen bei der Endoskopie des oberen Gastrointestinaltraktes. *Leber Magen Darm* 1987;17:299–304.
12. **Stevenson JG. Incidence of complications in pediatric transesophageal echocardiography: experience in 1650 cases. *J Am Soc Echocardiogr* 1999;12:527–532.**
13. **Kallmeyer I, Collard C, John A. Fox J, et al. The safety of intraoperative transesophageal echocardiography: A case series of 7200 cardiac surgical patients. *Anesth Analg* 2001;92:1126–1130.**
14. Savino JS, Hanson CW, Bigelow DC, et al. Oropharyngeal injury after transesophageal echocardiography. *J Cardiothorac Vasc Anesth* 1994;8:76–78.
15. **Urbanowicz JH, Kernoff RS, Oppenheim G, et al. Transesophageal echocardiography and its potential for esophageal damage. *Anesthesiology* 1990;72:40–43.**
16. Kharasch ED, Sivarajan M. Gastroesophageal perforation after intraoperative transesophageal echocardiography. *Anesthesiology* 1996;85:426–428.
17. **O'Shea JP, Southern JF, D'Ambra MN, et al. Effects of prolonged transesophageal echocardiographic imaging and probe manipulation on the esophagus—an echocardiographic-pathologic study. *J Am Coll Cardiol* 1991;17:1426–1429.**
18. Savino JS, Weiss S. Safety of transesophageal echocardiography is still unclear. *Anesthesiology* 1990;73:366–367.
19. Sheony MM, Dhala A, Khanna A. Transesophageal echocardiogram in emergency medicine and critical care. *Am J Emerg Med* 1999;9:580–587.
20. Massey SR, Pitis A, Mehta D, et al. Oesophageal perforation following perioperative transesophageal echocardiography. *Br J Anaesth* 2000;84(5):643–646.
21. Muhiudeen-Russell IA, Miller-Hance WC, Silverman NH. Unrecognized esophageal perforation in a neonate during transesophageal echocardiography. *J Am Soc Echocardiogr* 2001;14:747–749.
22. Spahn DR, Schmid S, Carrel T, et al. Hypopharynx perforation by a transesophageal echocardiography probe. *Anesthesiology* 1995;82:581–583.
23. Badaoui R, Choufane S, Riboulot M, et al. Esophageal perforation after transesophageal echocardiography. *Ann Fr Anesth Reanim* 1994;13(6):850–852.
24. **Brinkman WT, Shanewise JS, Clements SD, et al. Transesophageal echocardiography: not an innocuous procedure. *Ann Thorac Surg* 2001;72:1725–1726.**
25. Lecharny JB, Philip I, Depoix JP. Oesophageal perforation after intraoperative transesophageal echocardiography in cardiac surgery. *Br J Anaesth* 2002;88(4):592–594.
26. Zalunardo MP, Bimmler D, Grob UC, et al. Late oesophageal perforation after intraoperative transoesophageal echocardiography. *Br J Anaesth* 2002;88(4):595–597.
27. Shapira MY, Hirshberg B, Agid R, et al. Esophageal perforation by a transesophageal echocardiogram. *Echocardiography* 1999;16:151–154.
28. Orihashi K, Hong Y, Sisto DA, et al. The anatomical location of the transesophageal echocardiographic transducer during a short axis view of the left ventricle. *J Cardiothorac Vasc Anesth* 1990;4:726–730.
29. Devries AJ, van der Maaten JM, et al. Mallory-Weiss tear following cardiac surgery: transesophageal echoprobe or nasogastric tube? *Br J Anaesth* 2000;84(5):646–649.
30. Laporta D, Kleiman S, Begin L, et al. Traumatic perforation of the cervical esophagus: a complication of endotracheal intubation [Letter]. *Intens Care Med* 1993;19:59–60.
31. Green MA, Alexander JA, Knauf DG, et al. Endoscopic evaluation of the esophagus in infants and children immediately following intraoperative use of transesophageal echocardiography. *Chest* 1999;116:1247–1250.
32. Muhiudeen IA, Roberson DA, Siverman NH, et al. Intraoperative echocardiography in infants and children with congenital shunt lesions: transesophageal versus epicardial echocardiography. *J Am Coll Cardiol* 1990;16:1687–1695.
33. Stevenson JG, Sorenson GK. Proper probe size for pediatric transesophageal echocardiography. *Am J Cardiol* 1993;72:491–492.
34. Ritter SB. Transesophageal real-time echocardiography in infants and children with congenital heart disease. *J Am Coll Cardiol* 1991;18:569–580.
35. Lawrence DR, Ohri SK, Moxon RE, et al. Iatrogenic oesophageal perforations: a clinical review. *Ann R Coll Surg Engl* 1998;80:115–118.
36. Bufkin BL, Miller JI, Mansour KA. Esophageal perforation: emphasis on management. *Ann Thorac Surg* 1996;61:1447–1452.
37. Flynn AE, Verrier ED, Way LW, et al. Esophageal perforation. *Arch Surg* 1989;124:1211–1215.
38. Fernandez FF, Richter A, Freudenberg S, et al. Treatment of endoscopic esophageal perforation. *Surg Endosc* 1999;13:962–966.

39. Attar S, Hankins JR, Suter CM, et al. Esophageal perforation: a therapeutic challenge. *Ann Thorac Surg* 1990;50:45–51.

40. Bladergroen MR, Lowe JE, Postlethwait RW. Diagnosis and recommended management of esophageal perforation. *Ann Thorac Surg* 1986;42:235–239.

41. Latham P, Hodgins L. A gastric laceration after transesophageal echocardiography in a patient undergoing aortic valve replacement. *Anesth Analg* 1995;81(3):641–642.

42. Kallmeyer I, Morse D, Body S, et al. Case 2-2000: Transesophageal echocardiography-associated gastrointestinal trauma. *J Cardiothorac Vasc Anesth* 2000;14(2):212–216.

43. Olenchock SA, Likaszczyk JJ, Reed J, et al. Splenic injury after intraoperative transesophageal echocardiography. *Ann Thorac Surg* 2001;72(6):2141–2143.

44. Chow MS, Taylor MA, Hanson CW. Splenic laceration associated with transesophageal echocardiography. *J Cardiothorac Vasc Anesth* 1998;12:314–316.

45. Hulyalkar AR, Ayd JD. Low risk of gastroesophageal injury associated with transesophageal echocardiography during cardiac surgery. *J Cardiothorac Vasc Anesth* 1993;7:175–177.

46. Krasna MJ, Flancbaum L, Trooskin SZ, et al. Gastrointestinal complications after cardiac surgery. *Surgery* 1988;104:773–780.

47. Egleston CV, Gorey TF, Wood AE, et al. Gastrointestinal complications after cardiac surgery. *Ann R Coll Surg Engl* 1993;15:52–56.

48. Zazharias A, Schwann T, Parenteau G, et al. Predictors of gastrointestinal complications in cardiac surgery. *Tex Heart Inst J* 2000;27:93–99.

49. **Hogue CW, Lappas GD, Creswell LL, et al. Swallowing dysfunction after cardiac operations. *J Thorac Cardiovasc Surg* 1995;110:517–522.**

50. **Rousou JA, Tighe DA, Garb JL, et al. Risk of dysphagia after transesophageal echocardiography during cardiac operations. *Ann Thorac Surg* 2000;69(2):486–489.**

51. Messina AG, Paranicas M, Fiamengo S, et al. Risk of dysphagia after transesophageal echocardiography. *Am J Cardiol* 1991;67:313–314.

52. Kawahito S, Kitahata H, Kimura H, et al. Recurrent laryngeal nerve palsy after cardiovascular surgery: relationship to the placement of a transesophageal echocardiographic probe. *J Cardiothorac Vasc Anesth* 1999;13(5):528–531.

53. Stayer SA, Bent ST, Andropoulos DA. Proper probe positioning for infants with compromised ventilation from transesophageal echocardiography. *Anesth Analg* 2001;92(4):1076–1077.

54. Andropoulos DB, Ayres NA, Stayer SA, et al. The effect of transesophageal echocardiography on ventilation in small infants undergoing cardiac surgery. *Anesth Analg* 2000;90(1):47–49.

55. Phoon CK. Airway obstruction caused by transesophageal echocardiography in a patient with double aortic arch and truncus arteriosus. *J Am Soc Echocardiogr* 1999;12(6):540.

56. Nakao S. Airway obstruction by a transesophageal echocardiography probe in an adult patient with a dissecting aneurysm of the ascending aorta and arch. *J Cardiothorac Vasc Anesth* 2000;14(2):186–187.

57. Cheitlin M, Alpert J, Armstrong W, et al. ACC/AHA guidelines for the clinical application of echocardiography: a report of the American College of Cardiology/American Heart Association Task Force on Practice Guidelines (Committee on Clinical Application of Echocardiography). *Circulation* 1997;95:1686–1744.

58. Saphir JR, Cooper JA, Kerbavez RJ, et al. Upper airway obstruction after transesophageal echocardiography. *J Am Soc Echocardiogr* 1997;10(9):977–978.

59. Sutton DC. Accidental transtracheal imaging with a transesophageal echocardiography probe. *Anesth Analg* 1997;85:760–762.

60. Vignon P, Gueret P, Chabernaud JM, et al. Failure and complications of transesophageal echocardiography. *Arch Mal Coeur Vaiss* 1993;86:849–855.

61. Ortega R, Hesselvik JF, Chandhok D, et al. When the transesophageal echo probe goes into the trachea [Letter]. *J Cardiothorac Vasc Anesth* 1999;13:114–115.

62. Cavero MA, Cristobal C, Gonzalez M, et al. Fatal pulmonary embolism of a right atrial mass during transesophageal echocardiography. *J Am Soc Echocardiogr* 1998;11(4):397–398.

63. Suriani RJ, Tzou N. Bradycardia during transesophageal echocardiographic probe manipulation. *J Cardiothorac Vasc Anesth* 1995;9:347.

64. Zwetsch G, Filipovic M, Skaravan K, et al. Transient recurrent laryngeal nerve palsy after failed placement of a transesophageal echocardiographic probe in an anesthetized patient. *Anesth Analg* 2001;92:1422–1423.

65. MacGowan SW. Intraoperative transesophageal echocardiography is a potential source of sepsis in intensive care. *Eur J Cardiothorac Surg* 2000;7:768–769.

66. Korsten HM, Cathinka H, Heesakkers P, et al. Sheath placement over transesophageal probes: a description of a "self-moving" method. *Anesthesiology* 2002;96(2):519–520.

67. Nikutta P, Mantey-Stiers F, Becht I, et al. Risk of bacteremia induced by transesophageal echocardiography: analysis of 100 consecutive procedures. *J Am Soc Echocardiogr* 1992;5(2):168–172.

68. Yasick A, Samra SK. An unusual complication of transesophageal echocardiography. *Anesth Analg* 1995;81(3):657–658.

69. Silvey SV, Stoughton TL, Pearl W, et al. Rupture of the outer portion of aortic dissection during transesophageal echocardiography. *Am J Cardiol* 1991;68:286–287.

70. Janelle GM, Lobato EB, Tang Y. AN unusual complication of transesophageal echocardiography. *J Cardiothorac Vasc Anesth* 1999;13(2):233–234.

71. Frommelt P, Stuth E. Transesophageal echocardiography in total anomalous pulmonary venous drainage drainage: hypotension caused by compression of the pulmonary venous confluence during probe passage. *J Am Soc Echocardiogr* 1994;7:652–654.

72. Bensky A, O'Brien W, Hammon J. Transesophageal echo probe compression of an aberrant right subclavian artery. *J Am Soc Echocardiogr* 1995;8:964–966.

73. Lunn R, Oliver W, Hagler D, et al. Aortic compression by transesophageal echocardiographic probe in infants and children undergoing cardiac surgery. *Anesthesiology* 1992;77:587–590.

74. Fleischer DE, Goldstein SA. Transesophageal echocardiography: what the gastroenterologist thinks the cardiologist should know about endoscopy. *J Am Soc Echocardiogr* 1990;3:428–434.

75. Chan KL, Cohen GI, Sochowski RA, et al. Complications of transesophageal echocardiography in ambulatory adult patients: analysis of 1500 consecutive examinations. *J Am Soc Echocardiogr* 1991;4:577–582.

76. Paiste J, Williams JP. Unsuccessful placement of transesophageal echocardiography probe because of esophageal pathology. *Anesth Analg* 2001;92:870–871.

77. Fry FJ. Biological effects of ultrasound: a review. *IEEE Trans Biomed Eng* 1979;67:604.

78. Weyman A. Physical principles of ultrasound. In: Weyman A, ed. *Principles and practice of echocardiography,* 2nd ed. Philadelphia: Lea & Febiger, 1994:3–28.

79. Hellman LM. Safety of diagnostic ultrasound in obstetrics. *Lancet* 1970;1:1133.

80. Feigenbaum H. Instrumentation. In: *Echocardiography,* 5th ed. Feigenbaum H, ed. Baltimore: Williams & Wilkins, 1993:1–67.

81. Flynn HG.Physics of acoustic cavitation in liquids. In: Mason WP, ed. *Physical acoustics.* New York: Academic, 1964.

82. Otto C. Principles of echocardiographic image acquisition and Doppler analysis. In: Otto C, ed. *Textbook of clinical echocardiography,* 2nd ed. Philadelphia: WB Saunders, 2000:1–28.

83. American Institute of Ultrasound in Medicine Bioeffects Report: bioeffects consideration for the safety of diagnostic ultrasound. *J Ultrasound Med* 1988;7(suppl):1–38.

84. **Weinger MB, Herndon OW, Gaba DM. The effect of electronic record keeping and transesophageal echocardiography on task distribution, workload, and vigilance during cardiac anesthesia. *Anesthesiology* 1997;87:144–145.**

THE COMPREHENSIVE INTRAOPERATIVE MULTIPLANE TRANSESOPHAGEAL ECHOCARDIOGRAPHIC EXAMINATION

STANTON K. SHERNAN
JACK S. SHANEWISE

Over the past two decades, perioperative transesophageal echocardiography (TEE) has become more recognized as a valuable hemodynamic monitor and diagnostic tool. In 1993, the American Society of Echocardiography (ASE) established the Council for Intraoperative Echocardiography (IOC), to address issues related to the rapidly increasing utility of TEE in the perioperative period and its important impact on anesthesia and surgical decision-making. In 1997, the board members of the IOC decided to create the "Guidelines for Performing a Comprehensive Intraoperative Multiplane TEE Examination," which included the collective endorsement of a recommended set of anatomically directed cross-sectional views and the corresponding nomenclature. These guidelines were adopted and then published by both the ASE and the Society for Cardiovascular Anesthesiologists (SCA) (1,2). They were established to:

1. Facilitate training in intraoperative TEE by providing a framework in which to develop the necessary knowledge and skills
2. Enhance and improve the technical quality and completeness of individual studies
3. Facilitate the communication of intraoperative echocardiographic data between centers to provide a basis for multicenter investigations
4. Encourage industrial development of efficient and rapidly acquiring labeling, storage, and analysis systems

The guidelines for the intraoperative TEE examination were not intended to be all encompassing, but rather to serve as a framework for a systematic and complete examination of cardiac and great vessel anatomy of the "normal patient and to serve as a baseline for later comparison." This examination may require 20 minutes to complete by the beginner, who must balance both comprehension and expedience in obtaining each two-dimensional image and sequentially view one structure at a time. The experienced and competent echocardiographer, however, should be able to complete this examination in less than 10 minutes in order to provide timely and relevant diagnostic information. A more thorough intraoperative TEE examination, including the delineation of detailed intra- and extracardiac anatomy, description of congenital heart defects, and qualitative/quantitative Doppler analysis is certainly recommended and warranted in appropriate patients. Ideally, a complete intraoperative TEE examination not only provides information that is relevant to the particular diagnosis in question, but also identifies unanticipated findings that may have a significant impact on perioperative management (e.g., patent foramen ovale, atrial thrombus, severe aortic atherosclerosis). The purpose of this chapter is to review the technique, anatomy, and clinical utility of the comprehensive intraoperative multiplane TEE examination.

REDUCING THE RISKS OF TRANSESOPHAGEAL ECHOCARDIOGRAPHY

When performed properly in appropriately selected patients, TEE is a very safe procedure, but on rare occasions serious complications can occur (3–5). The first step in a comprehensive TEE examination is a search for factors that increase the risk of the procedure (Table 5.1). The patient should be interviewed whenever possible and the medical record reviewed. The patient is asked about any history of esophageal or stomach problems and specifically questioned about dysphagia and hematemesis. The risks of performing

S. K. Shernan: Department of Anesthesiology, Perioperative, and Pain Medicine, Brigham & Women's Hospital, Harvard Medical School, Boston, Massachusetts.

J. S. Shanewise: Department of Anesthesia, Emory University, Atlanta, Georgia.

TABLE 5.1. RISK FACTORS FOR TRANSESOPHAGEAL ECHOCARDIOGRAPHY

Absolute contraindications
  Recent esophageal or gastric surgery, involving an
    anastomosis (<6 wk)
  Symptomatic esophageal stricture
  Esophageal diverticulum
  Esophageal tumor or abscess
  Acute lye ingestion
  Esophageal fistula

Probable increased risk
  Esophageal varaces
  Symptomatic hiatial hernia
  Mediastinal radiation
  Thoracic aortic aneurysm
  Vascular ring (double aortic arch)
  Coagulopathy
  Unexplained UGI bleed
  Osteophytic cervical spine disease
  Remote esophageal or gastric surgery

TEE in a patient with a positive history or symptoms must be weighed against the possible benefit of the information to be gained. The decision to proceed should be documented in the medical record with an acknowledgment of any increased risk and the informed consent of the patient. Consultation with a gastroenterologist for diagnostic esophagoscopy may be considered if the need to perform the TEE is great in a patient at increased risk. If the problem is confined to the distal esophagus or stomach, it is possible to limit the TEE examination to the middle and upper esophagus, avoiding the areas of concern. Symptomatic esophageal stricture, esophageal diverticulum, recent esophageal surgery, or esophageal tumor are generally considered absolute contraindications to TEE. Also, caution should be used in patients with a history of mediastinal radiation, aneurysms of the thoracic aorta, or a remote history of esophageal or gastric surgery.

INSERTING THE TRANSESOPHAGEAL ECHOCARDIOGRAPHY PROBE

The probe is usually inserted into the esophagus after induction of general anesthesia and tracheal intubation for intraoperative echocardiography. The stomach is first emptied by inserting and suctioning an orogastric tube. This improves TEE image quality by removing any air from the esophagus and the stomach. The TEE probe is inserted gently into the posterior pharynx in the midline. Excessive force should never be used to insert the probe, and on rare occasions the procedure must be abandoned simply because of the inability to insert the probe into the esophagus. The mandible is displaced anteriorly with a jaw lift or thrust and then gentle attempts are made to insert the probe blindly in the midline. Laryngeal bulging to one side or the other can be seen if the probe is not passing in the midline. If the probe does not

pass into the esophagus after a few attempts, a laryngoscope is used to displace the mandible anteriorly and ensure that the probe is being inserted in the midline.

OPTIMIZING THE MACHINE CONTROLS

Properly adjusting the echocardiography machine controls is necessary to obtaining high-quality images. However, images are much better in some patients than in others, and one of the challenges of learning TEE is to know when the image has been optimized, even if of poor quality, and that further efforts to improve the image are a waste of time. Overall image gain is adjusted so that the blood in the chambers appears to be almost black, with the echoes barely visible, and the tissues appear as a range of grays. Time gain controls are adjusted so that there is a uniform level of brightness from the near field to the far field of the image. Dynamic range (compression) varies the range of grays displayed and is adjusted to provide contrast between the blood and the tissues. The depth of the image is adjusted so that the entire extent of the structure of interest is included and centered in the image. The frequency of the imaging ultrasound is adjustable in most TEE probes. Higher frequencies have higher resolution but less penetration than lower frequencies, and the highest frequency with enough penetration to provide a clear image of the structure being examined is selected. Color flow Doppler gain is adjusted by increasing the gain until noise appears in the color sector, and then by backing it off just until the noise disappears. The color sector is adjusted to be as small as possible while including the entire area of interest so that the frame rate, or temporal resolution of the image, is maximized.

MULTIPLANE TRANSESOPHAGEAL ECHOCARDIOGRAPHY PROBE MANIPULATION: DESCRIPTIVE TERMS AND TECHNIQUE

The process of obtaining a comprehensive intraoperative multiplane TEE examination begins with a fundamental understanding of the terminology and technique for probe manipulation (Fig. 5.1). Efficient probe manipulation minimizes esophageal injury and facilitates the process of acquiring and sweeping through two-dimensional image planes. Horizontal imaging planes are obtained by moving the TEE probe up and down (proximal and distal) in the esophagus at various depths relative to the incisors [upper esophageal, 20–25 cm; mid-esophageal (ME), 30–40 cm; transgastric, 40–45 cm; deep transgastric, 45–50 cm]. Vertical planes are obtained by manually turning the probe to the patient's left or right. Further alignment of the imaging plane can be obtained by manually rotating one of the two control wheels on the probe handle, which flexes the probe tip to the patient's

TABLE 5.2. THE COMPREHENSIVE INTRAOPERATIVE MULTIPLANE TRANSESOPHAGEAL ECHOCARDIOGRAPHIC EXAMINATION

Probe Tip Depth: Upper esophageal (20–25 cm)

View: aortic arch (long axis)

Multiplane angle range	0 degrees
Anatomy imaged	Aortic arch; left brachiocephalic vein.
	Left subclavian and carotid arteries; right brachiocephalic artery
Clinical utility	Ascending aorta and arch pathology: atherosclerosis, aneurysms and dissections
	Aortic CPB cannulation site evaluation

View: aortic arch (Short Axis)

Multiplane angle range	90 degrees
Structures imaged	Aortic arch; left brachiocephalic vein;
	Left subclavian and carotid arteries; right brachiocephalic artery
	Main pulmonary artery and pulmonic valve
Clinical utility	Ascending aorta and arch pathology: atherosclerosis, aneurysms and dissections
	Pulmonary embolus; pulmonary valve evaluation (insufficiency, stenosis, Ross procedure)
	Pulmonary artery catheter placement

Probe Tip Depth: Mid-esophageal (30–40 cm)

View: four-chamber

Multiplane angle range	0–20 degrees
Anatomy imaged	Left ventricle and atrium
	Right ventricle and atrium
	Mitral and tricuspid valves
	Interatrial and interventricular septa
	Left pulmonary veins (slight probe withdrawal and turning to left)
	Right pulmonary veins (slight probe withdrawal and turning to right)
	Coronary sinus (slight probe advancement and turn to right)
Clinical utility	Ventricle Function: global and regional
	Intracardiac chamber masses: thrombus, tumor, air; foreign bodies
	Mitral and tricuspid valve evaluation: pathology, pathophysiology
	Congenital or acquired interatrial and ventricular septal defects evaluation
	Hypertrophic obstructive cardiomyopathy evaluation
	Ventricular diastolic evaluation via transmitral and pulmonary vein Doppler flow profile analysis
	Pericardial evaluation: pericarditis; pericardial effusion
	Coronary sinus evaluation: coronary sinus catheter placement; dilation secondary to persistent left superior vena cava

View: Mitral commissural

Multiplane angle range	60–70 degrees
Anatomy imaged	Left ventricle and atrium
	Mitral valve
Clinical utility	Left ventricle function: global and regional
	Left ventricle and atrial masses: thrombus, tumor, air; foreign bodies
	Mitral valve evaluation: pathology, pathophysiology
	Ventricular diastolic evaluation via transmitral Doppler flow profile analysis

View: two-chamber

Multiplane angle range	80–100 degrees
Anatomy imaged	Left ventricle, atrium and atrial appendage
	Mitral valve
	Left pulmonary veins (turning probe to left)
	Coronary sinus (short axis or long axis by turning probe tip to left)
Clinical utility	Left ventricle function: global and regional
	Left ventricle and atrial masses: thrombus, tumor, air; foreign bodies
	Mitral valve evaluation: pathology, pathophysiology
	Ventricular diastolic evaluation via transmitral and pulmonary vein Doppler flow profile analysis
	Coronary sinus evaluation: coronary sinus catheter placement; dilation secondary to persistent left superior vena cava

View: long axis

Multiplane angle range	120–160 degrees
Anatomy imaged	Left ventricle and atrium
	Left ventricular outflow tract
	Aortic valve
	Mitral valve
	Ascending aorta

(continued)

TABLE 5.2. (*continued*)

Clinical utility	Left ventricle function: global and regional
	Left ventricle and atrial masses: thrombus, tumor, air; foreign bodies
	Mitral valve evaluation: pathology, pathophysiology
	Ventricular diastolic evaluation via transmitral Doppler flow profile analysis
	Aortic valve evaluation: pathology, pathophysiology
	Ascending aorta pathology: atherosclerosis, aneurysms, dissections
	Hypertrophic obstructive cardiomyopathy evaluation
View: right ventricular inflow–outflow	
Multiplane angle range	60–90 degrees
Anatomy imaged	Right ventricle and atrium
	Left atrium
	Tricuspid valve
	Aortic valve
	Right ventricular outflow tract
	Pulmonic valve and main pulmonary artery
Clinical utility	Right ventricle and atrial masses and left atrial: thrombus, embolus, tumor, foreign bodies
	Pulmonic valve and sub–pulmonic valve: pathology; pathophysiology
	Pulmonary artery catheter placement
	Tricuspid valve: pathology; pathophysiology
	Aortic valve: pathology; pathophysiology
View: aortic valve (short axis)	
Multiplane angle range	30–60 degrees
Anatomy imaged	Aortic valve
	Interatrial septum
	Coronary ostia and arteries
	Right ventricular outflow tract
	Pulmonary valve
Clinical utility	Aortic valve: pathology; pathophysiology
	Ascending aorta pathology: atherosclerosis, aneurysms and dissections
	Left and right atrial masses: thrombus, embolus, air, tumor, foreign bodies
	Congenital or acquired interatrial septal defects evaluation
View: aortic valve (long axis)	
Multiplane angle range	120–160 degrees
Anatomy imaged	Aortic valve
	Proximal ascending aorta
	Left ventricular outflow tract
	Mitral valve
	Right pulmonary artery
Clinical Utility	Aortic valve: pathology; pathophysiology
	Ascending aorta pathology: atherosclerosis, aneurysms and dissections
	Mitral valve evaluation: pathology, pathophysiology
View: Bicaval	
Multiplane angle range	80–110 degrees
Anatomy imaged	Right and left atrium
	Superior vena cava (long axis)
	Inferior vena cava orifice: advance probe and turn to right to visualize inferior vena cava in the long axis, liver, hepatic and portal veins
	Interatrial septum
	Right pulmonary veins (turn probe to right)
	Coronary sinus and Thebesian valve
	Eustachian valve
Clinical utility	Right and left atrial masses: thrombus, embolus, air, tumor, foreign bodies
	Superior vena cava pathology: thrombus, sinus venosus atrial septal defect
	Inferior vena cava pathology: thrombus, tumor
	Femoral venous line placement
	Coronary sinus catheter line placement
	Right pulmonary vein evaluation: anomalous return, Doppler evaluation for left ventricular diastolic function
	Congenital or acquired interatrial septal defects evaluation
	Pericardial effusion evaluation

(continued)

TABLE 5.2. (*continued*)

View: ascending aortic (short axis)	
Multiplane angle range	0–60 degrees
Anatomy imaged	Ascending aorta
	Superior vena cava (short axis)
	Main pulmonary artery
	Right pulmonary artery
	Left pulmonary artery (turn probe tip to left)
	Pulmonic valve
Clinical utility	Ascending aorta pathology: atherosclerosis, aneurysms and dissections
	Pulmonic valve: pathology; pathophysiology
	Pulmonary embolus/thrombus evaluation
	Superior vena cava pathology: thrombus, sinus venosus atrial septal defect
	Pulmonary artery catheter placement
View: ascending aorta (long axis)	
Multiplane angle range	100–150 degrees
Anatomy imaged	Ascending aorta
	Right pulmonary artery
Clinical utility	Ascending aorta pathology: atherosclerosis, aneurysms and dissections
	Anterograde cardioplegia delivery evaluation
	Pulmonary embolus/thrombus
View: descending aorta (short axis)	
Multiplane angle range	0 degrees
Anatomy imaged	Descending thoracic aorta
	Left pleural space
Clinical utility	Descending aorta pathology: atherosclerosis, aneurysms and dissections
	Intraaortic balloon placement evaluation
	Left pleural effusion
View: descending aorta (long axis)	
Multiplane angle range	90–110 degrees
Anatomy imaged	Descending thoracic aorta
	Left pleural space
Clinical utility	Descending aorta pathology: atherosclerosis, aneurysms and dissections
	Intraaortic balloon placement evaluation
	Left pleural effusion
Probe Tip Depth: Transgastric (40–45 cm)	
View: basal (short axis)	
Multiplane angle range	0–20 degrees
Anatomy imaged	Left and right ventricle
	Mitral valve
	Tricuspid valve
Clinical utility	Mitral valve evaluation ("fish-mouth view"): pathology, pathophysiology
	Tricuspid valve evaluation: pathology, pathophysiology
	Basal left ventricular regional function
	Basal right ventricular regional function
View: mid–short axis	
Multiplane angle range	0–20 degrees
Anatomy imaged	Left and right ventricle
	Papillary muscles
Clinical utility	Mid left and right ventricular regional and global function
	Intracardiac volume status
View: two-chamber	
Multiplane angle range	80–100 degrees
Anatomy imaged	Left ventricle and atrium
	Mitral valve: chordae and papillary muscles
	Coronary sinus
Clinical utility	Left ventricular regional and global function (including apex)
	Left ventricular and atrium masses: thrombus, embolus, air, tumor, foreign bodies
	Mitral valve: pathology and pathophysiology

(*continued*)

TABLE 5.2. (*continued*)

View: long axis
  Multiplane angle range   90–120 degrees
  Anatomy imaged   Left ventricle and outflow tract
                                  Aortic valve
                                  Mitral valve
  Clinical utility   Left ventricular regional and global function
                                  Mitral valve: pathology and pathophysiology
                                  Aortic valve: pathology and pathophysiology
View: Right ventricular inflow
  Multiplane angle range   100–120 degrees
  Anatomy imaged   Right ventricle and atrium
                                  Tricuspid valve: chordae and papillary muscles
  Clinical utility   Right ventricular regional and global function
                                  Right ventricular and atrium masses: thrombus, embolus, tumor, foreign bodies
                                  Tricuspid valve: pathology and pathophysiology

Probe Tip Depth: Deep transgastric (45–50 cm)
  View: long axis
    Multiplane angle range   0–20 degrees (anteflexion)
    Anatomy imaged   Left ventricle and outflow tract
                                  Interventricular septum
                                  Aortic valve and ascending aorta
                                  Left atrium
                                  Mitral valve
                                  Right ventricle
                                  Pulmonic valve
    Clinical utility   Aortic valve and subaortic pathology and pathophysiology
                                  Mitral valve pathology and pathophysiology
                                  Left and right ventricle global function
                                  Left and right ventricle masses: thrombus, embolus, tumor, foreign bodies
                                  Congenital or acquired interventricular septal defect evaluation

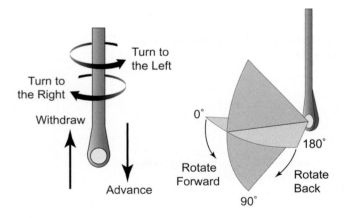

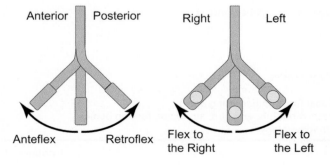

FIGURE 5.1. Terminology used to describe manipulation of the probe and transducer during image acquisition.

left or right (small wheel) or anteriorly and posteriorly (large wheel). Multiplane probes may further facilitate interrogation of complex anatomic structures, such as the mitral valve (MV), by allowing up to 180 degrees of axial rotation of the imaging plane without manual probe manipulation.

The published guidelines for performing a comprehensive intraoperative TEE recommend obtaining 20 views of the heart and great vessels, including all four chambers and valves of the heart, as well as the thoracic aorta and the pulmonary artery (PA) (Table 5.2) (Fig. 5.2). There are two conceptual approaches to performing a comprehensive TEE examination. One is to focus on the structures being examined, developing the views needed to examine each structure following a logical sequence moving from structure to structure (e.g., left atrium (LA), aortic valve (AV), MV, left ventricle (LV), etc.). The other approach is to focus on the views, developing each in a sequence, looking at the various structures displayed in each view. It is most practical to combine the two approaches, focusing on some of the structures in one part of the examination and some of the views in another. This may be done in many ways, and each individual should develop a set sequence that makes sense to them and follow it so that no structures are skipped.

There should be an administrative procedure for archiving the recorded images, and a method for keeping track of the studies performed for medical record purposes and to allow access to the study at a future date should the need arise. These records are especially important if charges are made for providing the intraoperative TEE services.

EXAMINATION OF SPECIFIC STRUCTURES

Left and Right Ventricle

The LV should be carefully examined for global and regional function using multiple transducer planes, depths, and rotational and angular orientations (Fig. 5.2). Regional assessment requires a systematic approach to evaluate each of the 16 individual LV segments: 6 basal, 6 middle, and 4 apical (Fig. 5.3). Analysis of segmental function is based on a qualitative visual assessment that includes the following grading system of both LV wall thickening and endocardial motion during systole: 1, normal (<30% thickening); 2, mild hypokinesis (10%–30% thickening); 3, severe hypokinesis (<10% thickening); 4, akinesis (no thickening); 5, dyskinesis (thinning and paradoxic motion). The ME four-chamber view at 0 to 20 degrees (Fig. 5.2A) and two-chamber view at approximately 80 to 100 degrees (Fig. 5.2B) enable visualization of the septal, lateral, inferior, and anterior segments at the basal, middle, and apical levels segments. The ME long-axis (LAX) view at 120 to 160 degrees (Fig. 5.2C) allows evaluation of the remaining anteroseptal and posterior LV segments. Because the apex of the LV is usually located inferior to the base, retroflexion of the probe tip may be required to minimize LV foreshortening. The

transgastric mid–short-axis view (TG mid-SAX) at 0 to 20 degrees (Fig. 5.2D) is the most commonly used view for monitoring LV function because it allows a mid-papillary assessment of the LV segments supplied by all three major coronary arteries: the right, left circumflex, and left anterior descending arteries (Fig. 5.4). This view also enables qualitative and quantitative evaluation of pericardial effusions. Advancing or withdrawing the probe at the transgastric depth enables LV evaluation at the respective apical and basal levels (TG basal SAX view) (Fig. 5.2F). Further evaluation of the LV can be obtained at the mid-papillary transgastric depth by increasing the multiplane angle to the TG two-chamber (80–100 degrees) (Fig. 5.2E) and TG LAX (90–120 degrees) views (Fig. 5.2J). Global LV function requires assessment of dilatation (LV diameter <6 cm at enddiastole), hypertrophy (LV wall thickness >1.2 cm at enddiastole), and contractility. A more extensive quantitative evaluation of ventricular performance can be acquired by planimetry measurements of end-diastolic and end-systolic areas from which ejection fractions, ventricular volumes, cardiac output, and mean circumferential shortening can be calculated.

Right ventricular (RV) regional and global function can be assessed from the ME four-chamber view (Fig. 5.2A), which allows visualization of the septal and free walls. Although a formal segmental scheme has not been developed for the RV free wall, regional assessment of the septum can be performed. Turning the probe to the right and advancing slightly from the ME depth allows visualization of the tricuspid valve (TV), coronary sinus (CS), and RV apex. Rotating the multiplane angle to 60 to 90 degrees until the right ventricular outflow tract opens up develops the ME RV inflow–outflow view (Fig. 5.2M), in which the right atrium (RA), TV, inferior RV free wall, right ventricular outflow tract (RVOT), pulmonic valve (PV), and main PA can be viewed "wrapping around" the centrally oriented AV. This view often allows optimal Doppler beam alignment to evaluate the TV and can also be helpful for directing PA catheter floating and positioning. The TG mid-SAX view displays the crescent-shaped, thinner-walled RV to the left of the LV in Fig. 5.2D. The TG RV inflow view (Fig. 5.2N) is developed by turning the probe to the right to center the RV at this depth and by rotating the multiplane angle forward to 100 to 120 degrees, thereby revealing the inferior RV free wall. Slight anteflexion, advancement, and rotation of the probe back toward 0 degrees often reveals the RVOT and PV. Despite the asymmetric shape of the RV, global function can still be assessed from the ME four-chamber, TG mid-SAX, ME RV inflow–outflow, and TG RV inflow views (Fig. 5.2A, D, M, and N) using a quantitative evaluation scheme similar to that previously delineated for the LV. Qualitative echocardiographic findings consistent with a diagnosis of global RV dysfunction include dilatation and hypertrophy, flattened or leftward shift of the atrial and ventricular septum, tricuspid regurgitation, and a dilated CS.

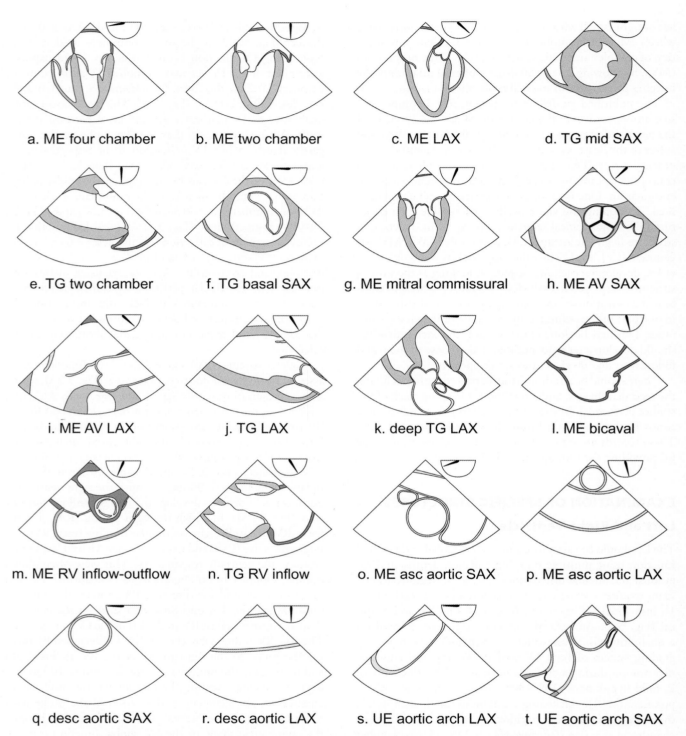

a. ME four chamber b. ME two chamber c. ME LAX d. TG mid SAX

e. TG two chamber f. TG basal SAX g. ME mitral commissural h. ME AV SAX

i. ME AV LAX j. TG LAX k. deep TG LAX l. ME bicaval

m. ME RV inflow-outflow n. TG RV inflow o. ME asc aortic SAX p. ME asc aortic LAX

q. desc aortic SAX r. desc aortic LAX s. UE aortic arch LAX t. UE aortic arch SAX

FIGURE 5.2. Twenty cross-sectional views comprising the recommended comprehensive transesophageal echocardiographic examination. Approximate multiplane angle is indicated by the icon adjacent to each view. *ME,* mid-esophageal; *TG,* transgastric; *UE,* upper esophageal; *SAX,* short axis; *LAX,* long axis; *AV,* aortic valve; *RV,* right ventricle; *asc,* ascending; *desc,* descending.

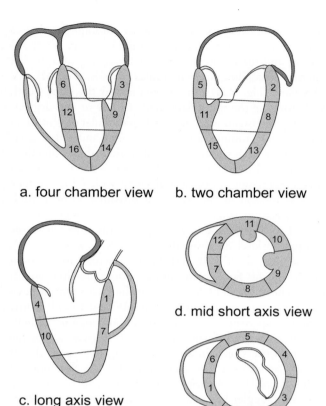

a. four chamber view   b. two chamber view

c. long axis view

d. mid short axis view

e. basal short axis view

FIGURE 5.3. Sixteen-segment model of the left ventricle. **A:** Four-chamber views show the three septal and three lateral segments. **B:** Two-chamber views show the three anterior and three inferior segments. **C:** Long-axis views show the two anteroseptal and two posterior segments. **D:** Mid–short-axis views show all six segments at the middle level. **E:** Basal short-axis views show all six segments at the basal level. The basal segments are as follows: *1,* basal anteroseptal; *2,* is basal anterior; *3,* basal lateral; *4,* basal posterior; *5,* basal inferior; *6,* basal septal. The middle segments are as follows: *7,* mid-anteroseptal; *8,* mid-anterior; *9,* mid-lateral; *10,* mid-posterior; *11,* mid-inferior; *12,* mid-septal. The apical segments are as follows: *13,* apical anterior; *14,* apical lateral; *15,* apical inferior; *16,* apical septal.

Mitral Valve

The echocardiographic evaluation of the MV requires a thorough assessment of its leaflets (anterior and posterior), annulus, and the subvalvular apparatus (chordae tendineae, papillary muscles, and adjacent LV walls) in order to locate lesions and define the cause and severity of the pathophysiology. The mitral leaflets can be further divided into posterior leaflet scallops—lateral (P1), middle (P2), and medial (P3)—that correspond with respective anterior leaflet sections—lateral third (A1), middle third (A2), and medial third (A3) (Figs. 5.5 and 5.6). The leaflets are united at the anterolateral and posteromedial commissures. The ME four-chamber view (Fig. 5.2A) displays the larger-appearing anterior leaflet to the left of the posterior leaflet. Anteflex-

ing the probe provides imaging of the anterior aspect of the MV while gradual advancement of the probe and retroflexion shifts the image plane to the posterior aspect of the MV. Maintaining the probe at the ME depth and rotating the multiplane angle forward to 60 to 70 degrees develops the ME mitral commissural view (Fig. 5.2G), in which A2 is flanked by P1 on the right of the image and P3 on the left, giving A2 the appearance of a "trapdoor" as it moves in and out of the imaging plane throughout the cardiac cycle. Further forward rotation of the probe to 80 to 100 degrees develops the ME two-chamber view (Fig. 5.2B), with the posterior leaflet now to the left of the image and the anterior leaflet to the right. Final forward probe rotation to 120 to 160 degrees reveals the ME LAX view (Fig. 5.2C), which images P2 on the left and A2 on the right. The TG basal SAX view (Fig. 5.2F) enables visualization of both MV leaflets ("fish-mouth view") if the probe is anteflexed and withdrawn slightly from the mid-papillary level of the LV. In this view, the posteromedial commissure is in the upper

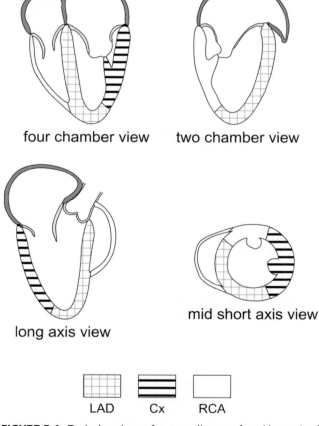

four chamber view   two chamber view

long axis view

mid short axis view

LAD   Cx   RCA

FIGURE 5.4. Typical regions of myocardium perfused by each of the major coronary arteries to the left ventricle. Other patterns occur due to normal anatomic variations or coronary disease with collateral flow. *RCA,* right coronary artery; *Cx,* circumflex; *LAD,* left anterior descending.

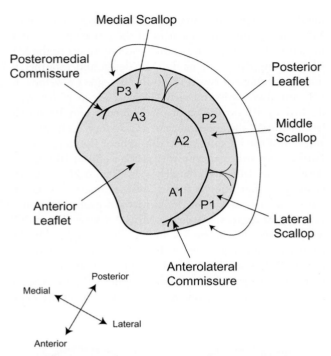

FIGURE 5.5. Anatomy of the mitral valve. *A1,* lateral third of the anterior leaflet; *A2,* middle third of the anterior leaflet; *A3,* medial third of the anterior leaflet; *P1,* lateral scallop of the posterior leaflet; *P2,* middle scallop of the posterior leaflet; *P3,* medial scallop of the posterior leaflet.

left, the anterolateral commissure to the lower right, the posterior leaflet to the right, and anterior leaflet to the left of the image. Rotation of the probe to 80 to 100 degrees develops the TG two-chamber view (Fig. 5.2E) that is especially useful for evaluating the chordae tendineae and corresponding papillary muscles. Further functional evaluation of the MV requires a quantitative Doppler evaluation [pulsed-wave Doppler (PWD), continuous-wave Doppler (CWD), and color flow Doppler (CFD)] of transmitral and pulmonary venous flow for assessing MV regurgitation, stenotic lesions, and LV diastolic function.

Aortic Valve: Aortic Root and Left Ventricular Outflow

The three cusps of the semilunar AV are best visualized simultaneously in the ME AV SAX view (Fig. 5.2H), which is obtained by centering the valve in the image and rotating the probe forward to 30 to 60 degrees until a symmetric view of all three cusps is seen. The noncoronary cusp is seen adjacent to the atrial septum, the right cusp is anterior and farthest from the transducer, and the left cusp is to the right in the image pointing in the direction of the LA appendage. This view permits planimetry of the AV orifice, evaluation of congenital anomalies of the AV (e.g., bicuspid AV), and qualitative assessment of aortic insufficiency when CFD is

used. Withdrawing the probe slightly through the sinuses of Valsalva allows for imaging the right coronary artery anteriorly, and the left main coronary branching into the left anterior descending and circumflex arteries. The ME AV LAX view (Fig. 5.2I) can be obtained at the same depth while rotating the multiplane angle to 120 to 160 degrees, allowing for visualization of the left ventricular outflow tract (LVOT), AV annulus and leaflets (right and either noncoronary or left), sinuses of Valsalva, sinotubular junction, and proximal ascending aorta. This view is particularly useful for evaluating aortic insufficiency with CFD, systolic anterior motion of the MV, and proximal aortic pathology (dissections, aneurysms). Decreasing the angle back to 90 to 120 degrees and advancing into the stomach to the transgastric level develops the TG LAX view (Fig. 5.2J). In this view, the LVOT and AV are oriented to the right and in the far field in the image, often allowing parallel alignment of the Doppler beam for the assessment of flows and pressure gradients through the AV and LVOT (aortic stenosis, hypertrophic obstructive cardiomyopathy). Rotating the angle back further to 0 to 20 degrees, advancing deep into the stomach, and anteflexing the tip so that it lies adjacent to the LV apex allows for the development of the deep TG LAX view (Fig. 5.2K), which also often provides Doppler beam alignment for measuring transaortic valve and LVOT flow velocities and may also provide an additional window for assessing flows through muscular ventricular septal defects and LV apical pathology (thrombus, aneurysms).

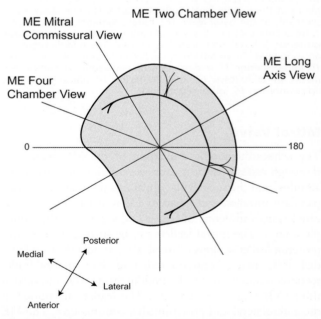

FIGURE 5.6. Short axis drawing of the mitral valve illustrating how it is transected by the mid-esophageal (*ME*) views. Rotating the multiplane angle from 0 to 180 degrees moves the imaging plane axially through the entire mitral valve.

Tricuspid Valve

The echocardiographic evaluation of the TV requires a thorough assessment of its three leaflets (anterior, posterior, and septal), annulus, chordae tendineae, papillary muscles, and the corresponding RV walls. In the ME four-chamber view (Fig. 5.2A), the septal TV leaflet is displayed on the right side of the image and the posterior or anterior TV leaflet on the left side, depending on the depth of the probe. Rotating the multiplane angle to 60 to 90 degrees develops the ME RV inflow–outflow view (Fig. 5.2M), which displays the posterior TV leaflet on the left side of the image and the anterior TV leaflet on the right side of the image adjacent to the AV. The TG RV inflow view (Fig. 5.2N) is obtained by advancing the probe into the stomach and rotating to 100 to 120 degrees. This view is ideal for visualizing the chordae tendineae and papillary muscles in the RV. Rotating back to the TG mid-SAX at 0 to 20 degrees and slightly withdrawing the probe provides a SAX view of the TV, displaying the anterior leaflet in the far field, the posterior leaflet to the left in the near field, and the septal leaflet on the right side of the image. A more extensive quantitative analysis of TV pathophysiology requires the use of Doppler echocardiography (PWD, CWD, and CFD) by aligning the beam parallel to trans-tricuspid flow in either the ME RV inflow–outflow or ME four-chamber view.

Pulmonic Valve and Pulmonary Artery

The pulmonic valve (PV) is a trileaflet, semilunar valve. The ME AV short axis view (Fig. 5.2H) displays the transition between the RVOT and PV. Rotating the angle back toward 0 degrees and withdrawing slightly develops the ME ascending aortic SAX view (Fig. 5.2O), displaying the transition between the PV and main PA and its bifurcation. Although the right PA is usually easy to visualize by turning the probe to the right, the left PA is often obscured by the interposing, air-filled, left main-stem bronchus. This view can be used in the Doppler echocardiographic assessment of PV flow disturbances because the Doppler beam can be aligned parallel to the flow. The ME RV inflow–outflow view (Fig. 5.2M) also can be used to assess the PV and main PA, which lie on the right side of the image adjacent to the AV, although the upper esophageal aortic arch SAX view (Fig. 5.2T), which displays the PV oriented to the left of the SAX view of the aortic arch, usually provides a more parallel Doppler beam alignment, facilitating the evaluation of pulmonic regurgitation or stenosis. Withdrawing the probe slightly in the deep TG LAX view (Fig. 5.2K) in combination with slight anteflexion and turning to the right can often allow visualization of the RVOT and PV to the left of the image in the far field, providing another imaging plane for Doppler evaluation in patients with subpulmonic and PV pathology.

Left Atrium, Left Atrial Appendage, Pulmonary Veins, and Atrial Septum

The LA is the closest cardiac structure to the TEE probe when positioned in the ME. Consequently, the LA is usually easily displayed in the top of the display at the vertex of the two-dimensional image sector. The ME four-chamber view (Fig. 5.2A) displays the LA almost in its entirety, with the LA appendage (LAA) oriented to its superior and lateral aspect when the probe is slightly withdrawn. The muscular ridges of the pectinate muscles within the LAA should not be confused with thrombi. Slight further withdrawal of the probe and turning it to the left brings the left upper pulmonary vein (LUPV) into view as it enters the LA from the anterior-to-posterior direction separated from the lateral border of the LAA by a prominent ridge of tissue. In contrast to the LUPV, which is usually reasonably parallel to the Doppler beam, the left lower pulmonary vein (LLPV) enters the LA just below the LUPV in a lateral-to-medial direction and is usually more perpendicular to the beam. Pulmonary venous Doppler flow velocity profiles are useful for the qualitative and quantitative assessment of LV diastolic function. Turning the probe to the right at this depth reveals the right upper pulmonary vein (RUPV) entering the LA in an anterior-to-posterior direction. The right lower pulmonary vein (RLPV) can sometimes be visualized as it enters perpendicular to the long axis of the LA by slightly advancing the probe. The interatrial septum (IAS), consisting of thicker limbus regions flanking the thin fossa ovalis, also can be imaged in the ME four-chamber view (Fig. 5.2A). Benign lipomatous hypertrophy of the IAS must be distinguished from pathologic lesions such as atrial myxomas. The presence of a patent foramen ovale or congenital atrial septal defect should be assessed with CFD and intravenous injections of agitated saline into the RA. Advancing the probe and rotating the angle to 80 to 100 degrees develops the ME two-chamber view (Fig. 5.2B), which allows for further imaging of the LA by turning the probe from left to right. The LAA and LUPV can be seen by turning the probe more to the left. Rotating the probe to the right at this level and adjusting the multiplane angle to 80 to 110 degrees develops the ME bicaval view (Fig. 5.2I), which shows the superior vena cava (SVC) entering the RA to the right of the image and the inferior vena cava (IVC) entering from the left. The IAS can be seen in the middle of the image separating the LA and RA. The RUPV and RLPV can usually be seen if the probe is turned further to the right just beyond the LAX view of the SVC. This transition of images also can be used in conjunction with CFD to identify sinus venosus atrial septal defects and anomalous pulmonary venous return.

Right Atrium and Coronary Sinus

The RA can be most easily visualized in the ME four-chamber view (Fig. 5.2A) by turning the probe to the patient's right side. In this view, the entire RA can be visualized for size, overall function, and the presence of masses (thrombi, tumors). Rotating the multiplane angle to 80 to 110 degrees develops the ME bicaval view (Fig. 5.2L), which displays the RA and its internal structures (eustachian valve, Chiari network, crista terminalis). The SVC can be imaged entering the RA on the right of the image, superior to the right atrial appendage, and the IVC enters the RA on the left. Advancing and turning the probe to the right allows for a qualitative evaluation of the intrahepatic segment of the IVC and hepatic veins. Pacemaker electrodes and central venous catheters for hemodynamic monitoring or cardiopulmonary bypass (CPB) can be easily imaged in this view.

The CS lies posteriorly in the atrioventricular groove, emptying into the RA at the inferior extent of the atrial septum. The CS can be viewed in LAX entering the RA just superior to the tricuspid annulus by advancing and slightly retroflexing the probe from the ME four-chamber view (Fig. 5.2A). The CS can be imaged in SAX in the ME two-chamber view (Fig. 5.2B) in the upper left of the display. Turning the probe to the left in this view often allows visualization of the CS in LAX as it traverses the lateral aspect of the atrioventricular groove. The CS and thebesian valve also can be visualized in the ME bicaval view (Fig. 5.2L) on the upper right of the image as it enters the RA at an obtuse angle, by turning the probe leftward simultaneously with retroflexion and leftward flexion. Echocardiographic visualization of the CS can be useful for directing the placement of CS catheters used during CPB for cardioplegia.

Thoracic Aorta

The proximal and mid-ascending thoracic aorta can be visualized in SAX in the ME ascending aortic SAX view (Fig. 5.2O). Advancing and withdrawing the probe should enable visualization of the thoracic aorta from the sinotubular junction to a point 4 to 6 cm superior to the AV and allow inspection for aneurysms and dissections. Rotating the multiplane angle to 100 to 150 degrees develops the ME ascending aortic LAX view (Fig. 5.2P), which optimally displays the parallel anterior and posterior walls for measuring proximal and mid-ascending aortic diameters. This view also can be obtained from the ME AV LAX view (Fig. 5.2I) by slightly withdrawing and turning the probe to the right.

Transesophageal echocardiographic imaging of the proximal and mid-aortic arch is often obscured by the interposing, air-filled trachea. Views of the aortic arch are obtained by withdrawing the probe from the ME ascending aortic SAX view at 0 degrees (Fig. 5.2O) and rotating leftward to obtain the upper esophageal aortic arch LAX view (Fig. 5.2S), which displays the proximal arch followed by the mid-arch, the great vessels (brachiocephalic, left carotid, and left subclavian artery), and distal arch before it joins the proximal descending thoracic aorta imaged in SAX. Alternatively, rotating the probe to 90 degrees develops the

upper esophageal aortic arch SAX view (Fig. 5.2T). Turning the probe to the left, this view delineates the transition of the distal arch with the proximal descending thoracic aorta. Turning the probe to the right and slightly withdrawing allows for the mid-arch and great vessels to be imaged on the right side of the screen, followed by the distal ascending aorta when the probe is subsequently advanced and rotated forward to 120 degrees (ME ascending aortic LAX view) (Fig. 5.2P). Epiaortic aortic scanning may be particularly useful for assessing the extent of ascending aortic and arch pathology (i.e., aneurysms, dissection, atherosclerosis) in order to determine cross-clamping and cannulation sites for CPB.

A SAX image of the descending thoracic aorta is obtained by turning the probe leftward from the ME four-chamber view (Fig. 5.4A) to produce the descending aortic SAX view (Fig. 5.2Q). Rotating the multiplane angle of the probe from 0 degrees to 90 to 110 degrees produces a LAX image, the descending aortic LAX view (Fig. 5.2R). The descending thoracic aorta should be interrogated in its entirety beginning at the distal aortic arch by continually advancing the probe and turning slightly to the left until the celiac and superior mesenteric arteries are visualized branching tangentially from the anterior surface of abdominal aorta when the probe is in the stomach. Thorough examination of the descending thoracic aorta may be necessary to evaluate the distal extent of an aneurysm or dissection. In addition, the descending aortic SAX and LAX views can be useful for confirming appropriate intraaortic balloon positioning.

CONCLUSION

We have presented an approach to performing a comprehensive intraoperative multiplane TEE examination based on the guidelines published by the ASE and the SCA. The exact way in which this examination is accomplished will vary from person to person, but the guidelines provide a framework for ensuring consistency and completeness. Performing the examination in a uniform way whenever possible will increase the practitioner's efficiency and reliability in using intraoperative TEE to help care for their patients.

KEY POINTS

- The complete examination provides maximal benefit of the technique for the patient.
- The complete examination provides a baseline for later comparison.
- The complete examination reveals unexpected, often important, findings.
- The complete examination facilitates learning of normal anatomy and variants.

■ The goal is not to get all 20 views in all patients. The goal is to elucidate the structure and function of the heart and great vessels

REFERENCES

1. Shanewise JS, Cheung AT, Aronson S, et al. ASE/SCA guidelines for performing a comprehensive intraoperative multiplane transesophageal echocardiography examination: recommendations of the American Society of Echocardiography Council for Intraoperative Echocardiography and the Society of Cardiovascular Anesthesiologists Task Force for Certification in Perioperative Transesophageal Echocardiography. *J Am Soc Echocardiogr* 1999;12(10):884–900.

2. **Shanewise JS, Cheung AT, Aronson S, et al. ASE/SCA guidelines for performing a comprehensive intraoperative multiplane transesophageal echocardiography examination: recommendations of the American Society of Echocardiography Council for Intraoperative Echocardiography and the Society of Cardiovascular Anesthesiologists Task Force for Certification in Perioperative Transesophageal Echocardiography [see comments]. *Anesth Analg* 1999;89:870–884.**

3. Daniel WG, Erbel R, Kasper W, et al. Safety of transesophageal echocardiography. A multicenter survey of 10,419 examinations. *Circulation* 1991;83(3):817–821.

4. Brinkman WT, Shanewise JS, Clements SD, et al. Transesophageal echocardiography: not an innocuous procedure. *Ann Thorac Surg* 2001;72(5):1725–1726.

5. **Kallmeyer IJ, Collard CD, Fox JA, et al. The safety of intraoperative transesophageal echocardiography: a case series of 7200 cardiac surgical patients. *Anesth Analg* 2001;92(5):1126–1130.**

6

ARTIFACTS AND IMAGING ERRORS IN TRANSESOPHAGEAL ECHOCARDIOGRAPHY

LINDA SHORE-LESSERSON

The utility of any technology such as echocardiography is limited by operator experience and ability to accurately interpret the results. For diagnostic purposes, it is important to be proficient in diagnosing that the image abnormalities observed are in fact abnormal. However, it is equally important to be skilled in recognizing when the "apparent" abnormalities observed are artifactual, and are in fact "normal." Artifacts are errors in interpretation of structures due to the inherent properties of the ultrasound technology itself (Table 6.1). When ultrasound travels through a medium of homogenous acoustic impedance, the sound wave travels in a straight line. When a medium of different acoustic impedance is encountered, the beam is either reflected or refracted. Dense objects such as calcium, prosthetic materials, and bone cause almost complete reflection of the transmitted wave. Bright echoes from the strong reflectors make it difficult, if not impossible, to image objects beyond the strong reflector. This leads to the property of acoustic shadowing (1). Commonly shadowing occurs at calcific areas of atherosclerosis or plaque (Fig. 6.1). This is most commonly seen at the sinotubular junction in the ascending aorta, where acoustic shadowing obliterates imaging beyond the plaque (Fig. 6.2). The acoustic impedance of the stentless valves, homograft valves, or the leaflets of bioprosthetic valves is similar to that of native valves. Acoustic shadowing will be seen in association with valvular prostheses that contain synthetic materials in their struts, supporting structures, and prosthetic leaflets (2–4) (Fig. 6.3).

Reverberations occur when the ultrasonic beam travels through fluid, strikes the far wall of the image and returns to the transducer. An image is displayed based on the time that it took for the signal to return to the transducer. If the near side of the transducer functions as another reflecting surface, the ultrasonic beam will retrace itself, hit the

far side of the image again, and return to the transducer. (The second reflecting surface may be the transducer or it may be another reflective surface within the body.) Thus, this added distance of travel produces another image at exactly twice the distance from the transducer as the original image. This second signal (image) is referred to as a reverberation. Reverberations can be single, in which case they are referred to as "mirror image" artifacts, or they can be multiple or countless. The most common depiction of a mirror image reverberation occurs in the descending thoracic aorta where the long or short axis of the aorta appears to be duplicated. This artifact may be confused with a true double-barrel aorta or even an aortic dissection. The application of Doppler echocardiography will distinguish these entities because the Doppler spectrum will be the same in the artifact as it is in the true structure (Fig. 6.4). The Doppler spectrum of a pathologic lumen will be either absent or qualitatively different from that of the true structure (Fig. 6.5). This mirror image artifact of the descending aorta does not occur when there is left pleural fluid because the fluid attenuates the reflection of the ultrasound waves that create the artifact (5).

Side lobe beams, more common with phased-array transducers, are weaker and are projected in a different direction from the central ultrasonic beam. When a side lobe beam contacts an object, the echocardiograph displays the resultant echoes in the center of the display, as if they were generated from the main beam (1). This is due to the fact that the transducer cannot discriminate the returning signal as having been generated from the main beam or from a side lobe. Generally side lobe artifacts do not confound because they are weaker signals and only result in artifactual images when there is no "real" echo in the same space occupied by the side lobe artifact. When a side lobe contacts an object that is a strong reflector, such as a prosthetic valve, the image can be misplaced in its location on the screen (2). It is important to rule out these artifacts by imaging in multiple planes. If a side lobe beam is emitted from an oscillating transducer, then a single object will create multiple side lobe artifacts displayed

L. Shore-Lesserson: Department of Anesthesiology, Mount Sinai School of Medicine; and Department of Anesthesiology, Mount Sinai New York University Medical Center, New York, New York.

TABLE 6.1. COMMON IMAGING PROBLEMS

Common Artifacts	Common Pitfalls
Shadowing	Left atrial appendage muscle
Reverberation (descending aorta)	Coumadin ridge
Reverberation (ascending aorta)	Lipomatous infiltration of interatrial septum
Side lobes	Left atrioventricular groove
Near field clutter	Eustachian valve, Chiari network
Lateral dropout	Innominate vein
Doppler aliasing	Oblique image of aortic wall
Doppler ghosting	Transverse/oblique sinus
Zero velocity line	Pleural space

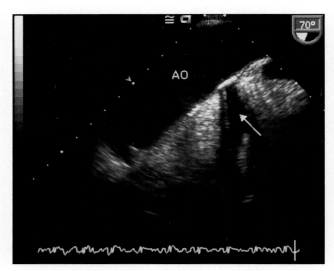

FIGURE 6.1. Shadowing is seen beyond a calcific plaque in the aorta. The image depicts the long axis of the descending aorta as it reaches the aortic arch, at a 70-degree imaging plane. The arrow points to the dark shadow cast by the aortic calcific plaque, beyond which no image is visible. *AO,* aorta.

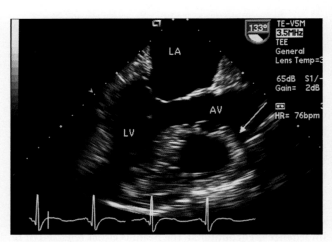

FIGURE 6.2. The arrow points to shadowing seen at the sino-tubular junction of the ascending aorta. Note the echolucent shadow that results from the plaque at the posterior wall of the sinotubular junction. *LA,* left atrium; *LV,* left ventricle; *AV,* aortic valve.

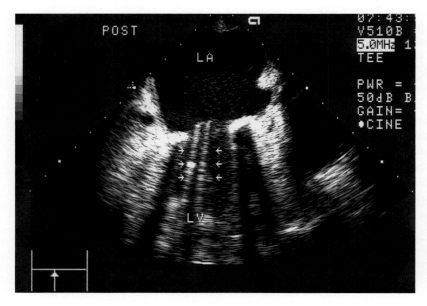

FIGURE 6.3. Transesophageal long-axis two-chamber view shows an implanted St. Jude mitral valve prosthesis. The echolucent areas distal to the valve are caused by shadowing from the valve (arrows). In this area, no image can be seen. The echodense linear densities distal to the valve represent reverberations from the St. Jude valve leaflets themselves. *LA,* left atrium; *LV,* left ventricle.

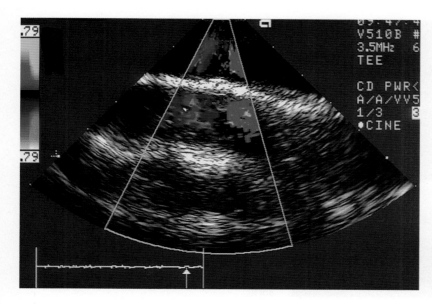

FIGURE 6.4. The long axis of the descending aorta is seen at a 90 degree imaging plane. Note the duplication of the image, which creates an artifact, a lumen of exactly the same size. The color Doppler spectrum in a reverberation artifact is the same as that in the true structure. This is a mirror image artifact as a result of reverberation. *DESC AO,* descending aorta.

as a curved line at the same level as the true object (Fig. 6.6). This side lobe is frequently seen with intracardiac catheters or cannulae and may mimic other structures or extracardiac spaces (6).

DOPPLER ARTIFACTS

Doppler echocardiography is integral to a complete echocardiographic examination. Common artifacts of Doppler imaging include "aliasing" and ghosting. Aliasing occurs with pulsed-wave and color Doppler modalities. It is the phenomenon whereby the frequency of the Doppler shift is higher than that which can be detected by the instrument. This frequency, known as the Nyquist limit, is defined by the pulse repetition frequency and can be altered using a number of manipulations that increase the frame rate. When the Nyquist limit is exceeded, the spectral display of pulsed-wave Doppler will "wrap around." For example, if blood is flowing away from the transducer at a high velocity, the spectral envelope will be below the baseline and will wrap around above the baseline to appear as if it is flowing toward the transducer. This is analogous to the original cartoons where the frame rate was so slow as to make the wheels of a car appear to be moving backward. This type of artifact, if not recognized, can cause the examiner to make an erroneous diagnosis about the direction of blood flow (1,7,8). Because color Doppler is a form of pulsed-wave Doppler, aliasing also may occur. When the Nyquist limit is exceeded, the color display will alias. For example, if blood is flowing away from the transducer at a high velocity, the initial display of blue color will change to red at the Nyquist limit and will thus

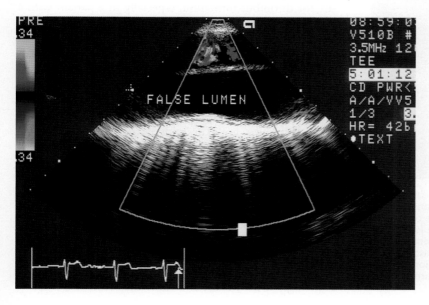

FIGURE 6.5. The long axis of the descending aorta is seen at a 90 degree imaging plane. True dissection of the descending aorta reveals two lumens of different size and caliber with different Doppler flow patterns. The appearance of the true lumen and false lumen side by side is much like that of a reverberation artifact.

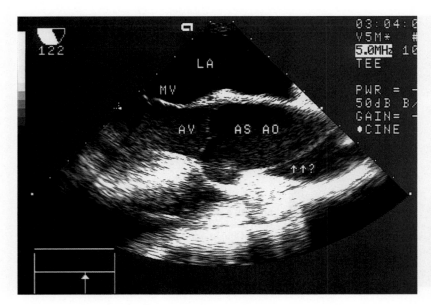

FIGURE 6.6. This mid-esophageal long-axis view of the ascending aorta (*122°*) reveals a curved structure within the lumen of the aorta (*arrows* and *?*). This curved image is a side lobe artifact from the echogenic plaque at the sinotubular junction. This plaque is also visualized in the image. *LA*, left atrium; *MV*, mitral valve; *AV*, aortic valve; *AS AO*, ascending aorta.

appear to be flowing toward the transducer. Similarly, when blood is flowing from left to right in a column perpendicular to a transducer, the flow will be red as it flows toward the transducer. At the point where blood flow is perpendicular to the ultrasonic beam, no color is recorded and the measurable velocity would be zero. As the flow passes the perpendicular, the flow away from the transducer will be displayed in blue (Fig. 6.7). Rapidly moving structures such as cardiac valves can produce flashes of color, a phenomenon known as "ghosting."

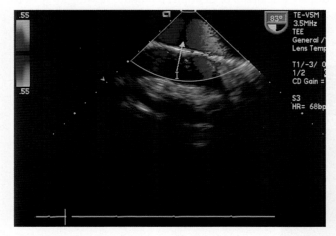

FIGURE 6.7. Blood flowing in a column can change color merely due to its changed position with respect to the transducer. As blood passes from right to left across the sector, the color is initially red when it flows toward the transducer. The color changes to blue when the blood flows away from the transducer. When the blood flow is exactly perpendicular to the ultrasonic beam (between the red and the blue), there will be no color recorded (black) and the recorded velocity will be zero. The arrow points to this zero velocity point.

PITFALLS IN IMAGING

Pitfalls are errors in diagnosis that arise as a result of normal structures mimicking pathologic entities and often can result in unnecessary clinical interventions. The novice echocardiographer is susceptible to misinterpretation of such structures; thus, familiarity with the normal examination is mandatory (9).

Left Atrial Pitfalls

The left atrial appendage (LAA) has pectinate muscles that may appear thick and hypertrophied. These can be visualized as parallel muscle ridges that protrude into the LAA and may mimic thrombus (3,10). Because the LAA is a common site for thrombus formation, especially in a patient with a large atrium or a rhythm of atrial fibrillation, the echocardiographer must be able to distinguish the appearance of thrombus from pectinate muscle ridges (11) (Fig. 6.8). Multiplanar imaging has improved our ability to image the LAA.

The tomographic slice of atrial tissue that separates the LAA from the left upper pulmonary vein appears as a globular mass that protrudes into the lumen of the left atrium (LA). This "mass" undulates with the cardiac motion and can mimic tumor or thrombus (11). Before advances in echocardiography and multiplanar scanning, this tissue was often confused with thrombus material and received the nickname the "coumadin ridge" (Fig. 6.9).

The region between the LA and left ventricle at the level of the mitral annulus is called the left atrioventricular (AV) groove. This region is abundant with potential diagnostic pitfalls (12). Normal structures that occur in this space include the true descending aorta or lipomatous infiltration. Pathologic structures are also commonly seen in this space.

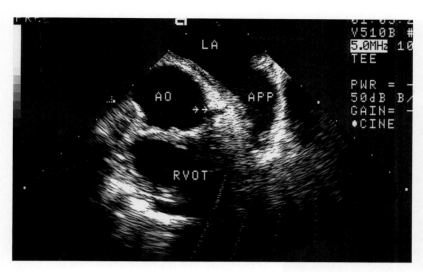

FIGURE 6.8. The left atrial appendage (LAA) is a common site for thrombus formation. The normal muscular structures of the LAA such as the pectinate muscles and false tendons have a similar echogenicity to that of thrombus and are shown in the figure. In this transverse 0 degree image from the mid-esophagus, the pectinate muscles appear as a gray mass lining the wall of the appendage. Differentiation from thrombus can be difficult and often is a diagnosis based on the clinical condition present. The arrows point to the left main coronary artery orifice. *LA,* left atrium; *AO,* aorta; *RVOT,* right ventricular outflow tract; *APP,* appendage (left atrial).

These include mitral annular abscesses, tumors, a hiatal hernia, and aneurysms of the pulmonary vein, coronary arteries, or descending thoracic aorta. A persistent left superior vena cava (LSVC) appears as an echolucent cavity in the left AV groove. This structure can be followed in its course posterior to the LA and into a large coronary sinus, into which it commonly drains (13,14) (Fig. 6.10). The diagnosis is confirmed by injection of echo contrast into a left-sided upper extremity intravenous line, which then opacifies the echolucent space. Left superior vena cava appears in 0.5% of the general population and in 3% to 10% of patients with congenital heart disease.

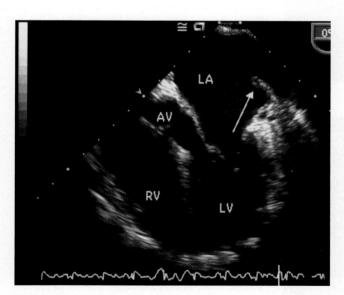

FIGURE 6.9. The insertion sites of the left upper pulmonary vein and the left atrial appendage into the left atrial wall share a ridge of tissue that invaginates into the left atrium. This ridge of tissue, denoted by the arrow, looks like a mass structure within the heart and has been named the "coumadin ridge." *LA,* left atrium; *LV,* left ventricle; *AV,* aortic valve; *RV,* right ventricle.

Right Atrial Pitfalls

The right atrium (RA), rich with embryologic remnants, frequently presents the echocardiographer with complex anatomic structures that mimic pathologic structures. The right and left venous valves of the sinoatrial orifice regulate the flow of blood from the sinus venosus to the atrium in amphibians and reptiles. In mammals, the venous valve loses its hemodynamic function and is identified only when related congenital anomalies occur. In approximately 2% of the population, a remnant of the right valve of the sinus venosus exists as the Chiari network. This lacelike structure is frequently elongated, highly mobile, and fibrinous in its appearance. Its fibers originate from the eustachian or thebesian valves and may attach to the crista terminalis of the atrial wall or to the RA floor (15–18). An autopsy study demonstrated that a Chiari network can be found in 1.3% to 4% of autopsy studies, which is consistent with its echocardiographic incidence. Although many clinicians believe that a Chiari network is of little clinical consequence, it has been shown to be more highly associated with atrial septal aneurysm and patent foramen ovale, and hence a risk for paradoxic embolism (19,20). Its unusual appearance also mandates that it be distinguished from a thrombus, vegetation, or other mass lesion (21).

At the junction of the inferior vena cava and RA, the eustachian valve is the embryologic remnant of the septum that directed inferior vena cava blood across the foramen ovale *in utero.* Familiarity with the appearance of the eustachian valve (22) and its characteristic position in the RA can help to rule out atrial pathology (23–30) (Fig. 6.11). A lipomatous interatrial septum also may be confused with an infiltrative process within the heart. A hypertrophied interatrial septum may give the appearance of an atrial septal defect in that the relative echodensity of the fossa ovalis is low and gives the appearance of a defect. Aneurysms of the interatrial septum have been associated with complications such as embolic phenomena and AV orifice obstruction. They appear

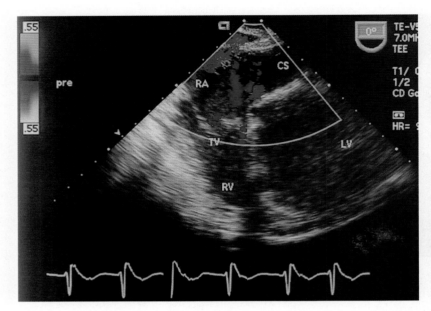

FIGURE 6.10. A left superior vena cava (LSVC) drains into the coronary sinus. In patients with an LSVC, the coronary sinus is often dilated, as shown in the figure. This is a result of the increased blood volume returning to the coronary sinus. *RA,* right atrium; *TV,* tricuspid valve; *RV,* right ventricle; *CS,* coronary sinus; *LV,* left ventricle.

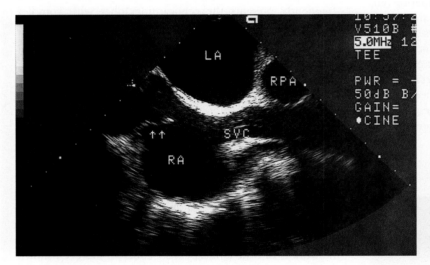

FIGURE 6.11. This mid-esophageal bicaval view of the right atrium (90 degree imaging plane) illustrates the eustachian valve at the junction of the inferior vena cava and the right atrium (*arrows*). It can be long and filamentous and can be confused with fibrinous mesh or a mass structure. *LA,* left atrium; *RA,* right atrium; *SVC,* superior vena cava; *RPA,* right pulmonary artery.

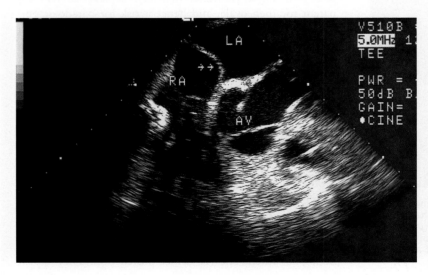

FIGURE 6.12. Aneurysms of the interatrial septum appear as thin, localized outpouchings of the atrial septum that vary in contour and protrude into the right or left atrium depending on the pressure difference. The arrows point to a small atrial septal aneurysm, which protrudes into the left atrium. *RA,* right atrium; *LA,* left atrium; *AV,* aortic valve.

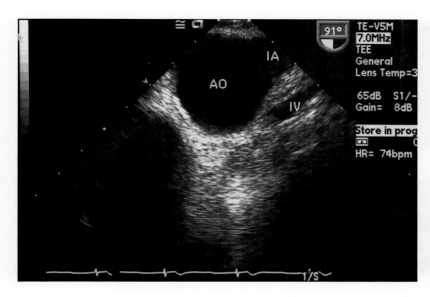

FIGURE 6.13. In this upper esophageal 90 degree image, the short axis of the aortic arch is seen as it gives rise to the innominate artery. The innominate vein is the small lucency beneath the wall of the aorta. *AO,* aortic arch; *IA,* innominate artery; *IV,* innominate vein.

as thin, localized outpouchings of the atrial septum that vary in contour and protrude into the right or LA depending on the pressure difference. They are differentiated from other structures by their relatively low reflectance, relationship to the atrial septum, and changes in their contour during the cardiac cycle (Fig. 6.12) (31).

Aortic Pitfalls

At the upper esophageal scanning plane of the transverse aorta, one can sometimes see a portion of the innominate vein as it courses across the mediastinum anterior to the transverse aorta (Fig. 6.13). When a large lumen of this vein is visible, its side-by-side position with the aorta can mimic the appearance of a dissection (32). The use of color flow and pulsed-wave Doppler spectral analysis can help to differentiate flow patterns and to rule out an aortic dissection. Another imaging pitfall in the aorta is at the distal transverse aorta when it curves to become the proximal descending aorta. A transverse image will yield an oblique slice through the aortic wall that often looks like a large atherosclerotic plaque extending into the lumen of the aorta.

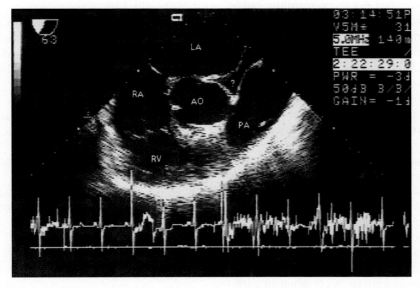

FIGURE 6.14. The space between the anterior left atrial wall and the posterior wall of the great vessels is a pericardial reflection called the transverse sinus. This space is visible only when the pericardium is filled with fluid as shown by the *?. RA,* right atrium; *LA,* left atrium; *RV,* right ventricle; *AO,* aorta; *PA,* pulmonary artery.

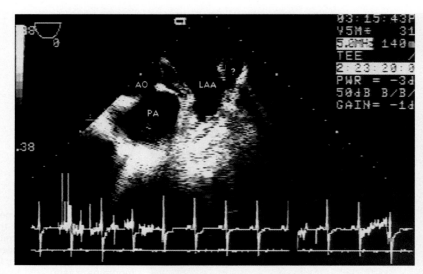

FIGURE 6.15. The space between the lateral left atrial wall and the left upper pulmonary vein is another pericardial reflection called the oblique sinus, shown by the *?*. This space is visible only when the pericardium is filled with fluid. Note that there is also a transverse sinus filled with fluid, between the aortopulmonary window and the LAA, in this figure. *AO*, aorta; *PA*, pulmonary artery; *LAA*, left atrial appendage.

Multiplanar scanning can better visualize this portion of the aorta (33).

Extracardiac Spaces

Various pericardial reflections, when fluid filled, may mimic abscess or cystic cavities. In patients without pericardial effusion, physiologic fluid collections can be found within these reflections, but usually cannot be detected echocardiographically. When a pericardial effusion is present, these spaces fill with fluid, and portions of the LAA and epicardium can be seen moving abnormally, in and out of the imaging plane. One such space, the transverse sinus, exists between the anterior LA and the posterior walls of the ascending aorta and pulmonary artery (6,34,35) (Fig. 6.14). Another pericardial reflection, the oblique sinus, exists between the posterolateral LA wall and the insertion site of the left upper pulmonary vein (Fig. 6.15). If these spaces are not appreciated as extracardiac, an intracardiac tumor or thrombus may be incorrectly diagnosed. Extracardiac spaces can be distinguished from true intracardiac spaces or blood vessels by color and spectral Doppler interrogation, which yields either an unidentifiable flow pattern, or more commonly, the absence of flow. The structure in Fig. 6.15 must be distinguished from the other structures that can occur in the left AV groove. The pleural space is another extracardiac space that can appear as an unknown cavity with abnormal masses within it (consolidated lung) when it is filled with fluid.

Pitfalls, or errors in interpretation, occur when an examiner is unfamiliar with normal anatomic variants that mimic pathologic conditions. For this reason, proper training and credentialing is essential for the echocardiographer whose recommendations directly affect patient care and clinical management.

KEY POINTS

- Artifacts are images that appear but are not present, or do not appear but are present. They arise as a result of the direct properties of ultrasound.
- Shadowing occurs when attempts are made to image objects with high echogenicity.
- Reverberation artifacts are most commonly seen in the descending aorta and in the ascending aorta when the size of the ascending aorta is enlarged.
- Pitfalls are images that appear abnormal but are actually normal structures.
- The most common RA pitfalls include the eustachian valve, Chiari network, and interatrial septal aneurysms.
- The most common LA pitfalls include the LAA and the coumadin ridge.
- The left atrioventricular groove is an area rich with anatomic pitfalls.
- Fluid in the extracardiac spaces makes the visualization of echocardiographic pitfalls more likely.

REFERENCES

1. Zabalgoitia M, Garcia M. Pitfalls in the echo-Doppler diagnosis of prosthetic valve disorders. *Echocardiography* 1993;10:203–212.
2. Bach DS. Transesophageal echocardiographic (TEE) evaluation of prosthetic valves. *Cardiol Clin* 2000;18:751–771.

3. **Alam M. Pitfalls in the echocardiographic diagnosis of intracardiac and extracardiac masses.** *Echocardiography* **1993;10:181–191.**

4. Rodrigues AG, Tardif JC, Dominguez M, et al. Transthoracic echocardiographic assessment of periprosthetic mitral regurgitation using intravenous injection of sonicated albumin. *Am J Cardiol* 1997;79:829–834.

5. **Appelbe AF, Walker PG, Yeoh JK, et al. Clinical significance and origin of artifacts in transesophageal echocardiography of the thoracic aorta.** *J Am Coll Cardiol* **1993;21:754–760.**

6. Walinsky P. Pitfalls in the diagnosis of pericardial effusion. *Cardiovasc Clin* 1978;9:111–122.

7. Ebrahimi R, Gardin JM. Pitfalls in the color Doppler diagnosis of valvular regurgitation. *Echocardiography* 1993;10:193–202.

8. Rudski LG, Picard MH. Artifacts, truths, and consequences. *Am J Med* 2000;108:589–591.

9. **Seward JB, Khandheria BK, Oh JK, et al. Transesophageal echocardiography: technique, anatomic correlations, implementation, and clinical applications.** *Mayo Clin Proc* **1988;63:649–680.**

10. Mihaileanu S, el Asmar B, Acar C, et al. Intra-operative transoesophageal echocardiography after mitral repair—specific conditions and pitfalls. *Eur Heart J* 1991;12(suppl B):26–29.

11. Kaymaz C, Ozdemir N, Kirma C, et al. Location, size and morphological characteristics of left atrial thrombi as assessed by echocardiography in patients with rheumatic mitral valve disease. *Eur J Echocardiogr* 2001;2:270–276.

12. **Zuber M, Oechslin E, Jenni R. Echogenic structures in the left atrioventricular groove: diagnostic pitfalls.** *J Am Soc Echocardiogr* **1998;11:381–386.**

13. Cohen BE, Winer HE, Kronzon I. Echocardiographic findings in patients with left superior vena cava and dilated coronary sinus. *Am J Cardiol* 1979;44:158–161.

14. Foale R, Bourdillon PD, Somerville J, et al. Anomalous systemic venous return: recognition by two-dimensional echocardiography. *Eur Heart J* 1983;4:186–195.

15. Mittal S, Bhise M, Mehta Y, et al. Chiari network: an interesting transesophageal echocardiographic finding. *J Cardiothorac Vasc Anesth* 1999;13:243.

16. Lewandowski B, Challender J, Dery R. Prolapsing Chiari malformation in tricuspid regurgitation: a moving filling defect in the inferior vena cava. *J Ultrasound Med* 1985;4:655–658.

17. Ducharme A, Tardif JC, Mercier LA, et al. Remnants of the right valve of the sinus venosus presenting as a right atrial mass on transthoracic echocardiography. *Can J Cardiol* 1997;13:573–576.

18. **Cujec B, Mycyk T, Khouri M. Identification of Chiari's network with transesophageal echocardiography.** *J Am Soc Echocardiogr* **1992;5:96–99.**

19. **Schneider B, Hofmann T, Justen MH, et al. Chiari's network: normal anatomic variant or risk factor for arterial embolic events?** *J Am Coll Cardiol* **1995;26:203–210.**

20. Kerut EK, Norfleet WT, Plotnick GD, et al. Patent foramen ovale: a review of associated conditions and the impact of physiological size. *J Am Coll Cardiol* 2001;38:613–623.

21. Victor S, Nayak VM. An anomalous muscle bundle inside the right atrium possibly related to the right venous valve. *J Heart Valve Dis* 1997;6:439–440.

22. Corno AF, Bron C, von Segesser LK. Divided right atrium. Diagnosis by echocardiography, and considerations on the functional role of the eustachian valve. *Cardiol Young* 1999;9:427–429.

23. **Alam M, Sun I, Smith S. Transesophageal echocardiographic evaluation of right atrial mass lesions.** *J Am Soc Echocardiogr* **1991;4:331–337.**

24. Bowers J, Krimsky W, Gradon JD. The pitfalls of transthoracic echocardiography. A case of eustachian valve endocarditis. *Tex Heart Inst J* 2001;28:57–59.

25. Georgeson R, Liu M, Bansal RC. Transesophageal echocardiographic diagnosis of eustachian valve endocarditis. *J Am Soc Echocardiogr* 1996;9:206–208.

26. **Limacher MC, Gutgesell HP, Vick GW, et al. Echocardiographic anatomy of the eustachian valve.** *Am J Cardiol* **1986;57:363–365.**

27. James PR, Dawson D, Hardman SM. Eustachian valve endocarditis diagnosed by transoesophageal echocardiography. *Heart* 1999;81:91.

28. Malaterre HR, Kallee K, Perier Y. Eustachian valve mimicking a right atrial cystic tumor. *Int J Card Imaging* 2000;16:305–307.

29. Palakodeti V, Keen WD Jr, Rickman LS, et al. Eustachian valve endocarditis: detection with multiplane transesophageal echocardiography. *Clin Cardiol* 1997;20:579–580.

30. Sawhney N, Palakodeti V, Raisinghani A, et al. Eustachian valve endocarditis: a case series and analysis of the literature. *J Am Soc Echocardiogr* 2001;14:1139–1142.

31. Gondi B, Nanda NC. Two-dimensional echocardiographic features of atrial septal aneurysms. *Circulation* 1981;63:452–457.

32. **Patel S, Alam M, Rosman H. Pitfalls in the echocardiographic diagnosis of aortic dissection.** *Angiology* **1997;48:939–946.**

33. Bartel T, Muller S, Nesser HJ, et al. Usefulness of motion patterns identified by tissue Doppler echocardiography for diagnosing various cardiac masses, particularly valvular vegetations. *Am J Cardiol* 1999;84:1428–1433.

34. Tjaik AJ. Echocardiography in pericardial effusion. *Am J Med* 1977;63:29–40.

35. Casarella WJ, Schneider BO. Pitfalls in the ultrasonic diagnosis of pericardial effusion. *Am J Roentgenol Radium Ther Nucl Med* 1970;110:760–767.

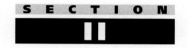

SECTION

II

CLINICAL APPLICATIONS: FUNDAMENTAL CONCEPTS

7

VENTRICULAR FUNCTION

MARTIN J. LONDON

When performing a perioperative transesophageal echocardiographic (TEE) examination, evaluation of global and regional ventricular function is usually the highest priority for the clinician. Clinically significant alterations of ventricular function (e.g., those that impact on the intensity of clinical care delivered or the ultimate outcome of the patient) are common and often very dynamic. The clinician must consider patient-specific factors [i.e., known cardiomyopathy, severe coronary artery disease (CAD) with easily inducible ischemia, hypertrophic cardiomyopathies and other causes of left or right outflow tract obstruction, significant stenotic or regurgitant valvular disease, pheochromocytoma, etc.]; the type of surgery (cardiac surgical procedures on or off pump, aortic vascular surgery, transplantation, major blood loss, large vascular tumor resection, etc.); and perioperative physiologic perturbations (e.g., air embolus, pulmonary embolus, etc.) that are commonly encountered in a busy clinical practice. The often acute, life-threatening nature of perioperative alterations in ventricular function mandate that the clinician make a TEE assessment at the same time he or she may be providing intensive clinical care.

Assessing ventricular function, whether on a qualitative or quantitative basis, requires consideration of global and regional function of both the left and right ventricles, and to a lesser but still important extent, the left and right atria. Although this approach should logically be broken down to a "four part" assessment, in reality, the interrelationships between each of these four chambers, whether by anatomic [i.e., septal interaction in which right ventricular (RV) failure reduces filling of the left ventricle (LV)] or physiologic interactions (e.g., regional ischemia decreasing diastolic distensibility of neighboring nonischemic segments), is often "more than the sum of the parts." Advances in integrative physiology, echo technology, and other imaging modalities [particularly cardiac magnetic resonance imaging (MRI)] and knowledge gleaned from diagnostic uses of echo (partic-

ularly assessment of myocardial viability using dobutamine stress echo) have increased the complexity of the literature at an intimidating pace. Fortunately, the basic foundations have not changed appreciably, and qualitative assessment of these parameters remains by necessity the most common approach and usually can be easily applied to clinical practice.

In this chapter, the basics of global and regional function are considered, along with the more complex and less clinical applicable evaluation of diastolic function.

CONTRACTION OF THE NORMAL LEFT AND RIGHT VENTRICLE

The normal LV approximates a truncated ellipsoid with a circular configuration increasing in area from the apex to the base. As ventricular function declines it assumes a more globular shape. The primary anatomic reference points for determination of ventricular dimensions are the apex, papillary muscles, and plane of the mitral valve (1). The long (major) axis (LAX) dimension runs from the LV (or RV) apex to the mid-plane of the mitral (or tricuspid valve) in the four-chamber view (Fig. 7.1). It is important to appreciate that the reference data for cardiac dimensions using normal reference groups were obtained using transthoracic echocardiography (TTE). Although resolution with TTE is generally inferior to TEE, the ability to obtain a wider variety of imaging planes by moving the transducer to different positions on the chest wall allows greater accuracy in obtaining a true LV (and RV) LAX. Foreshortening of the LAX view with TEE is a definite limitation, but this can be minimized by careful attention to technique. Although simultaneous studies comparing two-dimensional (2D) TEE with TTE have not been reported, a comparison of TEE with LV ventriculography measurements documented that TEE underestimates LV volumes, primarily by underestimating LAX length (approximately 2 cm) (2). However, it also must be appreciated that angiography may slightly overestimate dimensions from filling of endocardial muscle trabeculations by contrast, leading to an

M. J. London: Department of Anesthesia and Perioperative Care, University of California, San Francisco; and Anesthesia Service, Veterans Affairs Medical Center, San Francisco, California.

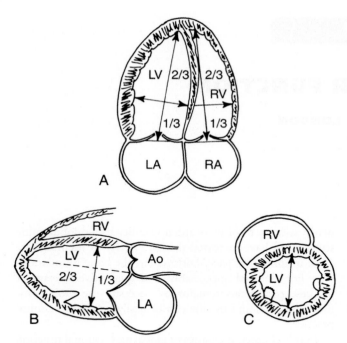

FIGURE 7.1. Standardized methods for measurement of intracardiac dimensions as recommended by the American Society of Echocardiography subcommittee on quantitation of two-dimensional echocardiograms in the apical four-chamber view **(A)**, parasternal short-axis view at the level of the chordae **(B)**, and parasternal LAX view **(C)**. The respective minor and major axes are represented by the double arrow lines. *Ao,* aorta; *LA,* left atrium; *LV,* left ventricle; *RA,* right atrium; *RV,* right ventricle. (Reprinted from Schiller NB, Shah PM, Crawford M, et al. Recommendations for quantitation of the left ventricle by two-dimensional echocardiography. American Society of Echocardiography Committee on Standards, Subcommittee on Quantitation of Two-Dimensional Echocardiograms. *J Am Soc Echocardiogr* 1989;2:360, with permission.)

underestimation of endocardial thickness. The apex of the ventricle is relatively fixed, with longitudinal shortening occurring primarily by descent of the mitral annulus (1). This "descent of the base" assessed by TTE has been shown to have prognostic value as a measurement of ventricular function following myocardial infarction (MI). However, perioperative measurement of this with TEE is not commonly performed.

The American Society of Echocardiography (ASE) recommends measuring short (minor) axis (SAX) dimensions at two-thirds the distance to the base (1). In clinical practice, an important and easily recognized anatomic reference, the insertion of the papillary muscles to the LV wall, is most commonly used.

Normal thickness of the LV walls is 6 to 12 mm; above this, hypertrophy is considered to be present. RV thickness is one third to half that of the LV, and over 5 mm is considered abnormal (Fig. 7.2). End-diastolic wall thickness should be measured at the onset of the QRS complex because atrial contraction can accentuate wall thinning.

The arrangement of the muscle layers across the LV wall is complex, with several obliquely oriented sheets running from apex to base. Ejection of blood from the LV occurs via a reduction in cross-sectional area during systole. Circumferential shortening is greatest in the endocardium, roughly twice that of the epicardium, with the mid-wall intermediate (3) (Fig. 7.3). Although cardiac MRI measurements suggest little variation in total circumferential shortening between different regions of the heart, tissue Doppler imaging (TDI) studies demonstrate a significant variation in myocardial velocity of contraction, with velocities at the base significantly greater than at the apex (4) (Fig. 7.4). Inward radial (e.g., SAX) movement is the primary mechanism, with only a small contribution from LAX contraction (5). This follows from the simple geometric rule that the volume of a cylinder decreases with the square of the radius and only linearly with a change in LAX length. The greater change in the radius of the ventricle forms the basis for using the transgastric (TG) SAX view for intraoperative monitoring of global LV function.

The complex muscle fiber orientation is responsible for the significant rotation and translation of the heart outward toward the chest wall that occurs during systole. This

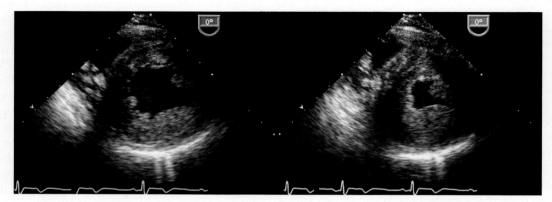

FIGURE 7.2. Concentric hypertrophy in a patient with severe aortic stenosis (left side, end-diastole; right side, end-systole). End-diastolic wall thickness exceeds 1.2 cm. Centimeter marks are along the sides of the sector.

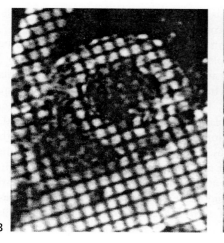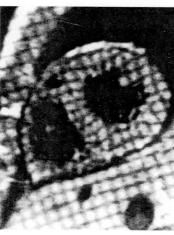

A,B

FIGURE 7.3. Cardiac magnetic resonance images depicting spatial modulation of magnetization (*stripes overlaying images*) at end-diastole **(A)** and end-systole **(B)**. Changes in the inter-stripe distance represent segment shortening. Note convergence of stripes at the endocardium during systole where circumferential shortening is maximal relative to the outer layers. (Reprinted from Clark NR, Reichek N, Bergey P, et al. Circumferential myocardial shortening in the normal human left ventricle. Assessment by magnetic resonance imaging using spatial modulation of magnetization. *Circulation* 1991;84:70, with permission.)

movement causes a changing frame of reference (e.g. an imaginary point at the center of the SAX view into which the endocardial border contracts) complicating attempts to analyze regional wall motion via automated methods. A variety of approaches to deal with this have been investigated, including "fixed" and "floating" frames of reference (the latter approach considered most accurate), along with an approach independent of a central reference point (the so-called "centerline" method, which relies on multiple chords drawn at right an-

gles to a centerline drawn between the endocardium and epicardium). Newer developments, particularly those using TDI, which encodes myocardial velocity in a specific region on interest, are less susceptible to translation but are still in their clinical infancy (4). Luckily for the clinician, human visual processing can deal with this movement more efficiently than computers, and observation by an experienced echocardiographer remains the gold standard for assessing wall motion.

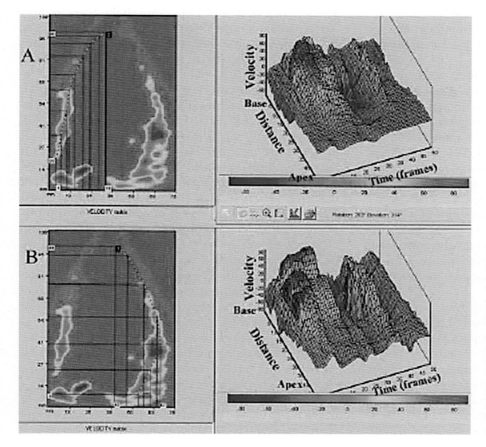

FIGURE 7.4. Three-dimensional reconstruction of myocardial velocity of the interventricular septum **(A)** and the lateral wall **(B)** along a curved line from the base to the apex obtained using high temporal resolution tissue Doppler imaging. The base–apex myocardial velocity gradient (highest at the base) during systole and diastole is depicted in the graphs. (Reprinted from Trambaiolo P, Tonti G, Salustri A, et al. New insights into regional systolic and diastolic left ventricular function with tissue Doppler echocardiography: from qualitative analysis to a quantitative approach. *J Am Soc Echocardiogr* 2001;14:93, with permission.)

ASSESSMENT OF GLOBAL VENTRICULAR FUNCTION

To assess systolic LV function, one must consider preload, afterload, and contractility. The interactions of these three parameters determine stroke volume, which along with heart rate determines cardiac output and ultimately oxygen delivery to the body. Clinical evaluation of each of these is possible using TEE, although only preload and contractility are easily assessed qualitatively (e.g. visually). Direct measurement of cardiac output using Doppler determination of stroke volume (based on measurement of the flow velocity integral) coupled with 2D measurement of aortic valve orifice area or LV outflow tract diameter can be performed with TEE and is discussed elsewhere (see Chapter 18) (6).

In routine clinical practice, LV systolic performance is assessed by the ejection fraction (EF), which is the end-diastolic volume (EDV) minus the end-systolic volume (ESV) divided by EDV, or [EDV − ESV]/EDV = EF. EF (and to a lesser extent ESV alone) are important independent prognostic indicators of outcome in patients with coronary artery or valvular heart disease in many clinical studies (7). The instantaneous relationship of ESV to end-systolic ventricular pressure over a wide range of volumes and pressures (usually assessed intraoperatively during cardiac surgery and obtained by a sudden preload reduction via inferior vena cava constriction) is considered a load-independent index of contractility (8). However, other physiologic factors must be considered, and routine clinical application of this approach remains impractical. End-diastolic volume alone is a less important predictor than ESV or EF.

Volumetric EF is a simple measurement to obtain using TEE and one that the clinician should spend time performing during training to properly "calibrate" their eyes because intraoperative clinical assessment is usually qualitative (visual). With the introduction of automated boundary detection technology in the early 1990s, which allows continuous real-time delineation of the endocardial–blood interface (based on the significant difference in the amplitude of low-energy backscattered echoes between the two interfaces), continuous intraoperative monitoring of the area-based analog of ejection fraction (fractional area change, or FAC) is now possible (9). Variability in the region of interest is an important technical factor that can limit its accuracy. Another limitation is its proprietary nature (limited to one vendor).

Ejection fraction is a load dependent index of LV function. It is primarily influenced by afterload (inverse relationship) and contractility (direct relationship). Within physiologic ranges, preload has little influence, although in the perioperative setting with its dramatic changes (particularly hypovolemia), it is more likely to be a factor. Anatomic factors, particularly valvular regurgitation and left-to-right intracardiac shunting, also must be considered. An EF of 50% or greater is considered the lower limits of normal, with most normal mean values in the high 60s to low 70s. Between 30–35% and 50% is considered moderate, and below 15% to 20% is usually considered severe dysfunction.

The paradigm of volumetric ejection fraction has been applied to simple chamber internal dimensions (with M-mode imaging) and cross-sectional areas (with single-plane 2D imaging) as fractional shortening (FS) and FAC, respectively (Fig. 7.5). To measure volumetric EF, two orthogonal LAX imaging planes are used and volume is calculated by the modified Simpson rule, otherwise known as the method of discs (Fig. 7.6). After tracing the endocardial border manually, a series of multiple discs (usually 20) are determined by the software at right angles to the LAX chord (assuming a prolate ellipsoid shape with the mitral plane at the base), and the area of each disk is computed ($\pi \times r^2$). Because two orthogonal views are measured, it is important that the LAX dimension be approximately equal in both views, and one must be particularly careful to avoid foreshortening of the apex. The single-plane area–length method can be used (particularly if a single LAX view is obtained), although it is more dependent on a symmetrically shaped ventricle without significant wall motion abnormalities. Likewise, in a normal ventricle, squaring the M-mode obtained internal diameters at the SAX level that were employed to determine FS (along with a small adjustment for apical contractility), can be used to calculate EF (10). This approach is based on TTE-derived M-mode diameters via the parasternal SAX view, which uses the septal and lateral walls as opposed to the inferior and anterior orientation with TEE, although this is not likely to have a significant impact.

Volumetric analysis of the RV is difficult and poorly standardized due to its crescent shape and the complex shape of the right ventricle output tract (RVOT). Most studies report volumes using a two-thirds (area) × (length) calculation in the LAX view, which geometrically has been modeled to an "ellipsoidal shell" (11). The four-chamber RV/LV volume ratio should approximate 0.6 in a normal ventricle. A straightforward anatomic observation is that the LV apex is the predominant point, and if the RV apex "shares" it, RV dilatation is likely present. Similar to the LV, depression of the descent of the RV base to the fixed apex is an accepted measure of dysfunction. More commonly, a dilated tricuspid valve annulus with tricuspid insufficiency and flattening of the LV septum are easily observed signs of dysfunction, particularly pressure overload.

The rate of LV (or RV) pressure change during isovolumic contraction (dp/dt) is another load-dependent index of contractility. It can be assessed by continuous-wave Doppler interrogation of either a mitral or triscupid regurgitant jet. Given its complexity of measurement, its load dependence, difficulty in obtaining precise imaging windows with TEE relative to TTE, and the easier visual analysis of volumetric changes, it is not a routine clinical measurement.

Load-independent measurements of contractility, as noted above, are complex and have limited, if any, current clinical applications (8). Although end-systolic pressure–volume measurements are now the most commonly described

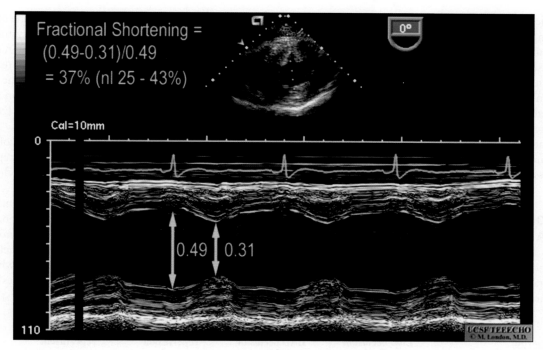

FIGURE 7.5. Fractional shortening in a normal left ventricle obtained by M-mode imaging of the transgastric short-axis view using end-systolic and end-diastolic internal dimensions (*arrows*). (Reprinted from *www.ucsf.edu/teeecho,* with permission.)

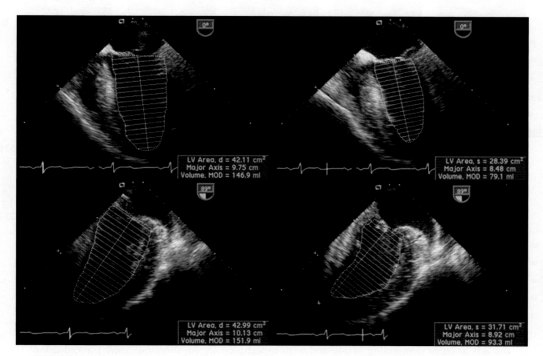

FIGURE 7.6. Determination of volumetric ejection fraction in the four- and two-chamber views using the method of discs on a commercial ultrasound unit. Notice the shortening of the long-axis chord, consistent with "descent of the base." The patient has marked left ventricular hypertrophy. The average ejection fraction from both views was 42%, although there is foreshortening in the two-chamber image.

method, older and simpler methods have been used. Of these, the simplest is the rate-corrected mean velocity of fiber (Vcf) shortening, which is the FAC divided by the LV ejection time (usually obtained from M-mode analysis of aortic valve opening and closing). Measurements of wall stress, either circumferential or meridional, are derived measures of systolic wall tension (approximating afterload). These require measurement of LV end-systolic pressure (although this is approximated clinically in several studies using systemic blood pressure alone), LV internal diameters, and posterior wall thickness.

PHYSIOLOGIC BASES FOR ISCHEMIA DETECTION

Animal and clinical data document the high sensitivity of echocardiographic methods for measuring the effects of myocardial ischemia on regional and global ventricular func-

tion. Most often this is assessed by 2D imaging alone, focusing on visually observed changes in regional systolic function at low temporal resolution (e.g., video frame rates). Newer methods can evaluate more complex changes (e.g., velocity of a particular myocardial segment throughout systole and diastole) at a much higher temporal resolution (as small as 5-msec increments for color M-mode TDI). Extensions of automated border detection technology (e.g. "color kinesis"), in which the magnitude and timing of color encoded endocardial excursion are displayed, are being reported at an increasing rate and starting to see substantial clinical use in echo laboratories (Fig. 7.7) (4,12).

Although these newer approaches are currently too cumbersome for the busy perioperative practitioner, it is inevitable that "technology creep" will occur, and familiarity with these methods is necessary. They are helping to redefine the physiologic meaning of ischemia with the term *myocardial asynchrony*, which refers to changes in wall velocity throughout the cardiac cycle instead of the previous

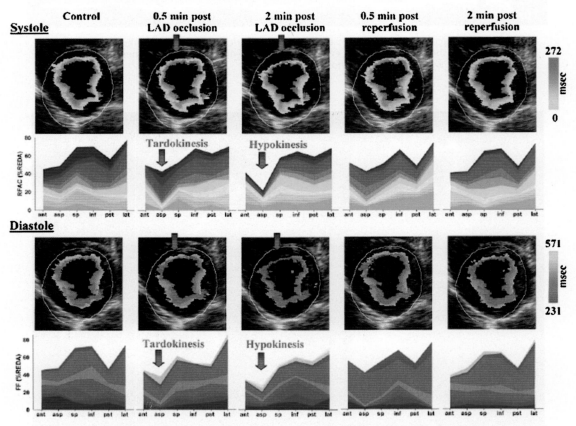

FIGURE 7.7. Changes in timing and extent of wall motion in a pig after complete occlusion of the left anterior descending artery and with reperfusion in the short-axis view tracked using color kinesis imaging. Left ventricular systolic and diastolic endocardial motion is encoded using different colors to represent consecutive time frames (indicated by the bars on the right side of the panel). Regional fractional area change (*RFAC*) or filling fraction (*FF*) of each of six regions (*ant*, anterior; *asp*, anteroseptal; *sp*, septal; *inf*, inferior; *pst*, posterior; *lat*, lateral) is displayed in the stacked histograms. The earliest change is tardokinesis, displayed as changes in the timing of the color bands in the anteroseptal region, followed by hypokinesis with thinning of the color bands. (Reprinted from Mor-Avi V, Collins KA, Korcarz CE, et al. Detection of regional temporal abnormalities in left ventricular function during acute myocardial ischemia. *Am J Physiol Heart Circ Physiol* 2001;280:H1772, with permission.)

arbitrary division into either systolic or diastolic periods. Thus, the phenomenon of postsystolic shortening, in which delayed wall thickening occurs after aortic valve closure caused by ischemia and which was previously detectable only by evaluation of pressure–volume loops, is now detectable directly and noninvasively (Fig. 7.8) (13–15). How this approach ultimately fits into clinical practice has yet to be determined.

The basic physiologic principle behind most forms of ischemia encountered perioperatively is the rapid reduction in regional myocardial function with acute reduction in myocardial blood flow in the affected coronary artery territory. These changes (termed regional wall motion abnormalities, or RWMAs) occur in a substantially shorter time frame than either ST-segment changes by electrocardiography (ECG) or increased filling pressures by pulmonary artery catheter (PAC), potentially allowing earlier diagnosis and therapy (16). Although ECG is superior for prolonged perioperative monitoring for obvious reasons, TEE is less influenced by a variety of physiologic factors that diminish ECG sensitivity and specificity (particularly left bundle branch block, pacing, Q waves or nonspecific ST-segment changes, catecholamine- and drug-induced changes in repolarization, etc.) (17). Anatomic interrogation allows instantaneous recognition of important factors (e.g., a chronically infarcted segment that is an unequivocal sign of a prior MI) in contrast to the "statistical probability" of a given ECG pattern.

The most sensitive changes with ischemia are reduction (hypokinesia) or cessation (akinesia) of systolic wall thickening (which normally thickens by 50% of the end-diastolic value) (18). With complete cessation of coronary flow, systolic wall thinning will occur (in a previously normal segment), causing outward bulging (dyskinesia). Because the function of the heart as a pump is to eject blood, requiring inward motion of the endocardial surface during systole to reduce cross-sectional area, a reduction in endocardial excursion is a more obvious visual sign of dysfunction, especially when compared with normal adjacent regions. Making this all the more obvious is the common response of the acutely ischemic ventricle to develop exaggerated endocardial excursion of the adjacent nonischemic regions (compensatory hyperkinesis), which offsets the adverse effects of regional dysfunction on stroke volume and cardiac output. Thus, changes in systemic hemodynamics are usually a late and ominous sign occurring with a large ischemic region [i.e., left main or proximal left anterior descending (LAD) stenosis] or with ischemia in multiple coronary distributions (including global subendocardial ischemia in the absence of CAD, as may occur with aortic stenosis) (19).

In the clinical setting, systolic wall thickening and endocardial excursion are assessed jointly to arrive at a wall motion "grade." These have been standardized by the ASE, may be easily learned, and are reproducible between practitioners for major changes in function (Table 7.1 and Fig. 7.9) (20).

Animal studies demonstrate that changes in endocardial excursion substantially overestimate the area of hypoperfused ischemic myocardium while systolic wall thickening more closely approximates it (Fig. 7.10) (21). This should come as no surprise because the former is not only the end result of the latter, but is also influenced by the adjacent nonischemic segments. Thus, "tethering" of the abnormal myocardium (either full thickness or involving the endocardium or epicardium) to adjacent segments imposes complex mechanical effects, either horizontally or vertically oriented within the cardiac muscle. Other factors (e.g., endocardial pacing, left bundle branch block, etc.) can reduce the specificity of abnormal endocardial excursion as a marker of ischemia. However, in these situations systolic wall thickening should

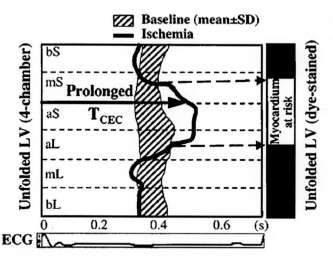

FIGURE 7.8. Demonstration of changes in postsystolic shortening (PSS) during left anterior descending artery occlusion in a pig assessed using strain rate imaging, calculated as the difference between two velocity points along the ultrasound beam divided by the distance (5 mm), allowing quantitation of ventricular compression or expansion. These data are used to calculate the time from the R wave to the occurrence of compression/expansion crossover (an index of PSS) in segments of an unfolded four-chamber left ventricle (*bS*, basal; *mS*, mid-septal; *aS*, apical septal; *aL*, apical lateral; *mL*, mid-lateral; *bL*, basal lateral). (Reprinted from Pislaru C, Belohlavek M, Bae RY, et al. Regional asynchrony during acute myocardial ischemia quantified by ultrasound strain rate imaging. *J Am Coll Cardiol* 2001;37:1144, with permission.)

TABLE 7.1. SCORING OF SEGMENTAL WALL MOTION ABNORMALITIES

Grade	Endocardial Excursion (%)	Wall Thickening (%)
Normal	>30	30–50
Hypokinesis		
Mild	10–30	30–50
Severe	<10	<30
Akinesis	0	<10
Dyskinesis	Outward bulging	Absent or systolic thinning
Hyperkinesis	Greater than "normal"	Greater than "normal"

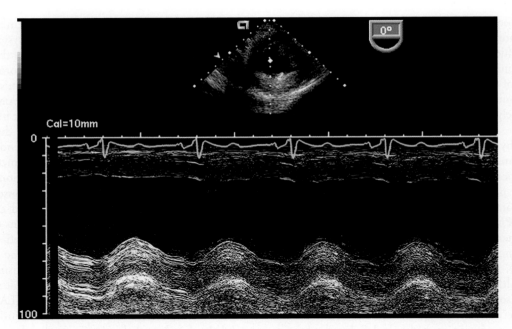

FIGURE 7.9. Severe hypokinesis to akinesis of the middle inferior segment of the transgastric short-axis view demonstrated using M-mode imaging (inferior segment on the upper portion, anterior segment on the bottom with normal systolic wall thickening and endocardial excursion). (Reprinted from *www.ucsf.edu/teeecho,* with permission.)

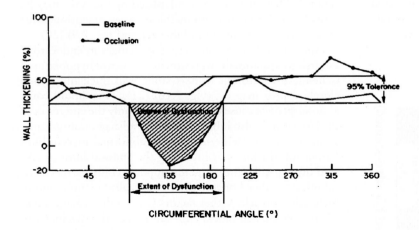

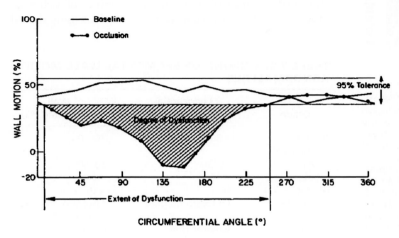

FIGURE 7.10. Circumferential extent and degree of dysfunction for systolic wall thickening (top plot) and endocardial excursion (bottom plot) in a single canine preparation during occlusion of the circumflex artery as measured by a circumferential plot of the transgastric short-axis view. The actual hypoperfused area (measured with radioactive microspheres) closely approximated the area delineated by the wall thickening abnormality but was markedly overestimated by the endocardial excursion plot. (Reprinted from Buda AJ, Zotz RJ, Pace DP, et al. Comparison of two-dimensional echocardiographic wall motion and wall thickening abnormalities in relation to the myocardium at risk. *Am Heart J* 1986;111:588, with permission.)

be normal. The magnitude of endocardial excursion and wall thickening varies between different regions of the heart and between different "normal" individuals. Thus, the patient's baseline status (if known) should serve as a control, which is particularly important when evaluating subtle changes (hypokinesia).

Abnormal loading conditions commonly encountered perioperatively, at either end of the volume or pressure spectrum, complicate interpretation of RWMAs. Wall motion can appear severely hypokinetic with hypervolemia or with elevated afterload accompanying severe hypertension. This is easily recognized when it affects all walls equally and motion returns to normal with reduction in pressure or volume. Hypovolemia accentuates the normal regional disparity in endocardial excursion and may cause gross disparity, particularly with abnormal baseline motion, producing dyskinetic motion in a previously akinetic segment. In this setting, wall thinning will not be present (22).

Interpreting wall motion in patients with severe left ventricular hypertrophy (LVH) is challenging because cross-sectional area may already be significantly reduced (particularly with concentric hypertrophy), making appreciation of subtle changes difficult. With hypertrophic cardiomyopathy, the ground glass appearance of the myocardium also complicates assessment. Ventricular pacing, particularly via endocardial wires during open chest cardiac procedures, can be problematic. Release of pericardial restraint with sternotomy has been reported to cause abnormal septal motion, which on occasion may be confused with ischemia.

With the rapid growth of off pump coronary artery bypass (OPCAB), using mechanical stabilization of the myocardium underlying the lesion being bypassed, neither endocardial excursion nor systolic wall thickening can be assessed during the anastomotic period. In addition, adjacent segments may be distorted from compression and other positioning effects. Detecting ischemia during this period is difficult using any modality (including ECG, since the electrical axis of the heart may be drastically altered). Ultimately cardiac output or other measures of systolic function are most important to guide therapy, at least while the stabilizer is used.

The numerical relationships between coronary blood flow and regional function are complex. Linear or exponential relationships have been reported. The differential transmural distribution of coronary blood flow from epicardium to endocardium is an important variable that must be considered. The subendocardium has a higher metabolic requirement, greater susceptibility to the adverse effects of elevated filling pressure (either intrinsic due to a reduction in diastolic distensibility with ischemia or extrinsic as with fluid overloading), is more sensitive to flow reduction and shows earlier change in thickening than the epicardium. The earlier alteration in subendocardial function is a complicating factor in newer studies of regional myocardial velocity and strain with TDI (14).

Regional function may start to deteriorate with only a 20% reduction in transmural flow. Thus, it is difficult to determine whether normal resting myocardium will deteriorate or, conversely, to predict the response of an RWMA in the resting state to revascularization. Myocardial viability is assessed using measures of metabolism (PET scanning), intact microvascular circulation (thallium imaging, perfusion contrast echocardiography), and mechanical contractile reserve (dobutamine stress echo testing). Although each of these measurements provides complimentary and additive information, perioperative clinicians should be familiar with the basic echocardiographic responses to dobutamine (Fig. 7.11) (23). With low doses of dobutamine, normal myocardium becomes hyperkinetic as coronary blood flow increases. Development of hypo- or akinesis in a previously normal segment represents an ischemic response. Chronic transmural infarction will not respond to either low or high doses. Improvement of function in a baseline akinetic segment at a low dose suggests contractile reserve. A biphasic response with improvement at a low dose followed by deterioration at higher doses, is characteristic of a hibernating myocardium. The end-diastolic wall thickness of 0.6 cm has been shown to virtually exclude the potential for functional recovery with myocardial revascularization (24). Development of short-term myocardial stunning during cardiopulmonary bypass (CPB) surgery complicates early post-CPB prediction of long-term viability (25). Older reports suggested that new RMWAs after CPB failing to respond to

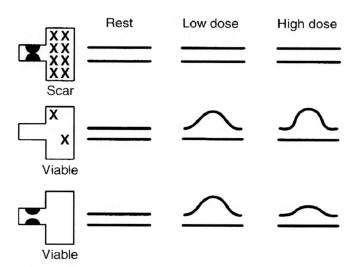

FIGURE 7.11. Response of a resting akinetic segment to dobutamine based on three different physiologic situations. At the top, a chronic infarction with scar shows no response; in the middle, viable myocardium with no scar or subtending stenosis increases continuously with a low and high dose; at the bottom, a normal segment subtended by a critical stenosis increases with a low dose but worsens with a high dose. This is termed a biphasic response and is characteristic of "hibernating myocardium." (Reprinted from Oh JK, Seward JB, Tajik AJ. *The Echo Manual,* 2nd ed. Philadelphia: Lippincott Williams & Wilkins, 1999:99, with permission.)

inotropic stimulation were an ominous sign. However, current clinical experience suggests that short-term stunning has a high rate of recovery, unless due to surgical technical difficulties/misadventures or anatomic abnormalities (i. e. intramyocardial vessel).

Localization of Ischemia: The 16- and 17-Segment System

Accurate anatomic classification of RWMAs is essential to guide clinical management, to localize coronary artery pathology, and to gauge therapy or the need for diagnostic intervention (i. e. cardiac catheterization). Documentation in the medical record using accepted terminology for quality improvement, billing, and communication with cardiologists and primary care providers is essential.

The 16-segment LV model adopted by the ASE in 1989 (a simplification of an older 20-segment model) was the basis of the Society of Cardiovascular Anesthesiologists' (SCA) comprehensive intraoperative protocol now in widespread clinical use (1,20). It is based on division of the left ventricle into apical, middle, and basal zones, with roughly equal mass, although anatomic studies demonstrate an expected decrease from base to apex. The basal and middle zones each contain six segments, whereas the apical zone with its smaller area has only four. To assess all 16 segments requires interrogation of five imaging planes: the mid-esophageal (ME) four-chamber, two-chamber, and LAX views along with two TG views: basal and middle.

A more recent American Heart Association (AHA)/ASE committee charged with standardizing myocardial nomenclature between radionuclear, echocardiographic, and magnetic resonance modalities adopted a 17-segment model in which an additional segment, located at the ventricular apex (devoid of direct contact with the ventricular cavity) has been added (Fig. 7.12) (26). The rationale for this "new" apical segment is the growth in echocardiographic assessment of myocardial perfusion using intramyocardial contrast, which should allow closer correlation with single-photon emission computed tomography nuclear cardiology studies, which routinely use this nomenclature. It will likely take time for this new segment to be accepted perioperatively given the relatively recent publication of the SCA 16-segment protocol. An additional change recommended is deletion of the term *posterior* from the segmental nomenclature because it is only used in echocardiography and not the other modalities. They recommend exclusive use of the term *inferior*.

Once wall motion has been assessed qualitatively in each of the 16 or 17 LV segments, an integer score for each grade of wall motion (increasing with worsening severity) can be assigned to each segment. The sum of the scores divided by the total number of segments visualized can be calculated to obtain a wall motion score index. This approach is used in research studies, especially those comparing echo data

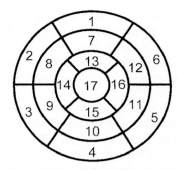

FIGURE 7.12. Circumferential polar plot of the revised nomenclature system in the transgastric views recently proposed by the American Society of Echocardiography. The circles, from outside to inside, represent the transgastric basal, mid-papillary, apical, and apex segments. Also noted is elimination of the term *posterior.* The numbers inside the circle are represented as follows: *1,* basal anterior; *2,* basal anteroseptal; *3,* basal inferoseptal; *4,* basal inferior; *5,* basal inferolateral; *6,* basal anterolateral; *7,* middle anterior; *8,* mid-anteroseptal; *9,* mid-inferoseptal; *10,* middle inferior; *11,* mid-inferolateral; *12,* mid-anterolateral; *13,* apical anterior; *14,* apical septal; *15,* apical inferior; *16,* apical lateral; *17,* apex. (Reprinted from Cerqueira MD, Weissman NJ, Dilsizian V, et al. Standardized myocardial segmentation and nomenclature for tomographic imaging of the heart: a statement for healthcare professionals from the Cardiac Imaging Committee of the Council on Clinical Cardiology of the American Heart Association. *J Am Soc Echocardiogr* 2002;15:466, with permission.)

to thallium or other radionuclear perfusion methods, and clinically for prognostication following MI. Although well validated in these settings, it is rarely used in the perioperative period.

The basal TG view can be problematic to obtain, and interpreting wall motion in this region adjacent to the fibrous atrioventricular skeleton can be difficult. As a result, the AHA/ASE group recommends scoring of basal segments containing myocardium in all 360 degrees around the ventricle (26). The clinician also must remember that to obtain a true ME four-chamber view, one must rotate the multiplane transducer approximately 10 degrees to "remove" the LV outflow tract (normally present in the neutral 0 degree orientation) (20). This allows visualization of the basal septal segment.

Assessment of the apex is accomplished nearly exclusively using the ME longitudinal orientations. A transverse apical image is sometimes possible below the TG SAX view (obtained by posteroflexion at that level) but not commonly. Given that the apex is in the "far field" of the image, it is important to optimize gain/time gain compensation settings in this region, place the transmit zone over the apex, and use as low a frequency as is consistent with optimal resolution (usually no higher than 5–6 MHz). In most new systems a "zoom" or RES feature also can help. Recognition by the clinician that apical RMWAs are commonly encountered in patients with significant CAD and that complications of infarction, particularly aneurysm and thrombus formation, are most commonly encountered

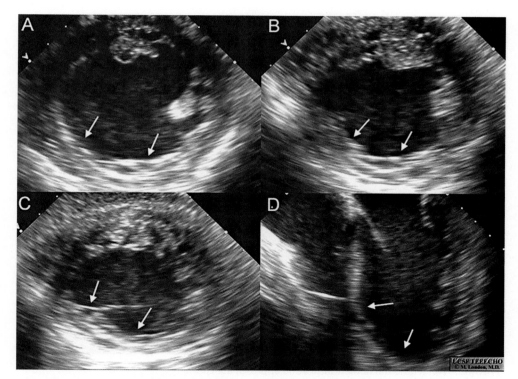

FIGURE 7.13. Chronic anteroseptal infarction in different imaging planes. A large area of infarction in the anteroseptal region characterized by wall thinning (approximately outlined by *arrows*) and akinesis is depicted. **A:** Basal transgastric short-axis view. **B:** Mid-transgastric short-axis view. **C:** Apical transgastric short-axis view. **D:** Mid-esophageal four-chamber view. A "hinge point" between normal and infarcted myocardium is easily visualized at the top arrow in frame **D**. Calcification of the anteromedial papillary muscle is present. (Reprinted from *www.ucsf.edu/teeecho*, with permission.)

in the apex, makes it an important area to evaluate (Fig. 7.13).

The TG LAX view can be helpful in assessing anterior and inferior segments in a complementary manner to the TG SAX view, especially when imaging from the ME planes is suboptimal. However, it is not possible to image the apex in this view.

Coronary Artery Perfusion Zones

The perfusion zones or territories of the three main coronary arteries, although potentially variable on an individual level, have been mapped to varying combinations of adjacent myocardial segments on a population basis (primarily using radionuclear perfusion imaging methods). The most important factor influencing this mapping is the origin of the posterior descending artery from the right coronary artery in a right dominant system (the common scenario) versus its origin from the circumflex in the less common left dominant system. There is usually some degree of overlap between territories, most commonly in the posterior segments and the inferior and lateral apical segments. The LAD artery usually perfuses these apical segments, although the posterior descending (inferoapical) or circumflex (lateral apical) artery

also may. In the newer 17-segment system, the highest degree of variability is encountered in the true apical segment (Fig. 7.14) (26).

The population-based uniformity of perfusion zones is one of the two main reasons for the popularity of the middle and basal TG SAX views for intraoperative monitoring (besides being easiest to continuously assess intracavitary area and volume); they are the only views in which a portion of the territories of all three main coronary arteries perfusing the LV are visualized. Usually the mid-papillary TG SAX view is used, although the basal view has similar anatomic characteristics. With reduction in flow in any (or all) of the three main coronary arteries, one will usually see a new RWMA. However, if stenosis occurs distal to this region (e.g. perfusing the apical segments), wall motion will usually remain normal in this view; thus, the clinician must periodically evaluate other imaging planes for a complete assessment. It should be pointed out that in the ME four-chamber view, right coronary artery perfusion of the RV free wall along with LAD arterial perfusion of the septum and left circumflex arterial perfusion of the lateral wall can be evaluated.

The right coronary artery perfuses the bulk of the RV, although the conus branch of the LAD artery may

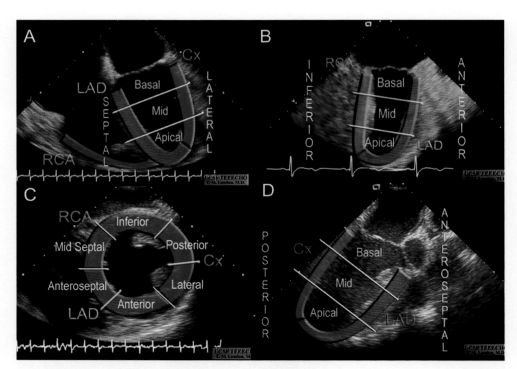

FIGURE 7.14. Segmental nomenclature and approximate coronary artery perfusion zones for the major imaging planes. **A:** Mid-esophageal (ME) four-chamber view. **B:** ME two-chamber view. **C:** Transgastric mix short-axis view. **D:** ME long-axis view. *RCA,* right coronary artery; *Cx,* circumflex; *LAD,* left anterior descending. (Reprinted from *www.ucsf.edu/teeecho.* Adapted from Shanewise JS, Cheung AT, Aronson S, et al. ASE/SCA guidelines for performing a comprehensive intraoperative multiplane transesophageal echocardiography examination: recommendations of the American Society of Echocardiography Council for Intraoperative Echocardiography and the Society of Cardiovascular Anesthesiologists Task Force for Certification in Perioperative Transesophageal Echocardiography. *Anesth Analg* 1999;89:870–884, with permission.)

supply a portion of the RV free wall. RV involvement during inferior LV infarction is common anatomically, but clinical manifestations (primarily RV failure manifested by systemic hypotension with clear lung fields) are infrequently observed. In the setting of inferior MI with RV ischemia, primary angioplasty with reperfusion of the right coronary artery is associated with significant recovery of RV function (27).

Ischemic Mitral Regurgitation

Acute or chronic mitral regurgitation is commonly associated with severe ischemia. Its recognition can provide information regarding severity and efficacy of therapy when it resolves completely. The regurgitant jet is usually central in origin and causes marked elevation of pulmonary artery pressures. Acute ventricular dilatation with incomplete leaflet coaptation, ischemic dysfunction of the papillary muscles, or hypokinesia of the underlying ventricular segment are suggested mechanisms. Acute annular enlargement with displacement of the papillary muscle tips, resulting in "loitering" (e.g., a slow response) of the leaflets to coapt properly in early systole is the functional mechanism (28).

With myocardial infarction, additional factors include LV cavity and annular dilatation, aneurysmal or pseudoaneurysmal changes (particularly of the basal segments), and, rarely, papillary muscle rupture. The latter most commonly involves the posteromedial muscle in the setting of either a right or circumflex infarction, because that papillary muscle is perfused by a single coronary artery in contrast to dual artery perfusion of the anteromedial muscle.

ASSESSMENT OF DIASTOLIC FUNCTION

Evaluation of diastolic function has become a rapidly growing and increasingly accepted area of investigation in cardiologic practice over the past decade. The codification of diastolic heart failure and the fact that perhaps one third of all heart failure cases are due to isolated diastolic failure has pushed this field from esoteric physiology to daily clinical practice (29,30). Echo evaluation relies primarily on spectral Doppler methods, most of which are straightforward and easy to perform [with the notable exception of accurately measuring isovolumic relaxation time (IVRT), a fundamental variable] (31). Newer reports have incorporated mitral annular velocity obtained used TDI, which is sensitive to changes in LV LAX dimension and volume.

Although qualitative analysis can yield useful information, the underlying research is nearly all quantitative, requiring measurement of spectral profiles, time durations, numerical correlation between different anatomic sites (e.g., mitral inflow velocity and pulmonary vein velocity); is based on serial evaluation of parameters over weeks or months; and requires adjustment for age and other pathophysiologic conditions (e.g., concurrent valvular pathology, LVH, different forms of cardiomyopathy, etc.). Thus, assessment is considerably more cumbersome than systolic function and of greatest importance; therapeutic interventions by the anesthesiologist in the perioperative period have not been investigated. Nevertheless, it can provide information helpful in estimating LV filling pressures (see hemodynamics chapter), and learning its basics will enhance the practitioners' appreciation of cardiac physiology and improve interpretation and integration of other types of echo data.

The physiology of diastole is complex enough that it has engendered a proposal to simplify the entire classical "Wiggers" cardiac cycle into three overlapping periods of contraction, relaxation, and diastolic filling (Fig. 7.15) (31). The basic purpose of diastole is to allow ventricular filling without abnormal elevation of LV pressure. In the initial phase, myocardial relaxation occurs. This is an active, energy-requiring event (and thus particularly susceptible to dysfunction with ischemia). As LV pressure falls below left atrium (LA) pressure, the mitral valve opens and early diastolic filling (diastasis) commences. Filling is driven primarily by elastic recoil (otherwise termed diastolic suction) and rate of active relaxation, not the LA pressure gradient. Diastasis accounts for approximately 80% of LV filling. As LV pressures rises during this phase, flow starts to decelerate as LV pressure approaches or even exceeds LA pressure. This is the downstroke of the A wave. Atrial systole occurs late in diastole, increasing the pressure gradient, augmenting filling by 15% to 20% in normal individuals and is recognized by the A wave. The ratio of percentage contribution between early and late filling is moderated by four key variables: rate of relaxation, elastic recoil, chamber compliance, and LA pressure. Each of these is influenced by numerous intrinsic and extrinsic factors.

Diastolic dysfunction is categorized into three ordinal categories of worsening dysfunction, the end result of which is irreversible, marked elevation of LV filling pressures leading

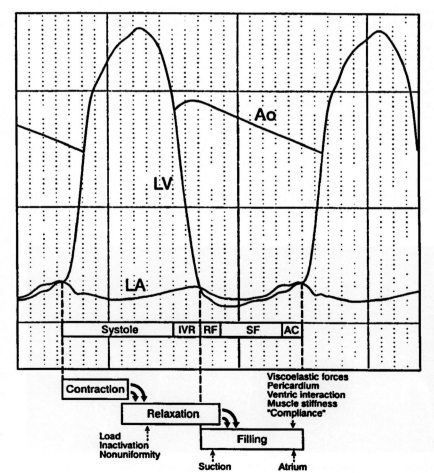

FIGURE 7.15. Diastolic filling of the left ventricle in a patient with hypertrophic cardiomyopathy. The cardiac cycle is depicted as the classic schema with systole and four phases of diastole (*IVR*, isovolumetric relaxation; *RF*, rapid filling; *SF*, slow filling; *AC*, atrial contraction) and as a proposed "simplified" functional system of contraction, relaxation, and filling. *LA*, left atrium; *LV*, left ventricle; *Ao*, aorta. Also noted are key variables influencing each of these phases. (Reprinted from Nishimura RA, Tajik AJ. Evaluation of diastolic filling of left ventricle in health and disease: Doppler echocardiography is the clinician's Rosetta stone. *J Am Coll Cardiol* 1997;30:9, with permission.)

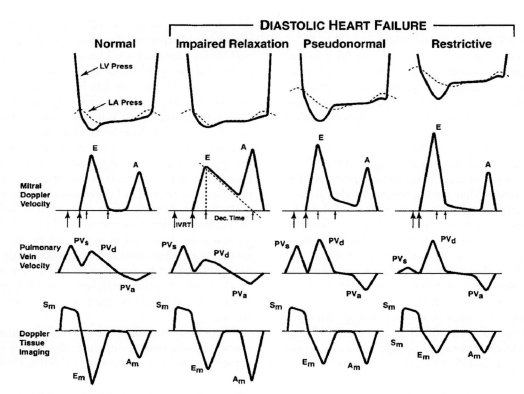

FIGURE 7.16. Assessment of diastolic function based on direct measurement of left ventricular and LA pressures with associated changes in echocardiographic parameters obtained using mitral Doppler velocity, pulmonary vein velocity, and Doppler tissue imaging. *IVRT,* isovolumic relaxation time; *Dec. time,* E-wave deceleration time; *E,* early left ventricular filling velocity; *A,* velocity of filling contributed by atrial contraction; *PVs,* systolic pulmonary vein velocity; *PVd,* diastolic pulmonary vein velocity; *Pva,* pulmonary vein velocity resulting form atrial contraction; *Sm,* myocardial velocity during systole; *Em,* myocardial velocity during early filling; *Am,* myocardial velocity during filling produced by atrial contraction. (Reprinted from Zile MR, Brutsaert DL. New concepts in diastolic dysfunction and diastolic heart failure. Part I: diagnosis, prognosis, and measurements of diastolic function. *Circulation* 2002;105:1391, with permission.)

to severe symptoms at rest or with minimal exertion (restrictive phase) (Fig. 7.16) (30). The earliest manifestation, commonly observed in adult practice and an extension or exaggeration of changes associated with normal aging, is impaired relaxation. This is easily recognized by widening of

the downslope of the A wave and reversal of the normal E/A ratio of greater than 1.0 (Fig. 7.17). The transitional phase between impaired relaxation and restrictive filling is more difficult to appreciate because the mitral inflow pattern approximates the normal pattern with a normal E/A

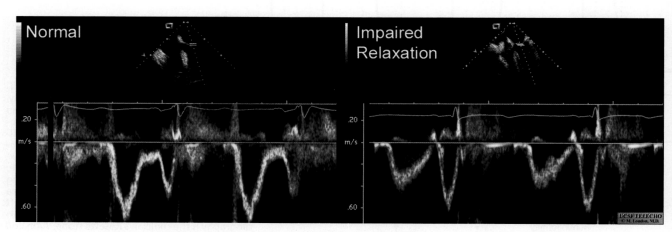

FIGURE 7.17. Grade 1 diastolic dysfunction (impaired relaxation). The deceleration time of the E wave is prolonged and the E/A ratio is less than 1.

ratio and deceleration time. This is termed pseudonormalization but in fact, LA pressure is now abnormally elevated. This can usually be distinguished from normal by evaluation of changes in pulmonary venous inflow (accentuation of diastolic predominance) and by reversal of the E/A ratio with acute preload reduction, although evaluation of other indices may be required. In the restrictive phase (often subdivided into reversible and irreversible phases), the increased LA pressure causes early opening of the mitral valve, reducing IVRT with a high transmitral gradient, causing a high E velocity. The early equalization of pressure shortens deceleration time. Atrial systole has less influence on filling because LV pressure is already increasing rapidly by this time; thus, the velocity of the A wave is decreased and the E/A ratio is greater than 2.0.

Changes in diastolic function of the RV can be assessed using analogs of the key anatomic sampling sites: tricuspid for mitral valve inflow and hepatic or superior vena caval velocities for the pulmonary veins (6). The respiratory variation in pressures associated with RV filling complicate interpretation, and considerably less information is available on this topic relative to LV diastolic function.

REFERENCES

1. **Schiller NB, Shah PM, Crawford M, et al. Recommendations for quantitation of the left ventricle by two-dimensional echocardiography. American Society of Echocardiography Committee on Standards, Subcommittee on Quantitation of Two-Dimensional Echocardiograms. *J Am Soc Echocardiogr* 1989;2:358–367.**
2. Smith MD, MacPhail B, Harrison MR, et al. Value and limitations of transesophageal echocardiography in determination of left ventricular volumes and ejection fraction. *J Am Coll Cardiol* 1992;19:1213–1222.
3. Clark NR, Reichek N, Bergey P, et al. Circumferential myocardial shortening in the normal human left ventricle. Assessment by magnetic resonance imaging using spatial modulation of magnetization. *Circulation* 1991;84:67–74.
4. **Trambaiolo P, Tonti G, Salustri A, et al. New insights into regional systolic and diastolic left ventricular function with tissue Doppler echocardiography: from qualitative analysis to a quantitative approach. *J Am Soc Echocardiogr* 2001;14:85–96.**
5. Vuille C, Weyman AE. Left ventricle I: general considerations, assessment of chamber size and function.In: Weyman AE, ed. *Principles and practice of echocardiography,* 2nd ed. Philadelphia: Lea & Febiger, 1994:575–624.
6. **Quinones MA, Otto CM, Stoddard M, et al. Recommendations for quantification of Doppler echocardiography: a report from the Doppler quantification task force of the nomenclature and standards committee of the American Society of Echocardiography. *J Am Soc Echocardiogr* 2002;15:167–184.**
7. Burns RJ, Gibbons RJ, Yi Q, et al. The relationships of left ventricular ejection fraction, end-systolic volume index and infarct size to six-month mortality after hospital discharge following myocardial infarction treated by thrombolysis. *J Am Coll Cardiol* 2002;39:30–36.
8. Poortmans G, Schupfer G, Roosens C, Poelaert J: Transesophageal echocardiographic evaluation of left ventricular function. *J Cardiothorac Vasc Anesth* 2000;14:588–598.
9. Liu N, Darmon PL, Saada M, et al. Comparison between radionuclide ejection fraction and fractional area changes derived from transesophageal echocardiography using automated border detection. *Anesthesiology* 1996;85:468–474.
10. Oh JK, Seward JB, Tajik AJ. Assessment of ventricular systolic function. In: *The echo manual,* 2nd ed. Philadelphia: Lippincott William & Wilkins, 1999:37–43.
11. Denslow S, Wiles HB. Right ventricular volumes revisited: a simple model and simple formula for echocardiographic determination. *J Am Soc Echocardiogr* 1998;11:864–873.
12. Koch R, Lang RM, Garcia MJ, et al. Objective evaluation of regional left ventricular wall motion during dobutamine stress echocardiographic studies using segmental analysis of color kinesis images. *J Am Coll Cardiol* 1999;34:409–419.
13. Derumeaux G, Ovize M, Loufoua J, et al. Doppler tissue imaging quantitates regional wall motion during myocardial ischemia and reperfusion. *Circulation* 1998;97:1970–1977.
14. Pislaru C, Belohlavek M, Bae RY, et al. Regional asynchrony during acute myocardial ischemia quantified by ultrasound strain rate imaging. *J Am Coll Cardiol* 2001;37:1141–1148.
15. Foex P, Leone BJ. Pressure-volume loops: a dynamic approach to the assessment of ventricular function. *J Cardiothorac Vasc Anesth* 1994;8:84–96.
16. Skidmore KL, London MJ. Myocardial ischemia. Monitoring to diagnose ischemia: how do I monitor therapy? *Anesthesiol Clin North Am* 2001;19:651–672.
17. London MJ. Multilead precordial ST-segment monitoring: "the next generation?" *Anesthesiology* 2002;96:259–261.
18. Vatner SF. Correlation between acute reductions in myocardial blood flow and function in conscious dogs. *Circ Res* 1980;47:201–207.
19. Gallik DM, Obermueller SD, Swarna US, et al. Simultaneous assessment of myocardial perfusion and left ventricular function during transient coronary occlusion. *J Am Coll Cardiol* 1995;25:1529–1538.
20. **Shanewise JS, Cheung AT, Aronson S, et al. ASE/SCA guidelines for performing a comprehensive intraoperative multiplane transesophageal echocardiography examination: recommendations of the American Society of Echocardiography Council for Intraoperative Echocardiography and the Society of Cardiovascular Anesthesiologists Task Force for Certification in Perioperative Transesophageal Echocardiography. *Anesth Analg* 1999;89:870–884.**
21. **Buda AJ, Zotz RJ, Pace DP, et al. Comparison of two-dimensional echocardiographic wall motion and wall thickening abnormalities in relation to the myocardium at risk. *Am Heart J* 1986;111:587–592.**
22. Seeberger MD, Cahalan MK, Rouine-Rapp K, et al. Acute hypovolemia may cause segmental wall motion abnormalities in the absence of myocardial ischemia. *Anesth Analg* 1997;85:1252–1257.
23. **Lualdi JC, Douglas PS. Echocardiography for the assessment of myocardial viability. *J Am Soc Echocardiogr* 1997;10:772–780.**
24. Cwajg JM, Cwajg E, Nagueh SF, et al. End-diastolic wall thickness as a predictor of recovery of function in myocardial hibernation: relation to rest-redistribution Tl-201 tomography and dobutamine stress echocardiography. *J Am Coll Cardiol* 2000;35:1152–1161.
25. Kloner RA, Jennings RB. Consequences of brief ischemia: stunning, preconditioning, and their clinical implications: part 1. *Circulation* 2001;104:2981–2989.
26. **Cerqueira MD, Weissman NJ, Dilsizian V, et al. Standardized myocardial segmentation and nomenclature for tomographic imaging of the heart: a statement for healthcare professionals from the Cardiac Imaging Committee of the Council on Clinical Cardiology of the American Heart Association. *J Am Soc Echocardiogr* 2002;15:463–467.**

27. Bowers TR, O'Neill WW, Grines C, et al. Effect of reperfusion on biventricular function and survival after right ventricular infarction. *N Engl J Med* 1998;338:933–940.

28. Glasson JR, Komeda M, Daughters GT, et al. Early systolic mitral leaflet "loitering" during acute ischemic mitral regurgitation. *J Thorac Cardiovasc Surg* 1998;116:193–205.

29. **Zile MR, Brutsaert DL. New concepts in diastolic dysfunction and diastolic heart failure. Part I: diagnosis, prognosis, and measurements of diastolic function. *Circulation* 2002;105:1387–1393.**

30. Zile MR, Brutsaert DL. New concepts in diastolic dysfunction and diastolic heart failure. Part II: causal mechanisms and treatment. *Circulation* 2002;105:1503–1508.

31. **Nishimura RA, Tajik AJ. Evaluation of diastolic filling of left ventricle in health and disease: Doppler echocardiography is the clinician's Rosetta Stone. *J Am Coll Cardiol* 1997;30:8–18.**

8

ECHOCARDIOGRAPHIC EVALUATION OF THE MITRAL VALVE

ANDREW MASLOW
A. STEPHANE LAMBERT

Among the many advances over the past two decades in the diagnosis of cardiac dysfunction, echocardiography has had the most dramatic impact on the evaluation of mitral valve (MV) disease. Yielding progressively clearer images of the MV apparatus in real time, echocardiography has facilitated accurate detection, understanding, and quantification of MV abnormalities (1–16). In addition, this diagnostic modality has been used to follow progression of valve disease with serial sonographic interrogation (15,17,18).

Transesophageal echocardiography (TEE) provides superior imaging of the MV when compared with transthoracic echocardiography (TTE) due to the use of higher frequencies, closer proximity to the heart, and less interference from tissues such as the chest wall and lung (7–12). Additional advances in TEE technology, such as multiplane imaging, increase the number of windows and angles from which the heart can be examined, exceeding the scope of older technologies and rivaling TTE (7–13). Furthermore, TEE can be a valuable adjunct to surgical decision making during cardiac surgery (1,2,12,19–27).

A comprehensive echocardiographic examination includes a complete evaluation of the cause and severity of MV dysfunction in addition to an assessment of the prognosis and requirement for treatment. Mitral valve dysfunction can be categorized as primary valve pathology (organic or nonfunctional), which may be stenotic or regurgitant, or secondary valve dysfunction (functional or nonorganic) due to changes in ventricular geometry and function, enlargement of the mitral annulus, or papillary muscle dysfunction. Because outcome is related to valve dysfunction or associated heart failure, early detection and treatment should improve outcome by limiting impairment (5,6,13,14,28). Persistent valve dysfunction, despite therapy, is associated with worse outcome, highlighting the need for reevaluation (1–6). The purpose of this chapter is to review the echocardiographic evaluation of the MV apparatus and discuss its impact on clinical decision making.

NORMAL MITRAL VALVE APPARATUS AND FUNCTION

The normal MV permits blood flow from the left atrium (LA) to the left ventricle (LV) during ventricular diastole, and prevents regurgitation during ventricular systole. Several variables affect blood flow through the left heart into the systemic circulation. These variables include (a) the pressure gradient between the LA and LV; (b) systolic and diastolic function of the cardiac chambers; and (c) MV mobility and competence, which depends on the interaction between the mitral leaflets, chordae, and papillary muscles (29–31).

The MV consists of an anterior and posterior leaflet made of fibrous tissue (Fig 8.1). Each is less than 3 mm thick (29–32). The MV area (MVA) ranges from 4 to 6 cm^2 (14). The anterior leaflet is semicircular or triangular in shape, and is divided into two or three segments or scallops, depending on the classification system (Table 8.1) (11). Compared with the posterior leaflet, the anterior leaflet is approximately twice as large, and covers two thirds of the mitral orifice during coaptation. The anterior leaflet has a smaller area of attachment to the mitral annulus, which is shared with the left and noncoronary cusps of the aortic valve. The posterior leaflet is shorter in height compared with the anterior leaflet, covers a third or less of the mitral orifice during coaptation and can be separated into three scallops (Table 8.1). In addition, the area of posterior leaflet attachment to the mitral annulus is more extensive in comparison with the anterior leaflet. The proximal two thirds of each leaflet is smooth, whereas the distal third of the leaflet and the area of chordal attachment on the ventricular side are rough. The chordae are numerous and arise from the anterolateral (ALPM) and posteromedial papillary muscles (PMPM).

A. Maslow: Department of Anesthesiology, Rhode Island Hospital; and Department of Anesthesiology, Brown University Medical School, Providence, Rhode Island.

A.S. Lambert: Department of Anesthesia, St. Michael's Hospital, University of Toronto, Toronto, Ontario, Canada.

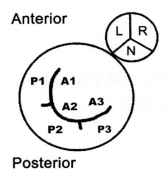

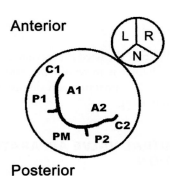

FIGURE 8.1. Schematic of the mitral valve displaying two commonly used systems to identify leaflet scallops. The two mitral valve leaflets (posterior and anterior) can be further divided into segments. The posterior leaflet is divided into three segments: *P1* (anterior; cephalad), *P2* (middle), and *P3* (posterior; caudad). Depending on which system of classification is used, the anterior leaflet is divided into two (Duran) or three (Carpentier) segments. In the Carpentier classification, the three segments correspond to those of the posterior leaflet (*A1, A2, A3*), whereas in the Duran classification the anterior leaflet is divided into anterior (*A1*) and posterior portions (*A2*). Furthermore, in the Duran classification there are two additional commissural (*C1, C2*) sections corresponding to the respective anterior and posterior commissures. Reprinted from Lambert AS, Miller JP, Merrick SH, et al. Improved evaluation of the location and mechanism of mitral valve regurgitation with a systematic transesophageal echocardiography examination. *Anesth Analg* 1999;11:966–971.

During ventricular diastole, the increasing atrioventricular gradient forces the mitral leaflets to open into the LV, while ventricular systole increases the ventriculo-atrial gradient, forcing the leaflets backward toward the mitral annular plane to facilitate coaptation. Papillary muscle contraction creates tension on the chordae to prevent the mitral leaflets from prolapsing past the mitral annular plane and into the LA. During mitral leaflet coaptation, a small portion of both anterior and posterior leaflets extends beyond the coaptation point. This "redundant" or residual tissue allows leaflet coaptation to be maintained even with changes in the mitral apparatus and/or ventricular geometry.

Additional roles of the mitral apparatus include maintenance of ventricular geometry and function. Chordae from the ALPM attach to the anterolateral portions of both leaflets, and those from the PMPM attach to the posteromedial portions of both leaflets (Fig. 8.2). Chordae may be

TABLE 8.1. TWO CLASSIFICATIONS OF MITRAL VALVE LEAFLET NOMENCLATURE TO IDENTIFY INDIVIDUAL SCALLOPS OF THE ANTERIOR (A) AND POSTERIOR (P) LEAFLETS

Classification	Anterior Leaflet Scallop	Posterior Leaflet Scallop
Carpentier, A	A1: cephalad, anteromedial	P1: cephalad, anterolateral
	A2: middle	P2: middle
	A3: caudad, posterolateral	P3: caudad, posterolateral
Duran, C	A1: anteromedial	P1: cephalad, anterolateral
	A2: posterolateral	PM: middle
	C1: anterior commissure	P2: caudad, posterolateral
	C2: posterior commissure	

divided into primary and secondary chordae (33). Detachment of the primary chordae may result in prolapse of the mitral leaflet and acute mitral regurgitation (MR), while detachment of the secondary chordae leaves a competent MV but results in reductions in ventricular function and systolic outflow. Understanding the role of the chordae and papillary muscles in maintaining ventricular geometry has influenced many surgeons' efforts to maintain the subvalvular apparatus during MV surgery (33).

The ALPM and PMPM appear echocardiographically as two single muscle bands or bundles of muscles that function in concert with the adjacent myocardium to exert a significant effect on dynamic LV geometry (Fig. 8.2). Normally, both papillary muscles insert toward the posterior aspect of the ventricular endocardium, resulting in optimal tension on the chordae during systole, while maintaining a posterior located leaflet coaptation point (34,35). This relationship is also important for directing transmitral flow toward the posterior aspect of the LV, which is subsequently followed by ventricular systolic outflow along the septum (35). Abnormal geometry may cause abnormal MV function. Anterior and inward displacement of the papillary muscles has been reported in patients with hypertrophied ventricles who are at risk for systolic anterior motion (SAM) and left ventricular outflow tract (LVOT) obstruction (35). Alternatively, posterior and apical displacement of the papillary muscles, seen with ventricular dysfunction and dilatation, increase leaflet tethering, which interferes with coaptation and causes MR (34).

A more thorough appreciation of mitral annular function has improved our understanding of MV dysfunction (36). The average annular diameter is no more than 3.0 cm, but the diameter may be as high as 3.8 cm. A normal indexed MV diameter is 1.7 to 1.8 cm/m^2 of body surface area (37,38). The position and geometry of the mitral annulus changes throughout the cardiac cycle and helps maintain normal blood flow. With the onset of systole, almost all of

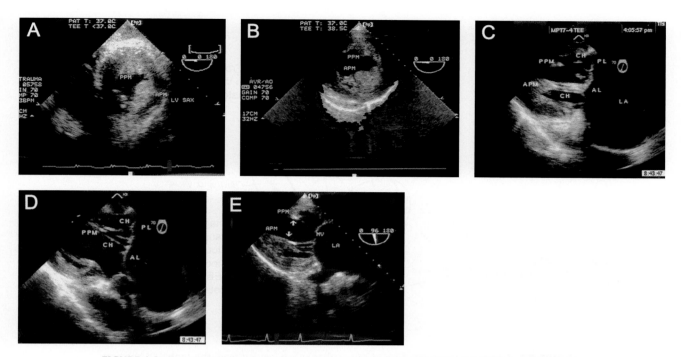

FIGURE 8.2. Transgastric imaging of the mitral valve (*MV*) subvalvular apparatus. **A and B:** Short-axis windows permit visualization of the anterior (*APM*) and posterior (*PPM*) papillary muscles. The PMs in *A* are normally positioned, whereas there is anterior displacement of the APM in *B*. In this latter patient, systolic anterior motion of the anterior MV leaflet was present. **C and D:** The APM, PPM, and chordae (*CH*) can be visualized with rotation of the transesophageal echocardiography probe to obtain the two-chamber (**C**) and long-axis (**D**) views. In the bottom middle panel, calcifications are seen along anterior and posterior chordae (*arrows*). **E:** Failure of the MV leaflets to return to the annular plane (*arrows*) due to the presence of a dilated cardiomyopathy and apical displacement of the papillary muscles that causes leaflet tethering. *AL,* anterior mitral leaflet; *PL,* posterior mitral leaflet; *LA,* left atrium.

the posterior segments of the mitral annulus contract. This results in posterior movement of these segments and reduces the mitral annular area. Two segments of the anterior annulus attached to the fibrous skeleton of the aortic valve lengthen and move upward. These movements of the MV annulus help maintain systolic outflow from the LV by widening the LVOT (36). Restricted MV annular movement seen with annular calcification, or rigid and complete annuloplasties, can interfere with LV systolic outflow. This insight has led to the development of annuloplasty techniques directed toward maintaining normal annular function.

GENERAL APPROACH TO THE ECHOCARDIOGRAPHIC EVALUATION OF THE MITRAL VALVE

Several investigations have described the utility of TEE in assessing the mitral apparatus (7–12). The echocardiographic examination typically begins with two-dimensional (2D) imaging to identify MV pathology and alterations in cardiac performance. After identifying areas of pathology, Doppler echocardiography is used to further assess direction of blood flow and quantify degree of dysfunction. The examination

consists of both transesophageal and transgastric imaging of the mitral apparatus. Due to variability in anatomic relationships among various patients, the MV should be viewed from as many windows as possible.

After inserting the multiplane probe to the mid-esophageal level, the transducer is rotated to 0 degrees (Figs. 8.3 and 8.4). From this level, the mid-esophageal four- or five-chamber view at the level of the LVOT is obtained to visualize the middle scallops of the anterior and posterior leaflets (A2; P2). By flexing the transducer tip or withdrawing the TEE probe, the mid-esophageal three-chamber view is obtained to evaluate the more anterior scallops (A1; P1), which can be found at the level of the superior aspect of the LVOT or above. By retroflexing the transducer or advancing the TEE probe, a four-chamber view below the LVOT at the level of the tricuspid valve (TV) is obtained to visualize the more posterior scallops (A3; P3). The TEE examination is continued by rotating the transducer angle from 0 to 180 degrees. Three more commonly described views include the mid-esophageal mitral commissural view, the mid-esophageal two-chamber view (50–90 degrees), and the mid-esophageal long-axis or LVOT view (110–145 degrees) (Figs. 8.3 and 8.4). In the two-chamber and mitral commissural views, it is also possible to visualize all the mitral

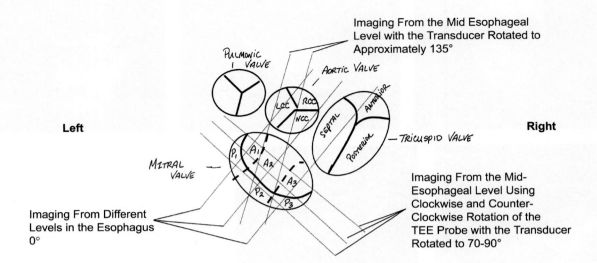

FIGURE 8.3. Schematic representation of the cardiac valves viewed from the cephalad position. Various lines are depicted demonstrating the interpretation used during this study. The mitral valve is described according to the Carpentier classification (*A1, A2,* and *A3* refer to the three segments of the anterior leaflet; *P1, P2,* and *P3* refer to the segments of the posterior leaflet). The drawn lines are based on imaging from three different transesophageal echocardiographic windows: 0, 90, and 135 degrees. The mid-esophageal mitral commissural view, seen at 90 degrees, also may be obtained using more acute angles. *LCC,* left coronary cusp; *RCC,* right coronary cusp; *NCC,* noncoronary cusp. Reprinted from Maslow AD, Schwartz C, Bert A. Pro: Single-plane echocardiography provides an accurate and adequate examination of the native mitral valve. *J Cardiothoracic Vasc Anesth* 2002;16:508–514.

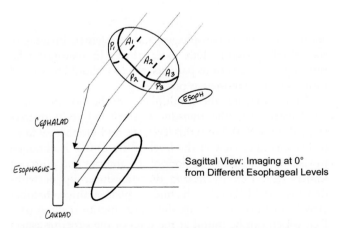

FIGURE 8.4. Schematic representation of the mitral valve (*MV*) as seen using single plane (0 degree) imaging from three different locations in the esophagus (*Esoph*). *A1, A2,* and *A3* refer to the three segments of the anterior leaflet. *P1, P2,* and *P3* refer to segments of the posterior leaflet. The three-dimensional structure of the MV shows that it does not lie in one plane. The dotted lines in the upper image, which shows the MV from above, refer to each of the three esophageal levels of imaging. In the lower image, the valve is shown in the sagittal plane and demonstrates that the valve extends from a cephalad to a caudad position. Echocardiographic beams from three different levels within the esophagus are depicted. Reprinted from Maslow AD, Schwartz C, Bert A. Pro: Single-plane echocardiography provides an accurate and adequate examination of the native mitral valve. *J Cardiothoracic Vasc Anesth* 2002;16:508–514.

scallops by rotating the TEE probe (Figs. 8.5–8.7). At the mitral commissural level, P1, A2, and P3 are seen. Rotation of the TEE probe to the patient's left allows visualization all three posterior scallops. Rotation of the TEE probe to the patient's right may allow visualization of the entire anterior leaflet. From the long-axis view (110–145 degrees), P2, P3, and A1 to A3 are seen most commonly.

Transgastric imaging of the MV begins at the base of the LV, permitting cross-sectional imaging of the MV. At this level both leaflets may be seen (Fig. 8.8). Valve area can be measured by planimetry, and the location of transvalvular flow can be identified. With further advancement of the TEE probe or retroflexion of the transducer, the mid-papillary short-axis view can be obtained. This view is useful to assess global ventricular function and to determine the position of the papillary muscles (Fig. 8.2A and B). Rotation of the ultrasound transducer to approximately 90 degrees allows further assessment of ventricular function, visualization of papillary muscles, and chordal pathology (Fig. 8.2). Additional transgastric windows for evaluating flow across the LVOT include the transgastric long-axis window (80–110 degrees with anterior rotation of the TEE probe), deep transgastric long-axis window (0 degrees), and other intermediary

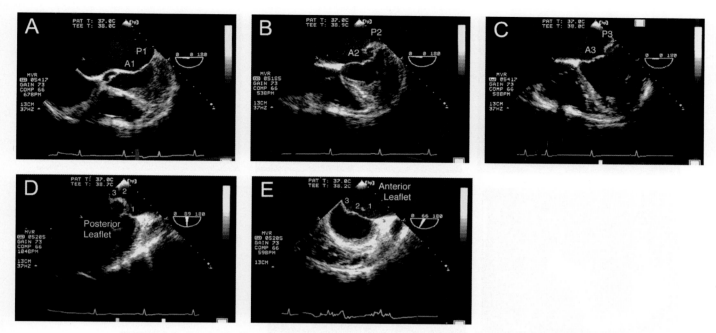

FIGURE 8.5. Esophageal imaging of the mitral leaflets permits identification of individual scallop morphology and function. This case demonstrates a flail of the middle posterior (*P2*) scallop with mild prolapse of *P3*. **A–C:** All segments of the anterior (*A1, A2, A3*) and posterior (*P1, P2, P3*) mitral leaflet can be visualized from various intermediary transesophageal echocardiographic windows using three levels of esophageal transverse imaging at 0 degree. Posterior **(D)** and anterior **(E)** rotation of the TEE probe allows visualization of the respective posterior and anterior leaflets.

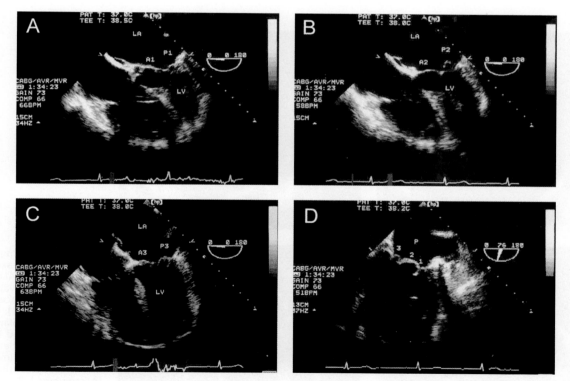

FIGURE 8.6. Transesophageal imaging of the mitral leaflets at the mid-esophageal depth. Although P1 appears normal **(A)**, prolapse of P2 and P3 is demonstrated in **B–D.** All three posterior segments are seen with posterior rotation. *LA,* left atrium; *LV,* left ventricle; *A1, A2, A3,* anterior mitral valve leaflet segments.

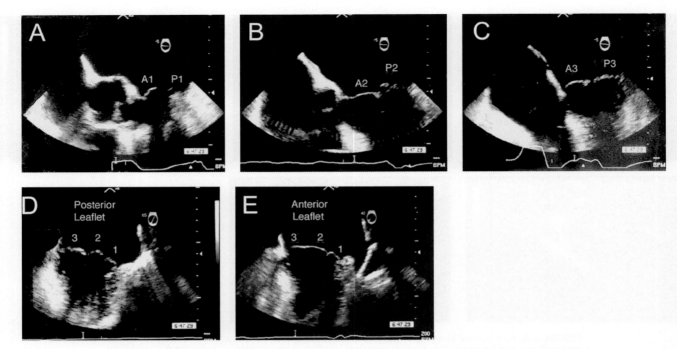

FIGURE 8.7. Transesophageal imaging at the mid-esophageal depth of a patient with mitral valve prolapse of A1 **(A and E)** and normal A2 and A3 **(B, C, and E)**. Borderline prolapse and thickening of the posterior leaflet segments is demonstrated in **A–D**. Small rotations of the transducer and turning the transesophageal echocardiography probe can alter the imaging plane from viewing all the segments of the posterior leaflet (P1, P2, P3: **D**) to all those of the anterior leaflet **(E)**. Reprinted from Maslow AD, Schwartz C, Bert A. Pro: Single-plane echocardiography provides an accurate and adequate examination of the native mitral valve. *J Cardiothoracic Vasc Anesth* 2002;16:508–514.

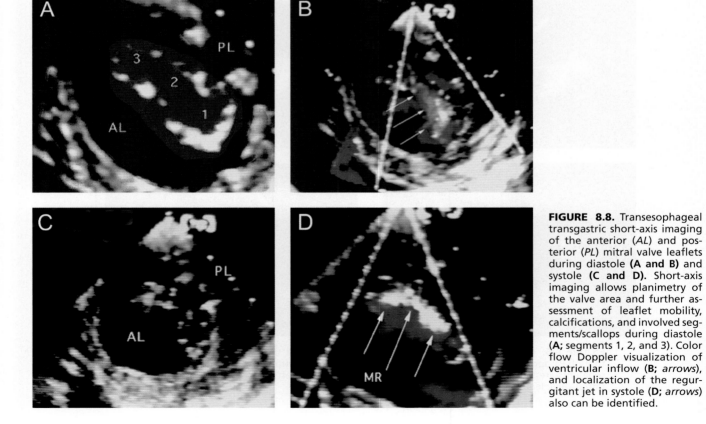

FIGURE 8.8. Transesophageal transgastric short-axis imaging of the anterior (*AL*) and posterior (*PL*) mitral valve leaflets during diastole **(A and B)** and systole **(C and D)**. Short-axis imaging allows planimetry of the valve area and further assessment of leaflet mobility, calcifications, and involved segments/scallops during diastole **(A;** segments 1, 2, and 3). Color flow Doppler visualization of ventricular inflow **(B;** *arrows*), and localization of the regurgitant jet in systole **(D;** *arrows*) also can be identified.

windows. After MV surgery, esophageal imaging of the LVOT may be obscured by artifact from the prosthesis. Transgastric images may allow visualization, Doppler assessment, and quantitation of LVOT blood flow, in the presence of limited esophageal windows.

After 2D imaging is performed, color flow Doppler (CFD) imaging should be used to assess blood flow and direction of flow across the MV. Turbulent ventricular inflow during CFD evaluation in diastole suggests mitral stenosis (MS), whereas turbulent flow into the LA during systole suggests MR. After CFD imaging is performed, pulsed-wave (PWD) and continuous-wave (CWD) Doppler can be applied to further quantify transvalvular flow. The PWD sample volume is placed at the leaflet MV tips to obtain maximum transvalvular velocities. Normal blood flow velocity across the valve varies with age. Passive inflow during early filling (E wave) is less than 80 to 100 cm/s, and is 0.75 to 1.5 times greater than the late transvalvular flow associated with atrial contraction (A wave; ϵ/A = 0.75–1.5) (Fig. 8.9A). Normal deceleration time of the E wave ranges from 150 to 200 msec. The isovolumic relaxation time (80–160 msec) is the interval from cessation of ventricular outflow to the beginning of ventricular inflow. Continuous-wave Doppler may be used in the presence of MS or an obstructing mass, when "alias-

ing" occurs during PWD sampling of ventricular inflow at velocities of greater than 1.4 m/s. For patients with severe MR or high-output states, ventricular inflow velocities may be elevated even in the absence of significant stenosis. These Doppler values are also affected by changes in ventricular and atrial diastolic function and aortic valve dysfunction.

During the TEE examination, the pulmonary venous flow should be analyzed using CFD and PWD (Fig. 8.9D and E). The PWD sample volume should be placed 1 to 2 cm into the pulmonary vein so that the ultrasound beam is aligned with blood flow within 20 degrees of parallel. The left pulmonary veins often can be seen using two transverse planes, but also may require rotation of the transducer from 0 to 90 degrees. The right pulmonary veins also may be seen using transverse plane imaging, but intermediary windows with the transducer rotated as much as 60 degrees may be necessary. The examination should begin with 2D imaging, and followed by CFD and PWD modalities. Normal pulmonary venous flows are not turbulent (<50 cm/s), with systolic (S) inflow being equal to or slightly greater than diastolic (D) flow. Blunting or reversal of the systolic venous flow (S/D <1) has been demonstrated for patients with moderate/severe and severe MR (Fig. 8.9E). Blunting of the systolic venous flow may also be seen in patients with atrial relaxation abnormalities.

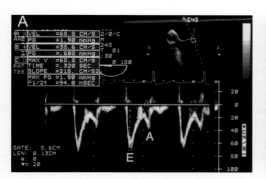
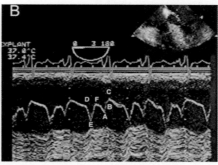
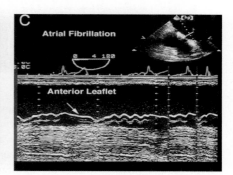
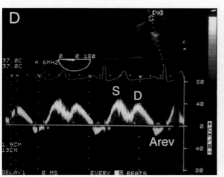
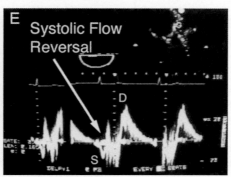

FIGURE 8.9. A: Normal transmitral Doppler flow velocity profile. **B:** M-mode echocardiogram of the anterior mitral leaflet (*D–E*, mitral leaflet opening in early diastole; *E–F*, mitral leaflet closing; *A*, mitral leaflet opening in late diastole; *B*, B segment; *C*, mitral leaflet closure at end diastole). **C:** Abnormal M-mode echocardiogram in a patient with atrial fibrillation demonstrating irregular anterior leaflet motion. **D:** Normal pulmonary venous Doppler flow velocity profile. **E:** Systolic flow reversal (*arrow*) of the left upper pulmonary vein consistent with severe mitral regurgitation. *E*, early transmitral filling; *A*, late transmitral filling (atrial contraction); *S*, systolic pulmonary venous flow; *D*, diastolic pulmonary venous flow; *A rev*, late diastolic reversal (atrial contraction).

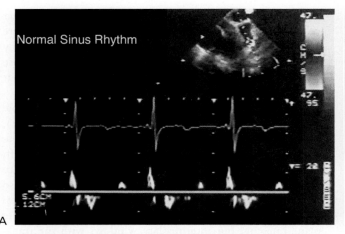

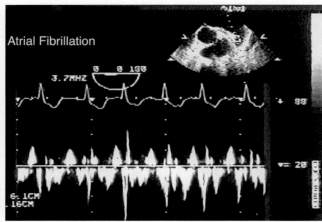

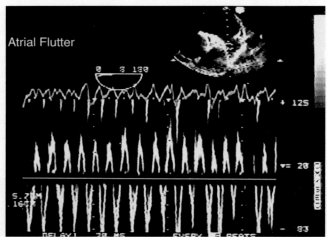

FIGURE 8.10. Doppler flow velocity profiles of the left atrial appendage in patients with normal sinus rhythm **(A)**, atrial fibrillation **(B)**, and atrial flutter **(C)**.

Because 24% of patients with MR may have some variability between the right and left pulmonary venous flow patterns, both right and left veins should be evaluated (39).

Imaging of the left atrial appendage (LAA) is important for the diagnosis of masses or "spontaneous echo contrast," a phenomenon associated with reduced atrial function, and increased risk of thromboembolic events. Patients with atrial tachydysrhythmia or MS are particularly prone to atrial dysfunction. Doppler assessment of the LAA also may be useful for diagnosing atrial dysrhythmias (Fig. 8.10).

M-mode echocardiography also may be useful during MV assessment. Application of M-mode echocardiography from the TEE four- or five-chamber or long-axis windows, where the M-mode cursor is perpendicular to MV leaflet motion, allows visualization of mitral leaflet intermediary motion and measurement of thickness. The normal M-mode mitral echogram is analyzed at several temporal points throughout the cardiac cycle (Fig. 8.9B and C). In early diastole the MV leaflets open (D–E segment). As LV and LA pressures equilibrate, flow diminishes and the MV closes (E–F segment). With the onset of atrial contraction, the leaflets open again (A wave) until ventricular pressure equals and exceeds atrial pressure, at which time the leaflets close (C).

Normally when there is minimal obstruction to ventricular inflow, the M-mode slopes (D–E, E–F, and A–C segments) are steep. However, when ventricular inflow is slowed or impeded, as is the case with ventricular diastolic dysfunction or MS, the slopes may be prolonged (40–42). Another sign of ventricular diastolic dysfunction is the presence of a "B bump" in the otherwise normally flat A–C segment (43,44). M-mode echocardiography of the MV and aortic valve leaflets from the mid-esophageal long-axis window may be useful in the evaluation of MV leaflet SAM and LVOT obstruction. Because intermediary positions can be seen with M-mode, the presence of MV leaflets in the LVOT during systole and premature closure of the aortic leaflets can be visualized.

MITRAL REGURGITATION

Etiology and Mechanisms

The etiology of MR can be categorized as functional (secondary) or nonfunctional (primary, organic) (Table 8.2). Nonfunctional MR is characterized by a primary abnormality of the MV apparatus. Conversely, functional MR is

TABLE 8.2. ETIOLOGIES OF MITRAL REGURGITATION

Classification by Mitral Valve Leaflet Mobility and Annular Dilation	Classification by Mitral Valve Morphology

Excessive leaflet mobility
  Myxomatous valve disease
    (leaflet and/or chordae)
  Torn chordae
  Torn/ruptured papillary
    muscle
  Endocarditis
  Prosthetic valve dysfunction
  Rheumatic valve disease
	Abnormality of Valve
	  Apparatus
	  Myxomatous valve
	    disease
	  Torn chordae
	  Torn/ruptured papillary
	    muscle
	  Endocarditis
	  Prosthetic valve
	    dysfunction

Restrictive leaflet mobility
  Rheumatic disease
  Ischemic papillary muscle
  Cardiomyopathy
  Calcific disease
  Prosthetic valve dysfunction
  Radiation associated valve
    disease
	Rheumatic disease
	  Cardiomyopathy
	  Calcific disease
	  Systolic anterior motion
	  Cleft
	  Endocarditis
	  Trauma
	  Radiation associated
	    valve disease

Annular dilation
  Cardiomyopathy
	Normal valve apparatus
	  Cardiomyopathy
	  Ischemia

Miscellaneous
  Systolic anterior motion
  Cleft
  Endocarditis
  Trauma	

associated with relatively normal MV morphology (1,29–31). A second classification is based on valvular motion, which may be restricted (cardiomyopathy, ischemia) or excessive (myxomatous disease, prolapse, torn chordae or papillary muscle) (Table 8.2). In addition, the MV annulus may be dilated (dilated cardiomyopathy) (30). Patients with functional MR often present with an MR jet that is centrally directed into the LA compared with an eccentrically directed jet seen in those patients with a primary MV abnormality (Fig. 8.11). The majority of patients presenting for surgical treatment of MR have excessive mobility most often due to myxomatous disease (1). Other specific etiologies include ischemia, rheumatic mitral disease, endocarditis, prosthetic valve dysfunction, and calcification of the mitral apparatus.

The etiologies of ischemic MR include papillary muscle dysfunction and ischemia-related changes in ventricular function and geometry (4,5,29–31). In the absence of papillary muscle rupture, leaflet mobility is restricted. Papillary muscle dysfunction is frequently associated with coronary artery disease (CAD) and ventricular dysfunction of the adjacent myocardium (1,29). The PMPM is affected more often than the ALPM, due to its coronary artery blood supply and limited collateral vessels in the presence of CAD. Papillary muscle rupture occurs within 3 to 4 days of myocardial infarctions (<1%) and rarely after chest trauma. The

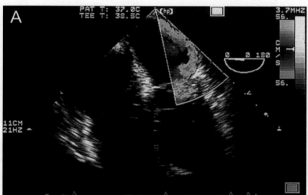
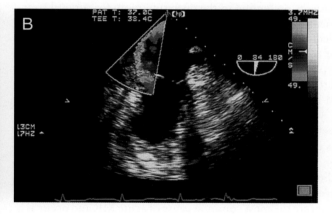
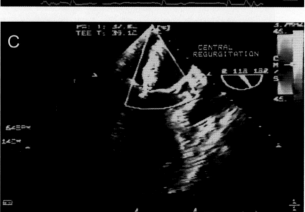

FIGURE 8.11. Color flow Doppler imaging of mitral regurgitant (*MR*) jets. **A:** Eccentric posterolateral MR jets. **B:** Eccentric MR jet along the inferior atrial wall. **C:** Centrally directed MR jet.

patient is usually acutely symptomatic, and if left untreated, the condition is fatal. A similar presentation may occur with chordal disruption; however, these patients are more likely to stabilize and not require emergent surgery.

In cases of dilated cardiomyopathies, several mechanisms affect MV leaflet coaptation and mobility, including an increased annular diameter, a reduction of systolic transmitral pressure (coapting pressure or force), an apical or posterior displacement of papillary muscles (local remodeling), and a decrease in the papillary muscle–annular angle, resulting in MV leaflet tethering (35,45–48). In patients with ventricular systolic dysfunction (LV ejection fraction <50%), the severity of MR may be less related to the degree of ventricular systolic dysfunction and more to local remodeling, resulting in apical or posterior displacement of papillary muscles (48). Although *in vitro* studies suggest that each of these mechanisms alone may cause MR, significant valve dysfunction often results from a combination of abnormalities. Calcification of the chordae or papillary muscles also decreases the mobility of the MV leaflets, resulting in tethering or tenting of the valve leaflets. These pathologies are not uncommon in elderly patients and may occur in the absence of ischemic cardiac disease.

Nonfunctional or organic causes of MR are associated with mitral apparatus abnormalities, including myxomatous degeneration, prolapse, chordal tears, severe calcification, endocarditis, rheumatic disease, prosthetic valve dysfunction, and clefts. Myxomatous changes are seen in the majority of patients presenting to the operating room for surgical treatment of MR, although only a small percentage of these patients (≤10%) ever require surgery (1,29,49,50). In a group of 86 patients presenting with MV prolapse requiring valve replacement, the development of moderate to severe MR occurred 25 years after the initial diagnosis (49,50). However, in the presence of severe MR, surgery was required within 1 year (49,50). Within this group of patients, those with leaflet thickening are at greater risk for complications such as endocarditis, severe MR, and the need for surgical repair or replacement. Excessive leaflet motion strains primary chordae, leading to chordal elongation, laxity, or tear with eventual MV leaflet prolapse and flail (1,49,50). Chordal tears are the most common cause of acute MR and occur as a result of myxomatous disease, rheumatic heart disease, calcification, endocarditis, myocardial infarction, or trauma. The posterior leaflet is most often involved. Rheumatic valvular disease more commonly causes MS or aortic insufficiency (13,14,16,17,29,51,52). Although MS or mixed MS/MR is more common, 10% to 30% of rheumatic valves may be primarily regurgitant, and are more likely to be present in younger patients within 10 to 20 years of the initial streptococcal infection. Endocarditis occurs after the introduction of microorganisms to an area of altered flow, usually around abnormal valves or valve prostheses. The infection causes MR because of destruction and perforations in the leaflets or surrounding tissues. Symptoms include a range of

TABLE 8.3. ECHOCARDIOGRAPHIC ASSESSMENT OF MITRAL REGURGITATION

Two-dimensional echocardiography
   Mitral morphology
   Mitral mobility
   Left atrial size
   Left ventricular size (diastole, systole)
   Right heart function
   Tricuspid valve morphology

Doppler echocardiography
   Pulmonary venous flows
   Color Doppler jet area
   Color Doppler jet/left atrial area or size
   Proximal jet width
   Proximal isovelocity surface area
   Continuity equation
   Pulmonary artery pressures

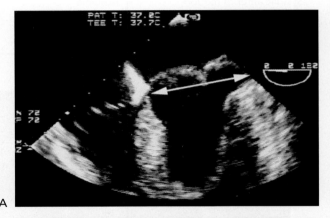

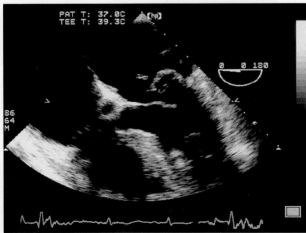

FIGURE 8.12. Mitral leaflet pathology associated with mitral regurgitation. **A:** Prolapse of both anterior and posterior leaflets. **B:** Flail posterior leaflet with ruptured chordae.

constitutional symptoms, signs, and cardiac complications such as arrhythmias and congestive heart failure (CHF). Depending on patient presentation, the report of a previous febrile episode may be remote. Radiation-associated valve disease, after treatment of thoracic cancers (e.g., lymphoma, breast cancer), may cause significant dysfunction of the MV, aortic valve, and/or TV (53–55). The incidence of radiation-associated valve disease may be increasing as a result of increased survival and longevity of cancer patients. Cardiac effects of radiation include pericarditis, CAD, myocardial fibrosis, and regurgitant valve dysfunction. The onset or detection of valve dysfunction has been reported in asymptomatic patients as young as 11.5 years and, for symptomatic patients, 16.5 years (53–55). Congenital MV clefts may result in focal MR, and occur more commonly in the anterior leaflet, but also may occur in the posterior leaflet.

Echocardiographic Assessment

Two-Dimensional Echocardiographic Evaluation

Two-dimensional echocardiography permits differentiation of the causes of MR by defining the mobility, morphol-ogy, and anatomic relationships of the mitral apparatus (Table 8.3) (7–10,12). Excessive leaflet mobility is consistent with myxomatous valve degeneration, chordal laxity or tear, or papillary muscle rupture. Myxomatous changes of the mitral leaflets can be further described as scalloping (or billowing), prolapsing, or flail. Flail refers to echocardiographic demonstration of the free leaflet edge in the LA above the annular plane (Fig. 8.12). Flail also may refer to chordae or papillary muscle seen freely mobile above the annular plane with attachment to the MV leaflet. Prolapse describes the displacement of the mitral leaflet above the annular plane by more than 2 mm. Scalloping (or billowing) describes excessive MV leaflet mobility and redundancy without prolapse or flail. Although the posterior leaflet (most commonly the middle leaflet; P2) is often the cause of MR, anterior leaflet pathology is not infrequently observed (7–10,12). In myxomatous degeneration there may be varying degrees of leaflet thickening (>3 mm), which increases the risk for endocarditis, severe MR, and the need for surgery (Fig. 8.13). In these patients, the MR jet is often eccentric, reflecting an organic etiology.

Ischemic papillary muscle dysfunction (without rupture) results in decreased leaflet mobility (45,46,56). Because the PMPM is more frequently affected, decreased mobility may

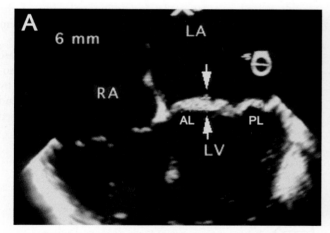

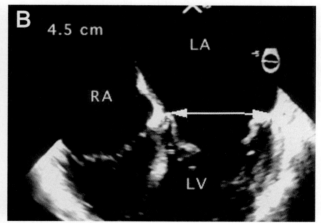

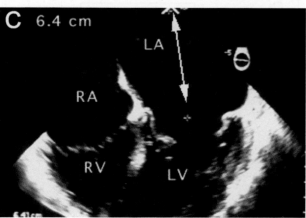

FIGURE 8.13. Myxomatous mitral valve degeneration and annular dilatation. **A:** Thickened anterior (*AL*) mitral leaflet (6 mm) (*arrows*). **B:** Enlarged mitral annulus (4.5 cm; *arrows*). **C:** Enlarged left atrium (*LA*) which measured approximately 6.4 cm in the anterior-posterior dimension (*arrows*). Chronic mitral regurgitation is associated with increases in cardiac chamber size. The posterior LA wall may be missed using transesophageal echocardiography, thereby leading to underestimation of the true atrial diameter. *PL,* posterior mitral leaflet; *LV,* left ventricle; *RA,* right atrium; *RV,* right ventricle.

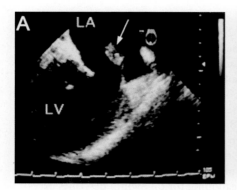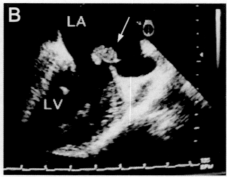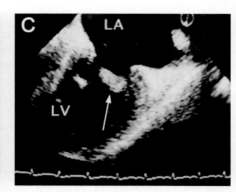

FIGURE 8.14. A–C: Transesophageal echocardiographic imaging at the mid-esophageal depth demonstrating a ruptured papillary in a patient who became acutely dyspneic 2 days after an inferior wall myocardial infarction. The mobile mass, seen in multiple views (*arrows*), is thick and freely mobile. *LA,* left atrium; *LV,* left ventricle.

be noted along the posteromedial segments of both leaflets (P2/3; A2/3). Dysfunction of the ALPM would be expected to cause anterolateral segment (P1/2; A1/2) restriction. Papillary muscle rupture is noted by a flail leaflet and visualization of a thick echodense mass (part of papillary muscle) attached to the chord and leaflet moving freely in the LV and LA (Fig. 8.14). Because papillary muscle rupture is an acute event, the ventricular cavity is usually not enlarged, compared with more chronic states of MR. Wall motion analysis demonstrates focal hypokinesis or akinesis of the myocardium surrounding the involved papillary muscle. Depending on the coronary anatomy, the remainder of the myocardium may appear normal to hyperdynamic. These findings are in contrast to chordal rupture, in which a thin echodense structure (chord) is freely mobile, and ventricular function becomes acutely hyperdynamic without wall motion abnormalities.

Patients with LV dilatation or dysfunction develop MR from decreased MV leaflet mobility and failure of the leaflet to coapt normally during ventricular systole. Although the leaflets may appear normal, there may be varying degrees of calcification appearing as echo-bright densities along the chordae or papillary muscles. Echocardiographic features of MR due to dysfunctional myocardium include a central MR jet, enlarged ventricular cavity, posterior and apical displacement of papillary muscles, a reduced papillary muscle–mitral annular angle, increasing tethering of the MV leaflet, and varying degrees of annular enlargement (Figs. 8.15–8.17) (35,45,46,56).

Rheumatic mitral disease is a chronic progressive disease of the mitral apparatus that, although more commonly associated with MS, also may cause MR. Leaflets are described by varying degrees of calcification, thickening, retraction, and decreased mobility, and in some cases prolapse and increased

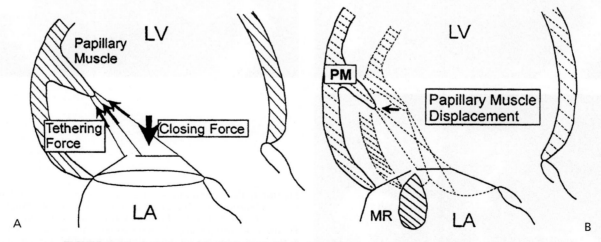

FIGURE 8.15. A: Forces of leaflet coaptation: closing force and tethering force. **B:** Effects of posterior or lateral papillary muscle (*PM*) displacement on mitral coaptation. In the presence of ventricular dysfunction and dilatation, papillary muscle displacement causes increased MV leaflet tethering and a reduction in coaptation force, resulting in reduction of coaptation and mitral regurgitation (*MR*). *LA,* left atrium; *LV,* left ventricle. Reprinted from Otsuji Y, Handschumacher MD, Schwammenthal E, et al. Insights from three-dimensional echocardiography into the mechanism of functional mitral regurgitation. *Circulation* 1997;96:1999–2008.

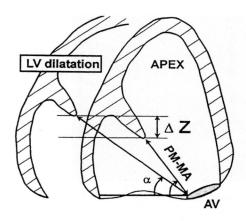

ΔZ = Apical PM shift

FIGURE 8.16. The effects of apical displacement (*Z*) of the papillary muscle in patients with dilated cardiomyopathy. Apical and lateral shift of the papillary muscle produces a decrease in the papillary muscle–annular angle (α) and an increased distance from the papillary muscle to the anterior mitral annulus (*PM–MA*), defined as the area of interaction (trigone) between the anterior mitral annulus and the aortic valve (*AV*). These changes increase tethering of the mitral leaflets. *LV,* left ventricle; *AV,* aortic valve. Reprinted from Otsuji Y, Handschumacher MD, Schwammenthal E, et al. Insights from three-dimensional echocardiography into the mechanism of functional mitral regurgitation. *Circulation* 1997;96:1999–2008.

mobility (Figs. 8.18A–C and 8.19) (13,14,29,51,52). These changes result in MR.

Two-dimensional evidence of endocarditis includes a range of findings depending on the timing, presentation, and location of the infection (Fig. 8.20) (29). Acute infections

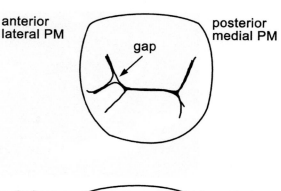

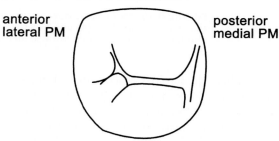

FIGURE 8.17. Annular dilatation results in a small gap (*arrow*) along the anterolateral commissure **(top panel).** With apical and posterior/lateral displacement of the papillary muscles (*PM*), the gap extends and includes the posterolateral commissure. The combination of annular dilatation and PM displacement causes significant mitral regurgitation. Reprinted from He S, Lemmon JD Jr, Weston MW, et al. Mitral valve compensation for annular dilation: *in vitro* study into the mechanisms of functional mitral regurgitation with an adjustable annulus model. *J Heart Valve Dis* 1999;8:294–302.

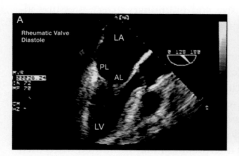

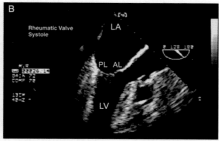

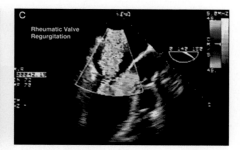

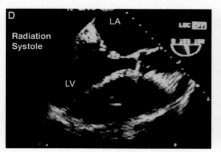

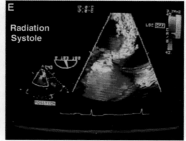

FIGURE 8.18. Mitral valve disease associated with rheumatic degeneration and radiation. **A–C:** Rheumatic mitral valve degeneration causes leaflet thickening, retraction (shortening), and restriction, resulting in severe mitral regurgitation. **D and E:** Radiation-induced changes of the mitral valve include leaflet thickening and retraction, resulting in severe mitral regurgitation. *AL,* anterior mitral leaflet; *PL,* posterior mitral leaflet; *LA,* left atrium; *LV,* left ventricle.

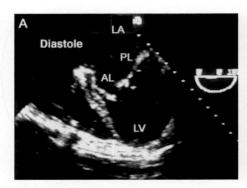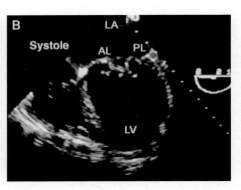

FIGURE 8.19. Mitral valve disease associated with rheumatic heart disease demonstrating diastolic leaflet restriction **(A)** and excessive systolic leaflet mobility and prolapse **(B)**. *AL,* anterior mitral leaflet; *PL,* posterior mitral leaflet; *LA,* left atrium; *LV,* left ventricle.

appear as mobile echodensities attached to the leaflets on the atrial side, or may less commonly appear on the chordae or papillary muscles. Acute infections are relatively homogenous in appearance. Delayed presentation manifests with varying degrees of leaflet calcification and mobility. The regurgitant jets may be singular or multiple, passing through large leaflet defects or smaller perforations. Abscesses appear as echolucent areas within or adjacent to the muscle atrial wall or along the papillary muscle tissue.

Radiation changes of the MV resemble rheumatic pathology (Fig. 8.18D and E) (53–55). Early changes involve thickening of the MV leaflets, which may progress to severe valvular fibrosis, shortening, and dysfunction. However, radiation changes do not result in the typical "doming" or hockey stick appearance seen with rheumatic valves.

Congenital mitral leaflet clefts occur more commonly on the anterior leaflet. Two-dimensional echocardiography demonstrates atypical breaks or acute bends in the leaflet, which permit regurgitation (Fig. 8.21) (29). Additional ab-

normal echocardiographic findings consistent with other congenital lesions may be seen, including ventricular septal defects.

Assessment of Regurgitant Severity

Although a number of echocardiographic measures of regurgitant severity are described, none are universally accepted as a gold standard to direct clinical practice (Table 8.4) (1,57–59). Therefore, echocardiographic measures of MR should be combined with clinical data to guide therapy. Echocardiographic measurements include assessment of pulmonary venous flow, CFD jet area, ratio of the regurgitant jet size to the LA size, proximal jet width (vena contracta), effective regurgitant orifice area (ROA), regurgitant volume (Rvol), and regurgitant fraction (RF). Measurement of LA and LV function/chamber size and pulmonary artery pressures allows assessment of the clinical impact of MR and perhaps the chronicity.

The incompetent MV allows blood to regurgitate into the LA during systole. The subsequent increase in LA pressure during ventricular systole impairs blood flow from the pulmonary veins, resulting in blunting or reversal of systolic pulmonary venous blood flow (Fig. 8.9E). However, because pulmonary venous blood flow is also affected by LA compliance, its interpretation may be limited when used alone. When compared with measures of ROA, Rvol, and RF, the correlation with pulmonary venous flows (S/D ratio) ranges from −0.66 to −0.74 (60). The normal pulmonary venous flow pattern has a sensitivity, specificity, and predictive value for moderate or less MR (ROA <0.3 cm^2) of 60%, 96%, and 94%, respectively (60). Blunting of pulmonary venous systolic flow has sensitivity, specificity, and predictive values for moderate/severe or severe MR of only 22%, 61%, and 30%, respectively (60). Pulmonary venous systolic flow reversal has a sensitivity, specificity, and predictive value of 69% to 86%, 98%, and 97%, respectively (39,60).

Color flow Doppler mapping of the regurgitant jet and measurement of the regurgitant jet area have been used to

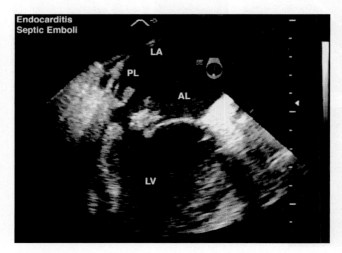

FIGURE 8.20. Transesophageal echocardiographic image of the mitral valve at the mid-esophageal depth demonstrating large, mobile masses on the posterior *(PL)* and anterior *(AL)* leaflets consistent with endocarditis nodules. *LA,* left atrium; *LV,* left ventricle.

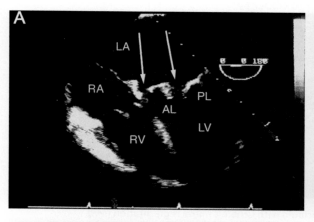

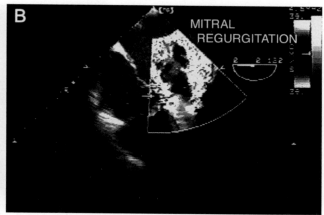

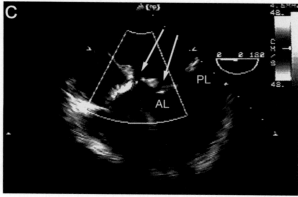

FIGURE 8.21. Mitral valve congenital clefts appear as dropout or areas of leaflet segmentation. More commonly, the anterior leaflet (*AL*) is involved, however, the posterior leaflet (*PL*) also may be involved. **A:** Cleft (*left arrow*) of the AL close to the annulus orifice (*right arrow*). **B:** Mitral regurgitation associated with the cleft. **C:** Ventricular septal defect (*left arrow*), and a second cleft (*right arrow*) of the AL. *RA*, right atrium; *RV*, right ventricle; *LA*, left atrium; *LV*, left ventricle.

assess MR volume (61,62). Mild regurgitation is said to be present when the size or length of the regurgitant jet is less than one third of the LA size or length. When this ratio is one third to one half, moderate MR is suspected, and when greater than one-half of the LA is filled with the regurgitant jet, moderate/severe or severe MR is diagnosed (Fig. 8.22). Attempts to correlate the CFD jet area with severity of regurgitation have demonstrated limited sensitivity and specificity. A CFD jet area of greater than 7.5 cm^2, and a jet area to LA size ratio of greater than 50% to 66% have been reported to be associated with greater than moderate/severe MR.

When compared with angiographic measures and to measurements of ROA and Rvol, the CFD jet area and the ratio of the jet area to the LA size may lead to overestimation of the severity of regurgitation in functional lesions characterized by a central jet. Only 6% to 11% of patients with functional regurgitation (centrally directed) and a large CFD jet area (>7.5 cm^2) were found to have severe MR, compared with 60% to 73% of patients with organic regurgitation (eccentrically directed) with a large CFD jet area (Fig. 8.22) (61,62). In contrast, assessment of the jet area may lead to underestimation of the severity of MR in patients with eccentrically directed jets (Fig. 8.23) (61,63).

TABLE 8.4. ECHOCARDIOGRAPHIC MEASURES OF MITRAL REGURGITATION SEVERITY

MR Grade	Jet Area (cm^2)	Jet/LA area (%)	Pulmonary Venous Flow	Proximal Jet Width (mm)	ROA (cm^2)	RVOL mL/beat	RF
0				2	<0.2		
1	<4	<20	S/D >1.00	3; <3	0.2–0.29; <1.5	<30; <20	9; <30
2	4–8	20–40	S/D >1.0	4.5; 3–5	0.3–0.39; ≤0.15	30–44; ≤25; 20–40	25; 30–39
3			S/D <1.0; systolic blunting	6.2; >5; ≥5.5	≥0.40; ≥0.3	45–49; ≥50; 40–60	47; 40–49; >40
4	7.8; >8.0	>40	systolic reversal	7.8; >6.0 or 6.5	≥0.6	≥60; ≥80	69; ≥50
References	53,54	51	39,51,54	54,55,56	51,52,54,57,60,62	50,51,57,58–59	50,57,62

MR, mitral regurgitation; LA, left atrium; S, pulmonary venous Doppler flow velocity profile systolic component; D, pulmonary venous Doppler flow velocity profile diastolic component; ROA, regurgitant orifice area; RVOL, regurgitant volume; RF, regurgitant fraction.

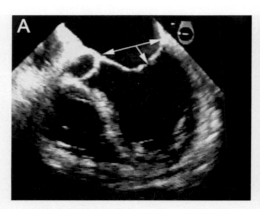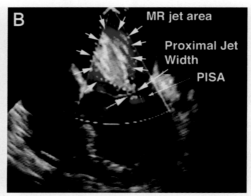

FIGURE 8.22. Restricted mitral leaflet mobility associated with ischemic mitral regurgitation (*MR*) or ventricular dilatation and dysfunction. **A:** Tethering is demonstrated by comparing the position of the coaptation point and the annular plane (*arrows*). **B:** The regurgitant jet is often centrally directed. Although the color Doppler jet area (*small arrows*) is consistent with severe MR (9.08 cm²), the jet width (*two arrows at valve orifice*; 0.27 cm) and regurgitant orifice area (0.12 cm²) measured by the proximal isovelocity surface area (*PISA*) technique, are consistent with mild to moderate or less regurgitation. Thus, MR severity using color Doppler jet area may be overestimated. *TVI,* time velocity integral; *ROA,* regurgitant orifice area; *Rvol,* regurgitant volume. MR jet peak velocity = 4.3 m/s; MR jet TVI = 125 cm; Nyquist limit = 57.7 cm/s; PISA radius = 0.38 cm; PISA flow rate = 52 cc/s; Rvol = 15 cc.

Several measures of MR assess both the size of the actual defect or orifice through which regurgitant flow passes, and the regurgitant volume (63,64). The simpler of these measures is the minimum proximal regurgitant jet width (vena contracta) at the site of regurgitation (Figs. 8.22 and 8.23). A jet width of at least 5.5 to 6.0 mm has been reported to have a high sensitivity, specificity, positive predictive value, and negative predictive value of 92% to 95%, 92% to 98%, 88% to 95%, and 95% to 98%, respectively, for grades 3 to 4+ MR measured with angiography (62–64). Grades 0, 1+, 2+, 3+, and 4+ MR have been correlated with proximal jet widths of 2 mm, 3 mm, 4.5 mm, 6.2 mm, and more than 7.8 mm, respectively (63). In another report, a jet width of 6.5 mm differentiated grade 1+ and 2+ from grade 3+ and 4+ with a sensitivity, specificity, positive predictive value, and negative predictive value of 90%, 83%, 79%, and 92%, respectively (62). Proximal jet width is a quick, simple, and accurate predictor of MR. However, researchers have noted that a clinician's ability to discern moderate regurgitation from severe regurgitation may reduce this method's predictive accuracy as compared with echocardiographic measurement of ROA and Rvol (59).

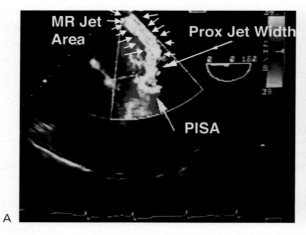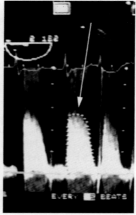

FIGURE 8.23. Assessment of mitral regurgitation (*MR*) severity in patients with eccentric regurgitant jets. **A:** Color Doppler jet area is only 3.61 cm²; however, the proximal jet width is 1.0 cm and the regurgitation orifice area (*ROA*) using the simplified formula is approximately 2.0 cm² [using a proximal isovelocity surface area (*PISA*) radius of 1.5 cm]. Both measures are consistent with severe MR, reflecting the potential for underestimating the regurgitant severity with eccentric jets when using color flow Doppler. **B:** MR Doppler flow velocity profile. *TVI,* time velocity integral; *Rvol,* regurgitant volume. MR jet peak velocity = 2.73 m/s; MR jet TVI = 33.8 cm; Nyquist limit = 39 cm/s; PISA flow rate = 480 cc/s; Rvol = 68 cc.

Mitral ROA, Rvol, and RF can be measured using the proximal isovelocity surface area (PISA) or proximal convergence area of the MR jet (Figs. 8.22 and 8.23) (59). As blood approaches the regurgitant orifice, flow becomes laminar, forming concentric isovelocity shells on the ventricular side of the MV. The radius and velocity of each shell or hemisphere can be used to measure the MR flow rate, which then allows measurement of the effective ROA, Rvol, and RF across the MV. The isovelocity can be seen by applying CFD to the MV during systole and adjusting the color map to obtain a uniform color with a discrete border where aliasing occurs. This border represents the Nyquist limit, from which the corresponding velocity can be obtained. The radius (r) of the isovelocity shell is used to calculate hemisphere area ($2\pi r^2$). When flow nears the orifice at an angle other than 180 degrees, an angle correction may be used to improve accuracy ($\alpha/180$). The flow rate (Flow$_H$) can be calculated by multiplying the product of the isovelocity of the Nyquist limit (Vel$_{NL}$) and $2\pi r^2$.

$$\text{Flow}_H = (\text{Vel}_{NL})(2\pi r^2)$$

According to the continuity equation, the flow rate though this shell is equal to the regurgitant flow rate across the MV.

$$\text{Flow}_H = \text{Flow}_{ORIFICE}$$

The effective regurgitant orifice area (ROA cm^2) of the regurgitant lesion can be calculated using the Flow$_{MR}$ and the peak velocity of the MR jet, measured with CWD (Vel$_{MR}$).

$$\text{ROAcm}^2 = \text{Flow}_{ORIFICE}/V_{MR}$$

Knowing the effective ROA, the Rvol can be calculated using the time velocity integral (TVI) of the regurgitant jet.

$$\text{Rvol cm}^3 = (\text{ROA})\text{cm}^2 (\text{TVI}_{MR})\text{cm}$$

Once the Rvol is known, the RV can be calculated if the forward stroke volume (SV) is known (LVOT; aortic valve; pulmonary artery or right ventricular outflow tract).

$$\text{RF\%} = \frac{(\text{Rvol (cc)})}{(\text{Rvol} + \text{SV})} = \frac{\text{Rvol (cc)}}{\text{SV}_{MV}}$$

The use of PISA or the proximal convergence area may be important in further quantifying moderate to severe MR (59). The amount of MR in patients with an ROA of less than 0.1 cm^2 is trace to mild, whereas ROAs of 0.2 to 0.3 cm^2, 0.3 to 0.4 cm^2, greater than 0.4 cm^2, and greater than 0.5 cm^2 are considered mild to moderate (2+), moderate (2 to 3+), moderate to severe (3+), and severe (4+), respectively (59,65). Regurgitant stroke volume and RFs based on PISA are defined as follows (59,65–67):

$$\text{Mild}(1+) = \text{Rvol} < 20\,\text{cc to } 30\,\text{cc (RF} < 30\%)$$
$$\text{Moderate}(2+) = \text{Rvol } 30\,\text{cc} - 44\,\text{cc (RF } 30 - 40\%)$$

$$\text{Moderate/Severe}(3+) = \text{Rvol} \geq 45\,\text{cc (RF} > 40\%)$$
$$\text{Severe}(4+) = \text{Rvol} \geq 60\,\text{cc (RF} \geq 50\%)$$

Although some variability exists, assessment of MR using PISA is believed to be more accurate and has been used as a reference for comparison (60,66). However, PISA is not routinely used in clinical practice due to the amount of time needed to perform the measurements and calculations. One simplified technique requires setting the aliasing velocity at 40 cm/s and assumes a peak velocity across the MV of 500 cm/s (100 mm Hg gradient) (68). With these assumptions:

$$\text{ROA cm}^2 = r^2/2$$

Although, several simplified formulas have been proposed, it remains to be seen whether or not the PISA technique will be used more routinely (68,69). Another problem using PISA to measure ROA involves the requirement to align the regurgitant jet in parallel with the ultrasound beam. Although this is possible with centrally directed jets, it may not be easily done with eccentric jets. For these latter patients, the simplified technique above may more easily apply, or one must rely on other quantitative methods.

Another method used to calculate Rvol and RF employs Doppler calculation of SV. By calculating the SV across the MV (VTI$_{MV}$ × A$_{MV}$) and across the aortic valve (or LVOT), one can measure regurgitant SV (SV$_{MV}$ − SV$_{AoV(LVOT)}$) and the RF (Rvol/(Rvol + SV$_{AoV(LVOT)}$ or Rvol/SV$_{MV}$). The SV also can be obtained by dividing the cardiac output (measured using either the thermodilution or Fick technique) by the heart rate. Although significant error may be introduced when measuring Doppler-acquired SV across the MV, RFs obtained by this technique have correlated well with angiographic measurements (70).

An MR index also has been proposed to evaluate severity by combining both Doppler and 2D echocardiographic measurements, including the extent of jet penetration into the LA, centricity of the regurgitant jet, PISA, CWD regurgitant jet profile, estimated pulmonary artery systolic pressure, pulmonary venous flow, and LA size (Table 8.5) (58). Each measurement is scored on a scale of 0 to 3, and the total is divided by the number of measurements. An index of 3.0 equals severe MR, and 0 equals no MR. The MR index is unaffected by the LV systolic function (ejection fraction). All patients with severe MR had an index greater than 1.83, and all patients with mild MR had an index less than 1.67. All patients with RF of greater than 60% had an index greater than 2.0, and an MR index greater than 2.17 identified 26 of 29 patients with severe MR, yielding sensitivity, specificity, positive predictive, and negative predictive values of 90%, 88%, 79%, and 94%, respectively (58). In addition to baseline assessment, stress testing may further elucidate the clinical significance of MR (57,71). Echocardiographic evaluation was performed at baseline and during exercise in 27 patients with varying degrees of functional MR. Regurgitant

TABLE 8.5. MITRAL REGURGITATION (MR) INDEX

MR Grade	Jet Penetration	PISA Radius (NL 50–64 cm/s)	CW Jet Profile	sPAP (mm Hg)	Pulmonary Vein	LA Size
0	None	None	No jet	<25	S/D >1	Normal
1	Central below PV	≤0.5 cm	Incomplete jet	25–30	S/D =1	Mild Enlg
2	Eccentric up to PV	0.5–1.0 cm	Complete jet 20%–50% density	31–45	S/D <1	Mild/Mod Enlg
3	Eccentric beyond PV	≥1.0 cm	Complete jet >50% density	>45	Systolic reversal	Mod/Sev Enlg

PIAS, proximal isovelocity area; NL, Nyquist limit; CW, continuous wave Doppler; PV pulmonary vein; sPAP, systolic pulmonary artery pressure; LA, left atrium; S/D, ratio of systolic to diastolic pulmonary venous flow velocities or time velocity integrals; Enlg, enlarged; Mod, moderate; Sev, severe.

Measure/Data	Mild MR	Moderate MR	Severe MR
Age (yr)	65	60	62
Regurgitant volume (mL)	12	31	59
Regurgitant fraction (%)	20	40	57
Left ventricular ejection fraction (%)	50	48	49
Mitral regurgitation index	1.1	1.8	2.4

Reprinted from Thomas L, Foster E, Hoffman JI, et al. The mitral regurgitation index: an echocardiographic guide to severity. *J Am Coll Cardiol* 1993;33:2016–2022, with permission.

volume measured by PISA increased with exercise from 21 to 39 mL (8–85 mL). There was good correlation between increases in Rvol and changes in proximal jet diameter (r = 0.82) and increase in pulmonary artery systolic pressure measured by trans-TV systolic gradient (r = 0.73), whereas a poor correlation was seen with CFD jet area (71). Ten patients with exercise-induced dyspnea had greater increases in the trans-TV gradient (48 vs. 20 mm Hg) and Rvol (34 vs. 11 mL) compared with other patients, including seven patients who stopped exercise due to fatigue, suggesting that larger increases in pulmonary artery pressure during stress signifies more significant valve dysfunction (71).

Effects of General Anesthesia on Mitral Regurgitation

The severity of MR made may be reduced after the induction of general anesthesia due to decreases in preload and afterload (5,72–74). This reduction in MR after general anesthesia is not seen in the presence of a flail mitral leaflet (62). In patients with CAD, a 46% discordance has been reported between ischemic MR assessed during cardiac catheterization compared with the evaluation performed after induction of general anesthesia (5). Seventy-nine percent of these patients were found to have some degree of instability during preoperative cardiac catheterization that was not present during the intraoperative examination prior to undergoing coronary artery bypass graft surgery (CABG) (5). Assuming hemodynamic stability following satisfactory revascularization, the intraoperative examination should be an accurate guide for the treatment of MR. In 246 patients scheduled for CABG with or without MV surgery, intraoperative echocardiography altered the surgical plan in 27 patients (11%) (75). Twenty-two patients scheduled for CABG and MV surgery had CABG only, and five patients scheduled for CABG had CABG and MV surgery. Mortality was zero in these latter five patients, and highest for patients who were scheduled for and underwent CABG and MV surgery (75). No patient required reoperation for MR.

Because the intraoperative quantitative assessment of MR may not reflect the preinduction state, accurate assessments of MV morphology and function are paramount. If questions regarding the treatment of MR persist, alterations in loading conditions (e.g., phenylephrine to increase afterload; Trendelenberg positioning to increase preload) may be useful to assess MV function under varying stress.

Echocardiographic Evaluation of Mitral Regurgitation as a Predictor of Outcome

The outcome of patients with MR depends on its cause and severity (1–6). Because ventricular remodeling can be halted and ventricular function restored with treatment of MR, early surgical intervention is suggested to improve patient outcome (1,2). Echocardiographic measurements that suggest ventricular remodeling include a left ventricular end-systolic diameter (LVESD) greater than 4.0 to 4.5 cm, a left ventricular end-diastolic diameter (LVEDD) greater than 6.0 to 6.4 cm, or an left ventricle ejection fraction (LVEF) from ≤40% to <60%, in the presence of at least moderate MR (1,19,76). These measures allude to the chronicity of MR and suggest that regression of MR is unlikely without surgery.

Other important signs include the elevation of pulmonary artery pressures and LA enlargement (57,58,71).

Although the progression and prognosis of MR are not clearly defined, patients with MR are likely to develop ventricular dilatation and dysfunction over variable periods of time (15). Increases in effective ROA of approximately 5.9 mm²/yr, Rvol of 7.4 cc/yr, and RF of 2.9% have been reported (15). There was, however, significant variability among those studied, with 11% demonstrating decreases of Rvol of more than 8 cc/yr, 38% showing no change, and 51% showing increases in Rvol of more than 8 cc/yr. Patients with restricted leaflet mobility did not change significantly, whereas patients with dilated annuli progressed more slowly, and those with flail leaflets progressed rapidly.

Patients with moderate to severe MR may remain asymptomatic for up to 10 years. However, when symptoms of CHF and arrhythmias develop, mortality rates may be as high as 5%/yr, and 8-year survival rates as low as 33% (1). Unless ventricular dysfunction or dilatation is present, medical therapy is unlikely to reduce the Rvol or improve cardiac function. Between 28% and 90% of patients with severe MR will require surgery within 5 to 10 years depending on the presence or absence of symptoms (1).

Outcome after MV surgery is related to preoperative ventricular dysfunction, functional status [New York Heart Association (NYHA) grade III/IV vs. grade I/II], and residual regurgitation despite treatment (2–6,77–79). In a study of 409 patients with isolated organic MR, the 5-year survival rate after MV surgery was highest for patients with LVEF of greater than 60%, intermediate for LVEF of 50% to 60%, and least for patients with LVEF of less than 50% (3). Operative mortality after combined CABG and MV surgery ranges from 8% to 20% and is significantly greater in patients with functional "ischemic" MR than in those with pure organic (nonfunctional) MR (<5%) (4,5,80–82). Operative mortality may be as high as 50% for combined CABG/MVR when the LVEF is less than 30% (2,3). These data highlight the importance of accurate MV assessment as well as patient selection for MV surgery with increased interest in performing an MV procedure prior to the development of ventricular dysfunction (75,83). Because outcome is also related to residual MR after surgery, the importance of an immediate post–cardiopulmonary bypass (CPB) echocardiographic assessment to determine the presence of significant (≥2+) residual MR cannot be overstated (2,6,77,78).

Mitral Regurgitation in Patients with Aortic Stenosis

The treatment of patients with moderate or severe MR in the setting of aortic stenosis (AS) is controversial. Conclusions regarding the regression of MR after aortic valve replacement (AVR) vary. In one study, MR decreased by one grade in 27%, was unchanged in 61%, and increased in 12% of patients (84). A similar percentage of patients was found

to have an increase in MR after AVR in a second study, while 60% had a reduction of one grade of severity (85). The amount of MR in patients with AS is partially related to changes in ventricular function and geometry (86–89). In a follow-up of 394 medical patients with AS, 36% had an increase in MR, 53% had no significant change, and 11% had a decrease (86). Patients with increased MR had a significant increase in transaortic valve gradient, an increase in end-systolic diameter, and a decrease in systolic function. Patients with stable MR had no change in end-systolic diameter or systolic function, and had an increase in ventricular hypertrophy (86). Patients without a significant increase in wall thickness were likely to have increases in ventricular diameter and MR (86). The researchers concluded that the normal adaptive response includes ventricular hypertrophy, which helps to maintain systolic function and prevent ventricular dilatation (86). Ventricular dilatation and reduction in systolic function are maladaptive forms of ventricular remodeling and are associated with significant increases in MR (86). Following AVR, a reduction in MR was seen when CABG was concurrently performed in patients with preoperative LVEF of no more than 40% and ventricular hypertrophy (thickness ≥15 mm) or enlarged ventricular cavities (LVEDD ≥6.0 cm; LVED length ≥9.0 cm) (87–89). For patients undergoing AVR/CABG, improvement in MR was seen in patients with a preoperative LVEF of 30%, LVEDD of 6.4 cm, and LVESD of 5.5 cm (87). Early and late follow-up showed significant reduction in chamber size and improvement in ventricular systolic function, both of which were associated with a reduction in MR.

The reduction in MR for patients with AS appears to be associated with improvement in ventricular function and geometry. Although one report demonstrated a greater reduction in MR for patients with normal mitral leaflet thickness, other reports have not demonstrated that mitral leaflet thickening or mitral annular calcification was associated with a change in MR after AVR for AS (84,85,87,89). For patients with AS scheduled for AVR, MV surgery should be considered when there is greater than moderate MR, especially when significant improvement is not expected or when primary (organic) mitral dysfunction is diagnosed.

Systolic Anterior Motion of the Mitral Valve and Left Ventricular Outflow Tract Obstruction

Systolic anterior motion of the mitral leaflets with LVOT obstruction is classically a dynamic process that results in MR and decreased ventricular output (90,91). Dynamic causes of SAM and LVOT obstruction have been reported in patients with ventricular hypertrophy, abnormalities of the mitral apparatus, after MV reconstruction, and after AVR for AS (20,21,90–93). Although this is a relatively uncommon cause of MR, its detection is important because the results of nonechocardiographic tests of cardiac

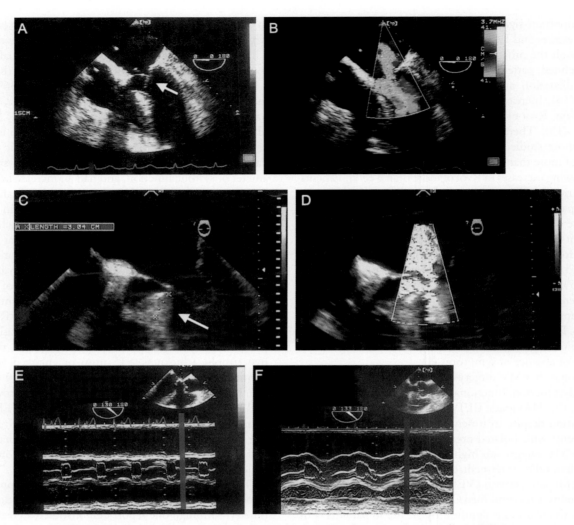

FIGURE 8.24. Transesophageal echocardiographic imaging demonstrating systolic anterior motion and left ventricular outflow tract obstruction (*SAM/LVOTO*). **A:** SAM of the anterior leaflet (*arrow*). **B:** Color flow Doppler shows aliasing in the LVOT and mitral regurgitation. **C:** A very prominent septal bulge (*arrow*) causes aliasing in the LVOT and mitral regurgitation **(D).** M-mode echograms of the aortic valve demonstrating normal **(E)** and premature closing **(F)** of the aortic valve leaflets.

performance will suggest a failing LV and may prompt therapy to increase contractility and reduce preload and afterload, all of which are likely to exacerbate dynamic LVOT obstruction.

Echocardiographic evidence of LVOT obstruction includes outflow tract narrowing and CFD aliasing during systole (Fig. 8.24). Two-dimensional echocardiography helps to identify the cause of LVOT obstruction. Findings of SAM include anterior displacement of the native mitral leaflets (anterior > posterior) causing impaired coaptation and MR. PWD or CWD profiles demonstrate an increased velocity (>1.4 m/s) with mid-systolic acceleration in the presence of LVOT obstruction. Aortic valve echogram shows mid-systolic or premature closure of the aortic valve leaflets (Fig. 8.24). The LV is often hypertrophic, with a small cavity and normal or hyperdynamic systolic function.

Earlier described mechanisms of LVOT obstruction causing MV leaflet SAM included the creation of high blood flow velocity and a Venturi effect associated with a disproportionately hypertrophied septum (asymmetric septal hypertrophy or idiopathic hypertrophic subaortic stenosis) (90,91). Although ventricular hypertrophy may be a contributing factor, currently proposed mechanisms are more complex and involve abnormalities of the mitral apparatus such as anterior and inward displacement of papillary muscles, which in turn displace the mitral apparatus and coaptation point closer to the LVOT (Figs. 8.24 and 8.25) (20,90–100). These changes also result in greater laxity of the chordae and increases in slack or residual leaflet segments that become susceptible to systolic outflow (90,91,98–100). The coapting lengths of the mitral leaflets also contribute to development of SAM and LVOT obstruction. Normally, the coapting distance (edges of the annulus to the coaptation

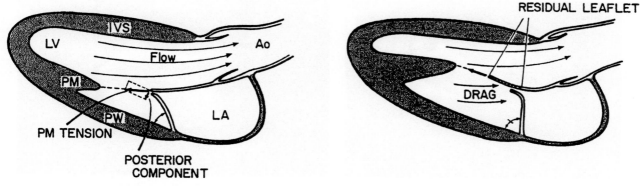

FIGURE 8.25. Schematic representation of the effects of anterior displacement of papillary muscles on left tension. Anterior displacement results in increased slack of residual leaflet segments, making them more susceptible to systolic outflow. *LA,* left atrium; *LV,* left ventricle; *IVS,* interventricular septum; *PW,* posterior wall; *PM,* papillary muscle; *Ao,* aorta. Reprinted from Levine RA, Vlahakes GJ, Lefebvre X, et al. Papillary muscle displacement causes systolic anterior motion of the mitral valve. *Circulation* 1995;91:1189–1195.

point or leaflet tips) of the anterior leaflet (AL) is significantly greater than the posterior leaflet (PL); however, in patients with SAM/LVOT obstruction this ratio is reduced, with both leaflets contributing equally to mitral coaptation (AL/PL ratio ≤1.1) (Fig. 8.26) (20,90). In this setting, the

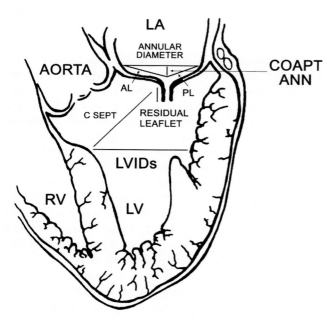

FIGURE 8.26. Schematic of the left ventricle (*LV*), left atrium (*LA*), and mitral valve (*MV*) apparatus depicting echocardiographic measurements that have been used to predict systolic anterior motion (*SAM*) in patients undergoing MV repair. Relative distances of the annulus to the coaptation point along the anterior (*AL*) and posterior (*PL*) leaflets, as well as the proximity of the coaptation point to the septum (*C-Sept*) have correlated with the occurrence and resolution of SAM. *RV,* right ventricle; *LVIDs,* left ventricular diameter during systole; *Coap-Ann,* distance from coaptation point to annular plane. Reprinted from Maslow AD, Regan MR, Haering JM, et al. Echocardiographic predictors of left ventricular outflow tract obstruction and systolic anterior motion of the mitral valve after mitral valve reconstruction for myxomatons valve disease. *J Am Coll Cardiol* 1999;34:2096–2104.

posterior leaflet coapts with the anterior leaflet closer to its base, increasing the amount of residual leaflet beyond the coaptation point, which is more susceptible to ventricular outflow (20). A distance of no more than 2.5 cm between the coaptation point and the ventricular septum (C-Sept) may predispose susceptible leaflets to systolic blood flow (20). These measurements have been demonstrated across different populations of patients, including those with ventricular hypertrophy and in patients after MV reconstruction (20,90,101). Resolution of SAM/LVOT obstruction is associated with increases in the AL/PL ratio and C-Sept.

Abnormalities of the mitral apparatus also alter ventricular inflow and outflow patterns (98). With a more posteriorly located coaptation point, ventricular inflow is directed along the posterior ventricular wall, and systolic outflow moves along the ventricular septum. When the mitral apparatus and coaptation point are displaced anteriorly and inward, ventricular inflow and outflow patterns may be reversed, thereby increasing the likelihood that systolic outflow will interact with the mitral apparatus, especially if there are residual or slack leaflet segments (98).

Other pathologic mechanisms that may predispose to development of SAM/LVOT obstruction include severe mitral annular calcification or anomalous insertion of the papillary muscle directly to the mitral leaflet. Mitral annular calcification reduces the normal function of the mitral annulus, which during systole helps to widen the LVOT, minimizing any resistance to the exit of blood from the ventricle. Impairment of annular function prevents the normal posterior movement of the mitral leaflets during systole (Fig. 8.27). Anomalous insertion of the ALPM into the anterior mitral leaflet impairs systolic leaflet motion, leaving greater amounts of slack leaflet in the LVOT. Outflow obstruction to a lesser degree also may be associated with subaortic membrane, cardiac masses, retained mitral leaflet during MVR, and obstructing struts of a bioprosthesis (102,103). Transesophageal imaging of the LVOT may be difficult after MV

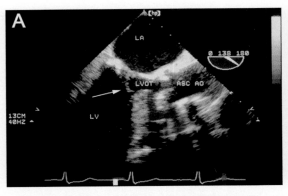

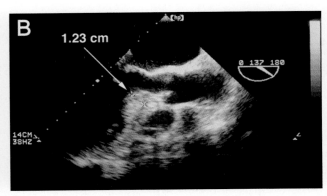

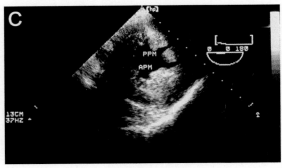

FIGURE 8.27. Systolic anterior motion and left ventricular out-flow tract (*LVOT*) obstruction in a patient with calcified mitral annulus (**A**; *arrow*), septal hypertrophy (**B**; *arrow*), and anteriorly displaced papillary muscle (**C**). All three pathologies may contribute to dynamic outflow tract obstruction. *LA,* left atrium; *LV,* left ventricle; *ASC AO,* ascending aorta; *APM,* anterior papillary muscle; *PPM,* posterior papillary muscle.

replacement due to shadowing of the LVOT; however, transgastric imaging of the LVOT is possible.

The medical management of LVOT obstruction involves discontinuation of inotropes, treatment of tachycardia, maintenance of preload and afterload, and ventricular pacing. Recently, pharmacologic alcohol infarction of the basal septum has been used to thin and widen the myocardial wall and LVOT, respectively. Surgical treatment for LVOT obstruction is infrequently needed, except for fixed lesions. Surgery for dynamic lesions may involve a combination of septal myomectomy and MV surgery, including a replacement with a low-profile valve or reconstruction of the native MV (91,94–97). The goal of MV reconstruction is to increase the AL/PL ratio and move the coaptation point posteriorly, resulting in a greater C-Sept distance (20,91,94–97,101).

Mitral Valve Reconstruction versus Mitral Valve Replacement

Mitral valve reconstruction has revolutionized the approach to patients with MR, perhaps increasing the likelihood that prophylactic surgery will be performed for patients with repairable anatomy (3,75,79,83). Although no randomized prospective study has been performed, the reported benefits of MV reconstruction compared with replacement include reductions in thromboembolic events, hemolytic anemia, anticoagulant related hemorrhagic events, and endocarditis (76,80,104–106). Another benefit of reconstruction is the maintenance of the subvalvular apparatus, which is believed

to help stabilize ventricular function and prevent ventricular remodeling immediately and later after MV surgery (106–108).

The feasibility of MV reconstruction is based on echocardiographic assessment and surgical inspection, the former having the benefit of assessing the MV apparatus and mobility during the normal cardiac cycle compared with a flaccid state during cardiopulmonary bypass and after atriotomy. The greatest success is reported for patients undergoing isolated MV reconstruction for myxomatous valve disease (prolapsed leaflet) primarily involving the posterior leaflet (81,108–112). Successful repair may be dependent on the mobility and length of the anterior leaflet because after repair, valve closure may primarily be a single (anterior) leaflet process, with the frozen posterior leaflet serving only as a buttress for closing (113). Compared with posterior leaflet repair, anterior leaflet surgery is more difficult and is likely to involve leaflet resection, chordal reattachment or transection, or procedures involving the papillary muscle (108,114,115). Several investigations report greater degrees of postoperative MR and reoperation following attempted repair of an anterior leaflet prolapse or flail (108,114,115). Valve repair for rheumatic MV disease is feasible when thickening, calcification, and restriction of the leaflet and subvalvular structures are minimal (81,104,111). Nevertheless, a 20% to 25% reoperation rate over 5 to 15 years has been reported and is probably related to progression of disease (77,81,104,111). Although the increased risk may be acceptable in young patients in order to avoid anticoagulation, MV replacement is the overall preferred procedure (111).

Mitral valve reconstruction has been advocated for patients with functional or ischemic MR (1,45–47,116). The mechanisms of functional MR include annular dilatation, reduced ventricular systolic function (reduced coapting force), ventricular dilatation, papillary muscle displacement, papillary muscle ischemia and dysfunction, and papillary muscle rupture (1,35,45–48,116). Although MV reconstruction has been reported after papillary muscle rupture, MV replacement with preservation of the subvalvular apparatus may be preferred (116). Because CABG and MV surgery is associated with increased mortality, the decision to perform valve surgery should be considered for patients with moderate or greater MR, especially if regression is unlikely. For patients with severe ventricular dysfunction (LVEF <26%) and cardiac dilatation, in which CAD is a contributing if not primary cause, revascularization and institution of medical therapy improves ventricular function and geometry, increases coapting force, reduces leaflet tethering, and significantly reduces MR (1,73,77). However, approximately half of the patients with moderate MR and preserved or mildly impaired ventricular function continue to have moderate MR despite myocardial revascularization and medical therapy (1,117). With increased understanding of the mechanism of functional MR, it is likely that a more aggressive surgical approach aimed at reducing regurgitation will follow, especially if MV reconstruction is feasible. Although leaflet resection, annuloplasty, and revascularization are currently more common repair techniques, it is possible that future reconstructive techniques may include ventricular resection, papillary muscle realignment, and chordal transection (35,45–48,118). These techniques would be directed at changing ventricular geometry, reducing leaflet tethering, and improving ventricular systolic function (45–47,116,118). Residual MR after MV reconstruction for patients with functional MR partially related to the pre-repair distance from the coaptation point to the annular plane (113,118,119). The incidence of residual MR was significantly greater when this distance was greater than or equal to 11 mm (119). When these data are considered in light of the increased role of the anterior leaflet after MV reconstruction, it may be reasonable to state that successful valve reconstruction depends on the length and mobility of the anterior leaflet, both of which can be assessed prior to the surgical procedure (113,118,119). For patients with organic valve dysfunction, more aggressive surgical treatments may occur with increased understanding of dysfunction, ability to predict progression and regression, and improved reconstructive techniques (81,83).

MITRAL STENOSIS

Obstruction of blood flow from the LA to the LV may be attributed to a several causes, including rheumatic MS, nonrheumatic calcification of the mitral annulus and leaflets, prosthetic valve dysfunction, a number of congenital lesions

TABLE 8.6. ETIOLOGIES OF LEFT VENTRICULAR INFLOW OBSTRUCTION

Abnormal valve apparatus
  Rheumatic valve
  Calcific stenosis
  Prosthetic valve dysfunction
  Parachute valve
  Mitral arcade
  Congenital mitral stenosis

Normal valve apparatus
  Thrombus
  Tumor (myxoma)
  Supravalvular ring
  Cor triatrium
  Severe left ventricular diastolic dysfunction
  Significant aortic valve insufficiency

(congenital MS, parachute MV, mitral arcade, supravalvular ring), and several nonvalvular lesions (tumor, cor triatrium, and thrombi) (Table 8.6) (13,14). Obstruction causes an increase in LA pressure, which results in LA dilatation, elevation in pulmonary vascular pressure and resistance, RV hypertrophy and failure, and secondary tricuspid regurgitation (13,14). The LV is often unaffected, except for cases of rheumatic myocarditis or when significant MR is present.

Except for infrequent cases of congenital anomalies, calcific disease, and prosthetic valve dysfunction, MS is almost always rheumatic in origin (Fig. 8.28) (13,14,120). Although it has been essentially eradicated from the Western world since the advent of antibiotics, rheumatic fever is still endemic in the developing world. Migrating populations provide an ongoing source of rheumatic valve disease in North America and Europe (51). Rheumatic fever is a disease of young people, and is recurrent in half of the cases (13,14,51,52). Typically, a streptococcal infection leads to an autoimmune reaction, which results in rheumatic fever. Acute pancarditis causes inflammation of all four cardiac valves, followed by progressive valvular damage of varying degrees. Symptoms from valve disease typically take 15 to 20 years to develop (13,14,51,52). Patients who present at a young age (within the first two decades) tend to have mostly MR, whereas older patients usually suffer from MS or mixed pathology (13,51). In North America, most patients presenting with rheumatic valve disease are older (>60 years) and display MS with varying degrees of MR. Younger patients may have been exposed to a greater inoculation of streptococcus and therefore display a more rapid progression of valve pathology, characterized by thickening, chordal laxity, leaflet prolapse, and MR; however, MS also may occur (51). Older patients are more likely to have been exposed to a smaller inoculation, resulting in a slower disease progression characterized by significant calcification and a greater degree of MS (51,52).

Nonrheumatic causes of MS are relatively uncommon (13,14). Nonrheumatic calcification of the mitral annulus

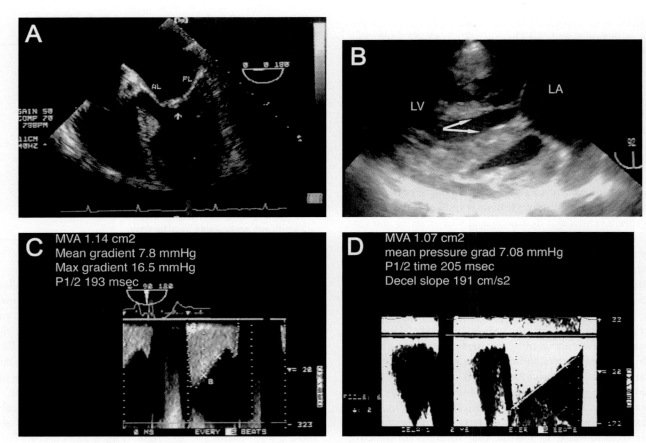

FIGURE 8.28. Transesophageal echocardiographic evaluation of rheumatic mitral stenosis. **A:** Mid-esophageal four-chamber view demonstrating commissural fusion and a hockey stick deformity (*arrow*) of the anterior leaflet (*AL*). **B:** Transgastric, two-chamber view demonstrating thickening of the subvalvular apparatus (*arrows*) in rheumatic stenosis. **C and D:** Doppler echocardiographic measurement of the maximum (*Max*), mean transmitral pressure gradient (*Mean PG*), pressure half time (*P 1/2*), and calculated mitral valve area (*MVA*) in patients with sinus rhythm (**C**; MVA = 1.14 cm²) and atrial fibrillation (**D**; MVA = 1.07 cm²). *PL,* posterior mitral leaflet.

and leaflets usually occurs in elderly patients and results in narrowing of the mitral annular area and reduced leaflet mobility (Fig. 8.29) (13). In these patients, there is an increased risk for cardiac rupture from excessive annular debridement during valve surgery (121). Causes of prosthetic valve stenosis include obstructing lesions (thrombus, infection), or in the case of mechanical valves, immobility of one or both leaflets (Fig. 8.30). Although initial treatment may include anticoagulation, thrombolysis, and antibiotics, surgery may be necessary.

Congenital stenotic lesions of the MV usually present at birth or during childhood and include a parachute valve and supravalvular ring (120). Congenital MS is characterized by fibrosis, thickening, and nodularity, but unlike rheumatic disease, does not contain calcification of the leaflets. A parachute valve is caused by the presence of only one functioning papillary muscle from which the chordae originate, resulting in limited leaflet opening. The leaflets and chordae are otherwise normal. A supravalvular ring is connective tissue that passes above the MV, causing obstruction to flow. In

contrast to cor triatrium, the supravalvular ring is low in the LA, extending from below the LAA to below the foramen ovale. Most cases of congenital MS present with additional cardiac defects, especially ventricular septal defect.

Echocardiographic Assessment

Two-Dimensional Echocardiography

The echocardiographic assessment of MS begins with a comprehensive 2D examination of the heart and MV, using all available views afforded by the current technology (Table 8.7). For patients with MS, the LV is typically small and the LA can be very large. This may cause rotation of the heart and distortion of the usual echocardiographic cross sections. Two-dimensional echocardiography is the imaging technique of choice to visualize the morphology and mobility of the mitral leaflets and subvalvular apparatus, as well as secondary changes in cardiac function (13,14,29). The hallmarks of rheumatic MS are commissural fusion along

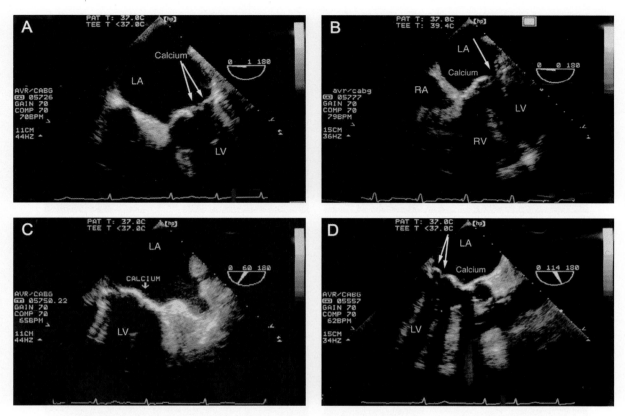

FIGURE 8.29. A–D: Transesophageal echocardiographic images at the mid-esophageal depth demonstrating nonrheumatic mitral valve (*MV*) morphologic changes. Severe annular, anterior, and posterior mitral leaflet calcification (*arrows*), which resulted in mild/moderate mitral regurgitation and mild mitral stenosis. *LA,* left atrium; *LV,* left ventricle; *RA,* right atrium; *RV,* right ventricle.

with thickening and calcification of the leaflets and chordae. Heavy calcification may make recognition of valvular structures difficult. In rheumatic MS, calcification begins at the leaflet tips and advances toward the annulus, contrasting the pattern seen in calcific MV disease in which calcification starts at the annulus and progresses toward the leaflet tips. The diastolic motion of the leaflets is affected by commissural fusion. Separation of the leaflet tips is impaired and the mid-portion of the anterior leaflet bends, with the leaflet appearing convex toward the septum and resembling a hockey stick (Fig. 8.28). When high LA pressures push the valve open in diastole, a pliable anterior leaflet takes on a characteristic curved appearance, referred to as doming. Normally the posterior leaflet motion is a mirror image of the anterior leaflet, but in rheumatic stenosis it parallels the anterior leaflet and is pulled anteriorly during diastole. The rate of leaflet closure during early diastole (E–F slope) depends on the atrioventricular gradient. With more severe stenosis, atrial emptying is further impaired, resulting in a prolonged atrioventricular gradient and E–F slope.

Examination of the subvalvular apparatus may demonstrate varying degrees of thickening and shortening of the

chordae. Because axial resolution is better than lateral resolution, chordae are best seen in the transgastric long-axis view. From the transgastric short-axis view at the base of the ventricle, the MV area can be measured using planimetry by tracing the inner borders of the mitral leaflets (Fig. 8.31) (122). Although this is a useful adjunct in the assessment of MS severity, there is a tendency to overestimate valve area (13,14). Calcifications of the MV annulus and leaflets may cause significant shadowing, making visualization of the orifice difficult. In 45 patients, planimetry during TEE was feasible in only 69% compared with 89% during TTE (122). Inability to perform planimetry was due to leaflet dropout (122). Furthermore, the stenotic MV orifice may not be planar, and attempts to locate the narrowest point may be difficult. Failure to adequately visualize the inner borders or locate the narrowest point reduces the accuracy and utility of planimetry during TEE examination. Two-dimensional imaging of prosthetic valves is hampered by artifact due to prosthetic material. However, it is possible to visualize leaflet mobility, leaflet thickening, and any echodense or echobright lesions along the valve. For calcific stenosis, echogenic lesions are seen along the MV annulus and extend onto the leaflets. Although relatively normal parts

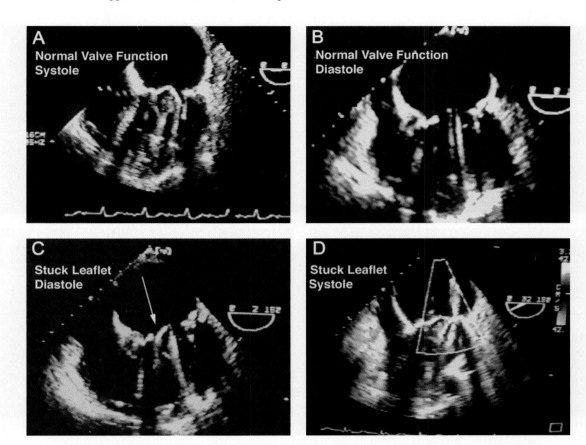

FIGURE 8.30. Transesophageal echocardiographic images at the mid-esophageal depth demonstrating a bi-leaflet mechanical valve (St. Jude Medical, Inc., St. Paul, MN) in the mitral position. **A:** Normal functioning bi-leaflet prosthetic valve in systole. **B:** Normal functioning bi-leaflet prosthetic valve in diastole. **C:** Immobility of the anterior mechanical leaflet during diastole associated with left ventricular inflow obstruction. **D:** Immobility of a mechanical leaflet during systole associated with mitral regurgitation.

TABLE 8.7. ECHOCARDIOGRAPHIC ASSESSMENT OF MITRAL STENOSIS

Two-dimentional echocardiography
  Mitral morphology
  Mitral mobility
  Echocardiography score
  Mitral valve area planimetry
  Left atrial size
  Left ventricular size (diastole, systole)
  Right heart function
  Tricuspid valve morphology
  Left atrial appendage flow, function, and masses

Doppler echocardiography
  Transvalvular gradient (mean and peak)
  Mitral valve area
    Pressure half time
    Deceleration time
    Continuity equation
    Color flow area
    Proximal isovelocity surface area
  Pulmonary artery pressures

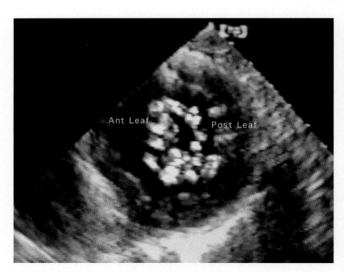

FIGURE 8.31. Transgastric echocardiographic cross-sectional image of the mitral valve demonstrating significant calcification of the anterior (*Ant*) and posterior (*Post*) leaflets. Direct planimetry of the valve can be performed by tracing the inner borders of the leaflets.

TABLE 8.8. SCORING SYSTEM TO ASSESS MITRAL VALVE MORPHOLOGY AND MOBILITY PRIOR TO PERCUTANEOUS MITRAL BALLOON VALVULOPLASTY

Grade	Mobility of Leaflets	Thickening of Leaflets	Calcification of Leaflets	Subvalvular Thickening
0	Normal	Normal (≤3 mm)	Normal	Normal
1	Highly mobile valve with only leaflet tips restricted	Leaflets near normal in thickness (4–5 mm)	Single area of increased echo brightness	Minimal thickness just below the mitral leaflets
2	Leaflet mid and base portions have normal mobility	Mid-leaflets normal, considerable thickening of margins (5–8 mm)	Scattered areas of brightness confined to leaflet margins	Thickening of chordal structures extending up to one third of the chordal length
3	Valve continues to move forward in diastole, mainly from the base	Thickening extending through the entire leaflet (5–8 mm)	Brightness extending into the leaflets	Thickening extending to the distal third of the chords
4	No or minimal forward movement of the leaflets in diastole	Considerable thickening of all leaflet tissue (>8–10 mm)	Extensive brightness throughout much of the leaflet tissue	Extensive thickening and shortening of all chordal structure extending down to the papillary muscles

Reprinted from Wilkins GT, Weyman AE, Abascal VM, et al. Percutaneous balloon dilatation of the mitral valve: an analysis of echocardiographic variables related to outcome and the mechanism of dilatation. *Br Heart J* 1988;60:299–308, with permission.

of mitral leaflet may be present, the overall annular diameter is significantly reduced.

An echocardiographic score for native valve stenosis has been described and has subsequently been shown to be predictive of disease progression and outcome after percutaneous balloon mitral valvuloplasty (Table 8.8) (16,22–24,51,122–129). A score of 0 to 4 is assigned to each of four measures based on the assessment of thickness and mobility of the mitral leaflets and subvalvular apparatus. A score of less than 8 was associated with a favorable result. The impact on progression was more related to changes in the mitral leaflets and not the subvalvular apparatus (16). In addition, the echocardiographic score was as good a predictor or a better predictor of progression and outcome after percutaneous balloon mitral valvuloplasty than measurement of initial MV area or other hemodynamic variables (16,22,23,123). Although correlation between echo score and outcome after surgical reconstruction or commissurotomy has not been extensively studied, investigators have noted that the success of surgical repair is higher for rheumatic patients with less annular and leaflet calcifications (25,26).

In order to assess the clinical impact of MS, additional 2D echocardiographic assessments, including measurement of LA and RV size and function, should be informed. An enlarged, hypokinetic RV is consistent with elevated pulmonary vascular resistance and afterload. Septal flattening in systole and diastole suggest pressure and volume overload, respectively. Left atrial dilatation is associated with increased dysfunction and risk of dysrhythmias, both of which increase the likelihood of thromboembolic events.

M-Mode Echocardiography

Although not used as frequently nowadays, M mode was once an important part of the echocardiographic assessment

of MS (29). The typical findings include MV thickening, anterior motion of the posterior leaflet, a decrease of the E–F slope, and a small A wave. The parallel motion of the mitral leaflets can be evaluated with M-mode echocardiography from the parasternal window during transthoracic examination. When compared with TEE, TTE is better able to examine both leaflets simultaneously using M mode.

Doppler Echocardiography

Continuous-wave Doppler can be used to quantitate the severity of MS (13,14,129,130). Transvalvular velocities are obtained by aligning the CWD cursor with transvalvular blood flow. From a tracing of the velocity time integral (VTI), the peak and mean transvalvular velocities are measured, which are then used to calculate pressure gradients using the Bernoulli equation (Fig. 8.28). In the majority of cases, transvalvular gradients correlate with MV area (Table 8.9). A mean gradient of less than or equal to 5 mm Hg is consistent with mild stenosis (MVA >1.5 cm^2), whereas mean gradients of 5 to 10 mm Hg and greater than 10 mm Hg are consistent with moderate (MV area 1.2–1.5 cm^2) and severe (MV area <1.2 cm^2) stenosis, respectively. The relationship between gradients and valve area diverge with decreases in blood flow, reductions in atrial and ventricular

TABLE 8.9. EXPECTED VALUES WITH VARIOUS DEGREES OF MITRAL STENOSIS

	Mild	Moderate	Severe
Mitral valve area (cm^2)	1.6–2.0	1.1–1.5	≤1.0
Mean transvalvular gradient (mm Hg)	<4.0	4.0–8.0	>8.0
Pressure half time (msec)	<150	150–220	≥220

chamber compliance, high or low heart rates, and irregular rhythms. Due to beat-to-beat variability of flow, the mean of 5 to 10 measurements is used to estimate the transvalvular gradient for patients with irregular rhythms (e.g., atrial fibrillation). Although the majority of transvalvular flows are directed centrally toward the ventricular apex, occasionally the jet may not be centrally directed, making it more difficult to align the CWD ultrasound beam with blood flow, thereby leading to underestimation of transvalvular velocities and gradients (130). Because of these limitations, further assessment of MS severity including MVA calculation is required.

Continuous-wave Doppler allows pressure half-time (PHT) measurement of the early ventricular filling (E-wave) deceleration slope, which in turn is used to calculate MV area (Figs. 8.28 and 8.32) (122). PHT is the time needed (in milliseconds) for the peak pressure gradient across the MV to decrease by half. If the MV orifice is small, it will take longer for the pressure gradient to equilibrate between the LA and LV, thus prolonging PHT. Conversely, for a large orifice, the gradient will dissipate quickly, yielding a lower PHT. The PHT is then used to estimate the MVA using the following formula:

$$MVA = 220/PHT$$

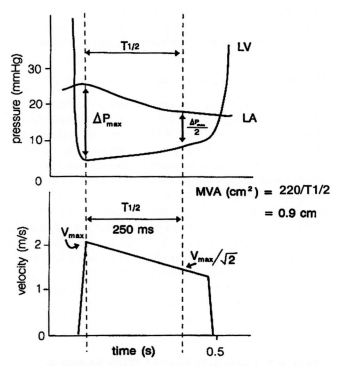

FIGURE 8.32. Schematic representation depicting the measurement of mitral valve pressure gradients (ΔP) and area (*MVA*) using pressure half-time (*T 1/2*). **A:** Graph of the change in transmitral pressure (ΔP) between the left atrium and left ventricle over time. **B:** *T* represents the time from ΔP max to ΔP max/2 and can be measured from the transmitral continuous-wave Doppler profile as the time from the maximum velocity (*V max*) to Vmax/1.414. *LV,* left ventricle; *LA,* left atrium.

where 220 is an empirically derived constant (5). The PHT can be obtained from the peak velocity (V_{MAX}). As shown below, the velocity ($V_{1/2}$) at which the pressure gradient is 1/2 Peak$_{GRADIENT}$ can be estimated from V_{MAX}. The time period (in milliseconds), from V_{MAX} to $V_{1/2}$ is equal to the PHT.

$$P_{GRADIENT} = 4V_{MAX}{}^2$$
$$1/2\ P_{GRADIENT} = 1/2\ (4\ V_{MAX}{}^2)$$
$$V_{1/2} = 0.7\ V_{MAX}\ or\ V_{MAX}/1.414$$
$$PHT = time\ between\ V_{MAX}\ and\ V_{1/2}$$

Calculation of the PHT also can be obtained from the measurement of the deceleration time (DT), which is the time from the peak early (E-wave) velocity to zero velocity (Doppler baseline). Deceleration time is related to the PHT by the following equation:

$$Area = 220/PHT$$
$$Area = 220/(0.29\ DT)$$
$$Area = 759/DT$$

Although poor alignment or increased angle of incidence between blood flow and the ultrasound beam underestimate transvalvular gradients, it does not affect the accuracy of MV area by PHT (130). Because the PHT and DT are measurements of trans-MV gradients, they are affected by conditions that affect ventricular filling or atrial emptying during diastole, such as aortic insufficiency and reduced LV compliance. These conditions may prolong the deceleration slope and underestimate MV area (overestimate severity). Conversely, the presence of an interatrial septal defect may shorten the deceleration slope, resulting in an overestimation of the MV area calculated by these methods.

The continuity equation assumes that in the absence of intracardiac shunting, flow and stroke volume [area × time velocity integral (TVI)] are constant throughout the heart. Using one of the following equations, one can calculate one variable if the other three are known (130):

$$A_1 \times TVI_1 = A_2 \times TVI_2$$

In the case of the MV, the equation translates into

$$MVA = (A_{LVOT} \times TVI_{LVOT})/TVI_{MV}$$

where

A_{LVOT} is the LVOT area, obtained by measuring LVOT diameter and calculating πr^2.

TVI_{LVOT} is the LVOT velocity distance, obtained by PWD in the deep transgastric long-axis view.

TVI_{MV} is the MV distance velocity, measured by CWD.

CFD provides a quick visual clue of significant obstruction (aliasing) to ventricular inflow and its direction, and helps identify other valvular pathology, including MR, tricuspid regurgitation, and aortic insufficiency, all of which

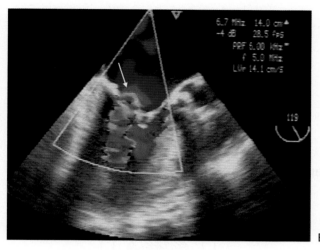

FIGURE 8.33. Mitral valve (*MV*) stenotic area measured by the proximal isovelocity surface area (*PISA*) technique. A: Schematic of a PISA associated with mitral stenosis. *r*, PISA radius; *black arrow,* mitral valve diameter. B: Transesophageal echocardiographic imaging of a stenotic MV at the mid-esophageal depth demonstrating PISA (*arrow*). C: PISA radius (*double-headed arrow*).

may have important prognostic and therapeutic implications. More importantly, two methods have used CFD to measure MV area: PISA and color flow area (Figs. 8.33 and 8.34). In a similar fashion in which PISA was used to calculate the ROA for patients with MR, it also can be used to calculate a stenotic orifice area using a similar series of concentric hemispheres (Fig. 8.33) (129,131). Based on the continuity equation, the flow at the level of any one of these hemispheres must be equal to the flow at the level of all the other hemispheres, and equal to the flow at the level of the stenotic orifice. The velocity at the level of the stenotic orifice is the peak MV velocity measured by CWD (V_{max}). One can then calculate the surface area of the MV orifice using the following equation:

$$MVA = \frac{2\pi r^2 \times V_{NL}}{V_{max}}$$

Because the PISA technique relates flow across only one orifice in one direction, the presence of other valve disease should not affect its accuracy in measuring the MV area. The above equation assumes that the orifice is round and

that it lies on one plane, neither of which may be true, and therefore may require an angle correction ($\alpha/180$ degrees). However, previous data suggest that this may not be necessary (129,131).

Color flow area assesses the margins of the CFD profile as blood passes through the MV orifice (Fig. 8.34) (29,129). This technique has been described during transthoracic examination, but it should be applicable during TEE study of the MV. During TTE examination, the apical four-chamber (a) and two- or three-chamber (b; achieved with 90 degree rotation of the transducer from a) windows are obtained. The maximal orifice diameters of the transmitral CFD profile are measured from the two perpendicular planes and used to calculate the MVA.

$$MVA = \pi/4 \, (ab)$$

The equation assumes an elliptical orifice. Because this technique measures MV area at the orifice, it is not affected by MR or aortic insufficiency.

The evaluation of the LA and LAA function and evidence of thromboemboli is an important part of the

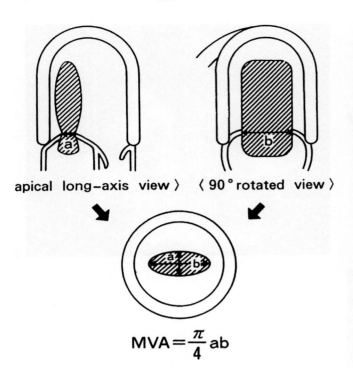

apical long–axis view ⟩   ⟨ 90° rotated view ⟩

$$MVA = \frac{\pi}{4}\,ab$$

FIGURE 8.34. Measurement of mitral valve area using diameters from two perpendicular views of transmitral, color flow Doppler profiles. *a*, diameter of color flow profile in the long-axis window; *b*, diameter of color flow profile 90 degrees from diameter *a*; *MVA*, mitral valve area. Reprinted from Kawahara T et al. Application of Doppler color flow imaging to determine valve area in mitral stenosis, *J Am Coll Cardiol* 1991:vol 18;87.

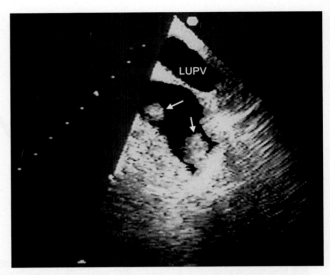

FIGURE 8.35. Transesophageal echocardiographic two-dimensional imaging of the left atrial appendage (*LAA*). Two masses (thrombi) are seen in LAA (*arrows*) in a patient with mitral stenosis, atrial fibrillation, and decreased atrial function and flow. *LUPV*, left upper pulmonary vein.

echocardiographic evaluation of MS for both medical and invasive therapy (Fig. 8.35). Swirling, smoke, or spontaneous echo contrast are precursors of thrombi and are associated with an increased risk for thromboembolic events. The presence of definite thrombi not only constitutes an increased risk for thromboembolism, but is also a contraindication for percutaneous balloon mitral valvuloplasty. There is an increased risk of developing thrombi when the LAA peak PWD velocity is less than or equal to 20 cm/s. These findings may support surgical evacuation of LAA thrombi and ligation (132).

Outcome

The onset of symptoms secondary to the obstruction of ventricular inflow depends on its cause. Congenital lesions present from infancy to early childhood (120). The survival rate for patients with congenital lesions is poor without surgery. However, with surgery, the 15-year survival rate is approximately 70% (120). Part of the morbidity and mortality may be related to the presence of additional congenital cardiac defects (120).

Rheumatic valve disease (MR, mixed MR/MS) presents from the second or third decade of life and beyond (52). Arguably, for rheumatic valve disease, the timing of presentation may be due to the quantity, severity, and treatment of the initial infection. Patients presenting later in life (>50 years of age) may have had a less severe initial infection or more aggressive treatment, resulting in slower progression. The amount of time from the initial presentation of rheumatic stenosis to being disabled may range from 5 to 20 years (14). Although the progression of disease for rheumatic stenosis is variable, morbidity and mortality increase significantly with the onset of symptoms and increasing disability. The progression of MS, defined by a reduction in valve area, is variable, with approximately 50% of patients having minimal change over 3 to 10 years (16,17). Two studies have reported a mean decrease in MV area of 0.09 cm²/yr (16,17). One study of 50 patients showed that progression over 3 years was related to the MV score and the transmitral gradients, and not initial valve area (16). Forty-two patients with a valve score of less than 8 had an average decrease in MV area of less than or equal to 0.06 cm²/yr, compared with a decrease of greater than or equal to 0.25 cm²/yr in patients with a valve score of greater than or equal to 8 (16). Progression was related to morphology and mobility of the leaflets and not the subvalvular apparatus. In another study of 100 patients with mild to moderate MS with mild to moderate leaflet thickening and calcification, the decrease in valve area over 2 to 3 years was 0.04 to 0.06 cm²/year (18). In contrast, a third study of 103 patients followed for 3 years with mild, moderate, and severe MS reported a greater decrease in MV area for patients with mild MS (0.12 cm²/yr) compared to patients with moderate MS (0.06 cm²/yr) and patients with severe MS (0.03 cm²/yr) (17). Valve score did not predict progression. There was, however, a greater decrease in MV area for patients with mild, moderate, or severe aortic insufficiency compared with trace or no aortic insufficiency (0.19 vs. 0.09 cm²/yr). In this study, 81% of patients did not demonstrate a significant change in grade of severity. Sixty-eight percent of patients demonstrated a decrease in valve area (<0.1 cm²/yr). From the available data, the rate of progression is variable, with a mean decrease in MV area of 0.9 cm²/yr. Decrease in MV area is probably related to several variables, including valve morphology and mobility, and the presence of aortic insufficiency. The latter may represent a marker of a greater initial infection and more rheumatic inflammation.

Ten-year survival rates for patients with rheumatic MS without symptoms or significant impairment (NYHA I) is greater than 80%, whereas survival is decreased to 50% for patients with mild to moderate symptoms (NYHA II), to 20% for moderate to severe impairment (NYHA III), and as low as 5% for severe impairment (NYHA IV) (13,14). Ten-year survival is improved with surgical therapy for categories III and IV to 80% to 90% and 65%, respectively (13,14).

Treatment

Because MS is a mechanical problem, medical therapy will not alter the progression of disease, but it may help temporarily stabilize heart function and prevent complications. Medical therapy is instituted for treatment of tachyarrhythmias, control of heart rate, treatment of CHF, and to prevent thromboembolic events. Periodic echocardiographic evaluation of the patient with MS is important to determine the timing of more invasive therapy such as percutaneous balloon mitral valvuloplasty, surgical repair, or surgical replacement.

Although there is little controversy regarding invasive therapy in disabled patients with severe MS, there is controversy in deciding the treatment of patients with mild to moderate MS, and of patients with or without symptoms who present for other cardiac surgical procedures (13,14). For asymptomatic patients with mild MS, MV procedures are more likely to increase the risk without any significant benefit. When no symptoms are present, patients are usually managed medically as needed, unless there is moderate MS (MVA $\leq$1.5 cm²) and evidence of cardiopulmonary changes (e.g., pulmonary artery systolic pressure of $\geq$50 mm Hg). When symptoms occur, and moderate or greater MS is present, then invasive therapy is warranted. For symptomatic patients with mild MS, the decision to perform invasive procedures is controversial because it may not be clear that the symptoms are related to mild MS. Stress testing to assess the changes in pulmonary artery systolic pressure, pulmonary capillary wedge pressure, and transvalvular gradient is useful to further qualify the clinical impact of valve disease. Results of the stress test are considered positive when the pulmonary artery systolic pressure rises beyond 60 mm Hg, pulmonary capillary wedge pressure surpasses 30 mm Hg, or the transvalvular gradient increases above 15 mm Hg (13,14). For these patients, an MV procedure may be warranted. The presence of LA enlargement, pulmonary hypertension, RV dysfunction, and tricuspid regurgitation are predictors of increased morbidity and mortality in patients with MS, and

may warrant more aggressive treatment earlier before these conditions occur (13,14,27,28,128).

Echocardiographic evaluation is not only important for determining the timing of invasive therapy, but also for predicting the outcome of percutaneous balloon mitral valvuloplasty or valve repair. Percutaneous balloon mitral valvuloplasty is the preferred technique for enlarging the MV orifice. Indications for percutaneous balloon mitral valvuloplasty include symptomatic patients with an MVA of less than or equal to 1.5 cm², mean transvalvular gradient greater than or equal to 10 mm Hg, LA pressure greater than or equal to 15 mm Hg, and NYHA class III or IV. Contraindications include patients with active endocarditis, LA or LAA thrombi, and significant mitral regurgitation ($\geq$2+). A successful percutaneous balloon mitral valvuloplasty is defined as an increase in MVA of 25% to 50% or a postprocedural valve area of greater than 1.5 cm² (ideally 2.0 cm²), a left-to-right cardiac shunt of less than 1.5, a decrease in mean transvalvular gradient of 25% to 50% or to less than 10 mm Hg, and a reduction in LA pressure to less than 15 mm Hg (22,24,123,124). Immediate postprocedural success occurs in as much as 90% in low-risk patients (normal to mildly decreased leaflet mobility and minimal calcification), and as low as 33% in high-risk cases, with 3- to 5-year event free survival rate reported as high as 84% in low-risk patients to as low as 13% in high-risk patients (122,127). Major procedural complications occur in less than 10% and more commonly include cardiac injury and tamponade, acute MR, and death (<1%) (13,14,22–24). Consistent echocardiographic predictors of poor outcome include an echocardiographic score of 8 to 10, increasing degrees of commissural and leaflet calcification, age 65 years or above, presence of tricuspid regurgitation ($\geq$2+), pulmonary hypertension [mean pulmonary artery pressure (PAP) >40 mm Hg], LV end-diastolic pressure greater than 10 mm Hg, and presence of atrial fibrillation (23,24,123–125,127,128).

If surgery is planned, then the decision to repair or replace the MV depends in part on the echocardiographic assessment of morphology and mobility of the MV apparatus, and the presence of secondary cardiac dysfunction. Repairs include open commissurotomy, debridement, leaflet resection, and a variety of procedures involving the chordae and papillary muscles. In one study, 327 patients underwent MV repair with a hospital mortality rate of 3.4% (27). The mean duration of follow-up was 8.6 years. Actuarial survival at 16 years was 84%, and the actuarial freedom from reoperation was 89.9% (27). There were 34 reoperations: 12 for MR, 18 for restenosis, and 4 for aortic valve disease. Outcomes were significantly worse if TV surgery was required, perhaps indicating more significant disease progression. In a long-term follow-up of 183 patients who underwent closed or open commissurotomy, the 10-year survival rate was 89% to 92% for closed and open procedures (25). Reoperations were more frequently associated with closed procedures (30% vs. 12%). Predictors of outcomes included NYHA class (I/II vs. III/IV), presence of MR, leaflet calcification, and atrial fibrillation (25). Although the incidence of reoperation is greater after repair of rheumatic valves (10%–20% at 5–15 years) than for other valve pathologies, outcome for selected patients (minimal calcification, good leaflet mobility, minimal additional cardiac dysfunction) is excellent (25–27). Valve replacement may be the definitive corrective procedure for MS, with a 10-year survival rate of greater than or equal to 90% for patients under the age of 60 years (28). Although morbidity and mortality for valve replacement is reported to be as high as 12%, with a 10-year survival rate as low as 64%, these patients tend to have greater severity of disease, and are poor candidates for other reparative procedures (13,14,28). Typically, valvuloplasty or valve surgery has been reserved for symptomatic patients with moderate or greater disease. Because short- and long-term morbidity are increased when secondary cardiac dysfunction is present, earlier valvuloplasty, or surgery may increase.

SUMMARY

Echocardiography is the diagnostic test of choice to assess MV function. Advances in ultrasound technology have increased our understanding of pathologic mechanisms and enabled echocardiographers to more efficiently assess valve function and determine the appropriate therapy. Intraoperative evaluation using TEE permits a comprehensive cardiac evaluation, assists surgical planning, and allows reevaluation after therapy has been instituted. As anesthesiologists become more facile with echocardiography, their role in this field will rapidly expand. Although this may help to further define the role of the cardiac anesthesiologist, it will require more complex multitasking. It is therefore important to establish an efficient method for performing a comprehensive echocardiographic global assessment of the heart and its individual components.

Although a number of techniques for assessing the MV have been delineated, their implementation is variable, depending on the individual case and the echocardiographer's experience. Two-dimensional and CFD echocardiography permit qualitative assessment of the morphology, mobility, origin, extent, and centricity of the MR jet. From these data, one can rapidly determine the cause of MV dysfunction and the need for further quantitative evaluation. This should include evaluation of the MR jet, measurement of the proximal jet width, and assessment of the pulmonary venous flows. A finding of normal pulmonary venous flow pattern or systolic flow reversal may help differentiate moderate from severe MR. Because this is often adequate to determine etiology, severity, and likelihood for regression or progression, other techniques are not commonly used. Although not commonly employed, measurements of ROA, Rvol, and PISA may be worthwhile to further clarify the severity of the MR. As echocardiographers become more adept, these techniques may be used more commonly, especially if they are simplified.

Similarly, the assessment of MS begins with 2D and CFD echocardiography to assess morphology, mobility, a valve score, and the origin, extent, and direction of the stenotic jet. Quantitative evaluation includes measurement of trans-MV gradients and valve area. The former is dependent on blood flow as well as MV area. Under anesthesia, blood flow may be significantly affected, potentially reducing the accuracy of this measurement alone. Therefore, the measurement of MV area using the PHT (or DT) is often employed. Due to 2D artifacts, planimetry of the MV is often difficult and may not be accurate. Methods such as PISA and the continuity equation are not frequently used.

For both MS and MR, a comprehensive cardiac evaluation is necessary to determine the clinical impact of valve dysfunction. For MR, LV dilatation and depression of systolic function suggest that MR may have greater clinical significance. For both MS and MR, LA enlargement, elevation of pulmonary artery pressures, or right heart dysfunction suggest that valve dysfunction is clinically significant. Finally, these data must always be coupled with the demographics and clinical evaluation of the patient to assess for symptoms of MV dysfunction (dysrhythmias, CHF, fatigue, dyspnea, etc.) to help determine the need for treatment. During the perioperative evaluation, the affects of anesthesia must be considered, and may require alteration of cardiac loading conditions in order to assess valve dysfunction under different degrees of cardiac stress.

Echocardiographic evaluation of the MV plays an important role in perioperative management of cardiac surgical patients. Consequently, the MV should be routinely assessed in all patients as part of the comprehensive examination. The information acquired during a comprehensive intraoperative TEE examination can assist in identifying high-risk patients, determining the definitive surgical approach, and in providing a timely post-CPB evaluation of the procedure, thereby allowing for the opportunity to immediately reintervene or to at least triage patients appropriately. In the near future, the role of intraoperative TEE in patients undergoing MV procedures will most certainly become even more important with the development of three-dimensional TEE and the further introduction of newer, minimally invasive approaches, including robotically assisted procedures in which direct visualization and inspection may be more limited.

KEY POINTS

- The AL of the MV is approximately twice as large as the PL, and covers two thirds of the mitral orifice during coaptation. The AL also has a comparatively smaller area of attachment to the mitral annulus, which is shared with the left and noncoronary cusps of the aortic valve. The PL is shorter in height compared with the AL, covers a third or less of the mitral orifice during coaptation, and can be separated into three scallops.
- The causes of MR can be categorized as functional

(secondary) or nonfunctional (primary; organic). Nonfunctional MR is characterized by a primary abnormality of the MV apparatus. Conversely, functional MR is associated with relatively normal MV morphology. A second classification is based on valvular motion, which may be restricted or excessive. In addition, the MV annulus may be dilated.

- Myxomatous changes of the mitral leaflets can be further described as scalloping, prolapsing, or flail. Ischemic papillary muscle dysfunction results in decreased leaflet mobility. Echocardiographic features of MR due to dysfunctional myocardium include a central MR jet, enlarged ventricular cavity, posterior and apical displacement of papillary muscles, a reduced papillary muscle–mitral annular angle, increasing tethering of the MV leaflet, and varying degrees of annular enlargement. Rheumatic mitral disease is characterized by varying degrees of leaflet calcification, thickening, retraction, and decreased mobility, and in some cases prolapse and increased mobility.

- Echocardiographic measurement of MR severity includes assessment of pulmonary venous flow, CFD jet area, ratio of the regurgitant jet size to the LA size, proximal jet width, effective regurgitant orifice area, regurgitant volume, and regurgitant fraction.

- Because the intraoperative quantitative assessment of MR may not reflect the preinduction state, accurate assessments of MV morphology and function are paramount. If questions regarding the treatment of MR persist, alterations in loading conditions may be useful to assess MV function under varying stress.

- Although ventricular hypertrophy may be a contributing factor to the development of SAM and dynamic LVOT obstruction, additional mechanisms involving abnormalities of the mitral apparatus including severe mitral annular calcification as well as anterior and inward displacement of papillary muscles, which in turn displace the mitral apparatus and coaptation point closer to the LVOT.

- Except for infrequent cases of congenital anomalies, calcific disease, and prosthetic valve dysfunction, MV stenosis (MS) is almost always rheumatic in origin. The hallmarks of rheumatic MS are commissural fusion along with thickening and calcification of the leaflets and chordae. In rheumatic MS, calcification begins at the leaflet tips and advances toward the annulus, contrasting the pattern seen in calcific MV disease in which calcification starts at the annulus and progresses toward the leaflet tips.

- Quantitative echocardiographic assessment of mitral stenosis severity includes Doppler acquired measurement of trans-MV pressure gradients and estimates of the stenotic MV area using a variety of techniques, including PHT, DT, PISA, continuity equation, and color flow area.

REFERENCES

1. Otto CM. Evaluation and management of chronic mitral regurgitation. *N Engl J Med* 2001;345:740–746.

2. Hausmann N, Siniawski H, Hotz H, et al. Mitral valve reconstruction and mitral valve replacement for ischemic mitral insufficiency. *J Cardiol Surg* 1997;12:8–14.

3. Enriquez-Sarano M, Tajik AJ, Schaff HV, et al. Echocardiographic predictors of survival after surgical correction of organic mitral regurgitation. *Circulation* 1994;90:830–839.

4. Dion R, Benetis R, Elias B, et al. Mitral valve procedures in ischemic regurgitation. *J Heart Valve Dis* 1995;9(suppl):124–131.

5. Sheikh KH, Bengston JR, Rankin JS, et al. Intraoperative transesophageal Doppler color flow imaging used to guide patient selection and operative treatment of ischemic mitral regurgitation. *Circulation* 1991;84:594–603.

6. Enriquez-Sarano M, Freeman WK, Tribouilloy CM, et al. Functional anatomy of mitral regurgitation. Accuracy and outcome implication of transesophageal echocardiography. *J Am Coll Cardiol* 1999;34:1129–1136.

7. Foster GP, Isselbacher EM, Rose GA, et al. Accurate localization of mitral regurgitant defects using multiplane transesophageal echocardiography. *Ann Thorac Surg* 1998;65:1025–1031.

8. Caldarera I, Van Herwerden AV, Taams A, et al. Multiplane transesophageal echocardiography and morphology of regurgitant mitral valves in surgical repair. *Eur Heart J* 1995;16:999–1006.

9. Stewart WJ, Currie PJ, Salcedo EE, et al. Evaluation of mitral leaflet motion by echocardiography and jet direction by Doppler color flow mapping to determine the mechanism of mitral regurgitation. *J Am Coll Cardiol* 1992;20:1353–1361.

10. Fehske W, Grayburn PA, Omran H, et al. Morphology of the mitral valve as displayed by multiplane transesophageal echocardiography. *J Am Soc Echocardiogr* 1994;7:472–479.

11. Lambert AS, Miller JP, Merrick SH, et al. Improved evaluation of the location and mechanism of mitral valve regurgitation with a systematic transesophageal echocardiography examination. *Anesth Analg* 1999;88:1205–1212.

12. Grewal KS, Malkowski MJ, Kramer CM, et al. Multiplane transesophageal echocardiographic identification of the involved scallop in patients with flail mitral valve leaflet: intraoperative correlation. *J Am Soc Echocardiogr* 1998;11:966–971.

13. Carabello RA. Timing of surgery in mitral and aortic stenosis. *Cardiol Clin* 1991;9:229–238.

14. Bruce CJ, Nishmura RA. Clinical assessment and management of mitral stenosis. *Cardiol Clin* 1998;16:375–403.

15. Enriquez-Sarano M, Basmadjian AJ, Rossi A, et al. Progression of mitral regurgitation. A prospective Doppler echocardiography study. *J Am Coll Cardiol* 1999;34:1137–1144.

16. Gordon SP, Douglas PS, Come PC, et al. Two-dimensional and Doppler echocardiographic determinants of the natural history of mitral valve narrowing in patients with rheumatic mitral stenosis: implications for follow-up. *J Am Coll Cardiol* 1992;19(5):968–973.

17. Sagie A, Freitas N, Padial LR, et al. Doppler echocardiographic assessment of long-term progression of mitral stenosis in 103 patients: valve area and right heart disease. *J Am Coll Cardiol* 1996;28(2):472–479.

18. Faletra F, DeChiara F, Crivellaro W, et al. Echocardiographic follow-up in patients with mild to moderate mitral stenosis: is a yearly examination justified? *Am J Cardiol* 1996;78:1450–1452.

19. Zuppiroli A, Rinaldi M, Kramer-Fox R, et al. Natural history of mitral valve prolapse. *Am J Cardiol* 1995;75:1028–1032.

20. Maslow AD, Regan MR, Haering JM, et al. Echocardiographic predictors of left ventricular outflow tract obstruction and systolic anterior motion of the mitral valve after mitral valve reconstruction for myxomatous valve disease. *J Am Coll Cardiol* 1999;34:2096–2104.

21. Freeman WK, Schaff HV, Khandheria BK, et al. Intraoperative evaluation of mitral valve regurgitation and repair by

transesophageal echocardiography: incidence and significance of systolic anterior motion. *J Am Coll Cardiol* 1992;20:599–609.

22. Cohen DJ, Kuntz RE, Gordon SPF, et al. Predictors of long-term outcome after percutaneous balloon mitral valvuloplasty. *N Eng J Med* 1992;19:1329–1335.

23. Palacios IF, Tuzcu ME, Weyman AE, et al. Clinical follow-up of patients undergoing percutaneous mitral balloon valvotomy. *Circulation* 1995;91:671–676.

24. Tuzcu EM, Block PC, Griffin B, et al. Percutaneous mitral balloon valvotomy in patients with calcific mitral stenosis: immediate and long term outcome. *J Am Coll Cardiol* 1994;23:1604–1609.

25. Detter C, Fischlein T, Feldmeier C, et al. Mitral commissurotomy, a technique outdated? Long-term follow-up over a period of 35 years. *Ann Thorac Surg* 1999;68:2112–2118.

26. Grossi EA, Galloway AC, Steinberg BM, et al. Severe calcification does not affect long-term outcome of mitral valve repair. *Ann Thorac Surg* 1994;58:685–687.

27. Bernal JM, Rabasa JM, Vilchez FG, et al. Surgery: mitral valve repair in rheumatic disease: the flexible solution. *Circulation* 1993;88:1746–1753.

28. Vincens JJ, Temizer D, Post JR. Long term outcome of cardiac surgery in patients with mitral stenosis and severe pulmonary hypertension. *Circulation* 1995;92(9 Suppl):II137–II142.

29. Weyman AE. Left ventricular inflow tract I. *The mitral valve in principles and practice of echocardiography*, 2nd ed. Philadelphia: Lea & Febiger, 1994:391–470.

30. Weiss SJ, Savino JS. What is the best way to assess mitral regurgitation. *Semin Cardiothorac Vasc Anesth* 1997;1:49–60.

31. Anmar T, Konstadt S. Intraoperative transesophageal echocardiographic evaluation of mitral regurgitation. *J Cardiothorac Vasc Anesth* 1996;10:397–405.

32. Crawford MH, Roldan CA. Quantitative assessment of valve thickness in normal subjects by transesophageal echocardiography. *Am J Cardiol* 2001;87:1419–1423.

33. Obadia JF, Casali C, Chassignolle JF, et al. Mitral subvalvular apparatus. Different functions of primary and secondary chordae. *Circulation* 1997;96:3124–3128.

34. Jiang J, Levine RA, King ME, et al. An integrated mechanism for systolic anterior motion of the mitral valve in hypertrophic cardiomyopathy based on echocardiographic observations. *Am Heart J* 1987;113:633–644.

35. He S, Lemmon JD Jr, Weston MW, et al. Mitral valve compensation for annular dilatation: *in vitro* study into the mechanisms of functional mitral regurgitation with an adjustable annulus model. *J Heart Valve Dis* 1999;8;294–302.

36. Glasson JR, Komeda M, Daughters GT, et al. Three dimensional regional dynamics of the normal mitral annulus during left ventricular ejection. *J Thorac Cardiovasc Surg* 1996;111:574–585.

37. Cohen GI, White M, Sochowski RA, et al. Reference values for normal adult transesophageal echocardiographic measurements. *J Am Soc Echocardiogr* 1995;8:221–230.

38. Drexler M, Erbel R, Muller U, et al. Measurement of intracardiac dimensions and structures in normal young adult subjects by transesophageal echocardiography. *Am J Cardiol* 1990;65:1491–1496.

39. Klein AL, Obarski TP, Stewart WJ, et al. Transesophageal Doppler echocardiography of pulmonary venous flow: a new marker of mitral regurgitation severity. *J Am Coll Cardiol* 1991;18:518–526.

40. Quinones MA, Gaasch WH, Waisser E, et al. Reduction in the rate of diastolic descent of the mitral valve echogram in patients with altered left ventricular diastolic pressure-volume relations. *Circulation* 1974;49:246–254.

41. Konecke LL, Feigenbaum H, Chang S, et al. Abnormal mitral valve motion in patients with elevated left ventricular diastolic pressures. *Circulation* 1973;47:989–996.

42. Hall R, Austin A, Hunter S. M-Mode echogram as a means of distinguishing between mild and severe mitral stenosis. *Br Heart J* 1981;46:486–491.

43. Kondo K, Shiina A, Tsuchiya M, et al. Hemodynamic significance of the A/E ratio and B-B′ step formation on the mitral valve echogram in patients with myocardial infarction. *J Cardiogr* 1982;12:861–867.

44. Saito T. Non-invasive assessment of left ventricular function and prognosis in acute myocardial infarction—clinical significance of B-B′ step of the mitral valve in M-mode echocardiography. *Jpn Circ J* 1982;46:1045–1050.

45. Otsuji Y, Handschumacher MD, Schwammenthal E, et al. Insights from three-dimensional echocardiography into the mechanism of functional mitral regurgitation. *Circulation* 1997;96:1999–2008.

46. He S, Fontaine AA, Schwammenthal E, et al. Integrated mechanism for functional mitral regurgitation. Leaflet restriction versus coapting force: *in vitro* studies. *Circulation* 1997;96:1826–1834.

47. Nielson SL, Nygaard H, Fontaine AA, et al. Papillary muscle misalignment causes multiple mitral regurgitant jets: an ambiguous mechanism for functional mitral regurgitation. *J Heart Valve Dis* 1999;8:551–554.

48. Yiu SF, Enriquez-Sarano M, Tribouilloy C, et al. Determinants of the degree of functional mitral regurgitation in patients with systolic left ventricular dysfunction: a quantitative clinical study. *Circulation* 2000;102:1400–1406.

49. Hanson EW, Neerhut RK, Lynch III C. Mitral valve prolapse. *Anesthesiology* 1996;85;178–195.

50. Devereux RB, Kramer-Fox R, Kligfield P. Mitral valve prolapse: causes, clinical manifestations, and management. *Ann Intern Med* 1989;111:305–317.

51. Carroll JD, Feldman T. Percutaneous mitral balloon valvotomy and the new demographics of mitral stenosis. *JAMA* 1993;270:1731–1736.

52. Marcus RH, Sareli P, Pocock WA, et al. The spectrum of severe rheumatic mitral valve disease in a developing country. Correlations among clinical presentation, surgical pathologic findings, and hemodynamic sequelae. *Ann Intern Med* 1994;120(3):177–183.

53. Carlson RG, Mayfield WR, Normann S, et al. Radiation-associated valvular disease. *Chest* 1991;99:538–545.

54. Gonzage AT, Antunes MJ. Post-radiation valvular and coronary artery disease. *J Heart Valve Dis* 1997;6:219–221.

55. Brand MD, Abadi CA, Aurigemma GP, et al. Radiation-associated valvular heart disease in Hodgkin's disease is associated with characteristic thickening and fibrosis of the aortic-mitral curtain. *J Heart Valve Dis* 2001;10:681–685.

56. Otsuji Y, Handschumacher MD, Liel-Cohen N, et al. Mechanism of ischemic mitral regurgitation with segmental left ventricular dysfunction: three-dimensional echocardiographic studies in models of acute and chronic progressive regurgitation. *J Am Coll Cardiol* 2001;37:641–648.

57. Schiller NB, Foster E, Redberg RF. Transesophageal echocardiography in the evaluation of mitral regurgitation. The twenty four signs of severe mitral regurgitation. *Cardiol Clin* 1993;11:399–408.

58. Thomas L, Foster E, Hoffman JI, et al. The mitral regurgitation index: an echocardiographic guide to severity. *J Am Coll Cardiol* 1999;33:2016–2022.

59. Thomas JD. How leaky is that mitral valve? Simplified Doppler methods to measure regurgitant orifice area. *Circulation* 1997;95: 548–550.

60. Pu M, Griffin BP, Vandervoort PM, et al. The value of assessing pulmonary venous flow velocity for predicting severity of mitral regurgitation: a quantitative assessment integrating left ventricular function. *J Am Soc Echocardiogr* 1999;12:736–743.

61. McCully RB, Enriquez-Sarano M, Tajik J, et al. Overestimation of severity of ischemic-functional mitral regurgitation by color Doppler jet area. *Am J Cardiol* 1994;74:790–793.

62. Flachskampf FA, Frieske R, Engelhard B, et al. Comparison of transesophageal Doppler methods with angiography for evaluation of the severity of mitral regurgitation. *J Am Soc Echocardiogr* 1998;11:882–892.

63. Grayburn PA, Fehske W, Omran H, et al. Multiplane transesophageal echocardiographic assessment of mitral regurgitation by Doppler color flow mapping of the vena contracta. *Am J Cardiol* 1994;74:912–917.

64. Tribouilloy C, Shen WF, Quere JP, et al. Assessment of severity of mitral regurgitation by measuring regurgitant jet width at its origin with transesophageal Doppler color flow imaging. *Circulation* 1992;85:1248–1253.

65. Dujardin KS, Enriquez-Sarano M, Bailey KR, et al. Grading of mitral regurgitation by quantitative Doppler echocardiography. *Circulation* 1997;96:3409–3415.

66. Pu M, Thomas JD, Vandervoort PM, et al. Comparison of quantitative and semiquantitative methods for assessing mitral regurgitation by transesophageal echocardiography. *Am J Cardiol* 2001;87:66–70.

67. Kolev N, Brase R, Wolner E, et al. Quantification of mitral regurgitant flow using proximal isovelocity surface area method: a transesophageal echocardiography perioperative study. *J Cardiothorac Vasc Anesth* 1998;12:22–26.

68. Pu M, Prior DL, Fan X, et al. Calculation of mitral regurgitation orifice area with use of a simplified proximal convergence method: Initial clinical application. *J Am Soc Echocardiogr* 2001;14:180–185.

69. Tokushima T, Reid CL, Hata A, et al. Simple method for estimating regurgitant volume with use of a single radius for measuring proximal isovelocity surface area: an *in vitro* study of simulated mitral regurgitation. *J Am Soc Echocardiogr* 2001;14:104–113.

70. Giesler M, Grossman G, Schmidt A, et al. Color Doppler echocardiographic determination of mitral regurgitant flow from the proximal velocity profile of the flow convergence region. *Am J Cardiol* 1993;71:217–224.

71. Lebrun F, Lancellotti P, Pierard LA. Quantitation of functional mitral regurgitation during bicycle exercise in patients with heart failure. *J Am Coll Cardiol* 2001;38:1685–1692.

72. Konstadt SN, Louie EK, Shore-Lesserson L, et al. The effects of loading changes on intraoperative Doppler assessment of mitral regurgitation. *J Cardiothorac Vasc Anesth* 1994;8:19–23.

73. Grewal KS, Malkowski MJ, Piracha AR, et al. Effect of general anesthesia on the severity of mitral regurgitation by transesophageal echocardiography. *Am J Cardiol* 2000;85:199–203.

74. Bach DS, Deeb GM, Bolling SF. Accuracy of intraoperative transesophageal echocardiography for estimating the severity of functional mitral regurgitation. *Am J Cardiol* 1995;76:508–512.

75. Flemming MA, Oral H, Rothman ED, et al. Echocardiographic markers for mitral valve surgery to preserve left ventricular performance in mitral regurgitation. *Am Heart J* 2000;140:476–482.

76. Christenson JT, Simonet F, Bloch A, et al. Should a mild to moderate ischemic mitral valve regurgitation in patients with poor left ventricular function be repaired or not. *J Heart Valve Dis* 1995;4:484–489.

77. Sheikh KH, De Bruijn NP, Rankin JS, et al. The utility of transesophageal echocardiography and Doppler color flow imaging in patients undergoing cardiac valve surgery. *J Am Coll Cardiol* 1990;15:363–372.

78. Tribouilloy CM, Enriquez-Sarano M, Schaff HV, et al. Impact of preoperative symptoms on survival after surgical correction of organic mitral regurgitation: rationale for optimizing surgical indications. *Circulation* 1999;99:400–405.

79. Enriquez-Sarano M, Schaff HV, Orszulak TA, et al. Valve repair improves the outcome of surgery for mitral regurgitation: a multivariate analysis. *Circulation* 1995;91:1022–1028.

80. Deloche A, Jebara VA, Relland JYM, et al. Valve repair with Carpentier techniques: the second decade. *J Thorac Cardiovasc Surg* 1990;99:990–1002.

81. Cosgrove DM, Chavez AM, Lytle BW, et al. Results of mitral valve reconstruction. *Circulation* 1986;74;I82–I87.

82. Smolens IA, Pagani FD, Deeb GM, et al. Prophylactic mitral reconstruction for mitral regurgitation. *Ann Thorac Surg* 2001;72:1210–1215.

83. Sheikh KH, Bengston JR, Rankin JS, et al. Intraoperative transesophageal Doppler color flow imaging used to guide patient selection and operative treatment of ischemic mitral regurgitation. *Circulation* 1991;84:594–603.

84. Adams PB, Otto CM. Lack of improvement in coexisting mitral regurgitation after relief of valvular aortic stenosis. *Am J Cardiol* 1990;66:105–107.

85. Tunick PA, Gindea A, Kronzon I. Effect of aortic valve replacement for aortic stenosis on severity on mitral regurgitation. *Am J Cardiol* 1990;65:1219–1221.

86. Brener SJ, Duffy CI, Thomas JD, et al. Progression of aortic stenosis in 394 patients: relation to changes in myocardial and mitral valve dysfunction. *J Am Coll Cardiol* 1995;25:305–310.

87. Christenson JT, Jordan B, Blaock A, et al. Should a regurgitant mitral valve be replaced simultaneously with a stenotic aortic valve. *Tex Heart Inst J* 2000;27:350–355.

88. Harris KM, Malenka DJ, Haney MF, et al. Improvement in mitral regurgitation after aortic valve replacement. *Am J Cardiol* 1997;80:741–745.

89. Brasch AV, Khan SS, DeRobertis MA, et al. Change in mitral regurgitation severity after aortic valve replacement for aortic stenosis. *Am J Cardiol* 2000;85:1271–1274.

90. Jiang L, Levine RA, King ME, et al. An integrated mechanism for systolic anterior motion of the mitral valve in hypertrophic cardiomyopathy based on echocardiographic observations. *Am Heart J* 1987;113:633–644.

91. Levine RA, Lefebvre X, Guerrero JL, et al. Unifying concepts of mitral valve function and disease: SAM, prolapse and ischemic mitral regurgitation. *J Cardiol* 1994;38:15–27.

92. Aurigemma G, Battista S, Orsinelli D, et al. Abnormal left ventricular intracavitary flow acceleration in patients undergoing aortic valve replacement for aortic stenosis. *Circulation* 1992;86:926–936.

93. Bartunek J, Sys SU, Rodriques AT, et al. Abnormal dynamic intraventricular flow velocities after valve replacement for aortic stenosis. Mechanisms, predictive factors, and prognostic significance. *Circulation* 1996;94:712–719.

94. McIntosh CL, Maron BJ, Cannon III RO, et al. Initial results of combined anterior mitral leaflet plication and ventricular septal myotomy-myectomy for relief of left ventricular outflow tract obstruction in patients with hypertrophic cardiomyopathy. *Circulation* 1992;86:II60–II67.

95. Joyce FS, Lever HM, Cosgrove DM III. Treatment of hypertrophic cardiomyopathy by mitral valve repair and septal myectomy. *Ann Thorac Surg* 1994;57:1025–1027.

96. Kofflard MJ, van Herwerden LA, Waldstein DJ, et al. Initial results of combined anterior mitral leaflet extension and myectomy

in patients with obstructive hypertrophic cardiomyopathy. *J Am Coll Cardiol* 1996;28:197–202.

97. Matsui Y, Shiiya N, Murashita T, et al. Mitral valve repair and septal myectomy for hypertrophic obstruction cardiomyopathy. *J Cardovasc Surg* 2000;41:53–56.

98. Lefebvre XP, He S, Levine RA, et al. Systolic anterior motion of the mitral valve in hypertrophic cardiomyopathy: An *in vitro* pulsatile flow study. *J Heart Valve Dis* 1995;4:423–438.

99. Lefebvre XP, Yoganathan AP, Levine RA. Insights from *in vitro* flow visualization into the mechanism of systolic anterior motion of the mitral valve in hypertrophic cardiomyopathy under steady flow conditions. *ASME* 1992;114:406–412.

100. Levine RA, Vlahakes GJ, Lefebvre X, et al. Papillary muscle displacement causes systolic anterior motion of the mitral valve. *Circulation* 1995;91:1189–1195.

101. Lee KS, Stewart WJ, Lever HM, et al. Mechanism of outflow tract obstruction causing failed mitral valve repair. Anterior displacement of leaflet coaptation. *Circulation* 1993;88:24–29.

102. Jett GK, Jett MD, Bosco P, et al. Left ventricular outflow tract obstruction following mitral valve replacement: effects of strut height and orientation. *Ann Thorac Surg* 1986;42:299–303.

103. Jett GK, Jett MD, Barnhart GR, et al. Left ventricular outflow tract obstruction with mitral valve replacement in small ventricular cavities. *Ann Thorac Surg* 1986;41:70–74.

104. Galloway AC, Colvin SB, Baumann FG, et al. A comparison of mitral valve reconstruction with mitral valve replacement: intermediate-term results. *Ann Thorac Surg* 1989;47:655–662.

105. Kay GL, Kay JH, Zubiate P, et al. Mitral valve repair for mitral regurgitation secondary to coronary artery disease. *Circulation* 1986;74:I88–I98.

106. Lee EM, Shapiro LM, Wells FC. Importance of subvalvular preservation and early operation in mitral valve surgery. *Circulation* 1996;94:2117–2123.

107. Goldman ME, Mora F, Guarino T, et al. Mitral valvuloplasty is superior to valve replacement for preservation of left ventricular function: an intraoperative 2-D echocardiographic study. *J Am Coll Cardiol* 1987;10:568–575.

108. Yu Y, Gao C, Li G, et al. Mitral valve replacement with complete mitral leaflet retention: operative techniques. *J Heart Valve Dis* 1999;8:44–46.

109. Fukui T, Yoshida K, Akasaka T, et al. Serial change of mitral regurgitation after mitral valve repair: comparison of anterior with posterior leaflet lesions. *J Cardiol* 1996;27:73–76.

110. El Khoury G, Noirhomme P, Verhelst R, et al. Surgical repair of the prolapsing anterior leaflet in degenerative mitral valve disease. *J Heart Valve Dis* 2000;19;75–81.

111. Skoularigis J, Sinovich V, Houbert G, et al. Evaluation of the long-term results of mitral valve repair in 254 young patients with rheumatic mitral regurgitation. *Circulation* 1994;90:II167–II174.

112. Ott DA. Repairing the mitral valve. *Circulation* 1995;91:1264–1265.

113. Green GR, Dagum P, Glasson JR, et al. Restricted posterior leaflet motion after mitral ring annuloplasty. *Ann Thorac Surg* 1999;68:2100–2106.

114. Mohty D, Orszulak TA, Schaff HV, et al. Very long-term survival and durability of mitral valve repair for mitral valve prolapse. *Circulation* 2001;104(12 Suppl 1):I1–I7.

115. Kuwaki K, Kiyofumi M, Tsukamoto M, et al. Early and late re-sults of mitral valve repair for mitral valve regurgitation. Significant risk factors of reoperation. *J Cardiovasc Surg* 2000;41:187–192.

116. David TE. Techniques and results of mitral valve repair for ischemic mitral regurgitation. *J Cardio Surg* 1994;9:274–277.

117. Aklog L, Filsoufi F, Flores KQ, et al. Does coronary artery bypass grafting alone correct moderate ischemic mitral regurgitation? *Circulation* 2001;104:168–175.

118. Messas E, Guerrero JL, Handschumacher MD, et al. Chordal cutting: a new therapeutic approach for ischemic mitral regurgitation. *Circulation* 2001;104:1958–1963.

119. Calafiore AM, Gallina S, Di Mauro M, et al. Mitral valve procedure in dilated cardiomyopathy: repair or replacement. *Ann Thorac Surg* 2001;71:1146–1152.

120. Serraf A, Joy Z, Belli E, et al. Congenital mitral stenosis with or without associated defects: an evolving surgical strategy. *Circulation* 2000;102:III166–III171.

121. Unal M, Sanisoglu, I, Konuralp C, et al. Ultrasonic decalcification of calcified valve and annulus during heart valve replacement. *Tex Heart Inst J* 1996;23:85–87.

122. Stoddard MR, Prince CR, Ammash NM, et al. Two-dimensional transesophageal echocardiographic determination of mitral valve area in adults with mitral stenosis. *Am Heart J* 1994;127:1348–1353.

123. Wilkins GT, Weyman AE, Abascal VM, et al. Percutaneous balloon dilatation of the mitral valve: an analysis of echocardiographic variables related to outcome and the mechanism of dilatation. *Br Heart J* 1988;60:299–308.

124. Sutaria N, Northbridge DB, Shaw TRD. Significance of commissural calcification on outcome of mitral balloon valvotomy. *Heart* 2000;84:398–402.

125. Gamra H, Zhang HP, Allen JW, et al. Factors determining normalization of pulmonary vascular resistance following successful balloon mitral valvotomy. *Am J Cardiol* 1999;83:392–395.

126. Eisenberg MJ, Ballal R, Heidenreich PA, et al. Echocardiographic score as a predictor of in-hospital cost in patients undergoing percutaneous balloon mitral valvuloplasty. *Am J Cardiol* 1996;78:790–794.

127. Zhang JP, Allen JW, Lau FY, et al. Immediate and late outcome of percutaneous balloon mitral valvotomy in patients with significantly calcified valves. *Am Heart J* 1995;129:501–506.

128. Sagie A, Schwammenthal E, Newell JB, et al. Significant tricuspid regurgitation is a marker for adverse outcome in patients undergoing percutaneous balloon mitral valvuloplasty. *J Am Coll Cardiol* 1994;24:696–702.

129. Degertekin M, Gencbay M, Basaran Y, et al. Application of proximal isovelocity surface area method to determine prosthetic mitral valve area. *J Am Soc Echocardiogr* 1998;11:1056–1063.

130. Stoddard MF, Prince CR, Tuman WL, et al. Angle of incidence does not affect accuracy of mitral stenosis area calculation by pressure half-time: application to Doppler transesophageal echocardiography. *Am Heart J* 1994;127:1562–1572.

131. Degertekin M, Basaran Y, Gencbay M, et al. Validation of flow convergence region method in assessing mitral valve area in the course of transthoracic and transesophageal echocardiographic studies. *Am Heart J* 1998;135:207–214.

132. Agmon Y, Khandheria BK, Gentile F. Echocardiographic assessment of the left atrial appendage. *J Am Coll Cardiol* 1999;34:1867–1877.

9

AORTIC VALVE

CHRISTOPHER A. TROIANOS

Transesophageal echocardiography (TEE) is a valuable clinical tool for the evaluation of aortic valve anatomy, function, and hemodynamics, providing quantitative assessment that prompts surgical intervention, correction of inadequate surgical repair, and reoperation for complications. Clinical information provided by TEE permits appropriate hemodynamic management for patients with aortic valve disease. Transesophageal echocardiography data are used for chronic clinical management and before, during, and after general anesthesia for patients undergoing aortic valve and non–aortic valve surgery. The application of Doppler echocardiography (pulsed-wave, continuous-wave, and color) with two-dimensional imaging allows for the complete evaluation of stenotic and regurgitant lesions. This chapter reviews the transesophageal echocardiographic anatomy, aortic valve disease etiology, and echocardiographic evaluation of the aortic valve, with particular emphasis on perioperative considerations. Indications for evaluation, implications for surgical intervention, and associated cardiovascular lesions are discussed and illustrative case scenarios are presented.

APPLICATIONS

The applications of preoperative TEE evaluation of an aortic valve include (a) imaging an aortic valve that has not been adequately imaged with transthoracic echocardiography (TTE), (b) determining the need for surgical intervention, (c) evaluating myocardial and valvular abnormalities that may be associated with aortic valvular lesions, and (d) determining the size of valve to be implanted. Valve sizing is an important consideration in deciding whether a valve should be replaced. Patients with small annular diameters may not derive a significant benefit from aortic valve replacement, particularly if they only have moderate aortic stenosis. Preoperative valve sizing is also important when valves of limited availability are to be implanted (i.e., homografts) (1).

High-resolution images obtained owing to the close proximity of the valve and the esophagus permit accurate diagnosis of the mechanism of valve dysfunction. Preoperative TEE evaluation of valve dysfunction allows discussion of therapeutic options with the patient before the patient is brought to the operating room. Discussion may include the feasibility of valve repair or available options for valve replacement such as a mechanical, bioprosthetic, or stentless valve and the Ross procedure (pulmonic autograft).

Intraoperative TEE is used in patients with known aortic valve disease undergoing valve replacement to confirm the preoperative diagnosis and determine the etiology of valve dysfunction, evaluate the feasibility of repair versus replacement, and determine the size of the valve to be implanted. The vast majority of aortic valves suitable for repair have regurgitant lesions rather than stenotic lesions. Valve repair for patients with aortic dissection involves resuspension of the cusps and is easily performed and highly successful in the absence of additional leaflet pathology. Valve repair techniques and pathology suitable for repair are further discussed later in this chapter. For patients undergoing aortic valve replacement for aortic stenosis, intraoperative TEE has been shown to alter the surgical plan in 13% (Table 9.1) (2).

Postoperatively, TEE is used to evaluate the success of repair or function of the prosthetic valve. The degree of residual aortic insufficiency (AI) is an important aspect of this evaluation and determines the need for further surgery and possible valve replacement. The number and area of regurgitant jets present after aortic valve replacement are less than after mitral valve replacement, but have a similar percentage decrease of regurgitant jet area after protamine administration (3). Patients undergoing the Ross procedure for autograft replacement of their aortic valve also require evaluation of the prosthetic pulmonic valve.

Left ventricular (LV) evaluation is important postoperatively because of the inherent low ventricular compliance present in patients with LV hypertrophy. Left ventricular volume is more accurately determined by two-dimensional echocardiographic assessment of LV cross-sectional area than by filling pressures measured with a pulmonary artery catheter. Characteristically, patients with decreased LV

C. A. Troianos: Department of Anesthesiology, Mercy Hospital of Pittsburgh, Pittsburgh, Pennsylvania.

TABLE 9.1. IMPACT OF INTRAOPERATIVE TEE DURING AORTIC VALVE REPLACEMENT IN 383 PATIENTS

	Surgical Impact
New Findings before Bypass	
7 PFO	2 closed
2 masses (TV fibroelastoma, LVOT accessory chordae)	2 removed
5 LAA thrombi	5 removed
10 homograft annular size measurements	10 sized
New Findings after Bypass	
1 new wall motion abnormality	No change

PFO, patent foramen ovale; LAA, left atrial appendage; TV, tricuspid valve: LVOT, left ventricular outflow tract obstruction.
From Nowrangi SK, Connolly HM, Freeman WK, et al. Impact of intraoperative transesophageal echocardiography among patients undergoing aortic valve replacement for aortic stenosis. *J Am Soc Echocardiogr* 2001;14:863–866, with permission.

compliance often require volume infusion despite high filling pressures. Accurate determination of optimal volume status requires TEE.

A comprehensive perioperative TEE examination performed in patients undergoing non–aortic valve surgery may reveal aortic valve disease in patients in whom a diagnosis of aortic valve disease was not previously apparent. It is important to identify aortic valvular disease because of the surgical and anesthetic implications associated with both aortic stenosis and regurgitation. The increased population of elderly patients presenting for surgery has increased the prevalence of calcific aortic stenosis. Identification of significant aortic stenosis is important for anesthetic management during noncardiac surgery and for surgical management during non–aortic valve cardiac surgery. Aortic valve replacement after previous coronary artery bypass grafting is associated

with a higher rate of mortality than combined aortic valve and coronary bypass surgery (4). It is therefore important to identify even moderate aortic stenosis during coronary bypass surgery and consider combination surgery to avoid the higher mortality rate associated with reoperation. Certain patients have a rapid progression of aortic stenosis, whereas others have a slower progression (Fig. 9.1). Patients with rapid progression tend to be elderly men who have associated coronary artery disease (5,6), a history of smoking, hypercholesterolemia, and elevated serum creatinine levels (7).

ECHO-ANATOMIC RELATIONSHIP

High-resolution images of the aortic valve provided by TEE result from the close proximity of the valve to the esophagus. The aortic valve is composed of three cusps that are associated with three bulges or pouchlike dilatations in the aortic wall called the sinuses of Valsalva (Fig. 9.2). The anatomic

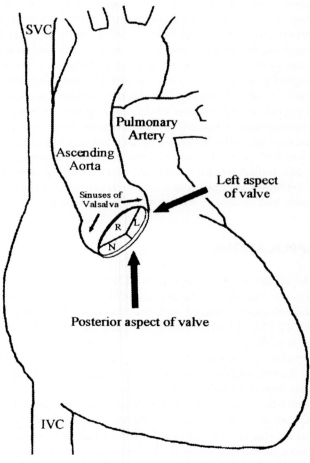

FIGURE 9.2. Illustration of the anatomic orientation of the aortic valve and sinuses of Valsalva within the heart. The aortic valve consists of three cusps: right (*R*), left (*L*), and noncoronary (*N*). The right and posterior aspects of the valve are inferior to the left and anterior aspects of the valve. *SVC,* superior vena cava; *IVC,* inferior vena cava.

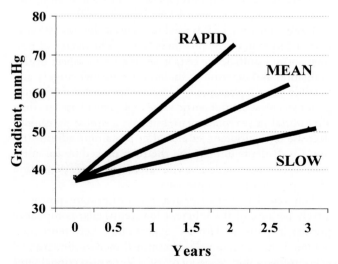

FIGURE 9.1. Progression of disease in patients with moderate aortic stenosis. Data derived from Peter M, Hoffmann A, Parker C, et al. Progression of aortic stenosis. *Chest* 1993;103:1715–1719.

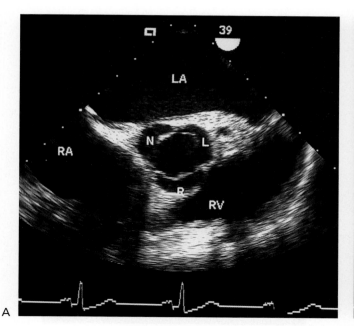
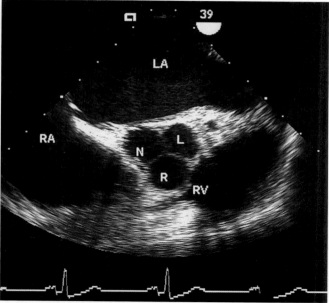

FIGURE 9.3. Transesophageal echocardiogram of the mid-esophageal aortic valve short-axis view during systole **(A)** and diastole **(B)**. A multiplane probe at 39 degrees provided this view in which all three aortic valve cusps are similar in size and appearance, indicating a true short-axis cross section. The aortic valve is identified by the right (*R*), left (*L*), and noncoronary (*N*) cusps. *LA,* left atrium; *RA,* right atrium; *RV,* right ventricle.

plane of the aortic valve is oblique compared with the plane of the esophagus, which is longitudinal within the body. The right, posterior aspect is inferior to the left anterior aspect of the valve (Fig. 9.2). The implication for TEE imaging is that the transducer must be flexed anteriorly and to the left from the transverse plane of the patient, to align the imaging plane with the plane of the aortic valve. Alternatively, a multiplane TEE probe is rotated forward 30 to 60 degrees with ante-flexion to develop the short-axis view of the valve (Fig. 9.3). This view is important for tracing the aortic valve orifice area using planimetry and for identifying the site of AI using color flow Doppler. Rotating the multiplane angle forward to 110 to 150 degrees (orthogonal to the short-axis view) develops the mid-esophageal (ME) aortic valve long axis (LAX) view (Fig. 9.4). This view provides imaging of the left ventricular outflow tract (LVOT), aortic valve, and aortic root to differentiate valvular from subvalvular and supravalvular pathology. Proximal to the aortic valve, the LVOT consists of the inferior surface of the anterior mitral leaflet, the ventricular septum, and the posterior LV free wall.

Hemodynamic assessment of antegrade and retrograde aortic valve flow requires a parallel orientation of blood flow and the Doppler beam. The ME views used for two-dimensional evaluation are inadequate for this assessment because blood flow is perpendicular to the Doppler beam. Conversely, the two transgastric (TG) views are more useful for the purpose of interrogating flow across the aortic valve, but not as useful for detailed two-dimensional anatomic assessment due to the far-field position of the aortic valve in

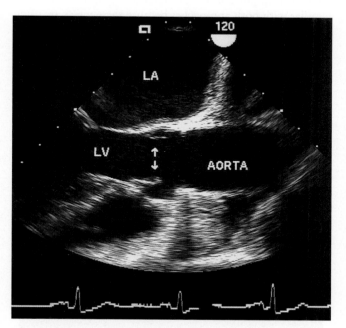

FIGURE 9.4. Transesophageal echocardiogram of the mid-esophageal aortic valve long-axis view during systole. A multiplane probe at 120 degrees provided this view of a normal aortic valve with leaflets (*arrows*) that open parallel to the aortic walls. The proximal ascending aorta is also imaged in this view. *LA,* left atrium; *LV,* left ventricle.

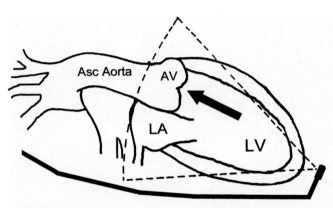

FIGURE 9.5. Illustration of the TEE probe position for the deep transgastric view of the aortic valve that allows a parallel orientation of blood flow through the aortic valve (*AV*) and left ventricular outflow tract (*arrow*). *LA*, left atrium; *LV*, left ventricle; *Asc*, ascending.

these views. The deep TG LAX view (Fig. 9.5) is developed from the TG mid short-axis view by advancing the probe and flexing it to the left until the aortic valve is viewed in the middle or left side of the image in the far field (Fig. 9.6). The TG LAX view is developed from the TG middle short-axis view by rotating the transducer forward from 0 degrees to 90 to 120 degrees until the aortic valve is viewed on the right side of the image in the far field (Fig. 9.7). Usually one or the other TG approach allows sufficient imaging to accomplish aortic valve flow measurement. It is important for the echocardiographer to become familiar with both approaches because these views are often difficult to obtain and require considerable practice and expertise. Stoddard et al. demonstrated 56% feasibility among

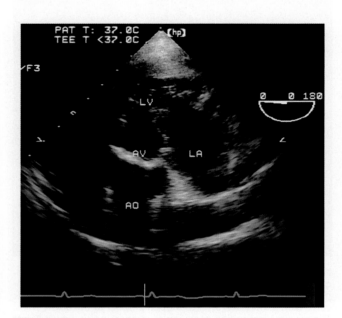

FIGURE 9.6. Transesophageal echocardiogram of the deep transgastric view. *AV*, stenotic aortic valve; *LA*, left atrium; *LV*, left ventricle; *AO*, ascending aorta.

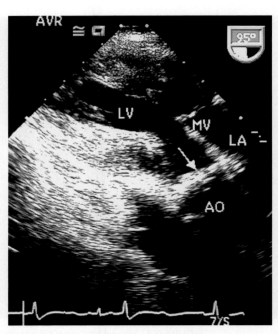

FIGURE 9.7. Transesophageal echocardiogram of the transgastric long-axis view. Arrow indicates direction of blood through the aortic valve. *AO*, aortic root; *LA*, left atrium; *MV*, mitral valve; *LV*, left ventricle.

the first 43 patients studied as compared with 88% feasibility among the latter 43 patients studied, suggesting a significant learning curve in measuring aortic valve blood flow velocity via the TG approach (8).

ETIOLOGY OF AORTIC STENOSIS

The most frequent causes of aortic stenosis are calcific stenosis of the elderly, as well as rheumatic and congenital causes (bicuspid, rarely unicuspid). Acquired stenosis occurs from calcification of the leaflets (calcific, rheumatic, or congenital) or commissural fusion (usually rheumatic). Subaortic stenosis (subaortic membrane or ridge, and asymmetric septal hypertrophy) and supravalvular stenosis (narrowed aortic root) mimic aortic stenosis but do not represent true valvular stenosis. Many of the echocardiographic techniques used for hemodynamic assessment of the aortic valve, however, also can be used to evaluate the severity of subvalvular and supravalvular pathology. Asymmetric septal hypertrophy or hypertrophic obstructive cardiomyopathy is discussed further in Chapter 25.

ECHOCARDIOGRAPHIC EVALUATION OF AORTIC STENOSIS

Two-Dimensional Ultrasound

A normal aortic valve appears as two thin lines that open parallel to the aortic walls in the ME aortic valve LAX view. The ascending aorta and LVOT are also inspected using this

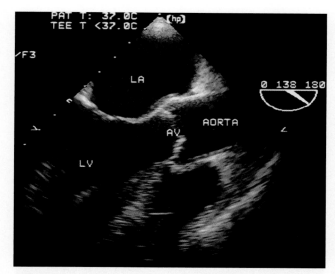

FIGURE 9.8. Transesophageal echocardiogram of the mid-esophageal aortic valve long-axis view during systole in a patient with aortic stenosis. A multiplane probe at 138 degrees provided this view of an aortic valve (*AV*) with doming leaflets. Leaflet doming is a qualitative sign of stenosis. The proximal ascending aorta is also imaged in this view. *LA*, left atrium; *LV*, left ventricle.

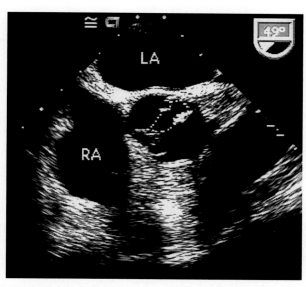

FIGURE 9.10. Transesophageal echocardiogram of the mid-esophageal aortic valve short-axis view in a patient with bicuspid aortic stenosis. Leaflet edges are traced to obtain a planimetry measurement of aortic valve orifice area. *LA*, left atrium; *RA*, right atrium.

view (Fig. 9.4). An important sign of stenosis is doming of the leaflets during systole (Fig. 9.8). The leaflets are curved toward the midline of the aorta instead of parallel to the aortic wall. Leaflet doming is such an important observation that this finding alone is sufficient for the qualitative diagnosis of aortic stenosis. Coincident with doming is reduced leaflet separation (<15 mm), which is appreciated in both the short- and long-axis views of the aortic valve. The short-axis view of the aortic valve permits evaluation of leaflet motion, as well as of calcification, commissural fusion,

and leaflet coaptation (Fig. 9.9). This short-axis view (30–60 degrees) allows measurement of aortic valve orifice area by two-dimensional planimetry (Fig. 9.10), which provides good correlation with other methods used for assessment of aortic stenosis (9). The probe is manipulated to provide the image with the smallest orifice to ensure that the cross section is of the leaflet tips. Assessment of a cross section that is oblique or inferior to the leaflet tips can lead to overestimation of the orifice size (Fig. 9.11). The valve appears

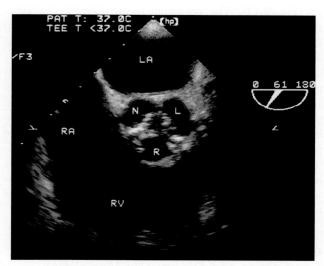

FIGURE 9.9. Transesophageal echocardiogram of the mid-esophageal aortic valve short-axis view during systole in a patient with aortic stenosis. *LA*, left atrium; *RV*, right ventricle; *RA*, right atrium; *N*, noncoronary cusp; *L*, left coronary cusp; *R*, right coronary cusp.

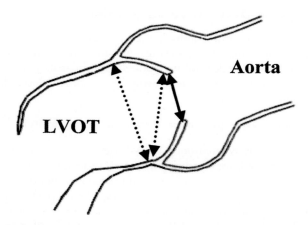

FIGURE 9.11. Illustration of various cross-sections that may be used to perform planimetry measurements of aortic valve orifice size. The solid line indicates the correct cross-section at the tips of the aortic cusps. The two dotted lines indicate an oblique cross section and a cross section that is inferior to the leaflet tips, assessment of both of which would result in an overestimation of aortic valve orifice size. *LVOT*, left ventricular outflow tract. (From Troianos CA. Perioperative echocardiography. In: Troianos CA, ed. *Anesthesia for the cardiac patient.* St. Louis: CV Mosby, 2002: page 155, with permission.)

TABLE 9.2. LIMITATIONS TO DETERMINATION OF AORTIC VALVE AREA PLANIMETRY

Limitation	Etiology	Consequence
Inadequate short-axis view	Leaflet edges not in sample plane	Over, or underestimation of area
Heavy calcification	Calcific degeneration of valve	Shadowing of anterior aspect of valve
"Pinhole" aortic stenosis	Advanced disease	Cannot identify valve orifice

circular in a true short-axis cross section, and all three cusps are viewed simultaneously and appear equal in shape; assessment via this approach prevents overestimation of the orifice size, as can occur with assessment of oblique cross sections of the valve (9). Multiplane TEE simplifies the location of the actual orifice by imaging the aortic valve, first in LAX to identify the smallest orifice at the leaflet tips. The orifice is centered on the image display screen and the transducer position is stabilized within the esophagus as the multiplane angle is rotated backward to the short-axis view. The smallest orifice is traced, and the two-dimensional cross-sectional area is displayed. Limitations of this technique are listed in Table 9.2 and include (a) the inability to obtain an adequate short-axis view; (b) heavy calcification, particularly posterior, that causes shadowing of the valve; and (c) the presence of "pinhole" aortic stenosis, in which the valve orifice cannot be identified. The short-axis view of the aortic valve identifies congenital abnormalities of the aortic valve, including bicuspid (Fig. 9.10) and unicuspid (Fig. 9.12) valves.

Doppler-Derived Valve Gradient

Doppler echocardiography is used to quantitate the severity of aortic stenosis by measuring the transvalvular blood velocity. The peak pressure gradient is estimated from the peak velocity measurement using the modified Bernoulli equation:

$$\text{aortic valve gradient} = 4 \times (\text{aortic valve velocity})^2$$

As previously mentioned, the ME views of the aortic valve are not suitable for measuring transaortic velocity because accurate Doppler measurements require a parallel alignment of the Doppler beam with the blood flow. The deep TG LAX view is developed by advancing the probe beyond the TG mid-papillary and apical short-axis views, maximally anteflexing the probe and flexing it to the left (Fig. 9.6). This places the probe at the LV apex, with the ultrasound beam directed toward the base of the heart (Fig. 9.5). The left atrium (LA) appears in the far field, to the right of the aortic valve and aortic root. A parallel alignment with blood flow in the LVOT and through the aortic valve is thus achieved.

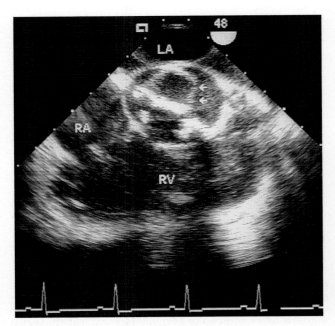

FIGURE 9.12. Transesophageal echocardiogram of the mid-esophageal aortic valve short-axis view in a patient with a unicuspid aortic valve as indicated by the arrows. *LA,* left atrium; *RA,* right atrium; *RV,* right ventricle. (From Troianos CA. Perioperative echocardiography. In: Troianos CA, ed. *Anesthesia for the cardiac patient.* St. Louis: CV Mosby, 2002: page 156, with permission.)

A parallel alignment of the ultrasound beam and aortic valve flow also can be obtained with the TG LAX view. This view is developed from the TG mid-papillary short-axis view by rotating the multiplane angle from 0 degrees to 90 to 120 degrees. The LA appears on the right side of the screen and the aortic valve is in the far field (Fig. 9.7).

Color flow Doppler and the audible Doppler signal are useful for identifying the location of the narrow high-velocity jet (Fig. 9.13). The continuous-wave Doppler cursor is placed within the narrow, turbulent jet and the spectral Doppler display is activated. Accurate localization provides a distinctive audible sound and a high-velocity (>3 m/s) spectral Doppler recording that exhibits a fine feathery appearance and a mid-systolic peak (Fig. 9.14). Normal aortic valves have peak velocities of 0.9 to 1.7 m/s in adults, and peak in early systole. More dominant and dense lower velocities are also evident on the spectral Doppler display of patients with aortic stenosis and represent the more laminar, lower velocities in the LVOT. Planimetry of the velocity over time spectral Doppler analysis of transaortic blood flow yields the velocity time integral (VTI) and an estimate of mean aortic valve gradient.

Gradient Discrepancies Between Different Conditions and Diagnostic Modalities

A gradient across a stenotic orifice is dynamic because of its dependence on flow. As the flow (or cardiac output) through

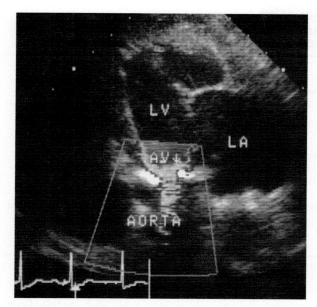

FIGURE 9.13. Transesophageal echocardiogram of the deep apical transgastric view with color flow Doppler applied over the stenotic aortic valve. The flow disturbance within the aortic valve (*AV*) identifies the stenotic orifice. *LA,* left atrium; *LV,* left ventricle. (From Troianos CA. Perioperative echocardiography. In: Troianos CA, ed. *Anesthesia for the cardiac patient.* St. Louis: CV Mosby, 2002: page 157, with permission.)

TABLE 9.3. LIMITATIONS TO ASSESSING THE SEVERITY OF AORTIC STENOSIS WITH TRANSVALVULAR VELOCITY MEASUREMENT

Etiology of Limitation	Consequence
Decreased transvalvular flow	Decreased pressure gradient
Severe LV dysfunction	
Severe mitral regurgitation	
Left to right intracardiac shunt	
Low cardiac output	
Increased transvalvular flow	Increased pressure gradient
Hyperdynamic LV function	
Sepsis	
Hyperthyroidism	

LV, left ventricular.

the valve decreases, the gradient also decreases. Conversely, as flow or the force of contraction increase, the gradient also increases (Table 9.3). Pressure gradients obtained preoperatively with transthoracic echocardiography use the same principles as intraoperative TEE. However, the intraoperative loading conditions, heart rate, and force of contraction may differ markedly from preoperative conditions, yielding disparate gradient data. Doppler-derived gradients also differ from gradients obtained in the cardiac catheterization laboratory, because of the differing techniques used for gradient determination. A catheter laboratory gradient is usually a "peak-to-peak" gradient, which represents the difference between the peak LV pressure and the peak aortic pressure. A Doppler gradient, however, is a "peak instantaneous" gradient, which is greater than the peak-to-peak gradient (Fig. 9.15). It is also important to correctly identify the origin of the gradient between the LV and aorta as either valvular, subvalvular, or supravalvular based on the two-dimensional anatomy. The shape of the spectral Doppler display differs, depending on the etiology of the outflow obstruction. Aortic stenosis produces a rounded pattern with a mid-systolic peak (Fig. 9.14), whereas LVOT obstruction produces a dagger-shaped pattern (Fig. 9.16).

Determination of Valve Area

Valve area is considered to be a more constant and less dynamic assessment of aortic stenosis. Recent evidence, however, indicates that the more pliable (moderately stenotic,

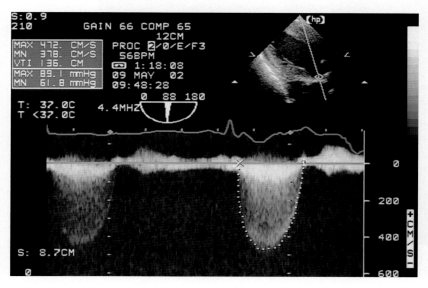

FIGURE 9.14. Continuous-wave spectral Doppler velocities through a stenotic aortic valve. The fine feathery appearance of the high (4.72 m/s) velocities with a mid-systolic peak indicates flow through a stenotic aortic valve. The denser lower velocities near the baseline indicate flow through the left ventricular outflow tract.

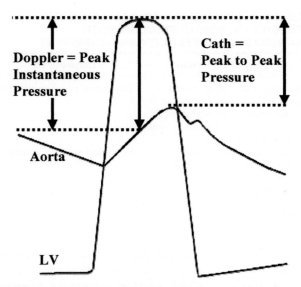

FIGURE 9.15. Illustration of the pressure tracings obtained during cardiac catheterization in a patient with aortic stenosis. The pressure gradient obtained with Doppler echocardiography is reflective of the peak instantaneous gradient. The cardiac catheterization gradient is the difference between the peak left ventricular and peak aortic pressures. *LV,* left ventricle. (From Troianos CA. Perioperative echocardiography. In: Troianos CA, ed. *Anesthesia for the cardiac patient.* St. Louis: CV Mosby, 2002: page 155, with permission.)

TABLE 9.4. LIMITATIONS TO DETERMINATION OF AORTIC VALVE AREA BY THE CONTINUITY EQUATION

Limitation	Etiology	Consequence
Inadequate transgastric view	Patient anatomy	Inability to position Doppler beam for velocity measurements
Inability to identify high-velocity jet	Pinhole aortic stenosis	Inability to measure transvalvular flow
Inability to measure an accurate LVOT diameter	Anatomic relation between LVOT and esophagus	Error in valve area calculations

LVOT, left ventricular outflow tract.

nonrheumatic) valves may open more with increased contractility (10). Nevertheless, with few exceptions, determination of aortic valve area with Doppler echocardiography is an important method of valve assessment that is not generally dependent on the state of LV function (Table 9.4). The continuity equation is used for calculation of valve area and is based on the assumption that blood flowing through sequential areas of a continuous, intact, vascular system must be equal. Blood flowing through the LVOT is thus equated with blood flow through the aortic valve:

$$\text{aortic valve}_{\text{BLOODFLOW}} = \text{LVOT}_{\text{BLOODFLOW}}$$

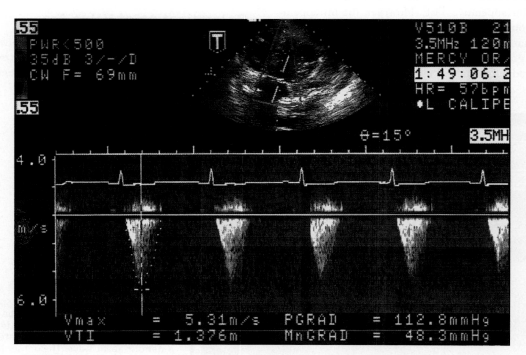

FIGURE 9.16. Continuous-wave Doppler recording in a patient with LVOT obstruction indicating a "dagger" appearance of the tracing.

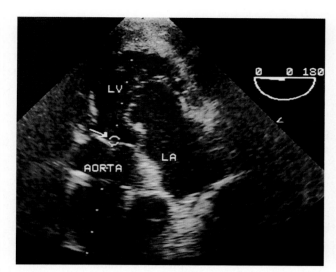

FIGURE 9.17. Transesophageal echocardiogram of the deep transgastric view with the pulsed-wave Doppler sample volume (*arrow*) placed in the LVOT just inferior to the aortic valve. *LA,* left atrium; *LV,* left ventricle.

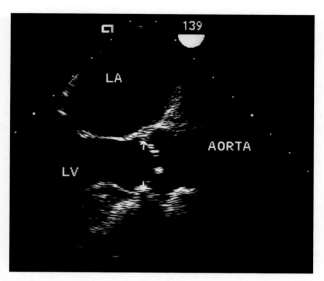

FIGURE 9.19. Transesophageal echocardiogram of the mid-esophageal aortic valve long-axis view during systole, indicating the site of measurement of the left ventricular outflow tract diameter (*arrows*). *LA,* left atrium; *LV,* left ventricle.

Substitution of blood flow with the product of velocity (VTI) and cross-sectional area yields:

$$\text{aortic valve area} \times \text{aortic valve}_{\text{VTI}} = \text{LVOT}_{\text{AREA}} \times \text{LVOT}_{\text{VTI}}$$

Aortic valve area is then calculated as:

$$\text{aortic valve area} = \frac{\text{LVOT}_{\text{AREA}} \times \text{LVOT}_{\text{VTI}}}{\text{aortic valve}_{\text{VTI}}}$$

LVOT_{VTI} is measured by placing the pulsed-wave Doppler sample volume in the LVOT just inferior to the aortic valve (Fig. 9.17) and tracing the spectral Doppler velocity over time (Fig. 9.18). Optimal sampling of LVOT velocity is performed by advancing the sample volume toward the aortic valve until "aliasing" occurs due to the high-velocity stenotic jet, then withdrawing the sample volume into the LVOT

until aliasing no longer occurs and the velocity tracing appears laminar (Fig. 9.18). Velocity is thus measured just beneath the aortic valve in the distal LVOT. $\text{LVOT}_{\text{AREA}}$ is determined using the ME aortic valve LAX view and measuring the LVOT diameter (*d*) near the aortic valve annulus (Fig. 9.19) to correspond to the same anatomic location as the pulsed-wave Doppler recording of LVOT velocity. $\text{LVOT}_{\text{AREA}}$ is calculated by assuming that the LVOT is circular and using the following formula:

$$\text{area} = \pi \times (d/2)^2$$

Calculation of $\text{LVOT}_{\text{AREA}}$ provides the greatest source of error in the continuity equation for valve area calculation. Erroneously foreshortened measurements of LVOT

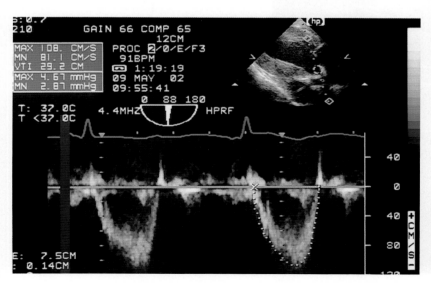

FIGURE 9.18. Planimetry of the pulsed-wave spectral Doppler velocities in the left ventricular outflow tract (*LVOT*) provides the velocity time integral (*VTI*) of LVOT flow. The laminar flow within the LVOT produces a pulsed-wave Doppler tracing with uniform velocities.

diameter are squared to significantly underestimate the true $LVOT_{AREA}$ and subsequently underestimate actual aortic valve area.

Another source of error with using the continuity equation for determination of aortic valve area is the patient with an irregular cardiac rhythm, such as atrial fibrillation. The equation is based on the conservation of mass and assumes that flow through the LVOT is equal to flow through the aortic valve. Different cardiac beats in a patient with an irregular rhythm have different stroke volumes. It is imperative to measure VTI for both the aortic valve and LVOT using the same cardiac beat. Using the continuous-wave spectral Doppler display of aortic valve flow, the aortic valve VTI is traced around the trailing edge of the higher velocity envelope as previously described. However, instead of using pulsed-wave Doppler to measure LVOT velocity, the $LVOT_{VTI}$ is traced from the same continuous-wave spectral Doppler display as the aortic valve VTI, except that the denser lower velocities within the same cardiac beat are traced (Fig. 9.20). This "double envelope" technique (11) circumvents the problem of different stroke volumes for different beats, but also can be used for patients with a regular rhythm. The author prefers using pulsed-wave Doppler for $LVOT_{VTI}$ measurements for patients with a regular rhythm because the continuous-wave Doppler beam used to measure aortic valve VTI may not precisely intercept the aortic valve jet and LVOT flow simultaneously. An alternative to measuring aortic valve and LVOT VTI from the same cardiac beat is to measure aortic valve and LVOT VTI of several (seven or more) cardiac beats and taking the average VTI for each in calculation of aortic valve area.

The stroke volume affects calculation of aortic valve area, even among patients with a regular sinus rhythm. Use of dobutamine to induce a larger stroke volume yields a slighter larger area that is related to the continuity equation rather than an actual change in valve area (12,13).

ECHOCARDIOGRAPHIC FINDINGS ASSOCIATED WITH AORTIC STENOSIS

Patients with aortic stenosis commonly have LV hypertrophy, which is an adaptive mechanism in response to the chronic pressure overload. Increased wall thickness reduces wall stress by distributing the pressure overload over greater myocardial mass, as indicated by La Place's Law:

$$\text{wall stress} = \frac{\text{pressure} \times \text{volume}}{\text{wall thickness}}$$

The major perioperative implication is that estimates of LV filling pressure are not reliable indicators of volume loading because of the associated decreased LV compliance. The second major concern is the development of systolic anterior motion (SAM) of the mitral valve because of the septal hypertrophy after aortic valve replacement for aortic stenosis. Although this condition is well recognized with asymmetric septal hypertrophy, SAM also can occur among patients with symmetric septal hypertrophy after aortic valve replacement. This is usually a manifestation of the abrupt reduction in LV afterload associated with an underfilled LV in patients with septal or concentric hypertrophy. The condition usually resolves with administration of volume,

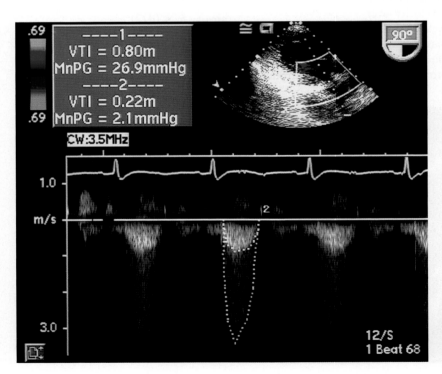

FIGURE 9.20. Planimetry of both the aortic valve and left ventricular outflow tract velocities is performed on the same cardiac beat using continuous-wave spectral Doppler.

phenylephrine, and discontinuation of inotropic and chronotropic medications.

Patients with aortic stenosis also manifest diastolic dysfunction with long-standing aortic stenosis. Mitral inflow and pulmonary venous flow patterns are examined with deceleration time. Systolic function is preserved until late in the disease progression, when LV dilatation develops. Systolic dysfunction due to aortic stenosis is usually reversible with valve replacement. Systolic dysfunction due to myocardial infarction may not improve and causes an underestimation of the severity of aortic stenosis by gradient determination.

Many patients with aortic stenosis also have AI. The diastolic regurgitation of blood into the LV increases transaortic blood flow during systole, yielding a higher gradient for a given aortic valve orifice. The presence of AI, however, does not affect continuity equation area calculations because the measurements of systolic flow in the LVOT and the aortic valve both account for the increased systolic flow.

Patients with aortic valve disease also may have mitral valve disease, manifested as mitral stenosis, regurgitation, or both. The presence of mitral stenosis causes an underestimation of the severity of aortic stenosis by gradient determination because of decreased transaortic blood flow.

CLINICAL CASE SCENARIOS
Aortic Stenosis and Normal Left Ventricular Function

A 55-year-old man with a bicuspid aortic valve presents for aortic valve replacement. The following echocardiographic data are obtained during the prebypass TEE evaluation:

> Aortic valve peak velocity 4.35 m/s
> Aortic valve velocity-time integral 0.978 m
> LVOT peak velocity 1.20 m/s
> LVOT velocity-time integral 0.283 m
> LVOT diameter 2.09 cm

This case scenario involving a patient with normal LV function allows for the diagnosis of severe stenosis to be made by velocity measurement alone. Normal aortic valve peak velocity in adults is 0.9 to 1.7 m/s. Although a velocity measurement of 4.35 m/s is an obvious indication of severe aortic stenosis to echocardiographers, the modified Bernoulli equation allows calculation of the pressure gradient for clinicians who prefer the pressure gradient to describe severity:

$$\text{aortic valve gradient} = 4 \times V^2 = 4 \times (4.35)^2 = 75.8 \text{ mm Hg}$$

Aortic valve area is determined by planimetry if the echocardiographic image allows adequate imaging of the leaflet edges in one imaging plane. Suboptimal imaging requires use of the continuity equation using the data provided:

$$\text{aortic valve (AV) flow} = \text{LVOT flow}$$
$$\text{AV area} \times \text{AV VTI} = \text{LVOT area} \times \text{LVOT VTI}$$

$$\text{AV area} = \frac{\text{LVOT}\left(\pi\left(\dfrac{d}{2}\right)^2\right) \times \text{LVOT VTI}}{\text{AV VTI}}$$
$$= \frac{3.45 \text{ cm}^2 \times 28.3 \text{ cm}}{97.8 \text{ cm}} = 1.00 \text{ cm}^2$$

Aortic Stenosis and Left Ventricular Dysfunction

A 78-year-old man with an acute myocardial infarction was found to have a 20 mm Hg aortic valve gradient, severe LV dysfunction (20% ejection fraction), and 2+ mitral regurgitation during cardiac catheterization. He is scheduled for coronary artery revascularization. The following echocardiographic data are obtained during the prebypass TEE evaluation:

> Aortic valve peak velocity 2.52 m/s
> Aortic valve velocity-time integral 0.582 m
> LVOT peak velocity 0.49 m/s
> LVOT velocity-time integral 0.111 m
> LVOT diameter 2.03 cm

This case scenario involving a patient with severe LV dysfunction and 2+ mitral regurgitation does not allow for the diagnosis of severe stenosis to be made by velocity measurement alone. The peak velocity measurement of 2.52 m/s is only slightly above normal (1.7 m/s). Given this value alone, the severity of aortic stenosis appears mild. The gradient calculated by the modified Bernoulli equation also indicates only mild stenosis:

$$\text{aortic valve gradient} = 4 \times V^2 = 4 \times (2.52)^2 = 25 \text{ mm Hg}$$

In contrast to the first case presented, determination of aortic valve area is required to determine the severity of aortic stenosis because the severe LV dysfunction and mitral regurgitation both cause decreased transaortic valvular flow during systole. Aortic valve area could not be determined by planimetry in this patient because of severe calcification. The posterior location of the calcification caused shadowing of the valve and did not allow area measurement by planimetry. The continuity equation is required to determine severity because the calculation is unaffected by the decreased transaortic blood flow:

$$\text{aortic valve (AV) flow} = \text{LVOT flow}$$
$$\text{AV area} \times \text{AV VTI} = \text{LVOT area} \times \text{LVOT VTI}$$

$$\text{AV area} = \frac{\text{LVOT}\left(\pi\left(\dfrac{d}{2}\right)^2\right) \times \text{LVOT VTI}}{\text{AV VTI}}$$
$$= \frac{3.23 \text{ cm}^2 \times 11.1 \text{ cm}}{58.2 \text{ cm}} = 0.62 \text{ cm}^2$$

This patient has severe aortic stenosis and may benefit from aortic valve replacement despite the increased cross-clamp time to replace the valve. The benefits derived from decreased LV afterload will likely improve LV function and possibly decrease the severity of mitral regurgitation. This decision requires considerable clinical judgment and must be weighed against the possibility that the increased aortic cross-clamp time may inhibit successful separation from cardiopulmonary bypass.

Measurement Errors when Using the Continuity Equation for Aortic Stenosis

Assuming a 10% error in the measured values obtained in the previous case, which measured value provides the greatest source of error in calculating aortic valve area using the continuity equation?

A 10% error in measurement of the velocity time integral of flow through the aortic valve yields the following results:

Aortic Valve VTI (cm)	LVOT VTI (cm)	LVOT Diameter (cm)	Aortic Valve Area (cm²)	% Error in Calculation
58.2	11.1	2.03 (3.23 cm² area)	0.62	Correct
64.0 (10% high)	11.1	2.03 (3.23 cm² area)	0.56	−10%
52.4 (10% low)	11.1	2.03 (3.23 cm² area)	0.68	+10%

A 10% error in measurement of the velocity-time integral of flow through the LVOT yields the following results:

Aortic Valve VTI (cm)	LVOT VTI (cm)	LVOT Diameter (cm)	Aortic Valve Area (cm²)	% Error in Calculation
58.2	11.1	2.03 (3.23 cm² area)	0.62	Correct
58.2	12.2 (10% high)	2.03 (3.23 cm² area)	0.68	+10%
58.2	10.0 (10% low)	2.03 (3.23 cm² area)	0.56	−10%

A 10% error in measurement of the diameter of the LVOT yields the following results:

Aortic Valve VTI (cm)	LVOT VTI (cm)	LVOT Diameter (cm)	Aortic Valve Area (cm²)	% Error in Calculation
58.2	11.1	2.03 (3.23 cm² area)	0.62	Correct
58.2	11.1	2.23 (10% high) (3.90 cm² area)	0.74	+19%
58.2	11.1	1.83 (10% low) (2.62 cm² area)	0.50	−19%

It is therefore most important that the LVOT diameter be measured carefully and accurately to avoid errors in aortic valve area determination using the continuity equation. As illustrated, a 10% error in the diameter measurement yields nearly a 20% error in aortic valve area calculation.

ETIOLOGY OF AORTIC INSUFFICIENCY

Aortic insufficiency is caused by either intrinsic disease of the aortic cusps or secondarily from diseases affecting the ascending aorta. Intrinsic valvular problems include rheumatic, calcific, and myxomatous valvular disease, endocarditis, traumatic injury, and congenital abnormalities. Conditions affecting the ascending aorta that lead to AI involve annular dilatation and include aortic dissection (secondary to blunt trauma or hypertension), mycotic aneurysm, cystic medial necrosis, Marfan syndrome, and chronic hypertension. The most common cause of pure AI is no longer postinflammatory, with the decreasing prevalence of rheumatic heart disease among cardiac surgical patients [14]. Aortic root dilatation is now the most common etiologic factor due to the increased prevalence of degenerative disease, followed by postinflammatory disease and bicuspid valve disease.

Two-Dimensional Ultrasound

The aortic valve, ascending aorta, and LVOT are inspected using the ME aortic valve LAX view (Fig. 9.4). A normal aortic valve appears as two thin lines that open parallel to the aortic walls during systole. Normal leaflets are often not visible during diastole, because they are parallel to the Doppler beam when closed. Stenotic leaflets that dome during systole often do not completely coapt during diastole, leading to AI. The diagnosis of leaflet prolapse is made when aortic leaflet tissue is imaged in the LVOT below the annular plane during diastole (Fig. 9.21). An aortic dissection in the aortic root causes disruption of leaflets from the aortic annulus and may cause leaflet prolapse. Two-dimensional echocardiography is used to determine the cause of the AI by identifying structural abnormalities of the leaflets or aortic root.

Although two-dimensional echocardiography is not useful for quantifying the severity of AI, there are several associated echocardiographic features. The LV is dilated and more spherical in shape with chronic AI, but not necessarily with acute AI. The mitral valve exhibits premature closure and fluttering of the anterior mitral leaflet during diastole. An eccentric AI jet directed toward the anterior mitral valve leaflet may cause doming of the anterior leaflet with convexity toward the left atrial side of the mitral valve (Fig. 9.22).

Color Doppler Echocardiography

Doppler echocardiography is used to quantitate the severity of AI by several techniques that involve color, pulsed-wave, and continuous-wave Doppler. These techniques are sensitive and reliable, but all have limitations. Color Doppler applied to the ME aortic valve short-axis view (30 to

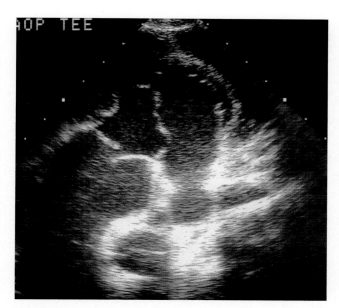

FIGURE 9.21. Deep transgastric echocardiogram of the aortic valve demonstrating leaflet prolapse.

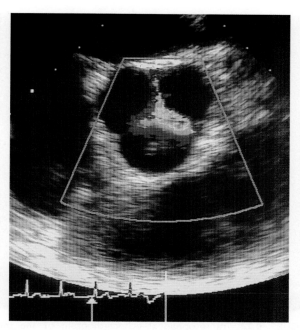

FIGURE 9.23. Transesophageal echocardiogram of the mid-esophageal aortic valve short-axis view with color flow Doppler in a patient with aortic insufficiency. The origin of the aortic insufficiency is predominantly between the right and left coronary cusps. (From Troianos CA. Perioperative echocardiography. In: Troianos CA, ed. *Anesthesia for the cardiac patient.* St. Louis: CV Mosby, 2002: page 160, with permission.)

50 degree multiplane angle) is useful for localizing the site of regurgitation (Fig. 9.23). Despite the orthogonal relationship between the aortic valve flow and Doppler beam in this short-axis view, the regurgitant orifice is identifiable because the AI jet is usually not completely orthogonal to the Doppler beam, particularly if the jet is eccentric. The ME aortic valve LAX view (120 to 150 degree multiplane angle) is the most useful for quantitating the severity of AI. Color Doppler reveals a flow disturbance in the LVOT originating from the aortic valve and directed into the LV (Fig. 9.24). A central jet is usually caused by aortic root dilatation, whereas

an eccentric jet usually implies a leaflet problem. The width of the jet at the orifice compared with the width of the LVOT correlates with angiographic determinants of AI (Table 9.5) (15).

Limitations of the use of color flow Doppler echocardiography to estimate the severity of AI are listed in Table 9.6.

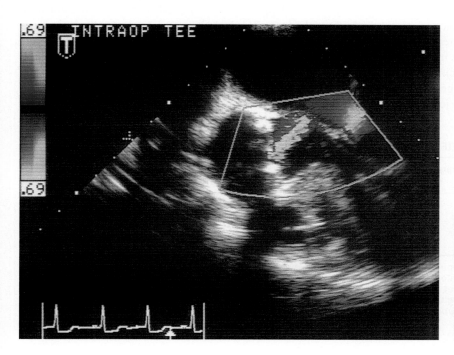

FIGURE 9.22. Transesophageal echocardiogram with a color flow Doppler in a patient with eccentric aortic insufficiency. The aortic insufficiency is identified by the color flow disturbance that originates from the aortic valve and directed toward the anterior mitral valve leaflet, creating a convexity in the mitral leaflet. (From Troianos CA. Perioperative echocardiography. In: Troianos CA, ed. *Anesthesia for the cardiac patient.* St. Louis: CV Mosby, 2002: page 160, with permission.)

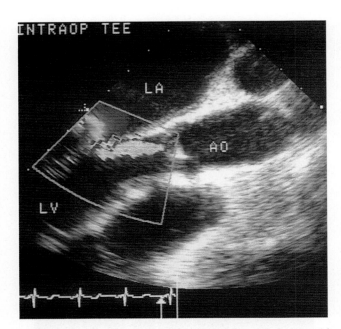

FIGURE 9.24. Transesophageal echocardiogram of the mid-esophageal aortic valve long-axis view with color flow Doppler in a patient with aortic insufficiency. *LA,* left atrium; *LV,* left ventricle; *AO,* ascending aorta.

One such limitation of this technique is that the regurgitant jet orifice and the true LVOT diameter (not foreshortened) may not be in the same imaging plane (16). This limitation is most apparent if "color M mode" is used to determine the jet/LVOT ratio. Color M mode refers to the application of M-mode imaging to a color flow Doppler image (Fig. 9.25). M-mode evaluation of the LVOT in the patient with AI is more useful for determination of the duration of AI into the diastolic phase rather than the jet/LVOT ratio. Another limitation of the jet/LVOT ratio method of assessing AI is that the shape of the regurgitant orifice may not be circular or symmetric. An irregularly shaped regurgitant orifice may cause the jet to appear wider in one imaging plane than another; hence the importance of examining multiple imaging planes (17). The AI jet also may be eccentric or converge with the mitral valve, rendering the jet particularly

TABLE 9.5. GRADING AORTIC INSUFFICIENCY

Severity of Aortic Insufficiency	Jet Width/LVOT Width Ratio	Average Regurgitant Fraction
1+	<0.25	28%
2+	0.25–0.46	33%
3+	0.47–0.64	53%
4+	>0.64	62%

From Perry GJ, Helmcke F, Nanda NC, et al. Evaluation of aortic insufficiency by Doppler color flow mapping. *J Am Coll Cardiol* 1987;9:952–959, and Kitabatake A, Ito H, Inoue M, et al. A new approach to noninvasive evaluation of aortic regurgitant fraction by two-dimensional Doppler echocardiography. *Circulation* 1985;72:523–529.

TABLE 9.6. LIMITATIONS TO ESTIMATING THE SEVERITY OF AORTIC INSUFFICIENCY WITH COLOR FLOW DOPPLER

Limitation	Etiology	Consequence
Shadowing of LVOT	Prosthetic aortic or mitral valve	Inability to image LVOT and AI jet
AI jet is wider in one plane versus another	Regurgitant orifice is three dimensional	Inaccurate estimate of AI jet width
Eccentric jet causing swirling of flow disturbance	Leaflet prolapse	AI jet appears wider than regurgitant orifice size

LVOT, left ventricular outflow obstruction; AI, aortic insufficiency.

difficult to evaluate in patients with mitral stenosis (18). If color Doppler cannot be applied to the LVOT from the ME aortic valve LAX view because of unusual anatomy or shadowing of the LVOT from a prosthetic mitral or aortic valve, a deep TG LAX or TG LAX view is used. The AI jet in this view appears red or mosaic in color, with the jet directed away from the aortic valve toward the LV cavity (Fig. 9.26). The length of the jet is not as important as the width of the jet at the orifice. Multiple imaging planes should be used to appreciate the three-dimensional character of the jet.

Continuous-Wave Doppler

Continuous-wave Doppler is also used to determine the severity of AI by measuring the deceleration slope of the regurgitant jet. A deep TG or TG LAX view aligns the regurgitant jet parallel to the Doppler beam. Color Doppler is useful for identifying the location and direction of the AI jet. The Doppler cursor is placed within the AI color flow Doppler jet and the continuous-wave spectral velocity profile is obtained (Fig. 9.27). The velocity of the regurgitant jet declines more rapidly in patients with severe AI because the larger regurgitant orifice allows a more rapid equilibration of the aortic and LV pressures. In other words, if the pressure difference between the aorta and LV approaches zero rapidly, the regurgitant jet velocity also approaches zero more rapidly, creating a steeper slope (Fig. 9.28). A regurgitant velocity slope of greater than 3 m/s^2 is indicative of advanced (3 or 4+) AI (19).

One limitation of this technique is that factors other than regurgitant orifice size influence the deceleration slope (Table 9.7). Systemic vascular resistance and LV compliance affect the rate of deceleration, irrespective of the regurgitant orifice size (20). Decreased systemic vascular resistance (sepsis) and reduced LV compliance (ischemia, cardiomyopathy, acute AI) cause a steeper deceleration slope because aortic and LV pressures equalize more rapidly with these conditions. Another limitation of this technique is that measurement of regurgitant jet velocity is difficult and unreliable in

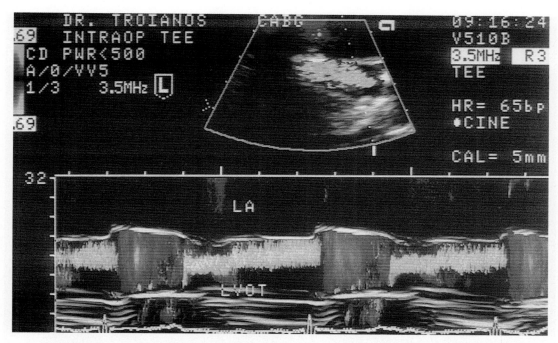

FIGURE 9.25. Color M-mode echocardiography of the left ventricular outflow tract in a patient with aortic insufficiency. *LA,* left atrium; *LVOT,* left ventricular outflow tract. (From Troianos CA. Perioperative echocardiography. In: Troianos CA, ed. *Anesthesia for the cardiac patient.* St. Louis: CV Mosby, 2002: page 161, with permission.)

patients with eccentric jets, because it is difficult to align the Doppler beam with the regurgitant jet.

Pulsed-Wave Doppler

Pulsed-wave Doppler is used to detect retrograde flow in the aorta during diastole. Holodiastolic flow in the abdominal aorta is both sensitive and specific for severe AI. Detection of holodiastolic retrograde flow in the proximal descending thoracic aorta and aortic arch is a sensitive indicator of AI, but is not specific for severe AI. Using the short-axis TEE view of the descending thoracic aorta, the pulsed-wave sample volume is placed as distal in the aorta as possible, near the diaphragm. Despite the orthogonal relationship between the aortic flow and Doppler beam in this short-axis view, the flow in the aorta is identifiable because the blood in the

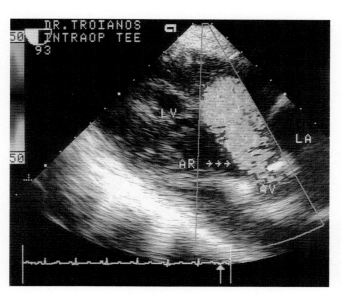

FIGURE 9.26. Transesophageal echocardiogram of the transgastric long-axis view with color flow Doppler in a patient with aortic insufficiency (*arrows*). *AV,* aortic valve; *LA,* left atrium; *LV,* left ventricle; *AR,* aortic regurgitation. (From Troianos CA. Perioperative echocardiography. In: Troianos CA, ed. *Anesthesia for the cardiac patient.* St. Louis: CV Mosby, 2002: page 155, with permission.)

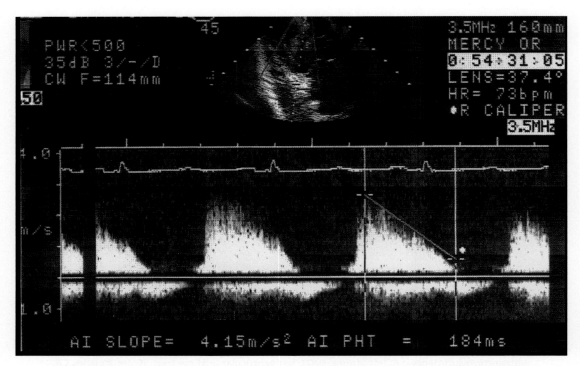

FIGURE 9.27. Continuous-wave spectral Doppler velocities within the left ventricular outflow tract in a patient with aortic insufficiency (AI). The slope of the velocity deceleration (AI slope = 4.15 m/s^2) indicates the severity of the AI. (From Troianos CA. Perioperative echocardiography. In: Troianos CA, ed. *Anesthesia for the cardiac patient.* St. Louis: CV Mosby, 2002: page 162, with permission.)

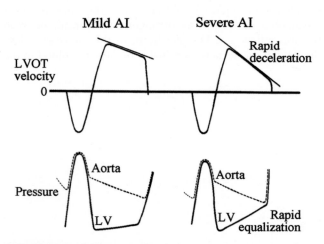

FIGURE 9.28. Illustration of the association between the left ventricular outflow tract (*LVOT*) deceleration slope and the pressure difference between the aorta and left ventricle (*LV*) during diastole. The deceleration slope is steeper and approaches zero velocity more rapidly with severe aortic insufficiency (*AI*) as the pressures in the aorta and left ventricle equalize more rapidly. (From Troianos CA. Perioperative echocardiography. In: Troianos CA, ed. *Anesthesia for the cardiac patient.* St. Louis: CV Mosby, 2002: page 162, with permission, and adapted from Feigenbaum H. *Echocardiography,* 5th ed. Philadelphia: Lea & Febiger, 1994:286, with permission.)

aorta tends to swirl as it travels down the aorta. The spectral Doppler display is examined for the duration of diastolic flow. Retrograde flow throughout diastole (holodiastolic) in the distal descending (21) or abdominal aorta (22) (Fig. 9.29) indicates severe AI.

Regurgitant Volume and Regurgitant Fraction

Regurgitant volume and regurgitant fraction also can be used to evaluate the severity of AI. Regurgitant volume is the difference between the systolic flow across the aortic valve and

TABLE 9.7. LIMITATIONS TO ESTIMATING THE SEVERITY OF AORTIC INSUFFICIENCY (AI) USING THE DECELERATION SLOPE

Limitation	Consequence
Increased systemic vascular resistance	Steeper slope overestimating AI
Decreased left ventricular compliance	Steeper slope overestimating AI
Eccentric AI jet	Cannot align Doppler beam with AI jet

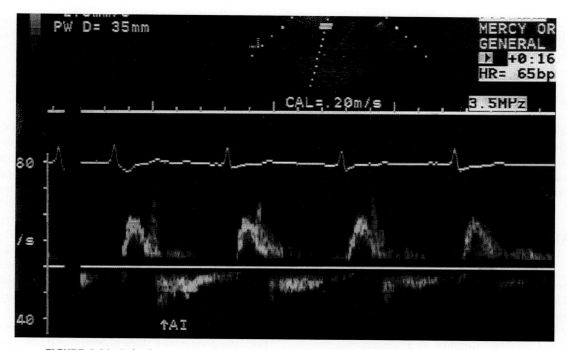

FIGURE 9.29. Pulsed-wave Doppler spectral velocity of blood flow in the descending thoracic aorta. The retrograde flow throughout diastole (*arrow*) is termed holodiastolic and is associated with severe aortic insufficiency. *AI,* aortic insufficiency. (From Troianos CA. Perioperative echocardiography. In: Troianos CA, ed. *Anesthesia for the cardiac patient.* St. Louis: CV Mosby, 2002: page 163, with permission.)

"net forward" cardiac output. In the absence of intracardiac shunts and mitral regurgitation, flow through the pulmonary artery or mitral valve is equivalent to (net) cardiac output. Pulmonary artery blood flow is reliably measured with TEE by measuring the pulmonary artery diameter (d), calculating its area [$\pi\,(d/2)^2$], and multiplying the area by the pulmonary artery VTI and heart rate (23). Aortic valve systolic flow is the product of aortic valve area and VTI. The aortic regurgitant volume is the difference between aortic valve systolic flow and pulmonary blood flow (cardiac output). Regurgitant fraction is expressed as the proportion of aortic valve systolic flow that is regurgitant volume and indicates the severity of AI (Table 9.5) (24).

$$\text{regurgitant volume} = \text{aortic valve systolic flow} - \text{cardiac output}$$

$$\text{regurgitant fraction} = \frac{\text{regurgitant volume}}{\text{aortic valve systolic flow}}$$

The continuity equation could be theoretically used to determine regurgitant orifice size. Diastolic velocities just above (aortic root–VTI) and through the aortic valve (aortic valve–VTI) are determined via Doppler echocardiography, and the cross-sectional area of the aortic root is determined via two-dimensional echocardiography (25,26). This technique, however, has not been widely accepted or validated:

$$\text{aortic valve regurgitant orifice} = \frac{\text{aortic root}_{\text{AREA}} \times \text{aortic root diastolic}_{\text{VTI}}}{\text{aortic valve regurgitant jet}_{\text{VTI}}}$$

ECHOCARDIOGRAPHIC FINDINGS ASSOCIATED WITH AORTIC INSUFFICIENCY

Chronic LV volume overload causes progressive LV dilatation over many years, whereas systolic function is preserved. Ejection fraction is initially normal, whereas end-diastolic dimensions are increased. In contrast to aortic stenosis, the ventricle remains relatively compliant until systolic dysfunction ensues late in the course of the disease process. Another contrasting feature is that the systolic dysfunction is not reversible. Acute AI is not associated with LV dilatation because the adaptive LV dilatation has not occurred. This lack of adaptation is associated with a decreased LV compliance and a rapid onset of symptoms. Other echocardiographic findings include premature mitral valve closure and fluttering of the mitral valve leaflets. Depending on the cause of the AI, aortic root abnormalities also may be present, including aortic dissection or aneurysm.

Aortic insufficiency causes an overestimation of mitral valve area by the pressure half-time method of determining mitral orifice size. The pressure half-time method exploits the relationship between mitral inflow deceleration and mitral valve area. Deceleration is based on the equalization of pressure in the LA and the LV and is prolonged as mitral orifice size decreases. In the absence of AI, LV volume (and subsequently left ventricular pressure) increases via mitral inflow alone. In the presence of AI, LV volume increases by both mitral inflow and aortic regurgitation, giving the impression that mitral inflow is better than actual inflow, thus underestimating the severity of mitral stenosis.

CLINICAL CASE SCENARIOS

Case 1

A 78-year-old man recovering from coronary artery bypass grafting 3 weeks before presentation of severe leg pain is brought emergently to the operating room for femoral embolectomy. Lack of proximal arterial flow prompts a change in the planned surgical procedure to a femoral-to-femoral artery bypass. Blood pressure measurement in the left upper extremity indicates progressive hypotension, while exploration of the contralateral femoral artery reveals lack of arterial perfusion. A TEE examination is performed to evaluate the causes of hypotension and lack of femoral arterial perfusion. Two-dimensional echocardiography reveals a large pericardial effusion compressing all four cardiac chambers. Color Doppler applied to the LVOT demonstrates an aortic valve diastolic jet width/LVOT width ratio of 0.7. An intimal flap imaged in the ascending aorta is also imaged in the arch and descending thoracic aorta. The origin of the left subclavian artery is identified in continuity with the true lumen and is not compromised.

Based on the above echocardiographic findings, the etiology of the hypotension is cardiac tamponade and associated impaired ventricular filling. In addition, a 0.7 jet/LVOT ratio is indicative of severe AI. These findings are explained by the presence of an aortic dissection imaged in the ascending aorta, arch, and descending aorta. Although an aortic dissection may cause decreased blood pressure measurements obtained from the left upper extremity due to compromised vascular flow, the etiology in this case is cardiac tamponade and severe AI. The aortic dissection has caused rupture of blood into the pericardial space and separation of the aortic leaflets from the annulus. The surgical procedure is altered again with institution of femoral artery–femoral vein cardiopulmonary bypass, replacement of the ascending aorta, and repair of the aortic valve. The feasibility of aortic valve repair is based on the appearance of the leaflets, which indicates whether the leaflets have intrinsic disease in addition to their separation from the annulus. Normal leaflets are resuspended to restore the competence of the valve.

Postoperatively, TEE is used to evaluate the success of repair and assess flow in the true and false lumens in the thoracic aorta. Restoration of flow within the true lumen provides adequate distal perfusion in the femoral vessels and decreases or eliminates flow in the false lumen, which is evident with echocardiography.

Case 2

A preoperative left ventriculogram was not performed because of renal insufficiency in a 72-year-old patient scheduled for coronary artery bypass grafting. Radiocontrast dye was also not injected into the aortic root. A blood pressure measurement of 150/50 mm Hg before cardiopulmonary bypass prompts a request for intraoperative TEE to evaluate the aortic valve and LV function. The LV TG short-axis view indicates increased diastolic dimensions and mild global LV dysfunction. A deep TG LAX view allows for the measurement of a regurgitant jet velocity slope of 5 m/s^2 in the LVOT. A pulsed-wave Doppler sample volume placed in the distal descending thoracic aorta near the diaphragm reveals holodiastolic flow reversal.

This intraoperative TEE evaluation indicates severe AI. Both the deceleration slope of 5 m/s^2 and holodiastolic flow reversal near the abdominal aorta are indicative of severe AI. LV dilatation suggests chronic insufficiency that has allowed adaptation by the patient's sedentary lifestyle. At a minimum, this diagnosis alters cardioplegia administration to a retrograde approach via the coronary sinus rather than antegrade into the aortic root. Aortic valve repair or replacement is also considered as an alteration of the planned surgical procedure.

AORTIC VALVE REPAIR

The vast majority of aortic valves suitable for repair have regurgitant lesions rather than stenotic lesions. It is important for the echocardiographer to understand the approaches to valve repair in order to recognize what valves are feasible for repair and to evaluate the repair intraoperatively after surgical intervention. Regurgitant lesions with anatomically normal leaflets and mobility are commonly caused by aortic root dilatation and have a characteristic central jet of insufficiency. Annular dilatation secondary to aortic root dilatation can be repaired if annular dilatation is limited and the leaflets are otherwise anatomically normal. The size and morphology of the aortic root is determined via TEE. A normal aortic root has sinuses of Valsalva that are symmetric and at most 2 to 3 mm larger than the valve annulus (27). Carpentier's technique of correcting annular dilatation employs continuous circumferential horizontal mattress sutures placed through the annulus (14,28). Cosgrove's technique places sutures at the commissures to advance the sinotubular ridge inward and allow central coaptation (Fig. 9.30) (14). This method provides selected plication to the most affected areas of the valve (usually the commissures).

Repair is a suitable option among patients with AI due to single-leaflet prolapse of either a tricuspid or congenitally

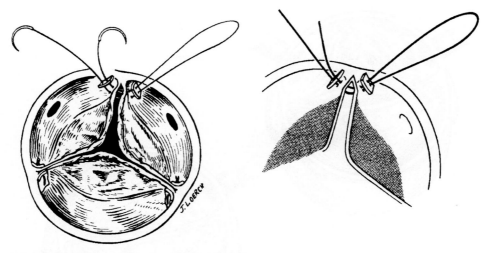

FIGURE 9.30. Aortic valve annuloplasty is performed by placing horizontal mattress sutures buttressed with Teflon felt at each commissure. Care is taken to avoid leaflet contact as the suture passes through the annulus, into the outflow tract, and back through the annulus. (From Cosgrove DM, Rosenkranz ER, Hendren WG, et al. Valvuloplasty for aortic insufficiency. *J Thorac Cardiovasc Surg* 1991;102:571–577, with permission.)

bicuspid valve. Although leaflet prolapse is observed in tricuspid aortic valves, this lesion most commonly affects bicuspid valves (14). The prolapsing area of the leaflet is resected and reapproximated with suture (Figs. 9.31 and 9.32). Annuloplasty is often performed in association with the triangular resection of the prolapsing leaflet. Calcification limits the

potential for valve reconstruction and is usually included in the resected portion of the leaflet.

Valve repair for patients with aortic dissection involves resuspension of the cusps and is easily performed and highly successful in the absence of additional leaflet pathology. Leaflet perforation caused by endocarditis can be repaired

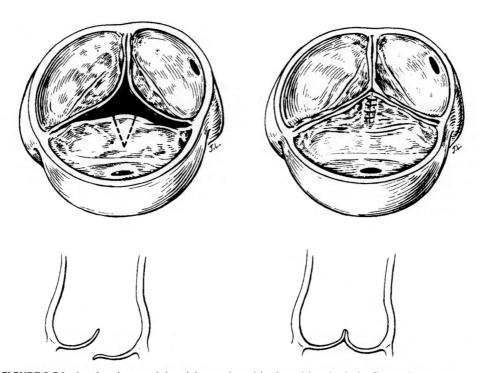

FIGURE 9.31. Aortic valve repair involving a tricuspid valve with a single-leaflet prolapse. Triangular resection of the free edge of the prolapsing cusp results in normal leaflet size and coaptation. (From Cosgrove DM, Rosenkranz ER, Hendren WG, et al. Valvuloplasty for aortic insufficiency. *J Thorac Cardiovasc Surg* 1991;102:571–577, with permission.)

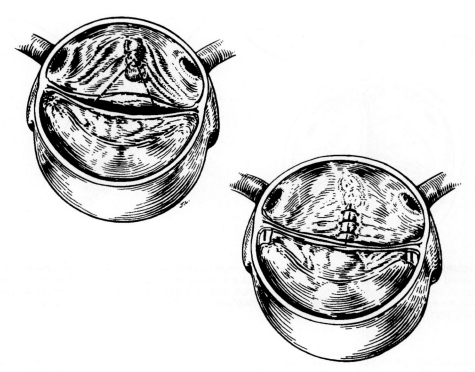

FIGURE 9.32. Aortic valve repair involving a bicuspid valve with leaflet prolapse involves resection of the raphe when present, triangular resection of prolapsing cusp, and annuloplasty. From Cosgrove DM, Rosenkranz ER, Hendren WG, et al. Valvuloplasty for aortic insufficiency. *J Thorac Cardiovasc Surg* 1991;102:571–577, with permission.)

by patch or primary closure if destruction is limited to a small perforation of a single leaflet.

SUMMARY

Transesophageal echocardiography is a valuable clinical tool for the evaluation of the aortic valve. High-resolution images obtained owing to the close proximity of the valve and the esophagus permit accurate diagnosis of the mechanism of valve dysfunction, valve sizing for replacement surgery, and identification of lesions associated with aortic valve pathology. The application of Doppler echocardiography provides a complete evaluation of stenotic and regurgitant lesions, leading to quantitative assessment that prompts initial surgical intervention, correction of inadequate repair, and reoperation for complications. It is important to identify aortic valvular disease because of the surgical and anesthetic implications associated with both aortic stenosis and regurgitation. The increased population of elderly patients presenting for surgery has increased the prevalence of calcific aortic stenosis. Because aortic valve replacement after previous coronary artery bypass grafting is associated with higher mortality than combined aortic valve and coronary bypass surgery (4), it is important to identify even moderate aortic stenosis during coronary bypass surgery and consider combination surgery to avoid the higher mortality associated with reoperation.

KEY POINTS

- The close anatomic proximity between the aortic valve and the esophagus permits accurate diagnosis of the mechanism of aortic valve dysfunction, valve sizing for valve replacement, and identification of associated lesions.
- Complete evaluation of the aortic valve uses two-dimensional imaging and pulsed-wave, continuous-wave, and color Doppler for quantitative evaluation of stenotic and regurgitant lesions.
- It is important to identify aortic stenosis among patients presenting for primary coronary artery surgery, because aortic valve replacement after previous coronary artery bypass grafting is associated with higher mortality than combined aortic valve and coronary bypass surgery.
- Velocity measurement of aortic valve flow provides an estimate of valve gradient using the modified Bernoulli equation. The force of ventricular contraction and transaortic blood flow determine transvalvular velocity in addition to the size of the stenotic orifice. The severity of aortic

stenosis is underestimated in patients with severe LV dysfunction. These patients require area determination to assess the severity of aortic stenosis.

- There is often a discrepancy between Doppler and cardiac catheterization derived gradient measurements.
- Aortic valve area is determined by planimetry or by using the continuity equation.
- Aortic insufficiency is caused by conditions affecting the aortic cusps or secondarily from diseases affecting the ascending aorta.
- Two-dimensional echocardiography is useful for identifying the causes of AI and associated lesions, but not for assessing the severity of regurgitation.
- Color, pulsed-wave, and continuous-wave Doppler are used to quantify the severity of regurgitation, but all techniques have limitations.
- The vast majority of aortic valves suitable for repair have regurgitant lesions rather than stenotic lesions.

REFERENCES

1. Oh CC, Click RL, Orszulak TA, et al. Role of intraoperative transesophageal echocardiography in determining aortic annulus diameter in homograft insertion. *J Am Soc Echocardiogr* 1998;11:638–642.
2. Nowrangi SK, Connolly HM, Freeman WK, et al. Impact of intraoperative transesophageal echocardiography among patients undergoing aortic valve replacement for aortic stenosis. *J Am Soc Echocardiogr* 2001;14:863–866.
3. Morehead AJ, Firstenberg MS, Shiota T, et al. Intraoperative echocardiographic detection of regurgitant jets after valve replacement. *Ann Thorac Surg* 2000;69:135–139.
4. Odell JA, Mullany CJ, Schaff HV, et al. Aortic valve replacement after previous coronary artery bypass grafting. *Ann Thorac Surg* 1996;62:1424–1430.
5. Peter M, Hoffmann A, Parker C, et al. Progression of aortic stenosis. *Chest* 1993;103:1715–1719.
6. Bahler RC, Desser DR, Finkelhor RS, et al. Factors leading to progression of valvular aortic stenosis. *Am J Cardiol* 1999;84:1044–1048.
7. Palta S, Pai AM, Gill KS, et al. New insights into the progression of aortic stenosis: implications for secondary prevention. *Circulation* 2000;101:2497–2502.
8. Stoddard MF, Hammons RT, Longaker RA. Doppler transesophageal echocardiographic determination of aortic valve area in adults with aortic stenosis. *Am Heart J* 1996;132:337–342.
9. Hoffmann R, Flachskampf FA, Hanrath P. Planimetry of orifice area in aortic stenosis using multiplane transesophageal echocardiography. *J Am Coll Cardiol* 1993;22:529–534.
10. Shively BK, Charlton GA, Crawford MH, et al. Flow dependence of valve area in aortic stenosis: relation to valve morphology. *J Am Coll Cardiol* 1998;31:654–660.
11. Maslow AD, Mashikian J, Haering JM, et al. Transesophageal echocardiographic evaluation of native aortic valve area: utility of the double-envelope technique. *J Cardiothorac Vasc Anesth* 2001;15:293–299.
12. Rask LP, Karp KH, Eriksson NP. Flow dependence of the aortic valve area in patients with aortic stenosis: assessment by application of the continuity equation. *J Am Soc Echocardiogr* 1996;9:295–299.
13. Lin SS, Roger VL, Pascoe R, et al. Dobutamine stress Doppler hemodynamics in patients with aortic stenosis: feasibility, safety, and surgical correlations. *Am Heart J* 1998;136:1010–1016.
14. Cosgrove DM, Rosenkranz ER, Hendren WG, et al. Valvuloplasty for aortic insufficiency. *J Thorac Cardiovasc Surg* 1991;102:571–577.
15. Perry GJ, Helmcke F, Nanda NC, et al. Evaluation of aortic insufficiency by Doppler color flow mapping. *J Am Coll Cardiol* 1987;9:952–959.
16. Reynolds T, Abate J, Tenney A, et al. The JH/LVOH method in the quantification of aortic regurgitation: how the cardiac sonographer may avoid an important potential pitfall. *J Am Soc Echocardiogr* 1991;4:105–108.
17. Taylor AL, Eichhorn EJ, Brickner ME, et al. Aortic valve morphology: an important *in vitro* determinant of proximal regurgitant jet width by Doppler color flow mapping. *J Am Coll Cardiol* 1990;16:405–412.
18. Masuyama T, Kitabatake A, Kodama K, et al. Semiquantitative evaluation of aortic regurgitation by Doppler echocardiography: effects of associated mitral stenosis. *Am Heart J* 1989;117:133–139.
19. Grayburn PA, Handshoe R, Smith MD, et al. Quantitative assessment of the hemodynamic consequences of aortic regurgitation by means of continuous wave Doppler recordings. *J Am Coll Cardiol* 1987;10:135–141.
20. Griffin BP, Flachskampf FA, Siu S, et al. The effects of regurgitant orifice size, chamber compliance, and systemic vascular resistance on aortic regurgitant velocity slope and pressure half-time. *Am Heart J* 1991;122:1049–1056.
21. Sutton DC, Kluger R, Ahmed SU, et al. Flow reversal in the descending aorta: a guide to intraoperative assessment of aortic regurgitation with transesophageal echocardiography. *J Thorac Cardiovasc Surg* 1994;108:576–582.
22. Takenaka K, Sakamoto T, Dabestani A, et al. [Pulsed Doppler echocardiographic detection of regurgitant blood flow in the ascending, descending and abdominal aorta of patients with aortic regurgitation]. *J Cardiol* 1987;17:301–309.
23. Savino JS, Troianos CA, Aukburg S, et al. Measurement of pulmonary blood flow with transesophageal two-dimensional and Doppler echocardiography. *Anesthesiology* 1991;75:445–451.
24. Kitabatake A, Ito H, Inoue M, et al. A new approach to noninvasive evaluation of aortic regurgitant fraction by two-dimensional Doppler echocardiography. *Circulation* 1985;72:523–529.
25. Reimold SC, Ganz P, Bittl JA, et al. Effective aortic regurgitant orifice area: description of a method based on the conservation of mass. *J Am Coll Cardiol* 1991;18:761–768.
26. Yeung AC, Plappert T, St. John Sutton MG. Calculation of aortic regurgitation orifice area by Doppler echocardiography: an application of the continuity equation. *Br Heart J* 1992;68:236–240.
27. Grimm RA, Stewart WJ. The role of intraoperative echocardiography in valve surgery. *Cardiol Clin* 1998;16:477–489.
28. Carpentier A. Cardiac valve surgery—"the French correction." *J Thorac Cardiovasc Surg* 1983;86:323–337.

SUGGESTED READINGS

Cosgrove DM, Rosenkranz ER, Hendren WG, et al. Valvuloplasty for aortic insufficiency. *J Thorac Cardiovasc Surg* 1991;102:571–577.

Maslow AD, Mashikian J, Haering JM, et al. Transesophageal echocardiographic evaluation of native aortic valve area: utility of the double-envelope technique. *J Cardiothorac Vasc Anesth* 2001;15:293–299.

Morehead AJ, Firstenberg MS, Shiota T, et al. Intraoperative echocardiographic detection of regurgitant jets after valve replacement. *Ann Thorac Surg* 2000;69:135–139.

Nowrangi SK, Connolly HM, Freeman WK, et al. Impact of intraoperative transesophageal echocardiography among patients undergoing aortic valve replacement for aortic stenosis. *J Am Soc Echocardiogr* 2001;14:863–866.

Odell JA, Mullany CJ, Schaff HV, et al. Aortic valve replacement after previous coronary artery bypass grafting. *Ann Thorac Surg* 1996;62:1424–1430.

Shively BK, Charlton GA, Crawford MH, et al. Flow dependence of valve area in aortic stenosis: relation to valve morphology. *J Am Coll Cardiol* 1998;31:654–660.

Stoddard MF, Hammons RT, Longaker RA. Doppler transesophageal echocardiographic determination of aortic valve area in adults with aortic stenosis. *Am Heart J* 1996;132:337–342.

Taylor AL, Eichhorn EJ, Brickner ME, et al. Aortic valve morphology: an important *in vitro* determinant of proximal regurgitant jet width by Doppler color flow mapping. *J Am Coll Cardiol* 1990;16:405–412.

10

ASSESSMENT OF THE TRICUSPID AND PULMONIC VALVES

REBECCA A. SCHROEDER
KATHERINE P. GRICHNIK
JONATHAN B. MARK

The tricuspid and pulmonic valves serve to separate the right heart structures and regulate the flow of blood from the periphery to the pulmonary vascular bed. Both valves are well assessed with transesophageal echocardiography (TEE) through multiple views and the full range of ultrasound. Detailed TEE assessment can elucidate the pathologic conditions and mechanisms that affect these cardiac structures.

STRUCTURE AND FUNCTION OF THE TRICUSPID VALVE

In contrast to the other cardiac valves, the tricuspid valve (TV) has three thin membranous leaflets that are not supported by a substantial fibrous annulus. The leaflets are less distinct than those of the other cardiac valves, separated more by indentations in a continuous sheet of tissue rather than true commissures. By standard designation, the TV consists of large anterior and septal leaflets and a smaller posterior leaflet. These three leaflets, attached to papillary muscles through their associated chordae tendineae and affixed to the annulus and a portion of the right ventricular (RV) free wall, make up the entire tricuspid apparatus (Fig. 10.1). The area of the TV is significantly greater than that of the mitral valve at 7 to 9 cm^2 (1).

The supporting structures of the TV tend to be more complex and variable than those of the mitral valve. The anterior papillary muscle is large and gives rise to the moderator band, a linear band of cardiac muscle that runs perpendicular to the papillary muscle, attaches to the septum near the apex of the RV, and may be mistaken for an intracardiac

mass. The posterior papillary muscle is frequently small and at times even absent.

The tricuspid annulus lies in a more apical position than that of the mitral valve, with its inferior margin adjacent to the junction of the inferior vena cava and coronary sinus. Beyond assessment of the anatomic structure and position of the tricuspid annulus, its systolic motion may be analyzed to provide important information about RV systolic function. Downward or apical movement of the annulus significantly augments RV stroke volume, even more than the corresponding effect of the mitral annulus on left ventricular ejection. With loss of annular motion, systolic shortening of the RV free wall decreases substantially, diminishing effective right heart function (2).

TRANSESOPHAGEAL ECHOCARDIOGRAPHIC EVALUATION OF THE TRICUSPID VALVE

Two-Dimensional and Color Flow Doppler

Evaluation of the TV, its supporting structures, and its function includes standard two-dimensional (2D) views, color flow Doppler (CFD), and spectral Doppler examination of the right-sided chambers, the TV, the venae cavae, and the hepatic veins. In some cases, TV images may be less well defined than typical mitral images because of the valve's distance from the probe and attenuation of the ultrasound signal by the fibrous mitral annular ring and the atrial septum.

The standard TEE imaging planes used for evaluating the TV have been well described by the Society of Cardiovascular Anesthesiologists/American Society of Echocardiography (SCA/ASE) TEE practice guidelines (Table 10.1) (3). The mid-esophageal (ME) four-chamber view is the most easily obtainable view of the TV (Fig. 10.2). In this view the atria and ventricles, the atrioventricular valves, and the atrial and ventricular septa are well seen. With regard to the TV, the ME four-chamber view displays the septal leaflet to

R. A. Schroeder and K. P. Grichnik: Department of Anesthesiology, Duke University Medical Center, Durham, North Carolina.

J. B. Mark: Department of Anesthesiology, Duke University Medical Center; and Department of Anesthesiology Service, Veterans Affairs Medical Center, Durham, North Carolina.

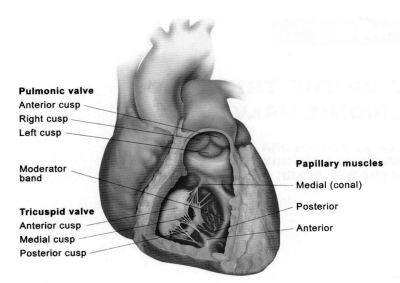

Pulmonic valve
Anterior cusp
Right cusp
Left cusp

Moderator band

Tricuspid valve
Anterior cusp
Medial cusp
Posterior cusp

Papillary muscles
Medial (conal)
Posterior
Anterior

FIGURE 10.1. Anatomic drawing of right ventricle, anterior view. Note the configuration of the leaflets of the pulmonic and tricuspid valves, the moderator band, and the tricuspid papillary muscles.

the right and either the anterior or posterior leaflets to the left, depending on the degree of TEE probe retroflexion. To image the TV in this view, it may be necessary to advance the probe slightly because the valve may be obscured by a calcified or prosthetic aortic valve. In this view, anatomic abnormalities of the TV are easily seen, as well as the relative sizes of the right atrium (RA) and ventricle that may result from tricuspid pathology. Color flow Doppler examination of the TV shows the presence of tricuspid regurgitation (TR). However, due to the complex three-dimensional structure of this valve, one should interrogate the valve with CFD throughout its superior-to-inferior aspect and across its transverse dimension (0, 30, and 60 degrees). Spectral Doppler examination of the valve may be attempted in the standard ME four-chamber view, but the angle of interception between blood flow and the ultrasound beam is frequently too high to yield an accurate result. At the same ME level, transducer rotation to 60 to 90 degrees displays

the RV inflow–outflow view (Fig. 10.3). In this view, the posterior leaflet of the TV appears to arise from the left side of the annulus and the anterior leaflet from the right (4).

Another imaging window for examining RV inflow may be developed easily beginning with the ME bicaval view (100–130 degrees of transducer rotation; Fig. 10.4A and B) and applying slight counterclockwise probe rotation (Fig. 10.4C and D). In this view, the basal RV and portions of the TV appear in the left far field and allow evaluation of TV inflow and possible regurgitation. One advantage of this view is that the ultrasound beam and the direction of flow are closely aligned, allowing accurate spectral Doppler measurements across the TV.

Transgastric (TG) views of the TV are useful, although slightly more difficult to obtain. The TG RV inflow view is developed from the TG short-axis (SAX) view of the left

(*text continues on page 143*)

TABLE 10.1. SUGGESTED VIEWS FOR IMAGING TRICUSPID VALVE

View	Transducer Position (degrees)	Structures Imaged
Mid-esophageal four-chamber	0–10	RA, RV, TV, IAS, IVS, LA, LV
Mid-esophageal RV inflow-outflow	60–90	TV, RV, RVOT, PV, AV
Mid-esophageal bicaval	100–120	RA, LA, IAS, SVC, IVC
Mid-esophageal RV inflow	110–130	RV, TV, RA
Transgastric TV (short axis)	0–20	TV (anterior, posterior, septal leaflets)
Transgastric RV inflow (long axis)	100–120	RV, TV, RA, chordae, papillary muscles
Transgastric hepatic	100–120	Hepatic veins

RA, right atrium; RV, right ventricle; TV, tricuspid valve; IAS, interatrial septum; IVS, interventricular septum; LA, left atrium; LV, left ventricle; RVOT, right ventricular outflow tract; PV, pulmonic valve; AV, aortic valve; SVC, superior vena cava; IVC, inferior vena cava.

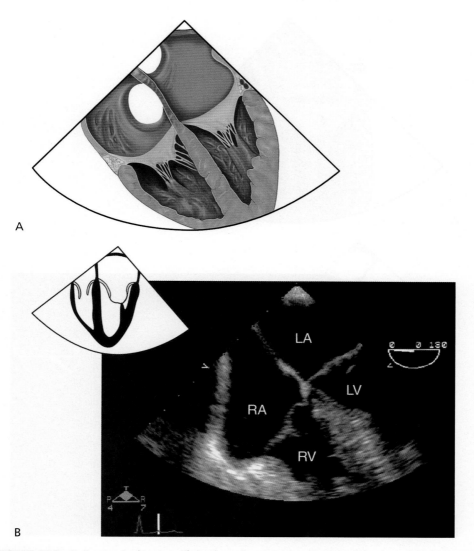

A

B

FIGURE 10.2. **A:** Anatomic drawing of the four-chamber view. **B:** TEE of the four-chamber view with corresponding schematic, and chambers labeled. *LA,* left atrium; *LV,* left ventricle; *RA,* right atrium; *RV,* right ventricle.

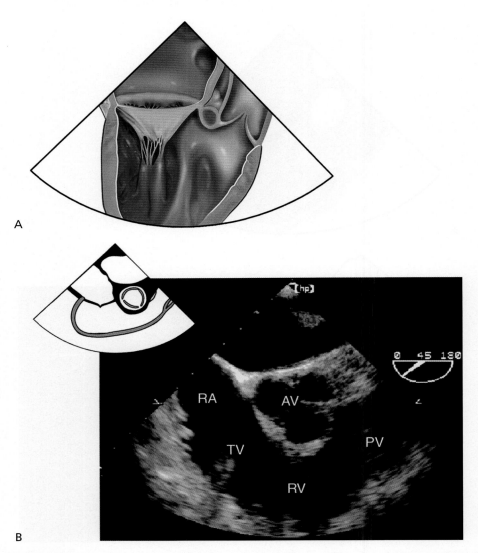

FIGURE 10.3. A: Anatomic drawing of right ventricular inflow–outflow view. **B:** Transesophageal echocardiography of the inflow–outflow view with corresponding schematic, chambers, and structures labeled. This is a good window through which to interrogate the tricuspid and pulmonic valves with color flow Doppler. *TV,* tricuspid valve; *RA,* right atrium; *RV,* right ventrium; *PV,* pulmonic valve; *AV,* aortic valve.

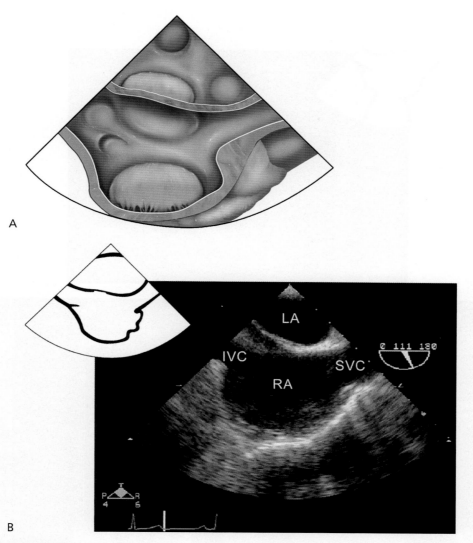

FIGURE 10.4. A: Anatomic drawing of the bicaval view. **B:** Transesophageal echocardiography (TEE) of the bicaval view with corresponding schematic, and chambers labeled.   (*Continued*)

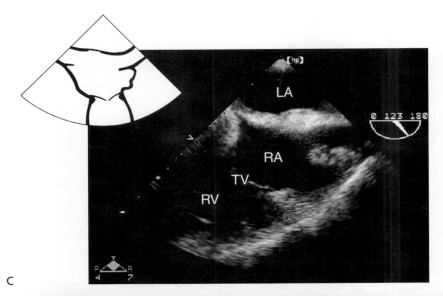

C

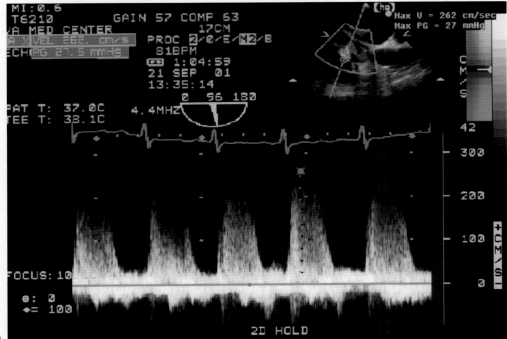

D

FIGURE 10.4. (*continued*). **C:** TEE of the modified bicaval view with corresponding schematic. This is an excellent view for Doppler interrogation of the tricuspid valve. Note prominent crista terminalis as a normal structure. **D:** Doppler interrogation of the tricuspid valve from the modified bicaval view. In this view the intersection of the direction of flow and the ultrasound beam is less than 20 degrees. *LA,* left atrium; *RA,* right atrium; *IVC,* inferior vena cava; *SVC,* superior vena cava; *RV,* right ventricle; *TV,* tricuspid valve.

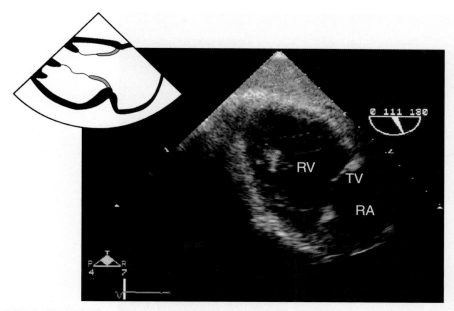

FIGURE 10.5. Transesophageal echocardiography of the deep transgastric right ventricular inflow view with corresponding schematic drawing, chambers, and structures labeled. *RA,* right atrium; *RV,* right ventricle; *TV,* tricuspid valve.

ventricle by turning the probe slightly clockwise, centering the RV on the display, and rotating the ultrasound beam to 100 to 120 degrees (Fig. 10.5). This scan plane displays the RV to the left and the RA to the right, and provides the best view of the TV supporting structures, including the chordae tendineae and papillary muscles. A TV SAX view is also possible by centering the RV in the middle of the screen and pulling back slowly (Fig. 10.6). This is the best technique for identification of specific leaflet pathology. Also, at this depth

the TEE probe can be rotated further clockwise to image the hepatic veins.

Spectral Doppler

Spectral Doppler examination of the TV is best performed using the bicaval tricuspid inflow view, the RV inflow–outflow view, or the ME four-chamber view, depending on which view provides the most parallel alignment of blood

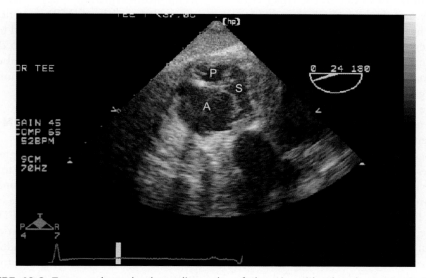

FIGURE 10.6. Transesophageal echocardiography of the tricuspid valve short-axis view with leaflets labeled. See text for details on obtaining view. *A,* anterior; *P,* posterior; *S,* septal.

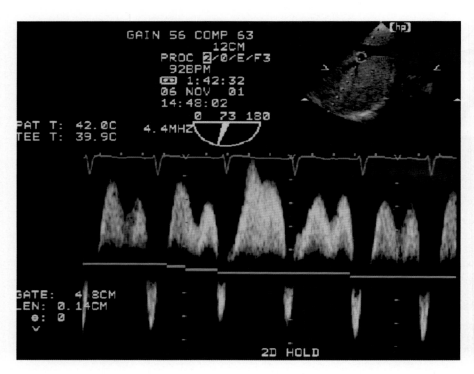

FIGURE 10.7. Transesophageal echocardiography of normal hepatic venous flow. Note the waveform deflections representing the systolic, diastolic, and atrial waves.

flow with the ultrasound beam. The sample volume should be placed between the leaflet tips during diastole to assess diastolic filling patterns. Characteristic early (E) wave and atrial (A) wave Doppler peaks correspond, respectively, to early ventricular filling and late diastolic filling from atrial contraction. Standard spectral Doppler measurements include isovolumic relaxation time (IVRT), E velocity, A velocity, E/A velocity ratio, and E-wave deceleration time. Typical patterns for TV inflow mirror those seen with mitral inflow and include impaired relaxation and restriction. Of note, tricuspid inflow patterns have lower absolute velocities than the corresponding mitral inflow waves due to the larger cross-sectional area of the TV and the lower pressures generated on the right side of the heart.

Analysis of hepatic venous flow patterns can provide useful information concerning TV and RV function. Normal venous flow in the hepatic veins is similar to pulmonary venous flow, with antegrade systolic (S) and diastolic (D) waves, and a retrograde A wave resulting from atrial contraction (Fig. 10.7). In addition, a small retrograde wave is sometimes observed at end-systole and designated a V wave, likely resulting from tricuspid annular recoil at end-systole. As RA pressure increases, the S wave and the S/D ratio decrease while the A wave increases. Severe TR obliterates the antegrade S wave and produces a reversed flow pattern during systole (Fig. 10.8B). In patients with atrial fibrillation, no A wave is seen in the hepatic venous or TV inflow patterns due to the lack of organized atrial contraction.

Spectral Doppler assessment of the TV can provide a significant amount of hemodynamic information. Pulmonary artery (PA) systolic pressure may be estimated by measuring the peak velocity of the tricuspid regurgitant jet. Use of the simplified Bernoulli equation yields the peak systolic RV-to-RA pressure gradient that, when added to an estimate of RA pressure, provides an estimate of peak PA systolic pressure. In turn, RA pressure is estimated by imaging the inferior vena cava (IVC) and measuring its respiratory variation in spontaneously breathing patients. The IVC is easily imaged in the ME bicaval view, appearing on the left side of the display (Fig. 10.4B). If the diameter decreases by 50% or more during inspiration (sniffing), RA pressure is less than 10 mm Hg. As for any quantitative Doppler assessment, it is critical to align the ultrasound beam parallel to the flow vector. Misinterpretation may occur when high-velocity jets of mitral regurgitation (MR) or aortic stenosis (AS) contaminate the TR jet signal. It is helpful to look for low-velocity antegrade flow through the TV to differentiate these flow patterns. Contrast enhancement also may help make the spectral Doppler signal envelope more visible.

TRICUSPID REGURGITATION

In the normal population, mild degrees of TR are extremely common. TR may be seen in up to 93% of patients over 70 years of age, and has an overall incidence of 65% (5). In these normal patients, however, the jet is turbulent, of high velocity, and appears small with CFD imaging. More severe TR arises in patients with rheumatic disease, endocarditis, carcinoid heart disease, tumors, endomyocardial fibrosis, or mechanical valve trauma resulting from severe deceleration injuries or iatrogenic mechanisms such as cardiac catheters (Fig. 10.8A). However, the most common cause of significant TR is annular dilatation and changes in RV anatomy

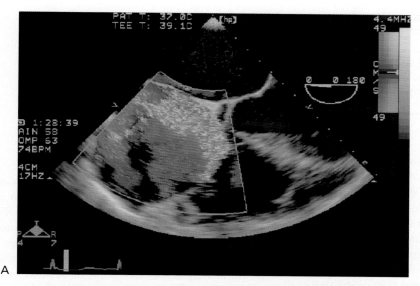

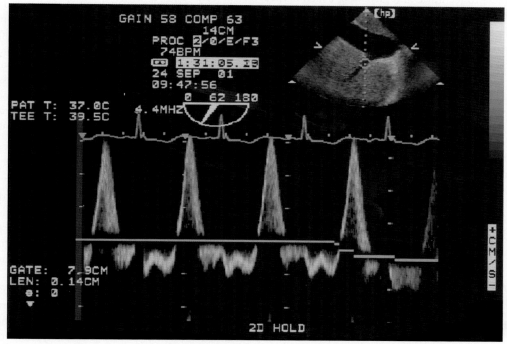

FIGURE 10.8. A: Transesophageal echocardiography of severe tricuspid regurgitation. Note the marked eccentricity of the regurgitant jet. **B:** Spectral Doppler evaluation of hepatic venous flow in the same patient with severe tricuspid regurgitation.

resulting from pulmonary hypertension, constrictive pericarditis, pulmonic stenosis (PS), and RV ischemia or infarct (6–8).

Assessing TR severity and deciding whether it is physiologic or pathologic may be difficult. Normal TR jet velocity is 2.0 to 2.5 m/s (9). Higher velocities may indicate pulmonary hypertension or PS, whereas lower measurements accompany more severe degrees of regurgitation.

Several methods are used to evaluate TR, and these should be viewed as complementary. On 2D examination, findings of RV volume overload suggest severe TR unless another cause is identified. These signs include RV and RA enlargement, flattening of the ventricular septum, dilatation of the tricuspid annulus, hepatic, or great veins, or leftward deviation of the atrial septum. The proximal isovelocity surface area (PISA) method of determining the size of the regurgitant orifice also may be useful in quantifying the degree of TR (10). In addition, pulsed-wave Doppler (PWD) analysis of hepatic vein flow may show reversed flow during systole (Fig. 10.8B). As always, clinical correlation is extremely important because chronic valvular disease can increase RA compliance and obviate many of these findings.

TABLE 10.2. GRADING TRICUSPID REGURGITATION

	Trace	Mild	Moderate	Severe
Distance from valve to most distal extent of jet (cm)	<1.5	1.5–3.0	3.0–4.5	>4.5
% of right atrium area		≤20	21–33	≥34
Area of jet (cm^2)	<2	2–4	4–10	>10

Several CFD grading systems for TR have been proposed. Two concentrate on estimation of the CFD regurgitant jet area, and the third focuses on the longitudinal extent of the jet into the RA (Table 10.2). All three systems classify TR into three or four grades that correspond to trace, mild, moderate, and severe regurgitation (11–13). Although these results correlate well with angiographic data, it is important to remember that all of these methods are semiquantitative at best, and subject to technical and physiologic factors that affect jet length and area.

TRICUSPID STENOSIS

Stenosis of the TV is most frequently of rheumatic etiology and in such cases invariably involves the mitral valve as well. Less common causes of tricuspid stenosis (TS) include methysergide toxicity, carcinoid heart disease, congenital anomalies, endocarditis, and endomyocardial fibrosis. Characteristic findings on 2D examination include doming of the leaflets during diastole, thickening of the leaflets, especially at their tips, restricted leaflet motion, and commissural fusion (Fig. 10.9). Spectral evaluation of TV inflow will show increased peak velocities (E waves >1.5 m/s) (10).

SPECIFIC PATHOLOGIC CONDITIONS OF THE TRICUSPID VALVE

Endocarditis

Transesophageal echocardiography is the most sensitive diagnostic test for detecting vegetations and perivalvular abscesses. Vegetations vary in appearance from flat, small, sessile lesions involving a single leaflet to large bulky, friable, echodense or oscillating masses that may obstruct flow through the valve (Fig. 10.10). The most common organisms are *Staphylococcus aureus* and *Pseudomonas aeruginosa*. Although endocarditis can affect any of the cardiac valves, tricuspid endocarditis is particularly common among intravenous drug abusers. It is important to evaluate the chordae tendineae and other supporting structures in any patient suspected of having endocarditis. Rather than the systemic manifestations commonly seen with left-sided endocarditis, tricuspid disease may be accompanied by pulmonary abscesses or infarcts (14–16).

Rheumatic Disease

Rheumatic heart disease may affect the TV in several ways. Rheumatic mitral stenosis or regurgitation eventually produce pulmonary hypertension, resulting in RV enlargement, tricuspid annular dilatation, and "functional" TR. Acute rheumatic carditis is characterized by edema and leukocyte infiltration with eventual erosion of the leaflet tips, leading ultimately to the formation of beadlike vegetations along the line of valve coaptation. Capillaries invade the vegetations during the healing phase, and fibrous nodules develop, frequently involving scarring and fusion of the chordae tendineae. At the site of healed vegetations, there is shortening of the free aspect of the cusps with chordal contracture and fusion between the cusps at the commissures. When this rheumatic process involves the TV, it usually results in TR rather than TS. Another distinguishing feature of primary rheumatic TV disease is that the RV is of normal size (4).

Ebstein's Anomaly

Ebstein's Anomaly of the TV is a congenital defect that occurs as an isolated malformation. The TV leaflets are displaced downward toward the RV apex, with the posterior, septal, and a portion of the anterior leaflets originating from the RV wall rather than the tricuspid annulus (Fig. 10.11A). The chordae are often missing altogether, and the leaflets are significantly redundant. The valve orifice itself is usually much smaller than normal and frequently incompetent. The "atrialized" portion of the RV remaining above the valve annulus is often thin and severely hypokinetic (Fig. 10.11B) (4,17). Clinical presentation is highly variable and related to the degree of TV displacement and the resulting distortion of RV anatomy and function. Generally speaking, the closer the valve is to the apex, the smaller the functional portion of the RV wall, and the more severe the hemodynamic derangement.

Carcinoid Heart Disease of the Tricuspid Valve

Carcinoid heart disease occurs almost exclusively in patients with hepatic metastases of their primary gastrointestinal tumors, or primary carcinoid tumors, such as ovarian, that do not drain into the portal circulation. Chronic

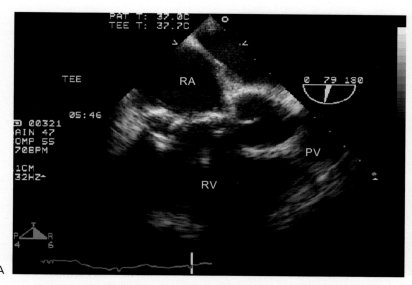

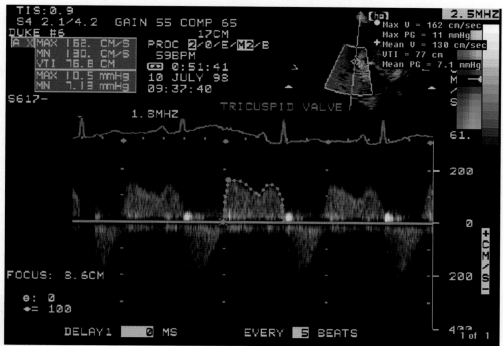

FIGURE 10.9. A: Transesophageal echocardiography (TEE) in a patient with severe tricuspid stenosis, chambers and structures labeled. **B:** 2-D *transthoracic echocardiogram* illustrating Doppler measurement of the tricuspid valve gradient in patient with severe tricuspid stenosis (and regurgitation) due to carcinoid heart disease. The tricupsid regurgitation can be seen as a mosaic of color flow in the right atrium. *RA*, right atrium; *RV*, right ventrium; *PV*, pulmonic valve.

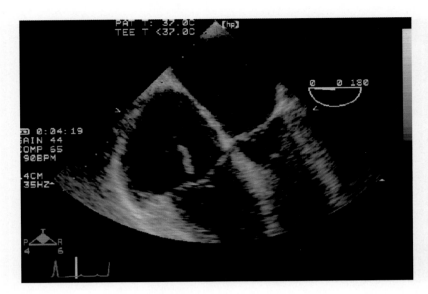

FIGURE 10.10. Transesophageal echocardiography of tricuspid vegetation in a patient with endocarditis.

right-sided cardiac valve involvement occurs in 50% of patients with carcinoid tumors and can be rapidly progressive (18). Chronic secretion of vasoactive amines such as serotonin and bradykinin leads to fibrosis of the endocardial surfaces of the right heart, including the ventricular surface of the TV and the pulmonary arterial surface of the pulmonic valve (PV). Echocardiographically, TV carcinoid disease results in short, thickened leaflets and eventually immobile, retracted cusps that may remain fixed in the open position (Fig. 10.12). TR is the most frequent lesion resulting from carcinoid heart disease, although the PV also can be involved. Of note, echocardiography has been used successfully to monitor patients being treated with somatostatin analogs. Cardiac surgical intervention is pursued in cases of severe valvular disease because carcinoid tumors are slow growing and carcinoid-related death more commonly results from cardiac failure than primary tumor growth (19).

Other Pathologic Conditions Affecting the Tricuspid Valve

Functional regurgitation of the TV results from annular dilatation, most frequently caused by chronic RV ischemia, cardiomyopathy, or volume overload (6–8). Enlargement of the annular ring causes relative displacement of the valve's supporting structures, leading to faulty coaptation of the leaflet tips and central regurgitation. Multiple jets are commonly seen.

Tricuspid valve prolapse is rare compared with mitral valve prolapse, and is remarkable if found in isolation. Prolapse of

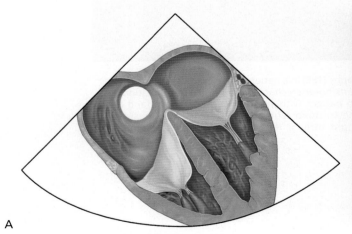

A

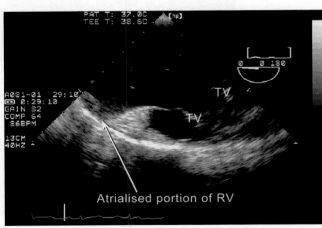

B

FIGURE 10.11. A: Anatomic drawing of valvular abnormalities in an Ebstein's Anomaly. **B:** Transesophageal echocardiography of a patient with an Ebstein anomaly. This was obtained from a four-chamber view with the probe turned to the right and advanced slightly. Note the thin portion of the right ventricular wall above the valve leaflet. *TV,* tricuspid valve.

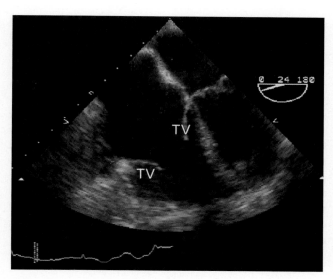

FIGURE 10.12. Transesophageal echocardiography of the tricuspid valve in a patient with carcinoid heart disease. The leaflets are fixed in the open position. *TV,* tricuspid valve.

the two atrioventricular valves usually coexists and is most commonly seen in patients with floppy valve syndromes such as Ehlers-Danlos syndrome, Marfan syndrome, Ebstein's Anomaly, or septum secundum atrial septal defects. Prolapse most frequently involves the anterior and septal leaflets and usually results in an eccentric TR jet. Diagnosis of TV prolapse is made by identifying displacement of valve leaflet tissue beyond the annular plane into the RA (Fig. 10.13) (4).

Heart disease accompanying systemic lupus erythematosus (SLE) is characterized by myocarditis, pericarditis, and endocarditis that may involve the TV. Lesions are small, berry-shaped excrescences that appear on both the atrial and

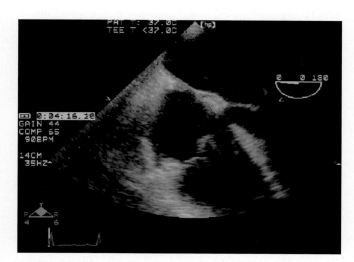

FIGURE 10.13. Transesophageal echocardiography in a patient with tricuspid valve prolapse. Note the prolapsed portion of the leaflet extending above the level of the valve annulus.

ventricular sides of the leaflets as well as on the chordae tendineae, papillary muscles, and the mural endocardium. Leaflets may become thickened and stenotic after multiple episodes of lupus endocarditis. The TV lesions of SLE may be differentiated from those caused by rheumatic disease based on the location of the vegetations. These appear only on the atrial side of the valve in rheumatic heart disease, but involve both sides in SLE (20).

Twenty percent of all cardiac myxomas occur in the right heart and frequently affect TV function by prolapsing into the TV annulus and causing dynamic valvular obstruction (10). Renal cell carcinomas may extend into the RA and TV, also causing obstructive symptoms. Papillary fibroelastomas may involve the TV and be difficult to differentiate from vegetations or clots (21). TV trauma, although rare, may result from deceleration injuries and blunt chest trauma, causing endothelial tears, hemorrhage into valvular cusps, or rupture of the papillary muscles and producing acute TR (22).

Artifacts

Many echocardiographic imaging artifacts may confound evaluation of the TV. In particular, pacing wires and intracardiac catheters may cause acoustic shadowing or be misinterpreted as intracardiac masses, clots, or vegetations (23).

STRUCTURE AND FUNCTION OF THE PULMONIC VALVE

The PV is trileaflet, similar in structure to the aortic valve, but has somewhat thinner leaflets because it functions in the lower-pressure ventriculoarterial system on the right side of the circulation. The three leaflets are designated the anterior, right, and left; the right and left cusps are both posterior to the anterior cusp (Fig. 10.1).

The basic semilunar valve structure of both the pulmonic and aortic valves consists of three cusps, associated sinuses of Valsalva, and a sinotubular junction. The structural similarity of these two valves results from their common embryologic origin. The annulus of the PV is ill defined compared with the aortic valve annulus. The pulmonary root is attached solely to RV muscle and forms the conus arteriosus. Thus, the pulmonic annulus is distensible because it is attached to ventricular muscle rather than to a stiff, fibrous annulus. The annular-sinotubular geometric relationships are assumed to be similar on the right and left sides of the heart, with the PA sinotubular junction 10% to 15% smaller than the PV annulus diameter (24). The anterior and right PV leaflets and their associated sinuses of Valsalva are minimally larger than the left. The area of the PV is about 2 cm^2/m^2 of body surface area, similar to that of the aortic valve (25). Additional shared anatomic features are the nodulus Arantii (small fibrous nodules on the free margin of the cusp) and the lunula (thin half moon–shaped areas along the free edge of each cusp that can have perforations not considered clinically important) (17).

TRANSESOPHAGEAL ECHOCARDIOGRAPHIC EXAMINATION OF THE PULMONIC VALVE

Transesophageal and transthoracic echocardiography are both used to visualize the right ventricular outflow tract (RVOT) and PV (26). TEE may provide additional helpful views when transthoracic echocardiography (TTE) is difficult or inadequate. However, the PV lies more anteriorly than the other cardiac valves, and thus also may be difficult to image with TEE due to its distance from the esophagus. Furthermore, visualization of all three leaflets of the PV is difficult with either TEE or TTE.

Transesophageal echocardiography of the PV relies on the standard imaging planes described by the SCA/ASE TEE practice guidelines (Table 10.3) (3). The first view is the ME aortic valve SAX view acquired at 30 to 60 degrees of probe rotation (Fig. 10.14). This scan plane displays the PV and the main PA to the right of the display, with the right posterior pulmonic leaflet appearing more posteromedial and the anterior pulmonic leaflet more lateral (26). Further rotation of the ultrasound beam to 60 to 90 degrees creates the ME RV inflow–outflow view, which demonstrates the RVOT, PV, and proximal PA on the right of the display (Fig. 10.3). Rotation of the probe to the right can improve the view and allow inspection of both the RVOT and a greater portion of the main PA. A third TEE view useful for PV imaging is the upper esophageal aortic arch SAX view, showing the PA and PV on the left side of the display (Fig. 10.15A). Turning the probe slightly to the left (counterclockwise) and retroflexing may improve the view of the PV. This is a good window in which to use spectral Doppler techniques to assess PS and pulmonary regurgitation (PR) because the ultrasound beamis aligned parallel to the PV flow vector (Fig. 10.15B).

Two other views can sometimes be useful in assessing the PV. Beginning with the TG RV inflow view at 100 to 120 degrees, adjustment of the multiplane angle back toward 90 degrees and anteflexing the probe can yield an image of the RVOT and the PV (Fig. 10.16) (3). A second view can be obtained from a deep TG view at 0 degrees. Turning the probe rightward (clockwise) and anteflexing can produce another window of the RVOT and PV. When assessing the PV using any of these scan planes, the RVOT and the main PA should always be assessed because abnormalities in either may influence PV function.

Color flow, PWD, and continuous-wave Doppler (CWD) echocardiography can be used to assess the PV. The orientation of blood flow through the PV is roughly perpendicular to flow through the aortic valve but is directed anterior-to-posterior and slightly right-to-left with respect to the patient. Color flow Doppler is used for qualitative assess-

ment of PR and PS in addition to defining the direction and velocity of flow, assisting in alignment of PWD or CWD measurements (Fig. 10.15).

In general, spectral Doppler measurements of antegrade peak PV velocities range between 0.5 and 1.0 m/s, with an average of 0.75 m/s (27). PS is defined as a gradient between the RV and the PA of 25 mm Hg, corresponding to a peak flow velocity of 2.5 m/s through the PV. Doppler flow patterns of retrograde flow through the PV may be used to estimate mean and end-diastolic PA pressures. The early peak gradient derived from the PR jet provides an estimate of mean PA pressure, whereas the late minimal gradient provides an estimate of PA diastolic pressure. In addition, PWD can be useful in assessing right-sided stroke volume and for calculating shunt or regurgitant fractions.

PULMONIC REGURGITATION

Pulmonic regurgitation can easily be evaluated using CFD to map the regurgitant jet in the RVOT (Fig. 10.17B). Trace to mild PR should be considered a normal variant when the CFD jet is less than 1 cm in length and not pandiastolic. Abnormal PR is diagnosed by a jet of greater than 1 cm in length that continues throughout diastole. Clinically significant PR is suggested by a color jet of greater than 2 cm into the RVOT or a regurgitant jet that extends to within 1 cm of the TV. Other features of significant PR include a peak jet velocity by PWD of greater than 2.5 m/s and holodiastolic flow (28,29). One cannot rely on turbulent flow to identify PR because moderate regurgitant jets may appear laminar owing to the small PA–RV pressure gradient. Furthermore, PR jet velocity may vary with respiration; several cardiac cycles may need to be averaged for accurate measurement of flow velocity. Jets of PR are usually central but may be eccentric as a result of a prolapsed leaflet. Color M-mode of the RVOT can confirm PR in the setting of tachycardia (30).

Pulmonic Stenosis

Pulmonic stenosis is characterized by leaflet doming, due to commissural fusion or leaflet thickening with restricted systolic motion. Associated echocardiographic findings include post-stenotic dilatation of the PA and its branches, with the left PA frequently appearing more dilated than the right (28,31). RV hypertrophy, a flattened ventricular septum (causing a D-shaped left ventricle), RA enlargement, and significant TR all suggest RV pressure overload. A search for coexisting congenital defects such as an atrial or ventricular septal defect should be performed.

Using CWD, the peak gradient across the PV is measured as an indicator of PS severity. A gradient of less than 25 mm Hg is considered mild and usually does not warrant intervention. A gradient of approximately 25 to 50 mm Hg reflects moderate stenosis, and greater than 50 mm Hg

TABLE 10.3. SUGGESTED VIEWS FOR IMAGING PULMONIC VALVE

View	Transducer Position (degrees)	Structures Imaged
Mid-esophageal right ventricular inflow–outflow	60–90	TV, RV, RVOT, PV, AV
Mid-esophageal aortic valve (short axis)	30–60	PV, main pulmonary artery
Upper-esophageal aortic arch (short axis)	0–20	PA, PV, aortic arch
Transgastric RV outflow	90	RVOT, PV
Deep transgastric outflow	0	RVOT, PV

TV, tricuspid valve; RV, right ventricle; RVOT, right ventricular outflow tract; PV, pulmonic valve; AV, aortic valve.

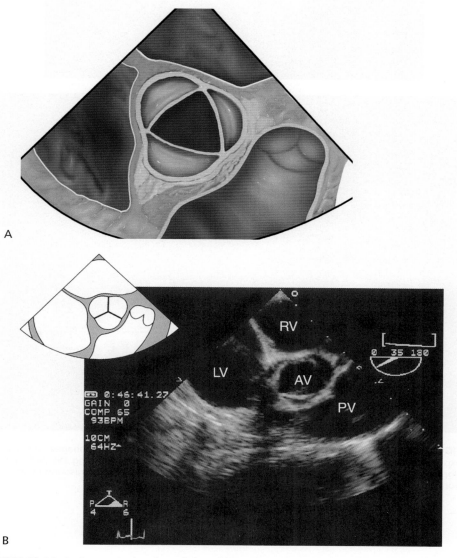

FIGURE 10.14. A: Anatomic drawing of the mid-esophageal aortic valve short-axis view showing the right ventricular outflow tract. Note the positional relationship between the aortic and pulmonic valves. **B:** Corresponding TEE with schematic drawing, chambers, and structures labeled. This is an excellent view in which to evaluate the pulmonic valve for the Ross procedure. *RV*, right ventrium; *PV*, pulmonic valve; *AV*, aortic valve; *LV*, left ventricle.

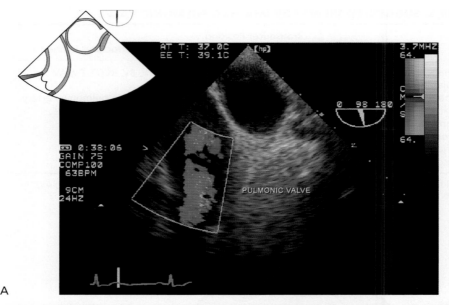

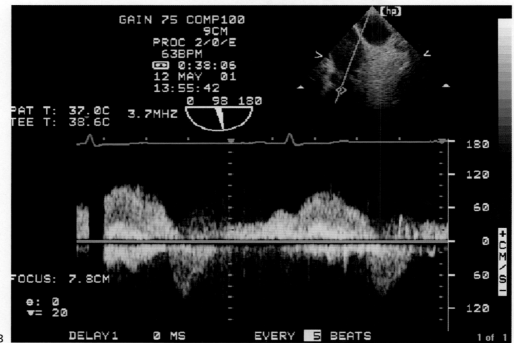

FIGURE 10.15. A: Transesophageal echocardiography (TEE) of the upper esophageal aortic short-axis view with color flow Doppler across the pulmonic valve. **B:** Corresponding TEE with spectral Doppler across the pulmonic valve. Note the alignment of blood flow and ultrasound beam direction.

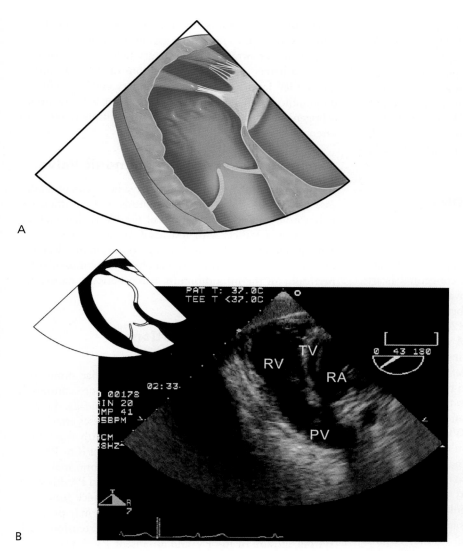

FIGURE 10.16. A: Anatomic drawing of transgastric right ventricular outflow view with pulmonic valve prominent. **B:** corresponding TEE with schematic drawing. Note that the right ventricular wall is well visualized. *TV,* tricuspid valve; *RV,* right ventricle; *PV,* pulmonic valve; *RA,* right atrium.

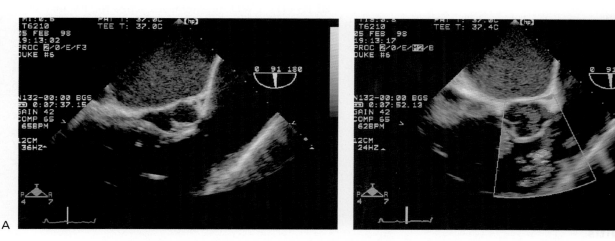

FIGURE 10.17. A: Transesophageal echocardiography (TEE) of right ventricular inflow–outflow view showing pulmonic valve and severely dilated ascending pulmonary artery in a patient with severe volume overload secondary to a long-standing atrial septal defect. **B:** TEE showing pulmonic regurgitation in the same patient.

is considered severe (28,29). Others have suggested that severe PS be defined by a gradient of 80 mm Hg and an RV systolic pressure of more than 100 mm Hg (25). The necessity for an intervention (balloon valvuloplasty or surgical repair/replacement) is determined by symptoms, such as exertional dyspnea, angina, or syncope, and documentation of severe stenosis by TEE or TTE. Stenotic PV lesions should be evident with CFD mapping as highly turbulent lesions with marked "aliasing" of the color signal within the proximal PA.

SPECIFIC PATHOLOGIC CONDITIONS OF THE PULMONIC VALVE

Congenital Diseases

Isolated RVOT obstruction in the adult population is rare and usually occurs as part of a complex congenital heart disease syndrome. Obstruction can be subvalvular, valvular, or supravalvular, with the most common being valvular PS. Supravalvular stenosis is characterized by PA narrowing, especially at the bifurcation of the main PA or its branches. It is often combined with other congenital abnormalities such as an atrial or ventricular septal defect or a patent ductus arteriosus. Subvalvular stenosis can be caused by infundibular or subinfundibular hypertrophy that results from primary valvular PS and often accompanies a ventricular septal defect (VSD). Unusual causes of RVOT obstruction include a right sinus of Valsalva aneurysm encroaching on the RVOT, postoperative mediastinal hematoma, sarcoma, or pericardial cyst. Outflow obstruction also may develop following repair of complex congenital heart disease (26,32). Complete RVOT obstruction, such as pulmonary atresia, presents in the neonate and never as an isolated lesion (33). Patients with pulmonary atresia or critical PS may require a shunt or other surgical procedure to repair or palliate this condition.

Valvular PS accounts for 10% to 12% of the congenital heart disease in the United States and is responsible for 90% of cases of RVOT obstruction (25). Congenital PS usually presents in newborns but may present in early adulthood after being asymptomatic for years. Other causes of valvular PS include commissural fusion, leaflet dysplasia, congenital bicuspid valve, rubella embryopathy, rheumatic heart disease, and senile calcification.

Transesophageal echocardiography is especially useful for monitoring patients during balloon valvuloplasty of the PV (34). Successful relief of PS is evidenced by laminar appearance on CFD and a reduced peak gradient by CWD across the valve.

Endocarditis

Isolated endocarditis of the PV is exceedingly rare, and the PV is the least commonly involved valve in cases of multivalvular endocarditis (35,36). PV endocarditis usually occurs in patients with predisposing factors such as a structurally abnormal valve, intravenous drug use, immunosuppression, or the presence of intravascular catheters such as PA and dialysis access catheters (37,38). Complications of PV endocarditis include RV failure and septic pulmonary emboli. Echocardiographically, PV endocarditis is seen as one or more mobile echogenic masses attached to the PV in multiple views, most often with coexisting PR.

Carcinoid Disease of the Pulmonic Valve

In a manner similar to tricuspid involvement, carcinoid disease affects the PV with both stenosis and insufficiency. Echocardiographically, carcinoid of the PV is characterized by thickened leaflets with restricted motion. Interestingly, acute palliation or relief of PS in this condition may lead to a hypercontractile RV with residual obstructing muscular hypertrophy in the infundibulum, parenthetically named the "suicide RV" (39).

Other Pathologic Conditions of the Pulmonic Valve

Papillary fibroelastoma is a rare benign cardiac tumor that occasionally involves the PV, although it more commonly affects the aortic valve (40). Echocardiographically, these tumors appear as small, mobile, echodense masses attached to the valve leaflets. They may be confused with vegetations from endocarditis but do not typically cause PR or PS.

Pulmonary hypertension also can cause abnormalities of PV structure and function. Secondary RV and PA dilatation stretch the PV muscular annulus and produce functional PR (Fig. 10.17). M-mode echocardiography may provide a useful clue for evaluation of pulmonary hypertension. Early systolic closure of the PV and an absent PV A wave occur with severe pulmonary hypertension, but not with valvular PS (41). PWD measurements across the PV may show rapid early systolic PA flow acceleration and mid-systolic slowing.

Prosthetic valves are rarely implanted in the pulmonic position. Prosthesis dysfunction, when it occurs, usually results in obstruction to flow. However, both PR and PS can be seen following the Ross procedure.

The PV may be injured iatrogenically during diagnostic or surgical procedures. Although PA catheterization has been incriminated as the cause of a flail anterior leaflet on the PV in one case, routine PA catheter placement does not cause significant PR (42).

SPECIAL PROCEDURES

The Ross Procedure

The PV can be harvested for use in another position, usually to replace the aortic valve in an operation known as the pulmonic valve autograft or Ross procedure (43). Early reports suggest that the PV also might serve as a mitral replacement (44). For these operations, intraoperative TEE is used to evaluate the structure of the PV as well as to measure the PV annulus and sinotubular junction dimensions (Fig. 10.14). The diameter of the PV annulus should be 10% to 15% larger than the diameter of the corresponding sinotubular junction. These measurements are compared with the aortic valve annular and sinotubular junction diameters. The aortic valve and PV measurements should be within 2 mm of each other to avoid dilation of either the sinotubular junction (causing commissural separation) or annular dilation; both conditions lead to autograft valvular incompetence. In a series of 81 patients undergoing the Ross procedure, David et al measured the range of aortic valve annulus diameters as 19 to 35 mm and the PV annulus diameters as 19 to 27 mm (24). In the situation of aortic valve and PV size mismatch, the aortic annulus can be reduced via plication and annuloplasty to achieve a geometric fit. It is also important to inspect the PV to be harvested for congenital abnormalities, incompetence, or stenosis, any of which would render it unsuitable for use as an aortic valve autograft. Furthermore, evaluation of PV size allows a homograft for the pulmonary outflow tract to be thawed in advance, shortening the cardiopulmonary bypass time (45). The harvested PV is then replaced with a PV cadaveric homograft.

After the procedure, suture lines from the PV homograft can be seen with few other differences noted compared to normal PV structure and function. Over time, though, PR or PS can develop, necessitating balloon valvuloplasty, PA stenting, or reoperation for PV replacement with a bioprosthetic or mechanical valve (46). Worsening aortic insufficiency is another primary cause of autograft failure. It is also important to evaluate LV wall function for new wall motion abnormalities because harvest of the PV may result in accidental ligation of a perforating septal coronary artery.

In a variation of the Ross procedure, the native aortic valve has been repaired and reinserted in the pulmonic position in a "semilunar valve switch" procedure. In one report, neopulmonic valvular stenosis was present in 54% of the patients undergoing this procedure (47).

KEY POINTS

- The TV apparatus is made up of a large anterior, small posterior, and small septal leaflets, a large anterior with small posterior and septal papillary muscles, an ill-defined annulus, and chordae tendineae.
- Primary TEE views to evaluate the TV include the ME four-chamber view, the ME RV inflow–outflow view, the ME bicaval tricuspid inflow view, and the TG RV inflow–outflow view.
- The best TEE view for estimating peak PA systolic pressure is the ME bicaval tricuspid inflow view because the

blood flow through the TV aligns with the Doppler signal. The best TEE view for estimating PA diastolic and mean pressures is the upper esophageal aortic arch view, in which the blood flow through the PV aligns with the Doppler signal.
- Tricuspid regurgitation is most often secondary to primary pulmonary or left-sided cardiac pathology.
- The peak flow of a TR jet, hepatic venous flow patterns, relative RA and ventricular size, and the appearance on CFD analysis of the regurgitant jet are all helpful in differentiating "physiologic" from pathologic TR.
- The PV apparatus consists of anterior, right posterior, and left posterior cusps with an ill-defined annulus, sinuses of Valsalva, and a sinotubular junction.
- Primary TEE views to evaluate the PV include the ME RV inflow–outflow view, the upper esophageal aortic arch view, and the TG RV inflow view.
- Multiple congenital conditions affect the PV, primarily to cause PS, but systemic diseases such as carcinoid and endocarditis can cause regurgitation or stenosis.
- The Ross procedure harvests the PV to place in the aortic position; the PV is replaced with a homograft.

REFERENCES

1. Hauck A, Freeman D, Ackerman D, et al. Surgical pathology of the tricuspid valve: a study of 363 cases spanning 25 years. *Mayo Clin Proc* 1988;63:851.
2. Isaaz K, Munoz L, Lee E, et al. Quantitation by Doppler echo of the motion of the cardiac base in normal man [Abstract]. *Circulation* 1989;80(suppl II):169.
3. **Shanewise JS, Cheung AT, Aronson S, et al. ASE/SCA guidelines for performing a comprehensive intraoperative multiplane transesophageal examination: recommendations of the American Society of Echocardiography Council for Intraoperative Echocardiography and the Society of Cardiovascular Anesthesiologists Task Force for Certification in Perioperative Transesophageal Echocardiography. *Anesth Analg* 1999;89:870–884.**
4. **Zaroff JG, Picard MH. Transesophageal echocardiographic (TEE) evaluation of the mitral and tricuspid valves. *Cardiol Clin* 2000;18:731–750.**
5. Klein AL, Burstow DJ, Tajik AJ, et al. Age-related prevalence of valvular regurgitation in normal subjects: a comprehensive color flow examination of 118 volunteers. *J Am Soc Echocardiogr* 1990;3:54.
6. Braunwald E. Valvular heart disease. In: Braunwald E, Zipes DP, Licina MG, eds. *A textbook of cardiovascular medicine.* Philadelphia: WB Saunders, 2001:1643–1722.
7. **Cohen SR, Sell JE, McIntosh CL, et al. Tricuspid regurgitation in patients with acquired, chronic, pure mitral regurgitation. I. Prevalence, diagnosis, and comparison of preoperative clinical and hemodynamic features in patients with and without tricuspid regurgitation. *J Thorac Cardiovasc Surg* 1987;94:481–487.**
8. Morrison DA, Ovitt T, Hammermeister KE. Functional tricuspid regurgitation and right ventricular dysfunction in pulmonary hypertension. *Am J Cardiol* 1988;62:108–112.
9. Oh JK, Seward JB, Tajik AJ. *The echo manual,* 1st ed. Boston: Little, Brown, 1994:178.

10. Otto CM.Echocardiographic evaluation of ventricular diastolic filling and function. In: *Anonymous textbook of clinical echocardiography.* Philadelphia: WB Saunders, 2000:358–359.

11. Miyatake K, Okamoto M, Kinoshita N, et al. Evaluation of tricuspid regurgitation by pulsed Doppler and two Dimensional Echocardiography. *Circulation* 1982;66:777.

12. Rivera JM, Vandervoort PM, Morris E, et al. Visual assessment of valvular regurgitation: comparison with quantitative Doppler measurements. *J Am Soc Echocardiogr* 1994;7:480.

13. Nagueh SF. Assessment of valvular regurgitation with Doppler echocardiography. *Cardiol Clin* 1998;16:405–419.

14. San Roman JA, Vilacosta I, Zamorano JL, et al. Transesophageal echocardiography in right-sided endocarditis. *J Am Coll Cardiol* 1993;21:1226–1230.

15. Clifford CP, Eykyn SJ, Oakley CM. Staphylococcal tricuspid valve endocarditis in patients with structurally normal hearts and no evidence of narcotic abuse. *Q J Med* 1994;87:755–757.

16. Ryan EW, Bolger AF. Transesophageal echocardiography (TEE) in the evaluation of infective endocarditis. *Cardiol Clin* 2000;18:773–787.

17. Netter FH. *Heart.* Summitt, NH: CIBA-GEIGY, 1981.

18. Moyssakis IE, Rallidis LS, Guida GF, et al. Incidence and evolution of carcinoid syndrome in the heart. *J Heart Valve Dis* 1997;6: 25.

19. Denney WD, Kemp WE, Anthony LB, et al. Echocardiographic and biochemical evaluation of the development and progression of carcinoid heart disease. *J Am Coll Cardiol* 1998;32:1017–1022.

20. Roldan CA, Shively BK, Crawford MH. An echocardiographic study of valvular heart disease associated systemic lupus erythematosus. *N Engl J Med* 1997;335:1424–1430.

21. Wolfe JT 3rd, Finck SJ, Safford RE, et al. Tricuspid valve papillary fibroelastoma: echocardiographic characterization. *Ann Thorac Surg* 1991;51:116–118.

22. Leszek P, Zielinski T, Rozanski J, et al. Traumatic tricuspid valve insufficiency: a case report. *J Heart Valve Dis* 2001;10:545–547.

23. Song MH, Usui M, Usui A, et al. Giant vegetation mimicking cardiac tumor in tricuspid valve endocarditis after catheter ablation. *Jpn J Thorac Cardiovasc Surg* 2001;49:255–257.

24. **David TE, Omaran A, Webb G, et al. Geometric mismatch of the aortic and pulmonary root causes aortic insufficiency after the Ross procedure. *J Thorac Cardiovasc Surg* 1996;112:1231–1239.**

25. **Brickner ME, Hillis LD, Lange RA. Congenital heart disease in adults: first of two parts. *N Engl J Med* 2000;342:256–263.**

26. **Shively BK. Transesophageal echocardiographic (TEE) evaluation of the aortic valve, left ventricular outflow tract, and pulmonic valve. *Cardiol Clin* 2000;18:711–729.**

27. Feigenbaum H. *Echocardiography,* 5th ed. Philadelphia: Lea & Febiger, 1994:101–675.

28. Kerut EK, McIlwain EF, Plotkin GD. *Handbook of echo-Doppler interpretation.* Armonk, NY: 1996.

29. Reynolds T, ed. The Echocardiographer's Pocket Reference, 2nd ed. Arizona: Arizona Heart Institute, 2000.

30. Savage RM, Aronson S, Shanewise JS, et al. Intraoperative echocardiography. In: Estafanous F.G., et al., eds. *Cardiac anesthesia.* Philadelphia: Lippincott, Williams & Wilkins, 1996.

31. Rumba MJ, Scott M, Walsh FW. Left hilar mass in a 62-year-old man: severe pulmonary valve stenosis with a poststenotic aneurysm. *South Med J* 1996;Aug 89(8):824–825.

32. Liau CS, Chu IT, Ho FM. Unruptured congenital aneurysm of the sinus of Valsalva presenting with pulmonic stenosis. *Cath Cardiovasc Interv* 1999;46:210–213.

33. Vargas-Barron J, Espinol-Zavaleta N, Rijlaarsdam M, et al. Tetralogy of Fallot with absent pulmonic valve and total anomalous pulmonary venous connection. *J Am Soc Echocardiogr* 1999;12:160–163.

34. Tumbarello R, Bini RM, Sanna A. Omniplane transesophageal echocardiography: an improvement in the monitoring of percutaneous pulmonary valvuloplasty. *Gior Ital Cardiol* 1997;27:168–172.

35. **Schaefer A, Meyer GP, Waldow A, et al. Images in cardiovascular medicine: pulmonic valve endocarditis. *Circulation* 2001;103:E53–E54**

36. Akram M, Khan IA. Isolated pulmonic valve endocarditis caused by group B streptococcus—a case report and literature review. *Angiology* 2001;52:211–215.

37. Kamaraju S, Nelson K, Williams DN, et al. *Staphylococcus lugdunnsis* pulmonary valve endocarditis in a patient on chronic hemodialysis. *Am J Nephrol* 1999;19:608.

38. Hearn CJ, Smedira NG. Pulmonic valve endocarditis after orthotopic liver transplantation. *Liver Transplant Surg* 1999;5:456–457.

39. *www.emedicine.com/emerg/topic/491.htm,* 2002.

40. Saad RS, Galvis CO, Bshara W, et al. Pulmonary valve papillary fibroelastoma. *Arch Pathol Lab Med* 2001;125:933–934.

41. *www.umdnj.edu//shindler,* 2002.

42. Sherman SV, Wall MH, Kennedy DJ, et al. Do pulmonary artery catheters cause or increase tricuspid or pulmonic regurgitation? *Anesth Analg* 2001;92:1117–1122.

43. Kouchoukos NT, Davila-Roman VG, Spray TL, et al. Replacement of the aortic root with a pulmonary autograft in children and young adults with aortic-valve disease. *N Engl J Med* 1994;330:1–60.

44. Kabbani SS, Jamil H, Hannoud A, et al. Mitral valve replacement with a pulmonary autograft: initial experience. *J Heart Valve Dis* 1999;8:367.

45. **Azari DM, DiNardo JA. The role of transesophageal echocardiography during the Ross Procedure. *J Cardiovasc Thorac Anesth* 1995;9:558–561.**

46. Hokken RB, Bogers AJ, Taams MA, et al. Does the pulmonary autograft in the aortic position in adults increase in diameter? An echographic study. *J Thorac Cardiovasc Surg* 1997;113:667–674.

47. Roughneen PT, DeLeon SY, Eidem BW, et al. Semilunar valve switch procedure: autotransplantation of the native aortic valve to the pulmonary position in the Ross procedure. *Ann Thorac Surg* 1999;67:745–750.

ECHOCARDIOGRAPHIC EVALUATION OF PROSTHETIC VALVES

SCOTT C. STRECKENBACH

An echocardiographer who is skilled at assessing prosthetic valves with transesophageal echocardiography (TEE) is in an optimal position to significantly impact perioperative patient care. TEE is critical for the diagnosis of prosthetic valve dysfunction due to endocarditis, thrombosis, dehiscence, or mechanical failure. However, prosthetic valve assessment is challenging for even the most experienced echocardiographers because each of the wide variety of manufactured valves has individual characteristic acoustic signals. In addition, the materials used in valve construction can create troubling acoustic shadows and reverberation artifacts that must be distinguished from real pathology.

The challenges involved in the echocardiographic assessment of prosthetic valves can be overcome if an echocardiographer can master the following three important objectives. First, the echocardiographer should develop a thorough understanding of the structure and mechanism of each of the commonly used prosthetic valves. Acquiring this knowledge initially requires reading, followed by direct experience through hands-on echocardiographic examination of different prosthetic valves. The best way to understand prosthetic valves is to inspect each one carefully and focus on the opening and closing mechanism. Accumulating this background knowledge will accelerate the rate at which each valve's acoustic signals can be recognized and understood. Second, the echocardiographer needs to develop a systematic examination for each prosthetic valve. The examination must include the appropriate views that will circumvent the prosthetic valve's acoustic shadows. In addition, the echocardiographic examination should include the use of zoom and slow-motion replay, both of which can be invaluable functions for detecting prosthetic valve dysfunction. Third, in order to become an expert at assessing prosthetic valve dysfunction, the echocardiographer should always compare the TEE findings with the surgical findings. Observing the sur-

gical procedure while the valve is being extracted provides an optimal learning opportunity not often gleaned by echocardiographic initiates.

This chapter focuses on the important features of performing a thorough intraoperative TEE examination of commonly encountered prosthetic valves. The structure, function, and characteristic acoustic signals of various prosthetic valves are reviewed. In addition, perioperative clinical case discussions are used to demonstrate the utility of TEE and its potential impact on perioperative surgical decision making.

STRUCTURE AND MECHANISM OF PROSTHETIC VALVES

The more commonly used prosthetic valves are listed in Table 11.1. The St. Jude Medical mechanical heart valve (St. Jude Medical, St. Paul, MN, U.S.A.) consists of an orifice ring, two semicircular leaflets, and a sewing cuff (Fig. 11.1). The two leaflets meet along a line that is outside the orifice ring. Two "pivot guards" are located on each side of the leaflet closure line and are designed to protect the leaflets. When closed, the leaflets lie 30 degrees to the plane of the orifice. When open, their position is 80 or 85 degrees relative to the orifice. The travel arc is therefore approximately 55 degrees. The open leaflets create one central and two lateral orifices that permit centrally directed flow (1). As the leaflets of a St. Jude valve close, a small amount of blood is forced into the proximal chamber, creating a transient regurgitant closing jet. All mechanical valves are associated with a small amount of transvalvular regurgitation. These closing jets are best appreciated during color flow Doppler (CFD) slow-motion replay. Bileaflet and single-leaflet mechanical valves also have washing jets that are designed to minimize the risk of thrombosis. These jets begin when the valve closes and persist until the valve reopens. Washing jets always originate from within the valve orifice. When the leaflets of the St. Jude valve are closed, washing jets originate at the orifice ring–leaflet interface and the leaflet–leaflet interface (2).

S. C. Streckenbach: Department of Anesthesia, Harvard Medical School; and Department of Anesthesia and Critical Care, Massachusetts General Hospital, Boston, Massachusetts.

TABLE 11.1. PROSTHETIC VALVE CLASSIFICATION

Mechanical valves
  Bileaflet valve
    St. Jude
    Carbomedics
  Monoleaflet valve
    Medtronic-Hall
    Bjork-Shiley
  Ball-Cage valve
    Starr-Edwards

Stented tissue valves
  Porcine aortic valve
    Carpentier-Edwards
    Hancock II
    Mosaic
  Pericardial-Edwards
    Carpentier-Edwards

Stentless tissue valves
  Toronto Stentless Porcine Valve
  Freestyle

Homograft
  Aortic
  Mitral

Valved conduit
  St. Jude
  Carbomedics
  Medtronic-Hall

The CarboMedics valve (Sulzer CarboMedics, Austin, TX, U.S.A.) differs slightly from the St. Jude valve (Fig. 11.2). First, the leaflet coaptation line lies within the orifice ring. Thus, pivot guards are absent. Second, the CarboMedics valve has a titanium ring between the orifice ring and the sewing cuff, making it more rigid. There are also similarities between the two valves. Both St. Jude and CarboMedics valves have a high orifice–to–sewing ring ratio and exhibit similar patterns of regurgitant washing jets. In addition, the CarboMedics valves and the later models of the St. Jude valve have the advantage of rotatability, implying that the leaflets and orifice ring can be rotated for optimal positioning after the valve is sewn into the annulus.

The Medtronic-Hall valve (Medtronics, Minneapolis, MN, U.S.A.) is the most commonly used single tilting disc valve. It consists of an orifice ring, a circular disc with a central aperture, and a sewing cuff (Fig. 11.3). The disc pivots on a central strut and actually elevates slightly as it opens to create a major and minor orifice. The leaflets move from 0 degrees to approximately 75 degrees in the aortic position, and 70 degrees in the mitral position during opening. The travel arc is therefore 70 or 75 degrees. The majority of antegrade flow passes eccentrically through the major orifice, the remainder through the minor orifice. Upon closure of the disc, a closing jet is created under the major orifice. While closed, small washing jets originate at the circular disc–ring interface, and a larger jet passes through the central aperture. The surgeon has the option of rotating this valve within the sewing ring.

The Bjork-Shiley valve (Shiley, Irvine, CA, U.S.A.) is no longer implanted in patients in the United States, although they may be encountered in some patients. This valve is slightly different from the Medtronic-Hall valve. It has a tilting disc that is held in place by inflow and outflow C-shaped struts. In early models, the disk only opened to 60 degrees. In an attempt to improve the hemodynamic profile of the valve, the Convexo-Concave model was created. Unfortunately, fractures in the C-shaped outflow struts that hold the disk in place have occurred. Some of these fractures have led to disk embolism and mortality (3,4). One way to differentiate the Bjork-Shiley valve from the Medtronic-Hall valve is to assess the regurgitant jets. Because the Bjork-Shiley valve does not have a central aperture, only peripheral jets are seen.

The Starr-Edwards valve (Baxter Healthcare, Edwards CVS Division, Santa Ana, CA, U.S.A.) is rarely implanted today, but because of its durability, many patients continue to present with this ball-and-cage valve. The orifice ring and stellite alloy cage constrain the up and down motion of a

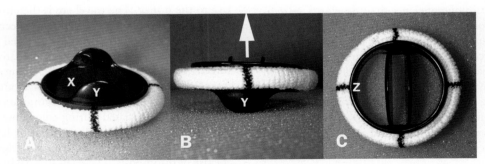

FIGURE 11.1. St. Jude mitral mechanical heart valve. **A:** Closed leaflets (*X*) and pivot guard (*Y*) viewed from the atrial perspective. Leaflets coapt above the plane of orifice ring at an angle. **B:** Open leaflets. The *arrow* defines the direction of flow. **C:** Open leaflets and orifice ring surrounded by sewing ring (*Z*) viewed from the ventricular perspective. Note one central and two lateral orifices. (Reproduced with permission from St Jude Medical, St. Paul, MN, U.S.A.)

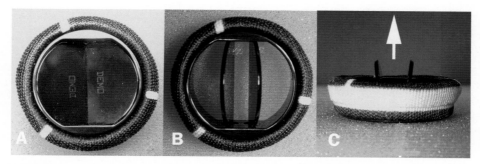

FIGURE 11.2. Carbomedics aortic valve. **A:** Closed leaflets from the aortic perspective. Leaflet coaptation line is within the orifice ring. **B:** Open leaflets from aortic perspective. **C:** Open leaflets demonstrating direction of flow (*arrow*). Note the absence of pivot guards.

silicone ball (poppet) (Fig. 11.4). The poppet moves to the top of the cage during ejection of blood. It returns to rest directly on the ring in diastole. Antegrade jets move around the circumference of the poppet and then converge downstream. A transient closing jet can be appreciated. Unlike the other mechanical valves, however, the Starr-Edwards valve does not have washing jets due to the direct contact of the poppet with the valve ring (Fig. 11.5). It is not surprising that the expected mean pressure gradient associated with this valve is higher than other mechanical valves. The combination of an increased mean transvalvular pressure gradient along with the valve's high profile (height) and the high risk of thrombus development have led to a decline in its use.

The stented porcine valve, as its name implies, consists of porcine aortic valve leaflets mounted on a stent (Fig. 11.6). The leaflets are treated to decrease antigenicity and the propensity to calcify. They open to a lesser degree than the leaflets in a native valve due to the leaflet treatment and the commissural supports (struts). The flow profile through the valve is similar to that through a native valve. Unfortunately, the sewing ring and struts decrease the effective orifice area, creating a nontrivial pressure gradient across most stented tissue valves. An important concept to remember is that valve sizes do not describe the internal orifice diameter but rather the outer diameter of the valve stent. For example, a 21-mm Hancock valve (Medtronics) has an orifice diameter

of 18.5 mm. This small orifice, coupled with the struts and slightly limited leaflet motion, significantly decrease the effective orifice area of any given valve. Stented tissue valves should have minimal regurgitation other than a brief closing jet. However, small and low-velocity regurgitant jets may be seen within the region of the commissures, particularly in the early post–cardiopulmonary bypass (CPB) period.

The pericardial valve consists of three leaflets constructed from bovine pericardium and mounted on a stent (Fig. 11.7). The sharp pericardial leaflet edges compared with the porcine valves can be demonstrated echocardiographically. Gross inspection of the pericardial valve reveals a central gap through which regurgitant flow is frequently seen in the early postoperative period, particularly during partial CPB. In addition, it is not uncommon with this valve to see small regurgitant jets more peripherally along the commissures. It is important to know that the majority of these jets decrease significantly, shortly after CPB.

Stentless valves have been designed to decrease the pressure gradient inherent in stented valves. The Toronto stentless porcine valve (SPV; St. Jude Medical) is an excised porcine aortic valve in which most of the sinus tissue has been removed. Consequently only enough aortic tissue remains to support the commissures and leaflets (Fig. 11.8A). A polyester (echoreflective) fabric around the base of the valve facilitates suturing, promotes tissue ingrowth, and

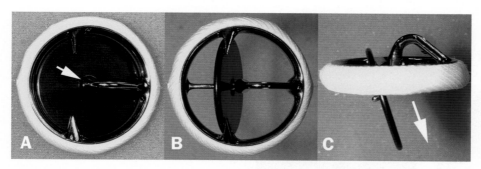

FIGURE 11.3. Medtronic-Hall aortic valve. **A:** Closed leaflet viewed from ventricular perspective. *Arrow* points toward central aperture with strut. **B:** Open leaflet. **C:** *Arrow* defines direction of flow through the major orifice.

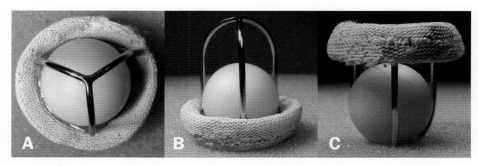

FIGURE 11.4. Starr-Edwards Valve. **A:** Closed valve viewed from above. **B:** Lateral view of closed valve. **C:** Open valve.

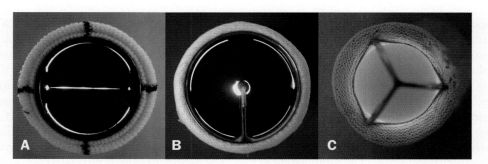

FIGURE 11.5. Mechanical valve regurgitant jet origin. A light source was projected through each valve in order to define the sites of washing jets. **A:** St. Jude valve. **B:** Medtronic-Hall valve. **C:** Starr-Edwards valve.

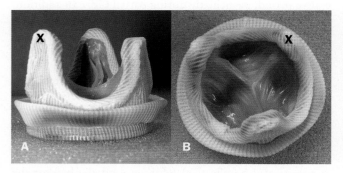

FIGURE 11.6. Stented porcine aortic valve designed for the mitral position (Hancock). **A:** Lateral view demonstrating commissural support component (strut) (*X*) of the valve frame. **B:** Viewed from above, a central gap is not present.

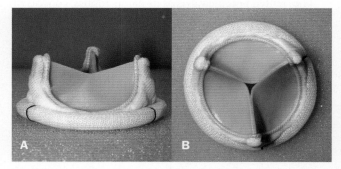

FIGURE 11.7. Pericardial valve (Carpentier-Edwards). **A:** Lateral view. **B:** View from above. Compared with a porcine valve, the leaflet edges are sharper, struts are smaller and a central gap is present.

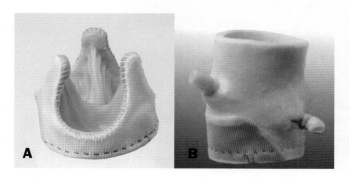

FIGURE 11.8. Stentless valves. **A:** Toronto stentless porcine valve. (Reproduced with permission from St. Jude Medical, St. Paul, MN, U.S.A.) **B:** Freestyle valve (Medtronics).

separates the xenograft from the patient's aortic wall. The valve is inserted with a subcoronary technique so there is no need for coronary reimplantation. Importantly, the patient's sinotubular junction must be small enough relative to the valve size to maintain leaflet coaptation.

The Freestyle valve (Medtronics) is an entire porcine aortic root (Fig. 11.8B) that also has an echoreflective polyester covering at the base of the valve. It provides the surgeon with more implantation flexibility (full root technique, root inclusion technique, complete subcoronary technique, and modified subcoronary technique) than the Toronto SPV (5). Depending on the technique used, coronary reimplantation may be necessary.

ECHOCARDIOGRAPHIC APPEARANCE OF PROSTHETIC VALVES

When the appropriate echocardiographic view of a bileaflet valve is obtained, two leaflets can be seen opening and closing. Where this view is obtained depends on the implanted valve position (e.g., mitral or aortic) and how the surgeon orients the valve within the annulus. When implanting a bileaflet valve in the mitral position, the surgeon can orient the valve such that the prosthetic leaflet commissure is parallel (anatomic) or perpendicular (antianatomic) to the native valve's commissure. Because diastolic blood flow through the native mitral valve (MV) is directed posteriorly, surgeons tend to insert a bileaflet MV prosthesis in the antianatomic position in order to increase the likelihood that both leaflets will open symmetrically, thus permitting flow to impact both leaflets equally. In the anatomic position, the anterior leaflet may not open as readily as the posterior leaflet. The orientation of the valve directly affects the multiplane angle at which one and two leaflets may be seen. When the ultrasound beam is perpendicular to the leaflet commissure or leaflet coaptation line (Fig. 11.9A), two leaflets are seen opening and closing. When parallel, only one leaflet is seen and its motion in the TEE image is limited. Figure 11.10 shows a St. Jude MV that was inserted in the antianatomic position with two-dimensional (2D) and CFD. When two leaflets are seen, several jets originate centrally and diverge laterally. In addition, small jets originate laterally and are directed perpendicular to the closed leaflet. When one leaflet is seen, two regurgitant jets originate laterally at the leaflet margins and converge toward the center of the valve.

Surgeons will generally orient a Medtronic-Hall valve in the mitral position such that the major orifice is directed posteriorly (6). The single leaflet of the Medtronic-Hall valve can be seen most optimally when the ultrasound plane is parallel to the strut (Fig. 11.9B). In this plane, the full excursion of the leaflet will be appreciated. A TEE deep transgastric (TG) and a mid-esophageal long-axis (ME LAX) view of a Medtronic-Hall valve in the aortic valve position is

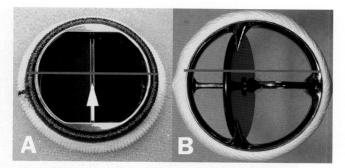

FIGURE 11.9. Transesophageal echocardiographic (TEE) viewing planes of mechanical valves. **A:** St. Jude valve. When the TEE plane is parallel to the red line, the two leaflets form an inverted V. Alternatively, when the plane is perpendicular to the red line or parallel to the closure line (*arrow*), only one leaflet will be seen. **B:** Medtronic-Hall valve. When the TEE plane is parallel to the red line and the strut, full leaflet excursion will be appreciated.

demonstrated in Figures 11.11 and 11.12, respectively. In both figures, the valve is aligned such that the major orifice is directed toward the noncoronary sinus. This alignment provides a flow profile that is as close to physiologic as possible for this prosthetic valve (7). The regurgitant jets associated with the Medtronic-Hall valve are distinctive. The predominant and distinguishing jet originates in the central aperture and is directed centrally. Two smaller lateral jets may be seen depending on how the ultrasound beam transects the valve. In the ME LAX view, only one jet will be seen if the ultrasound beam transects the central aperture because the strut will create an acoustic shadow (Fig. 11.12C). Both jets are more likely seen in the deep TG view (Fig. 11.11C).

A Starr-Edwards valve is echocardiographically distinct. Figure 11.13 demonstrates a Starr-Edwards valve in the mitral position. A significant acoustic shadow is created by the poppet and the sewing ring. The regurgitant CFD jet associated with the Starr-Edwards valve is a short-lived closing jet. There is no washing jet. The antegrade flow pattern consists of blood streaming around the poppet before converging downstream.

The TEE appearances of stented porcine and pericardial valves are similar. The leaflet motion in both valves approximates that of the native valve except for the slightly limited excursion. Figure 11.14 demonstrates a porcine valve (Hancock II) and a pericardial valve (Carpentier-Edwards) in the aortic valve position. In the ME aortic valve short-axis (SAX) view, the pericardial leaflets are more evident than those of the porcine valve. Struts can be recognized in the ME aortic valve SAX view, making it easy to differentiate a stented from a stentless valve. CFD may reveal occasional trivial regurgitant jets either centrally or peripherally at the commissures.

The stentless valve appearance varies with the implantation technique. In general, it is difficult to differentiate

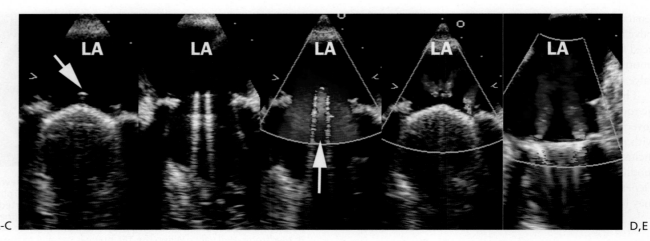

A-C   D,E

FIGURE 11.10. Transesophageal echocardiographic (TEE) views of a St. Jude mitral valve. **A:** Two-leaflet view, closed. The arrow defines the pivot guard. *LA,* left atrium. **B:** Two-leaflet view, open. **C:** Two-leaflet view, open with color flow Doppler (CFD). The arrow points to the central orifice. **D:** Two-leaflet view, closed, demonstrating regurgitant jets: three central jets that seem to diverge slightly, and one peripheral jet that is perpendicular with the closed leaflet. A second regurgitant jet originating on the other side of the valve also may be seen. **E:** St. Jude valve visualized with the TEE plane parallel to the closure line, and CFD demonstrating two laterally originating and centrally directed regurgitant jets.

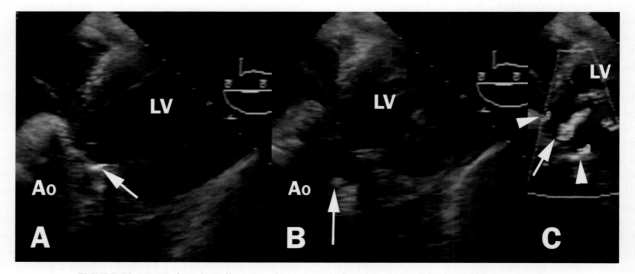

FIGURE 11.11. Medtronic-Hall aortic valve, transesophageal echocardiographic deep transgastric view. **A:** Closed valve. The *arrow* points to the closed leaflet near the noncoronary cusp. *Ao,* aorta; *LV,* left ventricle. **B:** Open valve. The *arrow* points to the open leaflet. Major orifice flow is directed toward the noncoronary sinus. **C:** Color flow Doppler reveals the predominant central jet (*arrow*) and small peripheral jets (*arrowheads*).

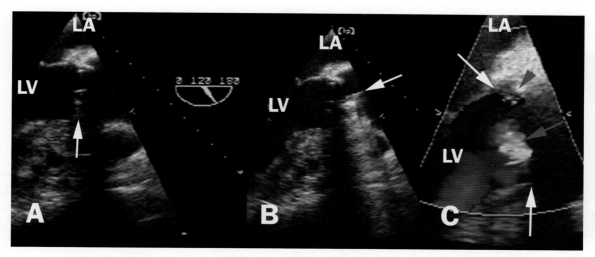

FIGURE 11.12. Medtronic-Hall aortic valve, transesophageal echocardiographic (TEE) mid-esophageal long-axis view. **A:** Closed valve. The *arrow* points to the leaflet at the level of the sewing ring. *LA,* left atrium; *LV,* left ventricle. **B:** Open valve. The *arrow* points to the distal edge of the open disc. Major orifice flow is directed toward the noncoronary sinus. Minor orifice is obscured by artifact. **C:** Color flow Doppler reveals a predominant central jet (*red arrow*) and a small peripheral jet (*red arrowhead*). White arrows define the sewing ring. Second peripheral jet is not seen at bottom of picture because of acoustic shadowing by strut. If TEE plane transects the valve off center, then two peripheral jets are seen without the central jet.

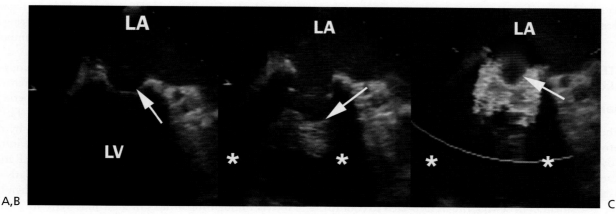

FIGURE 11.13. Starr-Edwards mitral valve visualized in a transesophageal echocardiographic mid-esophageal four-chamber view. **A:** Closed valve. *LA,* left atrium; *LV,* left ventricle. The *arrow* points to the poppet border. **B:** Open valve. The *asterisks* define acoustic shadows. **C:** Color flow Doppler reveals flow acceleration (*arrow*) around the poppet.

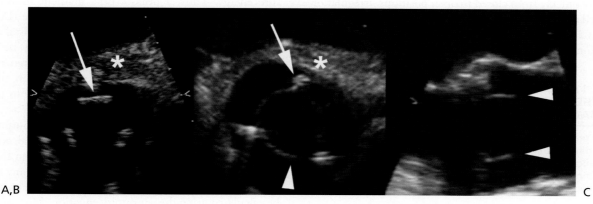

FIGURE 11.14. Transesophageal echocardiographic views of stented tissue valves. **A:** Porcine valve (Hancock II), mid-esophageal aortic valve short-axis view. Struts (*arrow*) are easy to see, but leaflets are not. The *asterisks* define postoperative edema. **B:** Pericardial valve, mid-esophageal aortic valve short-axis view. Struts (*arrow*) and leaflets (*arrowhead*) are easily visualized. **C:** Pericardial valve, TEE mid-esophageal aortic valve long-axis view demonstrating only leaflets (*arrowheads*).

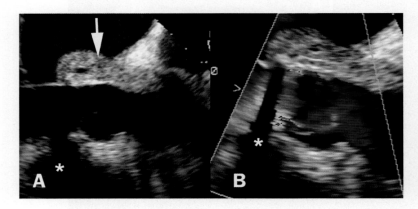

FIGURE 11.15. Freestyle (Medtronics) aortic valve visualized in the transesophageal echocardiographic midesophageal aortic valve long-axis view. **A:** The *arrow* defines the periaortic thickening consistent with postoperative edema. The *asterisk* defines acoustic shadow. **B:** Color flow Doppler accentuates the acoustic shadow.

a stentless valve from a native valve. However, increased echodensity present at the suture lines and the acoustic shadow created by the sewing cloth permit distinction. Figure 11.15 demonstrates a Freestyle valve that was inserted in a patient who presented with an infected porcine aortic valve prosthesis. A stentless valve can be differentiated from a homograft because the homograft does not create an acoustic shadow. No significant regurgitation is expected in the stentless valves.

SYSTEMATIC ECHOCARDIOGRAPHIC EVALUATION OF PROSTHETIC VALVES

General Concepts

Whether assessing a prosthetic valve in the immediate postoperative period or in the setting of suspected prosthetic valve dysfunction, performance of a systematic and thorough echocardiographic examination is essential (Table 11.2). The TEE examination typically begins with a 2D echocardiographic assessment. The sewing ring is inspected to confirm that it is well seated. A well-seated valve does not rock relative to the rest of the heart, nor does it have areas of circumferential echocardiographic lucency. The occluding mechanism should be evaluated to assure that the leaflets, discs, or poppet move quickly from closed to open positions. Irregular or restricted motion of one leaflet or disc at any time other than during CPB is abnormal. Low flow states, including partial separation from CPB, may be associated with asymmetric

TABLE 11.2. ESSENTIAL COMPONENTS OF A PROSTHETIC VALVE ECHOCARDIOGRAPHIC EVALUATION

1. Valve seating assessment
2. Occluding mechanism evaluation
3. Identification of any valvular or paravalvular regurgitation
4. Identification of any prosthetic valve stenosis
5. Identification of any unexpected mass on the sewing ring or leaflets
6. Evaluation of collateral cardiac structural involvement

leaflet opening. While studying the sewing ring and leaflets, abnormal echodensities representing sutures, fibrin strands, pannus, thrombus, or vegetation from endocarditis may be noticed (8–12).

Color flow Doppler is used to confirm the presence of normal antegrade flow, demonstrate expected washing jets (2,13), and rule out the presence of pathologic valvular or paravalvular jets. When looking for pathologic regurgitation, the entire circumference of the valve's sewing ring must be assessed. Perfunctory examinations can miss important pathology.

Pulsed-wave Doppler (PWD) and continuous-wave Doppler (CWD) are used to assess prosthetic transvalvular pressure gradients, and if necessary, the prosthetic valve area. In general, the mean gradient determined by TEE correlates well with the mean gradient determined by direct pressure measurement (14). However, the peak instantaneous prosthetic valve gradient determined by TEE may be higher than the gradient measured directly, particularly in the aortic position, due to pressure recovery (15). When blood travels through the orifices of a St. Jude valve for example, there is significant conversion of pressure energy to kinetic energy. This localized increase in blood velocity translates into a higher local pressure gradient. Downstream in the aorta, some of this kinetic energy is converted back to pressure energy. Thus, a peak-to-peak gradient measured directly [the difference between the left ventricle (LV) pressure and the aortic pressure measured in the distal ascending aorta using the cardioplegia catheter] may be significantly less than a TEE-determined peak instantaneous gradient, particularly for the St Jude valve. Both numbers are accurate, but the difference is due in part to pressure recovery.

In general, if the patient has a good cardiac output, if results of the 2D and CFD examination are normal, and if the pressure gradients are within normal limits, then the effective orifice area will be acceptable. However, if any of these three conditions are not met, the effective orifice area should be calculated using the continuity equation. Most prosthetic valves have an effective orifice area (EOA) that is less than a native valve, particularly when the valve size is small (16). The expected prosthetic valve EOA varies considerably with valve type, size, and position.

Whenever a prosthetic valve has been inserted and especially when it is dysfunctional, a search for involvement of other cardiac structures is necessary, particularly those contiguous with the valve in question. Insertion of a prosthetic MV can inadvertently cause aortic valve dysfunction. An abscess affecting a prosthetic aortic valve may extend into the anterior MV leaflet (17). Prosthetic MV endocarditis can seed the aortic valve. All of these findings may be critical to the patient's outcome.

Prosthetic Mitral Valves

The same TEE views used to assess a native MV also should be used to assess a prosthetic valve (18). Occasionally the TG basal SAX or deep TG views may be advantageous in some patients with a suspected prosthetic valve mass or thrombosis. Via the deep TG view, the LV side of the mitral prosthesis can be inspected. However, MV assessment should generally commence by obtaining an ME four-chamber view and centering the MV in the screen. The ultrasound beam is moved slowly and methodically from 0 to 180 degrees to scan the valve with 2D echo in order to assess the integrity of the suture line and the motion of the discs or leaflets. A search for abnormal masses on the leaflets or the sewing ring occurs concomitantly. Zoom and slow-motion replay should be used. Multiplane angle rotation from 0 to 180 degrees while applying CFD also should be used while searching for evidence of pathologic regurgitation. The CFD sector needs to be wide enough to see paravalvular jets but small enough to maintain a high frame rate. If a paravalvular leak is noted, its location should be identified. Figure 11.16 depicts a prosthetic MV mapping technique that helps describe the location of the paravalvular leak to the surgeon (19). This technique requires the echocardiographer to begin the examination with the prosthetic valve centered in the ME four-chamber view, and the echocardiographer to move in 10 degree increments looking for the regurgitant jet. If a jet is seen, the multiplane degree is noted. If the jet is on the left side of the valve as it appears on the screen, the jet should be mapped between 0 and 180 degrees. If the jet appears on the right side of the screen, the jet is mapped between 180 and 360 degrees (multiplane angle plus 180 degrees). After mapping the findings in the reference view (Fig. 11.16A), the view is transposed into the standard surgical view (Fig. 11.16B).

Next, the hemodynamic function of the valve should be assessed. The peak and mean gradients across the valve can be measured using CFD-guided PWD or CWD. The pressure half-time can be used as an index of valve function, but it does not accurately estimate prosthetic valve area (20). Alternatively, the continuity equation may be used to cal-

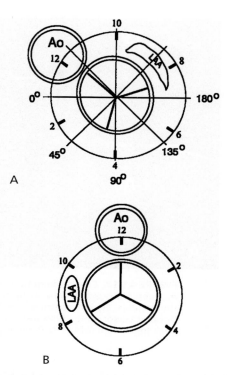

FIGURE 11.16. Prosthetic tissue mitral valve (MV) regurgitant jet mapping diagrams. **A:** Transesophageal echocardiographic perspective of the MV from the apex of the left ventricle. *Ao,* aorta; *LAA,* left atrial appendage. **B:** Surgeon's view of the MV from the right side of the patient. (Reprinted from Foster GP, Isselbacher EI. Accurate localization of mitral regurgitant defects using multiplane TEE. *Ann Thorac Surg* 1998;65:1025, with permission.)

culate the prosthetic MV area, albeit with some restrictions (21–23):

$$A_{PV} = \frac{0.785\ D^2_{LVOT} \times TVI_{LVOT}}{TVI_{PV}}$$

where A is area, D is diameter, PV is prosthetic valve, TVI is time velocity integral, and LVOT is left ventricular outflow tract. The LVOT may be used as the site for measuring forward stroke volume, assuming there is neither significant aortic insufficiency (AI) nor mitral regurgitation (MR). The presence of the former would lead to an overestimation of the prosthetic valve area, whereas significant MR would lead to an underestimation.

Prosthetic Aortic Valves

Inspection of the aortic valve requires two transesophageal views and at least one TG view. The ME aortic valve SAX view should be evaluated first to permit evaluation of bioprosthetic leaflet anatomy and excursion. All three leaflets should move symmetrically. Color flow Doppler can be used to identify valvular or paravalvular regurgitation. An ME aortic valve LAX view should be evaluated next. Rotation of the probe will provide a scan of the entire circumference

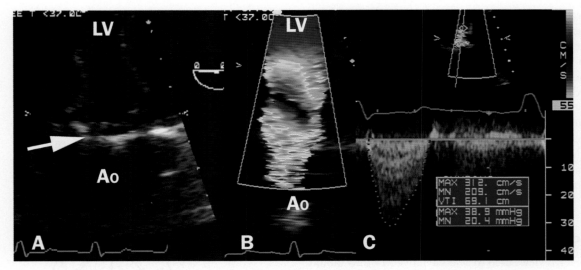

FIGURE 11.17. Echocardiographic measurement of a prosthetic transvalvular pressure gradient. **A:** Deep transgastric view of Starr-Edwards valve in the aortic position. The *arrow* points to the annulus. *LV,* left ventricle; *Ao, aorta.* **B:** Color flow Doppler used to align continuous-wave Doppler cursor. Color flow must be visualized distal to the annulus. **C:** Measured transvalvular peak [maximum (*MAX*) 38.9 mm Hg] and mean (*MN,* 20.4 mm Hg) pressure gradients.

of the valve's sewing ring. Although the proximal portion of a regurgitant jet will be masked due to acoustic shadowing (unless homograft has been implanted), a jet of pathologic significance will be appreciated in the LVOT. Assessment of a prosthetic aortic valve's disc motion and regurgitant jet anatomy is most optimally visualized in the ME aortic valve LAX, TG basal SAX, or deep TG views. Zoom and slow-motion replay functions can be particularly helpful. These same views should be obtained to determine the prosthetic valve pressure gradients and area.

The peak and mean pressure gradients should be determined in all patients (Fig. 11.17). Acceptable gradients depend on the valve size and the cardiac output. If the gradient is elevated (a mean of >20 mm Hg), or if the cardiac output is

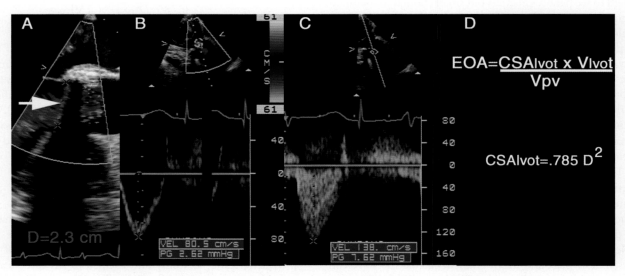

FIGURE 11.18. Continuity equation for measuring prosthetic aortic valve area. **A:** Transesophageal aortic valve long-axis view is obtained for measuring left ventricular outflow tract (LVOT) diameter in early systole (*D* = 2.3 cm) (*arrow*). **B:** LVOT peak velocity measured with pulsed-wave Doppler (*VEL* = 80.5 cm/s). **C:** Prosthetic AV peak velocity measured with continuous wave Doppler (138 cm/s). **D:** Continuity equation used to calculate effective orifice area (*EOA*).

low, the valve area should be measured (18). The continuity equation is valid in this setting (24,25):

$$A_{PV} = \frac{0.785 \, D^2_{LVOT} \times V_{LVOT}}{V_{PV}}$$

where V is peak velocity, and all other elements defined before. The peak velocity may be used in place of the TVI because the flow rate and prosthetic valve velocity are being measured in close proximity. Typically the LVOT diameter is measured in early systole, and the peak velocities are measured individually. The LVOT peak velocity is determined with PWD, and the prosthetic valve peak velocity with CWD. Figure 11.18 demonstrates the TEE images required to determine bioprosthetic valve area. If the LVOT is difficult to visualize, substituting the valve size as the LVOT diameter has been shown to correlate reasonably well with the actual orifice size (24).

An alternative to determining the peak velocities individually is to use the double envelope technique (26). With this technique, the peak LVOT and the peak prosthetic valve velocities are obtained in a single CWD envelope. Finally, a more simple but clinically useful method of assessing prosthetic valve area uses the Doppler velocity index (DVI), which is the calculated ratio of the LVOT peak velocity over the prosthetic valve peak velocity (24,26). The DVI obviates the need to determine the LVOT diameter, which is the measurement associated with greatest error in the continuity equation. In general, if the DVI is less than 0.25, the valve is considered to be significantly stenotic (26).

TRICUSPID AND PULMONIC VALVES

The echocardiographic assessment of the tricuspid valve (TV) is similar to that of the MV in that the transesophageal views usually provide enough information for a full evaluation unless there is concern of a possible mass on the right ventricular (RV) side of the valve. The pulmonic valve is rarely replaced but may be assessed in a similar manner to that for the aortic valve. In addition, an ME ascending aorta SAX view can be used to direct a CWD beam parallel to flow through the pulmonic valve to obtain a transvalvular pressure gradient.

PROSTHETIC VALVE COMPLICATIONS

In general, prosthetic valve malfunction can be associated with one of three problems: excessive regurgitation, reduced EOA, or valvular masses (e.g., thrombus or vegetation) (27). Excessive regurgitation can lead to hemolysis or, when se-

TABLE 11.3. PROSTHETIC VALVE COMPLICATIONS

Regurgitation
  Valvular
    Valve structural defect
    Surgical complication
    Bioprosthetic leaflet failure
    Mechanical leaflet malfunction
    Endocarditis
  Paravalvular (paraprosthetic)
    Severely calcified or diseased annulus
    Surgical complication
    Disrupted suture
    Endocarditis and abscess

Stenosis (decreased effective orifice area)
  Mechanical
    Inadequate leaflet opening
      Retained chordae tendinae
      Structural defect
      Thrombus
    Pannus formation
  Bioprosthetic
    Calcification
    Thrombus
    Pannus formation

Valvular mass
  Endocarditis
  Thrombus
  Pannus

vere, congestive heart failure (CHF). Patients with prosthetic valves that have a reduced EOA typically present with dyspnea on exertion. A mass on the valve may be associated with bacteremia (endocarditis) or stroke (thrombus or endocarditis). Table 11.3 summarizes the causes of valve dysfunction.

PROBLEM-ORIENTED CASE DISCUSSIONS
Preoperative Transesophageal Echocardiography Diagnoses

Case 1. Aortic St. Jude Valve Thrombosis

A 46-year-old patient presented in CHF, 13 years after receiving a St. Jude aortic valve prosthesis for severe AI of a congenital bicuspid valve. She had recently stopped taking coumadin. By TEE, one leaflet appeared immobile in a semi-open position. The second leaflet did not appear to open fully, but closed appropriately (Fig. 11.19A and B). This resulted in both AI and aortic stenosis (AS) (Fig. 11.19C). TEE revealed a transvalvular peak pressure gradient of 145 mm Hg. The surgeon found thrombus encasing the anterior leaflet and restricting the posterior leaflet. The valve was replaced with another St. Jude valve, and the dilated ascending aorta was replaced with a tube graft.

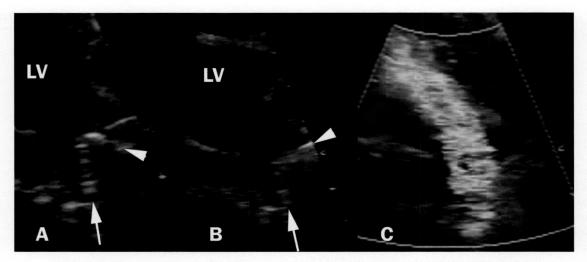

FIGURE 11.19. Case 1. Transgastric long axis views of a St. Jude valve in the aortic position during systole **(A)** and diastole **(B)**. One leaflet is fixed (*arrow*) while the other has restricted motion (*arrowhead*). *LV,* left ventricle. **C:** Severe aortic insufficiency demonstrated with color flow Doppler.

Comment

The patient's history was pivotal in the early diagnosis of this life-threatening situation. There are several reasons why patients might stop taking their prescribed anticoagulant therapy. When such a patient has a mechanical valve, TEE can confirm the diagnosis of thrombosis and expedite emergent surgery. An elevated transvalvular pressure gradient can be associated with prosthetic valve stenosis or severe regurgitation. The use of zoom and slow-motion replay were helpful in allowing the echocardiographer to identify the inhibited motion of one of the leaflets.

Case 2. Mitral Bioprosthetic Stenosis

A 74-year-old patient presented in CHF 12 years after undergoing mitral valve replacement (MVR) using a porcine aortic valve. The TEE examination revealed thickened and calcified leaflets (Fig. 11.20). Leaflet motion was severely restricted. Doppler assessment revealed moderate prosthetic mitral stenosis (MS) with a mean transvalvular pressure gradient of 7 mm Hg. The calculated MV area was not determined. There was mild MR but no paravalvular leak. There was also mild to moderate AI and a widely patent

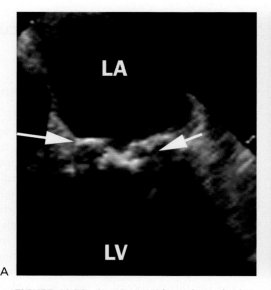
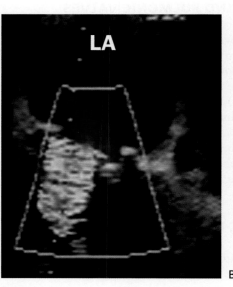

FIGURE 11.20. Case 2. **A:** Mid-esophageal echocardiographic view of a prosthetic porcine aortic valve in the mitral position with severe leaflet calcification. Arrows approximate the sewing ring. *LA,* left atrium; *LV,* left ventricle. **B:** Turbulent diastolic flow through narrowed orifice.

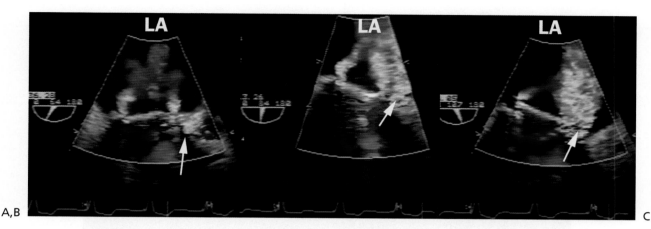

FIGURE 11.21. Case 3. **A:** Mid-esophageal view of a St. Jude mitral valve. The arrow defines the paravalvular leak. The two washing jets appear normal. *LA*, left atrium. **B and C:** The arrow defines a more significant paravalvular leak visualized after further multiplane rotation.

foramen ovale (PFO). Due to the patient's symptoms, the echocardiographic appearance of the valve, and the increased transvalvular pressure gradient, replacement of the dysfunctional prosthetic valve was recommended.

Comment

In a symptomatic patient with an MV bioprosthesis, the degree of leaflet immobility and calcification on 2-D echo is probably enough to warrant surgical intervention. Pressure gradient determination is also helpful. Using the pressure half-time method to estimate the MV area in this situation poses two problems. First, the pressure half-time method overestimates the true valve area of prosthetic valves (mechanical more than bioprosthetic). Second, the presence of a PFO will also lead to an overestimation of the true valve area since the PFO will allow faster decay in the left atrioventricular diastolic pressure gradient. Mitral valve area calculation using the continuity equation in this situation would be susceptible to error as well. The presence of AI and MR can lead to an error in the area calculation if the LVOT were used as the site of forward flow determination.

Case 3. Mitral St. Jude Valve Paravalvular Leak

An 81-year-old patient with a St. Jude valve in the MV position presented with a new murmur and anemia. Transesophageal echocardiography evaluation revealed a large paravalvular leak that spanned approximately 20% of the valve circumference (Fig. 11.21). The paravalvular leak was mapped to the 9 through 11 o'clock positions using the mitral prosthetic valve mapping technique (Fig. 11.22) (19).

Comment

In this case, the color jet appeared when the multiplane angle reached 54 degrees. The jet is on the right side of the valve as

the echocardiographer looks at the monitor (Fig. 11.21A). Any jet that is on the left side of the monitor is mapped between 0 and 180 degrees. Any jet on the right side of the screen is mapped between 180 and 360 degrees. Thus, a jet seen at 54 degrees on the right side of the monitor begins at a location that is mapped directly across from the 54 degree

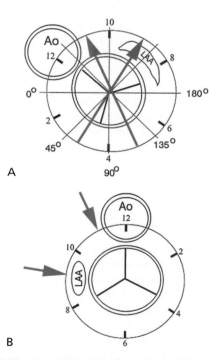

FIGURE 11.22. Case 3 (continued). Technique for mapping mitral prosthetic paravalvular regurgitant leaks. **A:** Transesophageal echocardiographic perspective of the mitral valve (MV) viewed from the left ventricular apex. *Red arrows* delineate the orientation of regurgitant leak determined from color flow Doppler. *Ao*, aorta; *LAA*, left atrial appendage. **B:** Surgeon's view of the transposed MV regurgitant leak orientation.

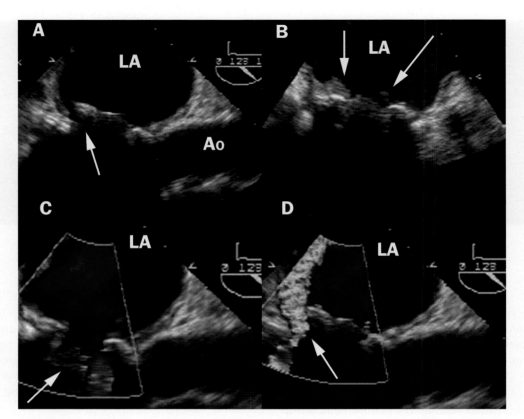

FIGURE 11.23. Case 4. **A:** Transesophageal echocardiographic mid-esophageal view of Starr-Edwards mitral valve endocarditis. The *arrow* defines the echolucent area consistent with partial dehiscence. *LA*, left atrium; *Ao*, aorta. **B:** *Arrows* point to vegetations. **C:** Color flow Doppler demonstrating diastolic flow around poppet (*arrow*). **D:** Posterior paravalvular regurgitation (*arrow*).

site, which is 234 degrees, or 9 o'clock. At 107 degrees the jet is still present on the right side of the screen. Therefore, the jet is localized to 287 degrees. or 11 o'clock (Fig. 11.21C). The area of regurgitation can then be translated into an image that represents the surgeon's view from the right side of the patient (Fig. 11.22B).

Case 4. Mitral Starr-Edwards Valve Dehiscence

A 42-year-old patient with MV prolapse experienced a bout of endocarditis and underwent a porcine MVR. The valve deteriorated several years later, at which time he received a Starr Edwards MVR. Thirteen years later he presented with left shoulder pain, fever, and shortness of breath. Blood cultures were positive for group B streptococcus. Transesophageal echocardiography revealed echogenic masses attached to the sewing ring (Fig. 11.23B). The echodensity of the masses was similar to that of the surrounding cardiac tissue. In addition, a paravalvular leak involving approximately one third of the annulus was demonstrated (Fig. 11.23D). Severe rocking of the prosthetic valve consistent with partial dehiscence was noted. Surgical inspection revealed large veg-

etations present on the sewing ring and around the valve annulus.

Comment

Because the echodensity of the masses was similar to that of surrounding cardiac tissue, thrombus or acute vegetation was more likely than chronic vegetation or pannus (11,12). Pannus and particularly chronic or "healed" vegetations typically have greater echodensity. The clinical setting and presence of paravalvular leak certainly supported the diagnosis of vegetations. This case also provides a good example of a significant area of echolucency indicative of partial valve dehiscence (Fig. 11.23A).

Case 5. Porcine Aortic Valve Destruction

A 63-year-old patient presented with CHF, 9 years after receiving a porcine aortic valve replacement (AVR). Her preoperative TEE revealed severe prosthetic valve AI due to apparent leaflet perforations (Fig. 11.24A and B). The surgeon found two torn leaflets (Fig. 11.24C) without evidence of sewing ring dehiscence or commissural separation from a strut.

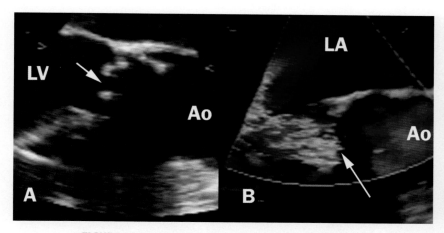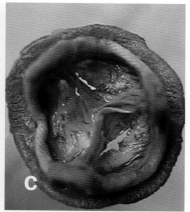

FIGURE 11.24. Case 5. Transesophageal echocardiographic mid-esophageal aortic valve long-axis view of a degenerated porcine aortic valve. **A:** The arrow points to an apparent hole in one of the leaflets. *Ao,* aorta; *LV,* left ventricle. **B:** Color flow Doppler demonstrating aortic regurgitation (*arrow*) filling approximately 60% of the left ventricular outflow tract. *LA,* left atrium. **C:** Gross specimen of explanted valve with leaflet perforations.

Comment

A common cause of tissue valve failure is leaflet destruction either by excessive calcification or perforation. Occasionally, one of the commissures will separate from the commissural support (strut), which creates flail of one or two leaflets. The color jet associated with perforation will usually be more central than the jet associated with a flail leaflet.

Case 6. Aortic Tissue Valve with Abscess

A 73-year-old patient underwent an AVR with a 23-mm porcine bioprosthesis. Twelve years later he presented with a febrile illness. A transthoracic echocardiogram (TTE) revealed evidence of valvular and paravalvular regurgitation. Intraoperative TEE revealed a rocking bioprosthetic valve with an abscess cavity in the intervalvular fibrosa (Fig. 11.25). The surgeon found a fluid-filled cavity in the posterior aortic root. The cavity extended into the base of the anterior MV leaflet. He elected to implant an aortic homograft and used the anterior leaflet component of the homograft to reinforce the area surrounding the abscess cavity.

Comment

This example of collateral damage demonstrates how an aortic root abscess can extend into the region of the adjacent MV via the intervalvular fibrosa. This region of mitral-aortic continuity is vulnerable to abscess extension or formation because it is the weakest segment of the aortic ring and contains mostly fibrous and relatively avascular tissue (27). It is critically important to diagnose the presence of an abscess in this region to avoid further devastating morbidity.

Case 7. Aortic Homograft Endocarditis

A 55-year-old patient with a homograft in the aortic valve position initially presented with vague symptoms. He was diagnosed with *Staphylococcus aureus* endocarditis. Antibiotics were started promptly, but his symptoms rapidly progressed. He developed myocardial ischemia in the right coronary artery distribution and suffered an embolic stroke. He was emergently taken to the operating room, where intraoperative TEE revealed a large anterior perihomograft space (Fig. 11.26). The surgeon therefore decided to cannulate the patient's femoral vessels prior to performing the sternotomy. The surgeon found a large nonhealing space between the noncoronary sinus and the homograft that was impinging on the right coronary artery. The repair included another homograft and coronary artery bypass grafts (CABGs).

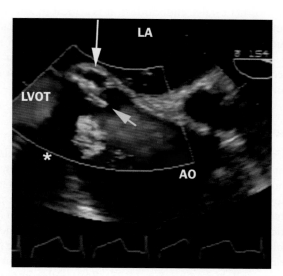

FIGURE 11.25. Case 6. Transesophageal echocardiographic mid-esophageal aortic valve long-axis view demonstrating porcine valve endocarditis with abscess. The *yellow arrow* depicts a strut. The *white arrow* points to an abscess cavity in the intervalvular fibrosa. *Asterisk,* acoustic shadowing; *Ao,* aorta; *LA,* left atrium; *LVOT,* left ventricular outflow tract.

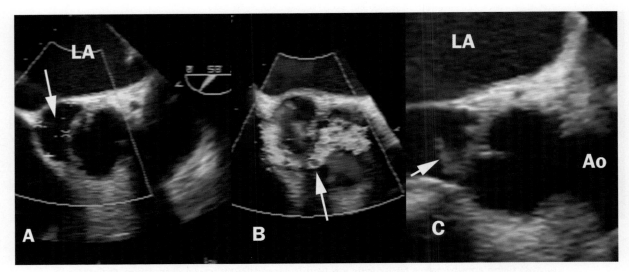

FIGURE 11.26. Case 7. Transesophageal echocardiographic views of aortic homograft endocarditis. **A:** Mid-esophageal aortic valve short-axis view. The *arrow* points to an abscess cavity. *LA,* left atrium. **B:** Color flow Doppler demonstrating communication between aorta and abscess cavity (*arrow*). **C:** Mid-esophageal aortic valve long-axis view. The *arrow* points to vegetation on the left ventricular side of the homograft leaflets. *Ao,* aorta.

Comment

Staphylococcus aureus endocarditis is rapidly destructive and requires immediate surgical intervention. It is important for the echocardiographer to communicate with the surgeon and become informed about the details of the operative procedure. In this situation, the surgeon chose to cannulate the femoral vessels due to the location of the abscess cavity, which was localized specifically by the echocardiographer prior to the incision. Whenever a patient presents with prosthetic valve endocarditis, it is critical to assess the circumferential cardiac tissue. An abscess cavity, fistula, or aneurysm may develop secondary to the infection. In this case, it is necessary to search for evidence of a fistula between the abscess cavity and the right atrium (RA) or left atrium (LA).

Case 8. Composite Root Fungal Endocarditis

A 67-year-old patient had a composite aortic root replacement with a St. Jude valve conduit. Four years later, an embolus to his lower extremity grew hyphae when it was removed and cultured. Despite antifungal therapy he presented with a perigraft aortic root abscess formation. An ME aortic valve SAX view revealed aortic root thickening and an echolucent area posterior to the valve sewing ring. The ME aortic valve LAX view confirmed the posterior echolucent area and wall thickening (Fig. 11.27). Both leaflets appeared free of endocarditis, and systolic flow seemed unimpeded. A 26-mm homograft was used to replace the composite root.

Comment

Echocardiographic evidence of abnormal thickening in the vicinity of the aortic root suggests the presence of an abscess, particularly when there is a contained echo-free area. Although vegetations can be found on tissue valve leaflets, they are infrequently found directly on mechanical valve leaflets. It is therefore not surprising that the leaflets appeared normal in the setting of a paravalvular abscess.

Case 9. Pericardial Mitral Valve with Leaflet Restriction

A 79-year-old patient underwent a pericardial MVR and a De Vega TV annuloplasty. The patient's postoperative period was complicated by pleural and pericardial effusions. One year later the patient presented with recurrent CHF. TEE assessment of the valve revealed focal leaflet thickening and impaired motion of one of the leaflets (Fig. 11.28A and B). Color flow Doppler revealed moderate MR (Fig. 11.28C). The mean transvalvular pressure gradient was 5 mm Hg. Surgical inspection revealed a white coating on part of the valve (Fig. 11.28D) consistent with pannus formation.

Comment

Pannus formation, also known as tissue ingrowth, can involve not only the annulus but also the tissue valve leaflets. The leaflet's edges in this case were also abnormal, possibly caused by the regurgitation previously initiated by pannus-induced leaflet restriction.

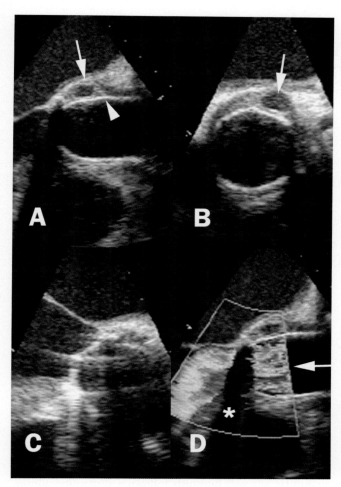

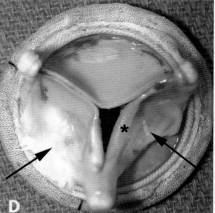

FIGURE 11.27. Case 8. Transesophageal echocardiographic views of a St. Jude valve conduit fungal endocarditis. **A:** Mid-esophageal aortic valve long-axis view. Abscess cavity (*arrow*) posterior to conduit (*arrowhead*). **B:** Mid-esophageal aortic valve short-axis view. Abscess (*arrow*) posterior to the conduit. **C:** Both St. Jude valve leaflets are free of apparent vegetation. **D:** Normal systolic flow demonstrated with color flow Doppler (*arrow*). *Asterisk*, acoustic shadow.

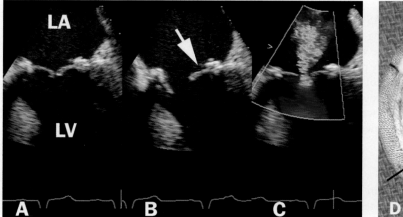

FIGURE 11.28. Case 9. **A and B:** Mid-esophageal echocardiographic views of a pericardial mitral valve. Both leaflets are thick. The arrow defines the restricted leaflet. *LA,* left atrium; *LV,* left ventricle. **C:** Color flow Doppler demonstrates central regurgitation. **D:** Explanted valve with pannus formation (*arrows*). Leaflet edges are thickened (*asterisk*).

Intraoperative Transesophageal Echocardiography Diagnoses

Case 10. Aortic Starr-Edwards Valve Paravalvular Leak

A 45-year-old patient with a history of repaired tetralogy of Fallot presented with symptoms of RV heart failure. At age 17, he had a ventricular septal defect repair and an RV outflow tract reconstruction. The original repair was complicated by injury to the aortic valve that required replacement with a Starr-Edwards valve. Over the ensuing years he developed severe pulmonary and tricuspid insufficiency along with trace to mild central AI diagnosed by TTE. He was consequently scheduled to undergo pulmonary valve replacement and TV reconstruction. In contrast to the preoperative TTE, intraoperative TEE revealed a large paravalvular leak around the aortic valve prosthesis. This echocardiographic finding significantly altered the operation by supporting the need for an unanticipated AVR (Fig. 11.29). Upon direct inspection of the aortic valve, the surgeon found a defect in the annulus at the site of the anatomic commissure between the noncoronary and right coronary cusps.

Comment

It is important to know what type of regurgitant jet is acceptable for each prosthetic valve. A Starr-Edwards valve should not ordinarily have significant central insufficiency with the exception of a closing jet. Although in this particular case the TEE was difficult due to the altered cardiac anatomy, the defect was further delineated after careful assessment using the Deep TG view.

Case 11. Aortic Pericardial Valve with Post-CPB Valvular Leak

An 85-year-old patient presented with severe AS due to a severely calcified, bicuspid aortic valve. Following extensive surgical debridement, a 23-mm pericardial valve with a reduced sewing ring was implanted. The immediate post-CPB TEE revealed regurgitant jets originating at each of the commissures (Fig. 11.30). Because the jets were of low velocity and had minimal LVOT penetrance, the valve was not replaced. A postoperative TTE 3 years later revealed no evidence of AI.

Comment

When assessing pericardial and porcine valves in the early post-CPB period, several small and low-velocity regurgitant color jets may be seen. These jets can occur in the central aspect of the valve, in the commissures peripherally, or along the sewing ring. Intravalvular jets typically are more significant prior to separation from CPB, and thereafter diminish. Those jets visualized along the sewing ring are usually due to suture holes, and diminish or even disappear after pro-

tamine administration. It is therefore important, when possible, to review the follow-up echocardiographic examination performed on patients who had questionable prosthetic valve insufficiency. In general, those jets that penetrate deep into the proximal chamber, those that demonstrate an area of visible proximal flow acceleration, and those that are of high velocity are more likely to require intervention. However, some regurgitant jets occur due to a heavily calcified annulus. In this situation the risk of valve revision may be excessive.

Case 12. Aortic Tissue Valve with Post-CPB Paraprosthetic Leak

A 78-year-old patient with three-vessel coronary artery disease (CAD) and severe AS underwent an AVR with a 25-mm porcine valve and a three-vessel CABG. The immediate post-CPB TEE revealed a regurgitant jet in the ME aortic valve SAX view that appeared to originate in the region of the right coronary cusp–noncoronary cusp commissure (Fig. 11.31A). A Deep TG view confirmed the presence of the jet that appeared to be paravalvular (Fig. 11.31B). After protamine administration, the regurgitant leak decreased significantly enough to convince the team that the degree of insufficiency was acceptable (Fig. 11.31C).

Comment

This particular regurgitant jet has some potentially worrisome characteristics, including high velocity, deep penetration, and wide vena contracta. However, many but not all similar jets will diminish following protamine administration. In the presence of a heavily calcified annulus, the surgeon may decide to accept the residual regurgitation. The surgeon also may wait, as in this case, with the expectation that the jet will diminish after protamine administration.

Case 13. Mitral St. Jude Leaflet Motion Impairment

A 57-year-old patient with rheumatic heart disease and a prior percutaneous mitral valvuloplasty presented for an MVR. Her preoperative TEE revealed severely calcified and thickened mitral leaflets and a high-velocity jet by CFD. Following native MV resection, a 25-mm St. Jude valve was inserted using Teflon pledgets on the LA side. The patient was successfully separated from CPB. Initial post-CPB TEE revealed normal movement of both leaflets (Fig. 11.32A and B), no paravalvular leak, and a normal transvalvular mean pressure gradient (3 mm Hg). Shortly after protamine was started, the pulmonary artery pressures (PAP) increased. Although a protamine reaction was initially suspected, TEE assessment in several imaging planes revealed that one of the leaflets was immobile (Fig. 11.32C). In addition, CFD

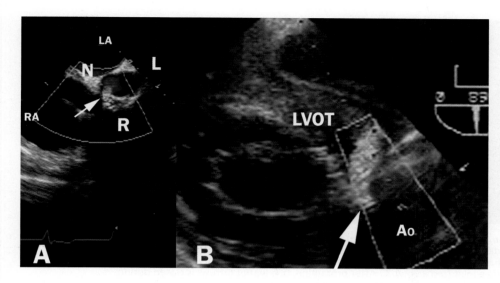

FIGURE 11.29. Case 10. Transesophageal echocardiographic views of a Starr-Edwards aortic valve. **A:** Mid-esophageal aortic valve short axis view. The *arrow* defines the origin of regurgitation at the annulus that corresponds to the commissure between the right (*R*) and noncoronary (*N*) cusps. *L,* left coronary cusp; *LA,* left atrium; *RA,* right atrium. **B:** Deep transgastric view with color flow Doppler demonstrating a wide, high-velocity and curved regurgitant jet that appears to originate outside of the sewing ring. *Ao,* aorta; *LVOT,* left ventricular outflow tract.

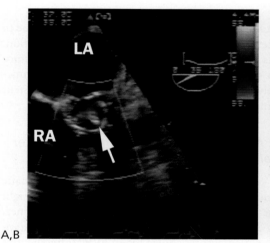

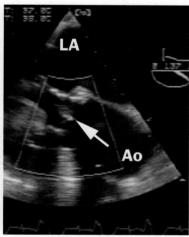

A,B

FIGURE 11.30. Case 11. Transesophageal echocardiographic views of a pericardial aortic valve. **A:** Mid-esophageal aortic valve short-axis view. Regurgitant jets (*arrow*) originate along each of the three commissures. *LA,* left atrium; *RA,* right atrium. **B:** Mid-esophageal aortic valve long-axis view. Regurgitant jet (*white arrow*) appears between the sewing ring borders. *Ao,* aorta.

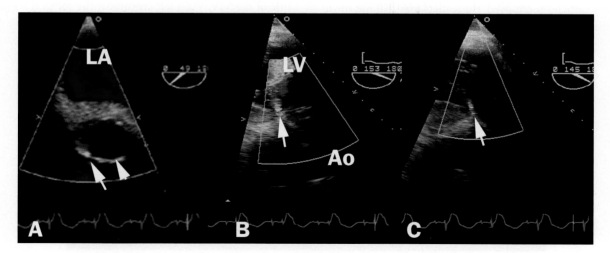

FIGURE 11.31. Case 12. Transesophageal echocardiographic views of a porcine aortic valve. **A:** Mid-esophageal aortic valve short-axis view. Small jet (*arrow*) appears to originate outside the sewing ring (*arrowhead*). *LA,* left atrium. **B:** Transgastric long-axis view. The regurgitant jet appears more significant demonstrating a higher velocity and deeper penetration (*arrow*). *Ao,* aorta; *LV,* left ventricle. **C:** After protamine, the jet is diminished (*arrow*).

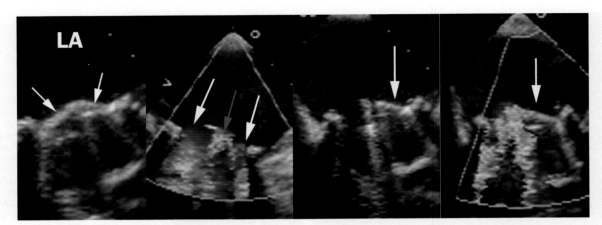

FIGURE 11.32. Case 13. Mid-esophageal views of a dysfunctional St. Jude mitral valve. **A:** Multiplane view at 60 degrees demonstrating bileaflet closure. *Arrows* define each leaflet. *LA,* left atrium. **B:** Normal diastolic flow in lateral orifices (*white arrows*). Transvalvular velocity is slightly higher in central orifice inlet (*red arrow*). **C:** After protamine, one leaflet (*arrow*) is closed during diastole. **D:** Transvalvular diastolic flow acceleration demonstrated with color flow Doppler.

revealed flow acceleration through the functioning side of the valve orifice (Fig. 11.32D). Furthermore, CWD was used to demonstrate an increased mean transvalvular pressure gradient (8 mm Hg). Cardiopulmonary bypass was reestablished to permit direct inspection of the prosthetic valve, which revealed small segments of the chordae tendineae between the sewing ring and the immobile leaflet. The chordae were carefully resected while the prosthetic valve was left undisturbed.

Comment

Direct inspection of a mechanical MV prior to left atriotomy closure may not guarantee normal function following separation from CPB. Prior to LA closure, the surgeon may keep the valve incompetent until intracardiac air is evacuated. Frequently this is accomplished using a Foley catheter. Once the Foley catheter is removed, the leaflets may still not move

properly. Often there is asynchronous leaflet opening due to inadequate flow through the valve. After CPB termination, the leaflets should begin to move normally. Rarely, immobility of a single leaflet may be observed, yet this dysfunction usually resolves spontaneously. Alternatively, persistent leaflet immobility may require surgical intervention.

Case 14. Mitral St. Jude Leaflet Immobility after Atrial Valve Replacement

A 66-year-old patient with a history of childhood rheumatic fever developed MS and underwent a St. Jude MVR. Eight years later she developed progressive exertional dyspnea. Following documentation of severe AS by cardiac catheterization, the patient was scheduled for an AVR. Intraoperative TEE revealed evidence of several small thrombi on the LA side of the MV. Via a left atriotomy, the surgeon removed a

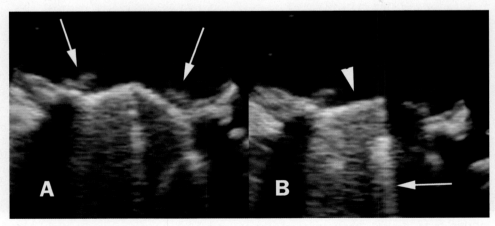

FIGURE 11.33. Case 14. Mid-esophageal views of St. Jude mitral valve thrombosis. **A:** Small mobile masses (*arrows*) on the left atrial side of the valve annulus. **B:** One leaflet is closed during diastole (*arrowhead*) while the other demonstrates adequate opening (*arrow*).

the venous lines transiently, which resulted in persistent moderate AI. After returning to full CPB, the valve was removed and inspected to reveal inadequate leaflet coaptation (Fig. 11.36C). A 23-mm Carpentier-Edwards porcine aortic valve was inserted and the patient recovered uneventfully.

Comment

Immediate echocardiographic evaluation of prosthetic valves is imperative. Hemodynamic stability does not guarantee proper valve function. In this case, the angle between the LVOT and the prosthesis was atypical. In addition, the eccentric and wide AI jet was enough to convince the surgeon to inspect the valve under direct vision.

Case 18. Porcine Mitral Valve Replacement Complicated by Aortic Insufficiency

A 74-year-old patient who had previously received a bioprosthetic MVR presented with MS and MR 12 years later. During resection of the prosthesis, the surgeon noticed an area beneath the aortic valve that appeared to have granulation tissue and fibrin, possibly representing a vegetation. The mitral prosthesis was subsequently replaced with a 27-mm porcine valve. Prior to separation from CPB, TEE revealed AI that had not been previously identified (Fig. 11.37). Close inspection while on partial CPB revealed apparent restriction of the left coronary cusp. The surgeon performed an aortotomy and noted that one of the MV reinforcement sutures had passed through the base of the left coronary cusp, restricting closure. A pericardial patch was used to facilitate a repair of the left coronary cusp. Postoperative TEE revealed only trivial residual AI.

Comment

Awareness of the surgical procedural details is imperative. It is critical to assess not only the prosthetic valve, but also to be cognizant of any potential collateral damage to the surrounding structures.

KEY POINTS

- A systematic echocardiographic examination sequence should be developed and followed during the assessment of every prosthetic valve.
- The zoom, slow-motion replay, and color suppress functions will facilitate the assessment of leaflet motion and valve regurgitation.
- All mechanical valves except the Starr-Edwards valve have specific washing jets. For any given valve, the washing jet appearance may be significantly different when viewing the valve in orthogonal planes.
- Most prosthetic valves are mildly stenotic. Transvalvular pressure gradients depend on valve size, valve position,

and cardiac output. In general, mean pressure gradients obtained echocardiographically correlate well with direct pressure measurements.

- It is imperative to understand the details of the surgical procedure prior to performing the post-CPB TEE evaluation. Direct communication with the surgeon throughout the operation is essential.

REFERENCES

1. Yoganathan AP, Chaux A, et al. Bileaflet, tilting disc and porcine aortic valve substitutes: in vitro hydrodynamic characteristics. *J Am Coll Cardiol* 1984;3(2):313–320.
2. **Flachskampf FA, O'Shea JP, et al. Patterns of normal transvalvular regurgitation in mechanical valve prostheses. *J Am Coll Cardiol* 1991;18:1493–1498.**
3. Khan SS, Gray RJ. Valvular emergencies. *Cardiol Clin* 1991;9:689–708.
4. Omar RZ, Morton LS, et al. Outlet strut fracture of Bjork-Shirley Convexo-Concave valve: can valve-manufacturing characteristics explain the risk? *J Thorac Cardiovasc Surg* 2001;121:1143–1149.
5. **Bach DS. Transesophageal echocardiographic evaluation of prosthetic valves. *Cardiol Clin* 2000;18:751–771.**
6. Fontaine AA, He S, Stadter R, et al. *In vitro* assessment of prosthetic valve function in mitral valve replacement with chordal preservation techniques. *J Heart Valve Dis* 1996;5:186–198.
7. Laas J, Kleine, P, Hasenkam, M. J, et al. Orientation of tilting disc and bileaflet aortic valve substitutes for optimal hemodynamics. *Ann Thorac Surg* 1999;68:1096–1099.
8. Orsinelli DA, Pearson AC. Detection of prosthetic valve strands by transesophageal echocardiography: clinical significance in patients with suspected cardiac source of embolism. *J Am Coll Cardiol* 1995;26:1713–1718.
9. Stoddard MF, Dawkins PR, et al. Mobile strands are frequently attached to the St. Jude Medical mitral valve prosthesis as assessed by two-dimensional transesophageal echocardiography. *Am Heart J* 1992;124:671–674.
10. Iung B, Cormier B, Dadez E, et al. Small abnormal echoes after mitral valve replacement with bileaflet mechanical prostheses: predisposing factors and effect on thromboembolism. *J Heart Valve Dis* 1993;2:259–266.
11. Barbetseas J, Nagueh SF, et al. Differentiating thrombus from pannus formation in obstructed mechanical prosthetic valves: an evaluation of clinical, transthoracic and transesophageal echocardiographic parameters. *J Am Coll Cardiol* 1998;32:1410–1417.
12. Piper C, Korfer R, et al. Prosthetic valve endocarditis. *Heart* 2001;85(5):590–593.
13. Lange HW, Olson JD, et al. Transesophageal color Doppler echocardiography of the normal St. Jude Medical mitral valve prosthesis. *Am Heart J* 1991;122:489–494.
14. Burstow, D, Nishimura RA, Bailey KR, et al. Continuous wave Doppler echocardiographic measurement of prosthetic valve gradients: a simultaneous Doppler-catheter correlative study. *Circulation* 1989;80:504–514.
15. VanAuker MD, Hla A, et al. Simultaneous Doppler/catheter measurements of pressure gradients in aortic valve disease: a correction to the Bernoulli equation based on velocity decay in the stenotic jet. *J Heart Valve Dis* 2000;9:291–298.
16. **Rashtian MY, Stevenson DM, et al. Flow characteristics of four commonly used mechanical heart valves. *Am J Cardiol* 1986;58:743–752.**

17. Pollak SJ, Felner JM. Echocardiographic identification of an aortic valve ring abscess. *J Am Coll Cardiol* 1986;7:1167–1173.

18. **Khandheria BK. Transesophageal echocardiography in the evaluation of prosthetic valves. *Cardiol Clin* 1993;11:427–436.**

19. **Foster GP, Isselbacher EI, et al. Accurate localization of mitral regurgitant defects using multiplane transesophageal echocardiography. *Ann Thorac Surg* 1998;65:1025–1031.**

20. **Dumesnil JG, Honos GN, et al. Validation and applications of mitral prosthetic valvular areas calculated by Doppler echocardiography. *Am J Cardiol* 1990;65:1443–1448.**

21. Chafizadeh ER, Zoghbi WA. Doppler echocardiographic assessment of the St. Jude Medical prosthetic valve in the aortic position using the continuity equation. *Circulation* 1991;83:213–223.

22. Leung DY, Wong J, et al. Application of color Doppler flow mapping to calculate orifice area of St. Jude mitral valve. *Circulation* 1998;98:1205–1211.

23. Bitar JN, Lechin ME, et al. Doppler echocardiographic assessment with the continuity equation of St. Jude Medical mechanical prostheses in the mitral valve position. *Am J Cardiol* 1995;76:287–293.

24. Rothbart RM, Castriz JL, et al. Determination of aortic valve area by two-dimensional and Doppler echocardiography in patients with normal and stenotic bioprosthetic valves. *J Am Coll Cardiol* 1990;15:817–824.

25. Bech-Hanssen O, Caidahl K, et al. Assessment of effective orifice area of prosthetic aortic valves with Doppler echocardiography: an *in vivo* and *in vitro* study. *J Thoracic Cardiovasc Surg* 2001;122:287–294.

26. Maslow AD, Haering MJ, Heindel S, et al. An evaluation of prosthetic aortic valves using transesophageal echocardiography: the double-envelope technique. *Anesth Analg* 2000;91:509–516.

27. **Barbetseas J, Zoghbi WA. Evaluation of prosthetic valve function and associated complications. *Cardiol Clin* 1998;16:505–530.**

NATIVE VALVE ENDOCARDITIS

GREGG S. HARTMAN

Endocarditis is defined as an inflammation of the endocardium. The formation of the intracardiac vegetations characteristic of the disease results from two etiologies, infectious and noninfectious. The echocardiographic appearance of either source can be similar and the diagnosis may only be confirmed at autopsy or surgery. The currently available imaging techniques can neither definitively diagnose an active infection nor completely exclude one when the clinical picture remains highly suspicious for an infective process. It is through the integration of the clinical picture, the echocardiographic images, and the microbiologic data that the presumptive diagnosis can be made.

INFECTIVE ENDOCARDITIS

Infective endocarditis (IE) is a microbial infection of the endocardial surfaces of the heart and can be classified as acute or subacute based on the severity and pace of the clinical picture and progression of disease (1). Despite progress in antimicrobial therapy and surgical management, IE continues to carry high morbidity and mortality risks. Rapid diagnosis, early appropriate treatment, and a cautious awareness of the potential complications are all essential to providing the best patient outcomes. Infective endocarditis represents one of the most serious of all clinical infections and describes the invasion or colonization of the internal cardiac structures (including the valves, mural endocardium, paravalvular tissue), leading to the formation of large friable aggregates called vegetations (Fig. 12.1). These vegetations can include the microorganism, fibrin, inflammatory (white) blood cells, and platelet aggregates. Depending on the virulence of the organism and the underlying anatomic site, there may be destruction of the tissue and extension into surrounding structures with abscess formation. The most common site of involvement is one of the heart valves, but

other sites include multiple valves, the chordae tendineae, other valvular supporting apparatuses, and the mural endocardium, with variable extension into the paravalvular tissues. Involvement of IE may extend beyond the heart itself to include the aorta, aneurysmal layers, other blood vessels, prosthetic devices, and the pericardial space.

Infective endocarditis can develop on normal native valves but more commonly occurs in the setting of several predisposing factors. Disruption of the endocardial surface of valves can occur either from mechanical factors due to high-velocity regurgitant jets or distal to obstructive, stenosed, native valves. This surface disruption can favor platelet and fibrin deposition on the denuded surfaces. Transient bacteremia provides microbial foci for infection of these sterile depositions. Virulence of the organisms, host immunologic factors, and properties of the native endothelial cells are also involved. Other host factors such as neutropenia, immunodeficiency, therapeutic immunosuppression, diabetes mellitus, and alcohol and intravenous drug abuse (IVDA) increase the likelihood of infection. In addition to depositions on native cardiac structures, indwelling intravascular catheters, pacing leads, intracardiac synthetic patches, and prosthetic valves are important factors leading to endocarditis.

EPIDEMIOLOGIC FACTORS

The most frequent cause of IE in developing countries is rheumatic fever. This occurs primarily in young patients. In contrast, epidemiologic factors are different in developed countries, secondary to longevity of the populations, increased nosocomial cases, and new predisposing factors. The incidence of IE is 1.7 to 6.2 cases per 100,000 person-years (2), with men more commonly affected than women. The median age range for infection has increased from 30 to 40 years in the preantibiotic era to 47 to 69 years more recently. This shift has been attributed to improving longevity, leading to an increase in degenerative valvular heart disease, an increased frequency of intravascular devices and prosthetic valves, and increased exposure to nosocomial bacteria (3). Patients with a history of IVDA have a high incidence

G. S. Hartman: Department of Anesthesiology, Dartmouth Medical School, Hanover, New Hampshire; and Department of Anesthesiology, Dartmouth-Hitchcock Medical Center, Lebanon, New Hampshire.

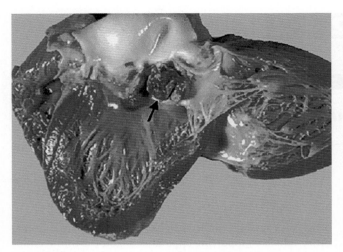

FIGURE 12.1. Gross specimen of mitral valve vegetations (*arrow*). (From Internet Pathologic Laboratory for Education, with permission.)

of IE at a rate of 150 to 2,000 per 100,000 patient-years and potentially higher in the setting of preexisting valvular heart disease (4).

Several general medical conditions predispose to IE. These include diabetes mellitus, long-term hemodialysis, and poor dental hygiene. Human immunodeficiency virus (HIV) infection also may increase the risk, but the increase is most pronounced in the setting of IVDA or advanced stages of the disease (5). The most common general cause of IE is mitral valve prolapse (MVP). This likely reflects the high prevalence of the condition in the general population, and only a modest increased risk secondary to the lesion. The risk is increased in the setting of MVP when associated with thickened mitral valve leaflets and moderate to severe mitral regurgitation (MR) (6).

Nosocomial IE accounts for 7% to 27% of all cases of IE in the setting of tertiary care hospitals, with the presence of infected intravascular prosthetic material in greater than 50% of the cases. Surgical wound infections and gastrointestinal and genitourinary tract procedures are common features of the other various sources (7).

MICROBIOLOGY OF INFECTIVE ENDOCARDITIS

Although fungi, rickettsiae (Q fever), and chlamydiae have at one time or another been responsible for these infections, most cases are bacterial; hence, the term *bacterial endocarditis* (BE) is often used interchangeably with *infective endocarditis*. Bacterial endocarditis can be further classified on clinical grounds into acute (ABE) and subacute (SBE) forms. This subdivision expresses the range of severity of the disease and the pace of the infection's progression, determined in large part by the virulence of the infectious microorganism in conjunction with the presence of underlying cardiac disease. Acute bacterial endocarditis describes a destructive, fulminant infection, usually in the setting of a previously normal heart valve with a highly virulent organism that leads in more than 50% of patients to death within days to weeks despite antibiotics and surgery. In contrast, low-virulence organisms can cause infection in a previously abnormal heart, particularly on deformed valves. In this setting, SBE may appear insidiously and, even untreated, pursue a protracted course of weeks to months.

The causative organisms vary with the clinical setting and underlying risk group. Previously α-hemolytic streptococci (viridans) was the most common cause of ABE, but this has recently been surpassed by the more virulent *Staphylococcus aureus*. *S. aureus* is commonly found on the skin and can infect either healthy or abnormal valves. It is responsible for 10% to 20% of cases overall and in a high percentage of patients with a history of IVDA. Coagulase-negative staphylococci infections are most commonly seen with prosthetic heart valve BE and only occasionally with native valve infections. Streptococci species BE is usually seen in the setting of damaged or otherwise abnormal valves (bicuspid aortic valves, MVP, etc.). Many forms of streptococci are isolated in patients with BE, including *S. bovis, S. sanguis, S. mutans,* and *S. mitis*. *S. bovis* is seen in BE of elderly patients in association with colonic neoplasms. Mouth and oral cavity flora make up the balance of remaining bacteria and include enterococci and the so-called HACEK group (Hemophilus, Actinobacillus, Cardiobacterium, Eikenella, and Kingella species). Polymicrobial infections are rare and when present are most often observed in the setting of IVDA. Fungi, rickettsiae, and chlamydiae are more rare than causative organisms.

In about 10% of all cases of endocarditis, the causative organism cannot be isolated from the blood (culture-negative endocarditis). This may be due to prior antibiotic therapy, difficulties in isolation and culturing of the microbe, or deep-seated infections with minimal or absent hematogenous seeding (8). Currently less than 10% of patients with the diagnosis of infective endocarditis according to strict criteria and who have not recently received antibiotics will have sterile blood cultures. Performing multiple blood cultures and adopting new diagnostic approaches (including isolation and identification techniques) have contributed to this low incidence (9). A technique of the polymerase chain reaction can be used for the identification of surgically excised vegetations resistant to culture techniques (10).

Clinical Presentation/Laboratory Data

The clinical presentation of IE typically includes both cardiac and noncardiac manifestations. Fever is the most common symptom, although it is not as prevalent with less virulent organisms, in the severely debilitated, among patients with chronic diseases like renal failure, or in the setting of

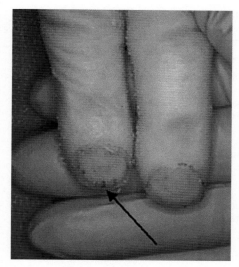

FIGURE 12.2. Peripheral manifestations of infective endocarditis. Splinter hemorrhages in distal nail beds of the fingers (*arrow*). (From Internet Pathologic Laboratory for Education, with permission.)

antibiotic therapy. Patients may experience generalized weight loss, malaise, and night sweats. In addition, classic peripheral signs such as splinter hemorrhages (Fig. 12.2) under nailbeds and conjunctival petechiae (Roth spots) may be present. Osler nodes are tender subcutaneous nodules on the fingers and Janeway spots are erythematous, hemorrhagic pustules on the soles of the feet. Cardiac findings include murmurs (often in the setting of preexisting murmurs) and congestive heart failure (CHF). A heightened level of suspicion should be maintained when a patient with a prosthetic heart valve has an unexplained fever because of the high frequency of invasive infections in this setting. New atrioventricular, fascicular, and bundle branch blocks should arouse suspicion because they may herald paravalvular extension of IE and invasion with associated increased morbidity and mortality (11).

Laboratory information can increase the level of suspicion for the diagnosis of IE. Nonspecific test abnormalities include anemia, as well as elevated white blood cell count, erythrocyte sedimentation rate, and C-reactive protein level.

DIAGNOSIS: CLINICAL CRITERIA

The classical Oslerian manifestations of IE include bacteremia or fungemia, evidence of active valvulitis, peripheral emboli, and immunologic vascular phenomena (12). When these findings are present, the diagnosis is uncomplicated. In other presentations, many or all of these criteria may be absent. In the setting of IVDA, IE often results from a *S. aureus* infection of the tricuspid or pulmonic valves. In this setting, the lungs may serve as a filter, limiting peripheral emboli and immunologic vascular events.

Because of the variable presentation of IE, diagnostic strategies have been proposed to improve both the sensitivity and specificity of detection. These criteria may be useful in ensuring appropriate and cost-effective use of diagnostic tests and antimicrobial treatment. In 1994, the Duke criteria were introduced and combined diagnostic factors with echocardiographic features in an attempt to integrate predisposing factors with clinical and laboratory information, thus increasing the yield in borderline cases (Table 12.1). The criteria stratified patients in three categories: definite, possible, and rejected. "Definite" cases were those in which microorganisms were identified by either pathologic grounds (IE documented at surgery or autopsy with culture or histology) or in which IE was diagnosed based on a collection of clinical criteria. The combination of two major criteria, or one major and three minor criteria, or five minor criteria were required. The classification of "possible" cases were those in which findings were not sufficient for the definite IE criteria. "Rejected" IE cases were those in which no pathologic findings were detected, there was a rapid resolution of clinical picture with minimal or no treatment, or a firm alternative diagnosis was made.

The utility of these criteria have been studied and validated in subsequent investigations, with a reported specificity of 99% and negative predictive value of >92% (14). The criteria rely heavily on echocardiographic findings. Although transthoracic echocardiography (TTE) can be useful in many cases, the improved resolution afforded by the esophageal approach has promoted transesophageal echocardiography (TEE) to the primary imaging modality.

Echocardiography

The importance of echocardiography in the diagnosis of IE has progressed as the quality of images has improved from M-mode echocardiography to TTE and finally TEE. The developments of two-dimensional imaging and the enhanced near-field resolution of TEE permit identification, localization, and characterization of potential vegetations. Extension of IE into paravalvular spaces also can be identified. Doppler color flow analysis of blood flow and valvular function permits the assessment of the hemodynamic sequelae of the IE invasion and subsequent valvular destruction. These have diagnostic and prognostic value and can serve as a mechanism for monitoring progression of disease or hopefully resolution. Echocardiography can therefore serve two major roles: quantification and characterization of the clinical diagnosis of IE, or as a "rule-out" modality when faced with a lower probability scenario. These aspects are summarized below from Otto and Pearlman:

In a patient with probable IE by clinical grounds, echocardiography can serve to:

1. Identify the presence, location, size and number of valvular vegetations.

TABLE 12.1. DUKE CRITERIA FOR DIAGNOSIS OF INFECTIVE ENDOCARDITIS (IE)

Major criteria
  Positive blood culture for infective endocarditis
    Typical microorganism for IE from two separate blood cultures: viridans streptococci[a],
      Streptococcus bovi, HACEK group[b]
    Community-acquired *Staphylococcus aureus* or entercocci, in the absence of primary focus
    Persistently positive blood culture, defined as recovery from a microorganism consistent
      with IE from:
      Blood cultures drawn more than 12 hours apart, or
      All of three or a majority of four or more separate blood cultures, with first and last
        drawn at least 1 hour apart
  Evidence of endocardial involvement
  Positive echocardiogram for IE
    Oscillating intracardiac mass, on value or supporting structures, or in the path of regurgitant
      jets, or on implanted material, in the absence of an alternative anatomical explanation, or
    Abscess, or
    New, partial dehiscence of prosthetic valve, or
  New valvular regurgitation (increase or change in pre-existing murmur not sufficient)
Minor criteria
  Predisposition: predisposing heart condition or intravenous drug use
  Fever: >38.0°C (100.4°F)
  Vescular phenomena: major arterial emboli, septic pulmonary infarcts, mycotic aneurysm,
    intracranial hemorrhage, conjunctival hemorrhages, Janeway lesions
  Immunological phenomena: glomerulonephritis, Osler nodes, Roth spots, rheumatoid factor
  Microbiologic evidence: positive blood culture but not meeting major criterion as noted
    previously[c], or serologic evidence of active infection with organism consistent with IE
  Echocardiogram: consistent with IE but not meeting major criterion as noted previously

[a]Including nutritional variant strains.
[b]HACEK, *Hemophilus species, Actinobacillus actinomycetemcomitans, Cardiobacterium hominis, Eikenella species,* and *Kingella kingae.*
[c]Excluding single positive cultures for coagulase-negative staphylococci and organisms that do not cause endocarditis.
From Durak DT, Luke AS, Bright DK, Duke Endocarditis Service. New criteria for diagnosis of infective endocarditis: utilization of specific echocardiographic criteria. *N Engl J Med* 1994;96:200–209, with permission.

2. Assess the functional abnormalities of the affected valve(s), especially valvular regurgitation.
3. Identify the underlying anatomy of the affected valve(s) and any coincident valvular disease
4. Quantify the effect of IE and accompanying valvular dysfunction of chamber size and function, especially the left ventricle.
5. Identify other complications of endocarditis (e.g., paravalvular abscesses, pericardial effusion).
6. Provide prognostic data on the anticipated clinical course, risk of systemic embolization, and potential need for surgical intervention.

When the likelihood of IE is low based on clinical grounds, echocardiography is often useful to "rule out" IE. In this setting, the echocardiographic goals include:

1. Documentation of the absence of valvular vegetations.
2. Assessment of anatomical and physiological variables which increase the likelihood of IE, including bicuspid aortic valve, myxomatous degeneration, etc. (15).

With two-dimensional ultrasound imaging, vegetations appear as irregular echogenic structures on the valve leaflets with motion that is dependent on the underlying valve movements but more irregular and chaotic. Additionally, the mo-

tion may lag behind that of the native structure. The lesions usually are located on the upstream side of the leaflets; thus, a mitral valve IE lesion will be on the left atrial (LA) surface of the valve and an aortic valve vegetation will be on the left ventricular surface of the aortic valve leaflets (Figs. 12.3 and 12.4). Although the vegetations may adhere anywhere on the valve surface, the lines of coaptation are the most common sites. The vegetation, if large enough, can prolapse across the orifice with antegrade blood flow and then backward into the upstream chamber with retrograde flow if valvular regurgitation, either preexisting or newly created, is present. M-mode recordings across the lesion can show rapid oscillations in diastole at rates greater than usual native valve motion, a finding of particular significance prior to routine two-dimensional imaging techniques. Valvular vegetations can be quite large, exceeding 3 cm in length (Fig. 12.5). Presentations can be that of isolated lesions or of multiple sites of involvement, either by direct extension or as a separate process. The vegetation process can be destructive (especially with highly virulent organisms) and erode into the underlying myocardium, leading to abscess formation. The characteristics of the IE vegetations can suggest the cause. Fungal endocarditis usually results in larger lesions

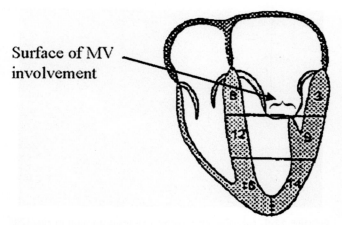

FIGURE 12.3. Schematic diagram of a mitral valve (*MV*) vegetation attached to the atrial side of the leaflet with prolapse into the left atrium in systole.

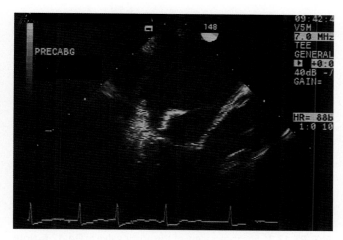

FIGURE 12.5. Large pedunculated infective endocarditis lesion on the posterior leaflet of the mitral valve.

when compared with those typical of bacterial infections. Highly virulent strains of bacteria usually result in more extensive and erosive lesions, with greater degrees of valvular destruction. The lesions themselves are composed of inert components (fibrin, platelet aggregates) and potentially infective elements (bacteria). Fragmentation and embolization of left-sided vegetations can lead to infarcts in the brain, liver, spleen, kidneys, and other tissues. Septic infarcts may occur secondary to the infective components.

It is important to remember that there are many other causes of abnormal ultrasound images of valves. Increased echogenicity can result from calcium deposition (Figs. 12.6 and 12.7), fibrosis, myxomatous changes, postrheumatic deformities, Lambl excrescences, and papillary fibromas, which are disrupted, flailed components of the valve itself. Healed vegetations cannot definitively be discerned from active lesions. Noninfectious lesions, including nonbacterial thrombotic endocarditis and cardiac lupus, can cause lesions with echocardiographic images similar to those of IE. However, an abnormal echogenic mass with independent motion, pedunculation, and location on the valve leaflet itself near the line of coaptation is most commonly a vegetation. Occasionally, M-mode tracings show rapid oscillatory motion.

Although TTE is commonly used in the initial workup of patients with suspected IE, TEE, because of its proximity to the cardiac structures and thus availability of higher frame rates (7 MHz), gives better resolution of small structures and spatial relationships. In many cases it has replaced TTE as the primary imaging modality. Development of three-dimensional ultrasonography will likely enhance the resolution and localization capacity of this modality.

Mitral Valve Imaging

The mitral valve is most frequently involved with IE of the four cardiac valves (16). Both the anterior and posterior

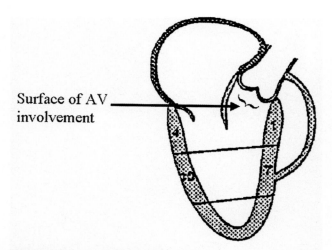

FIGURE 12.4. Schematic diagram of an aortic valve (*AV*) vegetation attached to the ventricular side of the leaflet with prolapse into the left ventricular outflow tract in diastole.

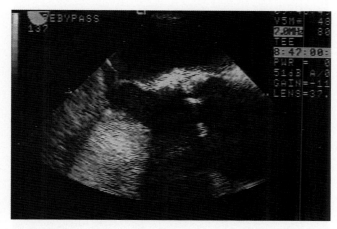

FIGURE 12.6. Long-axis view of the aortic valve with calcium on the leaflets. Note strong echogenic images and shadowing.

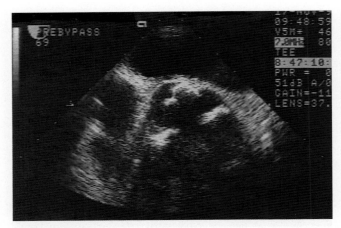

FIGURE 12.7. Short-axis view of the aortic valve in Fig. 12.6. Note prominent calcium deposits on multiple leaflets.

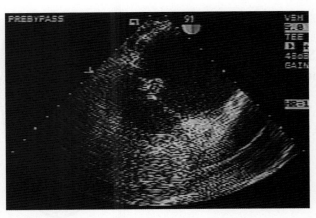

FIGURE 12.9. Infective endocarditis vegetation seen in Fig. 12.8 from the mid-esophageal two-chamber view.

leaflets can be involved either independently or simultaneously, and usually the lesion is attached to the atrial rather than the ventricular surface (Figs. 12.8 and 12.9). Lower pressure and forces in the atrial cavity probably are factors favoring atrial side attachment. Mitral valve involvement may result from extension of an aortic valve infection, because the two valves share annular attachment sites. Large pedunculated mitral valve vegetations may prolapse across the valve orifice during diastole, and if large enough can cause obstruction to flow with the clinical picture similar to that of mitral stenosis. More commonly, destruction of leaflets, disruption of the lines of coaptation, or rupture of supporting chordae tendineae results in MR (Fig. 12.10).

Degenerative changes common to the mitral valve can make the diagnosis of IE difficult. Myxomatous degeneration leading to leaflet thickening and fusion and chordal disruption can simulate findings of IE. Aragam et al. points out that the degree of leaflet involvement is key to differentiating between the two entities. Myxomatous degeneration

usually involves the leaflets diffusely and can lead to leaflet redundancy, whereas vegetations are typically more localized and involve the leaflet tips (17). Examination of the other valves for myxomatous changes (tricuspid involvement) can be helpful because simultaneous IE involvement of left- and right-sided valves is uncommon.

Thickening of the rheumatic mitral valve leaflets can resemble IE, although leaflet motion, particularly the posterior leaflet, is usually more pronounced in the setting of rheumatic disease. The differential diagnosis for IE also must include LA tumors such as pedunculated myxomas, and primary leaflet masses such as fibroelastomas. Serial echocardiographic imaging may be required to document any changes in size supportive of the diagnosis of IE.

Infective endocarditis can lead to extensive destruction of the valve and supporting structures. Flail leaflets and MR are the rule, with leaflet fusion and stenosis as a result of IE being rare occurrences. Flail leaflets whip back and forth

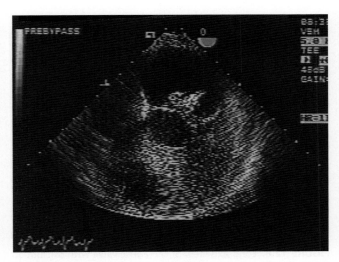

FIGURE 12.8. Infective endocarditis vegetation on the posterior mitral leaflet from the mid-esophageal four-chamber view.

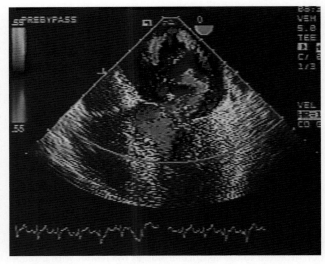

FIGURE 12.10. Laterally directed mitral regurgitation jet from infective endocarditis.

from the atrium to the ventricle during systole and diastole, with the leaflet tip and body moving in unison. This pattern of motion is different from that seen with prolapsing mitral leaflets, in which the central portion is bowed or concave. Doppler color flow studies are useful for quantifying the severity of MR. Findings of severe MR are a large regurgitant jet, systolic pulmonary vein flow reversal, and early systolic closure of the aortic valve.

Aortic Valve Imaging

The aortic valve is the most common valve involved with IE requiring surgical intervention. Simultaneous involvement of the mitral valve is not uncommon. Aortic involvement typically occurs in the setting of preexisting aortic valve abnormalities, including rheumatic changes, senile calcification, and bicuspid aortic valve. Aortic valve vegetations typically attach on the ventricular side of the valve and may flop back and forth across the outflow tract with systole and diastole. Size and degree of fixation can be quite variable (Figs. 12.11 and 12.12). As with mitral valve IE, identification relies on the location of the mass on the valve, underlying valvular defects, size, changing appearance, and associated valvular destruction. Typical of all IE lesions, exaggerated motion of a pedunculated mass with friable components are highly suggestive of the diagnosis.

Because of the high pressures on the aortic valve cusps during diastole, small fenestrations secondary to IE destruction of leaflet tissue can result in significant aortic insufficiency (AI) (Fig. 12.13). Mechanical forces then contribute to the destructive process. Completely disrupted flail leaflets result. Early in the process, there may be high-frequency diastolic fluttering of the valve caused by the regurgitant stream of blood flowing from the aorta through the leaflet defect. This may be regarded as pathognomonic for IE of the aortic valve. Doppler color flow will reveal a large regurgitant jet in AI,

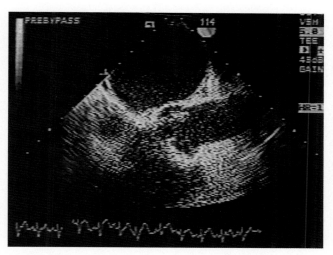

FIGURE 12.12. Mid-esophageal long-axis view of the aortic valve lesion in Fig. 12.11.

with the width of the base corresponding to the severity of the disease. Other echocardiographic findings consistent with severe disease include left ventricular volume overload, reversal of flow in the thoracic aorta, and premature closure of the mitral valve with diastolic MR. The finding of moderate to severe AI with IE suggests the need for urgent surgical intervention.

Right-Sided Imaging

Right-sided involvement with IE involves the tricuspid valve much more frequently that the pulmonic valve. Tricuspid IE is usually seen in the setting of IVDA, with the causative organism often being *S. aureus,* and presents as an acute rather than a subacute process (18). IVDA can predispose to involvement of an otherwise normal valve, whereas right-sided IE in the absence of IVDA is typically associated with congenital lesions or postsurgical repairs. Fragmentation of the

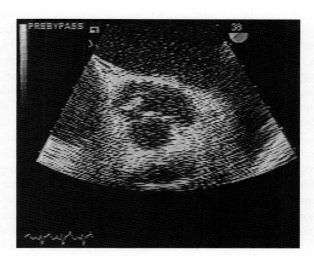

FIGURE 12.11. Echogenic lesion on the noncoronary cusp of the aortic valve from the mid-esophageal aortic valve short-axis view.

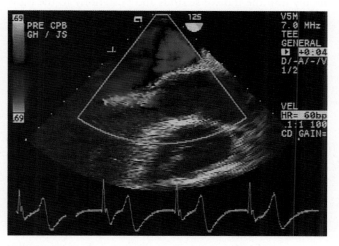

FIGURE 12.13. Regurgitant jet of aortic insufficiency through a hole in the aortic valve leaflet secondary to aortic insufficiency.

vegetations can lead to seeding of the lung from the septic emboli. Thus, the presentation of multiple lung lesions, IVDA, and fever is highly suggestive of IE (19). Cardiac findings, such as a murmur, can be subtle or absent despite severe valvular destruction from IE most likely due to the lower pressure of the right side of the heart. Vegetations of tricuspid IE can be large and can attach on either the atrial or ventricular surfaces. They are described as being more exophytic than left-sided lesions. As with left-sided lesions, the differential diagnosis of right-sided masses includes IE and tumors. Valvular attachment and synchrony of motion are distinguishing characteristics. Pulmonic valve IE is rare and usually a finding at autopsy. Underlying congenital heart disease is the common feature.

PARAVALVULAR ABSCESSES

Acute IE, especially with virulent organisms such as staphylococci or enterococci, can lead to paravalvular abscess formation. In addition to fever and echocardiographic findings for IE, extension of the infectious process can disrupt the native conduction pathways and result in high-grade atrioventricular block (20). Aortic root abscesses are most common following aortic valve replacements for endocarditis. On echocardiographic examination, the abscess appears as an echo-free space surrounding the valve and aortic wall or between the aortic annulus and ventricular septum. Extension is usually adjacent to the leaflet primarily involved with IE. Typically, extension of IE from the left coronary cusp progresses into the base of the anterior mitral leaflet and adjacent annulus. Further involvement can spread into the intraatrial septum. Right coronary cusp involvement can spread through the aortic root into the membranous and muscular portions of the interventricular septum and on to the right ventricular outflow tract. Rupture of the extension cavity into the interventricular septum can result in a ventricular septal defect (21). Noncoronary cusp infections extend locally into the transverse sinus and posteriorly to the right atrium, or the right ventricle.

Intracardiac fistulous tracts can occur. Although sometimes seen with advanced progression of native valve IE, a more common setting is a history of prosthetic valve replacement. Hemodynamic and clinical pictures will depend on the cardiac chambers involved and the direction of the resultant shunt flow. Severe hemodynamic collapse and pulmonary edema may be the clinical presentation (22).

PROGRESSION/RESOLUTION OF INFECTIVE ENDOCARDITIS LESIONS

Serial echocardiographic examinations can be helpful to determine the course of disease with either resolution or progression of the IE lesions. Typically lesions become smaller and more echodense, with the healing process corresponding to the pathologic findings of fibrosis, collagen, and calcium deposition (23). Complete resolution of lesions is atypical. New febrile episodes in the clinical setting of "healed" IE can be a difficult diagnosis.

The significance of the echocardiographic findings in IE remains controversial. There is common acceptance of the increased risk for complications (such as emboli and CHF) and the need for surgical intervention when the clinical picture and echocardiographic data are consistent with IE. Size, consistency, location, and degree of mobility can be useful in identifying patients at increased risk for complications. Although not universally applicable, size does relate to risk for systemic embolization. Infective endocarditis vegetations of greater than 10 mm in diameter increase the risk for emboli, CHF, the need for surgical intervention, and death (24). Although probably at increased risk for complications, the presence of vegetations is not necessarily an indication for surgery. Traditionally, the presence of two or more embolic events was an indication for surgery. Surgery is most beneficial early in the course of IE, because systemic embolization is most likely in the early phase of antibiotic therapy. Surgery is also beneficial in the setting of CHF, aggressive antibiotic-resistant organisms, and prosthetic valve IE. Failure of an IE vegetation to diminish in size on serial examinations or at least stabilize during appropriate antimicrobial therapy may be an indication for surgical intervention.

NONINFECTIVE THROMBOTIC VEGETATIONS

Nonbacterial thrombotic endocarditis (NBTE) and the endocarditis of systemic lupus erythematosus (SLE), called Libman-Sacks endocarditis, are characterized by vegetations on cardiac valves, but lack many of the other clinical features of IE. Like IE, the masses represent depositions of fibrin, platelets, and other blood components, but lack microorganisms and thus are sterile and noninflammatory. Nonbacterial thrombotic endocarditis is seen in cancer patients and patients with sepsis. This formerly had been called marantic endocarditis. Unlike IE, the valvular involvement of NBTE is usually of little consequence, with the morbidity resulting from systemic embolization of debris to the brain, heart, and other organs. Echocardiographically the lesions are small (usually <5 mm in diameter) and located on the lines of coaptation.

Because NBTE occurs in the setting of pulmonary embolisms and deep venous thromboses, alterations in the coagulation state are thought to be the origin. Underlying disease states such as cancer, particularly mucinous adenocarcinomas, are common. Other hypercoagulable states predisposing to NBTE include sepsis, burns, and hyperestrogenic states. Indwelling vascular catheters can cause endocardial damage and may be the etiology of NBTE seen in their presence.

Libman-Sacks endocarditis is an unusual finding and describes the vegetations seen commonly on both the tricuspid and mitral valves in patients with SLE. Similar to NBTE, these lesions are sterile and nondestructive. Circulating antiphospholipid antibodies can be isolated and are likely involved in the venous and arterial thrombosis seen in this clinical syndrome.

CONCLUSION

In his Gulstonian lectures in 1885, Osler made the following observations with respect to IE: Few diseases present greater difficulties in the way of diagnosis, difficulties which in many cases are practically insurmountable. Advances in echocardiography, particularly in TEE, have enabled clinicians to better diagnose this disease. IE can be better confirmed and equally ruled out with more certainty through the use of modern imaging modalities. Differentiation of vegetations from other more benign valvular abnormalities remains the challenge. Use of multiple imaging planes, various ultrasound modalities, and integration of the echocardiographic findings with clinical and laboratory data are still essential to making the accurate diagnosis of IE and thus direct appropriate therapy to best benefit the patient.

KEY POINTS

- Infective endocarditis continues to carry high morbidity and mortality risks.
- The most common site of involvement is one of the heart valves.
- Fever is the most common symptom.
- Vegetations appear as irregular echogenic structures that usually are located on the upstream side of the leaflets on the valve leaflets.
- Additional complications include abscess, fistula formation, septal defects, and heart block.
- Alternative possibilities include calcium deposition fibrosis, myxomatous changes, postrheumatic deformities, Lambl excrescences, and papillary fibromas.

REFERENCES

1. **Mylonakis E, Calderwood SB. Infective endocarditis in adults. *N Engl J Med* 2001;345:1318–1330.**
2. Berlin JA, Abrutyn E, Strom BL, et al. Incidence of infective endocarditis in the Delaware Valley, 1988–1990. *Am J Cardiol* 1995;76:933–936.
3. Watanaunakorn C, Burkert T. Infective endocarditis at a large community teaching hospital 1980–1990: a review of 210 episodes. *Medicine (Baltimore)* 1993;72:90–102.
4. **Frontera JA, Gradon JD. Right-sided endocarditis in injection drug users: review of proposed mechanisms of pathogenesis. *Clin Infect Dis* 2000;30:374–379.**
5. Ribera E, Miro JM, Cortes E, et al. Influence of human immunodeficiency virus 1 infection and degree of immunosuppression in the clinical characteristics and outcome of infective endocarditis in intravenous drug users. *Arch Intern Med* 1998;158:2043–2050.
6. Zuppiroli A, Rinaldi M, Kramer-Fox R, et al. Natural history of mitral valve prolapse. *Am J Cardiol* 1995;75:1028–1032.
7. Fernandez-Guerrero ML, Verdejo C, Azofra J, et al. Hospital-acquired infective endocarditis not associated with cardiac surgery: an emerging problem. *Clin Infect Dis* 1995;20:16–23.
8. Ramzi SC, Vinay K, Tucker C, eds. In: *Robbins Pathological basis of disease,* 6th ed. Philadelphia: WB Saunders, 1999.
9. Brouqui P, Raoult D. Endocarditis due to rare and fastidious bacteria. *Clin Microbiol Rev* 2001;14:177–207.
10. Goldenberger D, Kunzli A, Vogt P, et al. Molecular diagnosis of bacterial endocarditis by broad-range PCR amplification and direct sequencing. *J Clin Microbiol* 1997;35:2733–2739.
11. DiNubile MJ, Calderwood SB, Steinhaus DM, et al. Cardiac conduction abnormalities complicating native valve active infective endocarditis. *Am J Cardiol* 1986;58:1213–1217.
12. **Bayer AS, Bolger AF, Taubert KA, et al. Diagnosis and management of infective endocarditis and its complications. *Circulation* 1998;98:2936–2948.**
13. **Durak DT, Luke AS, Bright DK, Duke Endocarditis Service. New criteria for diagnosis of infective endocarditis: utilization of specific echocardiographic criteria. *N Engl J Med* 1994;96:200–209.**
14. Perez-Vazquez A, Farinas MC, Garcia-Palomo JD, et al. Evaluation of the Duke criteria in 93 episodes of prosthetic valve endocarditis: could sensitivity be improved? *Arch Intern Med* 2000;160:1185–1191.
15. Otto CM, Pearlman AS. *Textbook of clinical echocardiography.* Philadelphia: WB Saunders, 1995.
16. Watanaunakorn C. Changing epidemiology and newer aspects of infective endocarditis. *Adv Intern Med* 1977;22:21.
17. Aragam JR, Weyman AE. Echocardiographic findings in infective endocarditis. In: Weyman AE, ed. *Principles and practice of echocardiography,* 2nd ed. Philadelphia: Lippincott Williams & Wilkins, 1994.
18. Bain RC, et al. Right-sided bacterial endocarditis and endoarteritis. *Am J Med* 1958;24:98.
19. Wright JS, Glennie JS. Excision of tricuspid valve with later replacement in endocarditis of drug addiction. *Thorax* 1978;33:518.
20. Wang K, Goberl F, Gleason DF, et al. Complete heart block complication bacterial endocarditis. *Circulation* 1972;46:939.
21. Mansur AJ et al. Acquired ventricular septal defect and tricuspid valve disruption as a complication of infective endocarditis of the aortic valve. *J Cardiovasc Surg* 1093;24:669.
22. **Schwartzbard A, Tunick PA, Kronzon I. Aorta-to-left atrium fistula: a complication of endocarditis. *Circulation* 1998;98:604.**
23. Stafford A, et al. Serial echocardiographic appearance of healing bacterial vegetations. *Am J Cardiol* 1079;44:754.
24. Buda AJ, Zotz RJ, Lemire MS, et al. Prognostic significance of vegetations detected by two-dimensional echocardiography in infective endocarditis. *Am Heart J* 1986;112:1291.

ECHOCARDIOGRAPHIC EVALUATION OF INTRACARDIAC MASSES AND SEPTAL DEFECTS

JAMES A. DINARDO

Transesophageal echocardiography (TEE) plays an indispensable role in the detection and delineation of intracardiac masses and defects. For many of these lesions TEE is the diagnostic procedure of choice. This chapter will systematically describe the masses (thrombi, tumors) and septal defects [atrial (ASD) and ventricular (VSD)] most likely to be encountered in an adult cardiac surgical patient.

ATRIAL ANATOMY

Atrial anatomy requires some discussion because normal atrial structures can be a source of confusion in the TEE evaluation of masses and defects. The plane of the intraatrial septum (IAS) deserves mention because it is commonly presented in illustrations as an anteroposterior structure. In reality, the IAS extends from the right posteriorly, toward the left anteriorly. The orientation of the inferiormost aspect of the septum is more directly anteroposterior, thus making it more difficult to accurately visualize. The fact that the plane of the IAS is neither truly anteroposterior nor mediolateral is clearly demonstrated in cardiac magnetic resonance images (Fig. 13.1). The IAS is thickest peripherally (the limbus) and gradually narrows toward the more centrally located fossa ovalis. Lipomatous hypertrophy of the IAS causes thickening (2–3 cm) of the limbus, but spares the fossa ovalis. This gives the IAS a characteristic dumb-bell appearance. The incidence of lipomatous hypertrophy increases with obesity and age.

The coronary sinus (CS) runs transversely in the atrioventricular groove behind the left atrium (LA) and drains into the right atrium (RA) posteriorly and inferiorly, medial to the inferior vena cava (IVC) orifice, and just superior to the

tricuspid valve (TV) orifice near its septal leaflet. The CS is most optimally imaged in long axis by advancing or retroflexing the probe from the mid-esophageal (ME) four-chamber view. It can also be seen in the short axis (SAX) behind the LA in the ME two-chamber view. A dilated CS should prompt a search for a persistent left superior vena cava (LSVC) or anomalous pulmonary venous drainage to the CS. The diagnosis of CS dilatation secondary to RA hypertension should be one of exclusion.

The SVC and IVC enter the RA posteriorly and medially. The SVC orifice does not have a valve at its entry point into the RA. In contrast, the eustachian valve (EV) may be visualized at the anterior rim of the IVC. The EV is an embryonic remnant of the right sinus venosus valve. *In utero,* this valve serves to direct oxygen-rich blood from the IVC (via the umbilical veins and ductus venosus) across the foramen ovale and away from the TV (1). The valve gradually regresses postpartum. The EV can be imaged by transthoracic echocardiography (TTE) in 85% of children under 1 month of age, but only in 62% of children with a mean age of 3.3 years. Despite the fact that the EV is seen in as many as 86% of adult autopsy examinations, it is visualized in only a minority of patients by TTE. It is much more commonly seen by TEE and is usually less than 1 cm in length.

The Chiari network is a remnant of the septum spurium and the right valve of the sinus venosus. *In utero,* the Chiari network also serves to direct IVC blood toward the foramen ovale. Incomplete reabsorption of these structures results in filamentous, lace-like projections from the remnants of the eustachian (IVC) valve and thebesian (coronary sinus) valve to the upper wall of the RA or IAS (2). A persistent Chiari network is differentiated from a prominent EV by the presence of attachments to the upper RA wall near the crista terminalis. A Chiari network can be detected in 2% to 3% of patients at autopsy or by TEE (3). Careful delineation of the EV and Chiari network are important because they can be mistaken for atrial masses (4).

J. A. DiNardo: Department of Anesthesia, Boston Children's Hospital, Harvard Medical School, Boston, Massachusetts.

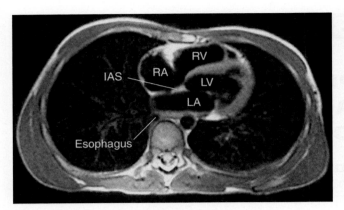

FIGURE 13.1. Cardiac magnetic resonance imaging demonstrating that the plane of the intraatrial septum (*IAS*) is neither truly anteroposterior nor mediolateral. *RA*, right atrium; *LA*, left atrium; *RV*, right ventricle; *LV*, left ventricle.

PATENT FORAMEN OVALE

The membrane of the fossa ovalis lies posterior to the superior aspect of the fatty limbus. Normally, there is fusion of the two structures within the first 2 years of life. When this fusion fails to occur, an oblique communication between the LA and RA known as a patent foramen ovale (PFO) persists (Fig. 13.2). A PFO can be detected at autopsy in approximately 27% of patients (3). However, a PFO is more common in some subsets of patients, including 83% of patients with a Chiari network and 55% of patients with an IAS aneurysm (2).

Transesophageal echocardiography is the diagnostic standard for detecting a PFO. A PFO is best visualized in a modified ME aortic valve SAX view by scanning between 30 and 60 degrees, or in the ME bicaval view. In many patients, shunting across the PFO (usually LA to RA) can be demonstrated with color flow Doppler (CFD) interrogation of the IAS. Saline contrast injection may be useful for opacifying the RA, especially when used in conjunction with a provocative maneuver (release of sustained positive airway pressure) to demonstrate right-to-left flow patency of a PFO. Agitated saline contrast is produced by vigorously transferring 10 mL of saline or albumin between two syringes connected by a stopcock. The agitated mixture can then be injected intravenously. It has been suggested that femoral vein (IVC) injection of contrast provides better sensitivity for PFO detection than antecubital vein (SVC) injection because IVC blood flow enhances impingement of contrast along the IAS (5). In anesthetized patients, release of sustained positive airway pressure will reverse the normal LA to RA pressure gradient and transiently elevate right atrial pressure (RAP) above left atrial pressure (LAP). In the presence of a PFO this will result in translocation of saline contrast from the RA to the LA. In order for the test to be reliable, the IAS must transiently bow into the LA. The amount of sustained positive airway pressure necessary to make this maneuver effective can be judged by observing the position of the IAS during and after release of the airway pressure. Contrast may appear in the LA in the absence of a PFO if pulmonary arteriovenous shunts exist. In this circumstance, appearance of contrast in the LA will be delayed (more than three cardiac cycles) and contrast will be seen traversing one or more of the pulmonary veins as they enter the LA. Contrast echocardiography and CFD have a sensitivity and specificity of nearly 100% for PFO detection (6–8).

A PFO is implicated in a variety of pathologic processes (3):

- Stroke from cardiac-derived emboli.
- Venous to arterial gas embolus associated with decom-

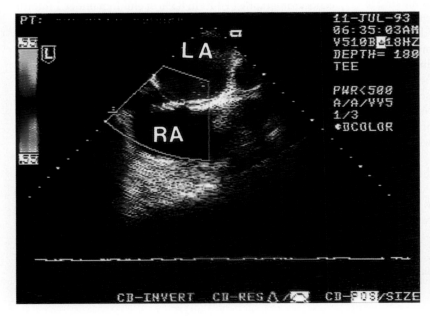

FIGURE 13.2. Patent foramen ovale. Modified mid-esophageal aortic valve short-axis view. Color flow Doppler demonstrates an oblique defect where the posterior fossa ovalis has failed to fuse to the superior aspect of the fatty limbus. Flow is left to right. *LA*, left atrium; *RA*, right atrium.

pression sickness in divers, high-altitude pilots, and astronauts.

- Platypnea-orthodeoxia syndrome, in which dyspnea and arterial hypoxemia are associated with upright position. A subset of these patients has an orthostatic increase in right-to-left shunting across a PFO as the underlying pathophysiology (9).
- Arterial hypoxemia when RAP exceeds LAP for all or part of the cardiac cycle in patients with pulmonary embolism, primary or secondary pulmonary hypertension, severe tricuspid regurgitation (TR), severe right ventricular (RV) dysfunction, or effective LA decompression following left ventricular assist device placement (10).

ATRIAL SEPTAL ANEURYSM

Atrial septal aneurysm (ASA) is classically defined as an aneurysmal protrusion of the IAS in which the base of the protrusion has a diameter 15 mm, and there is either protrusion of the aneurysmal portion of the IAS 15 mm beyond the plane of the remainder of the IAS, or phasic excursion of the aneurysmal portion of the IAS during the respiratory cycle 15 mm in total amplitude (11) (Fig. 13.3). Others have defined ASA using 10-mm dimensions rather than 15-mm (12). Dimensions are obtained with TEE in the ME four-chamber and bicaval views.

An ASA can be detected by TEE in 2.2% of the general population and in 24% of patients with a Chiari network (2,11). An ASA is associated with intraatrial shunting in approximately 55% of patients via an ASD (39%) or a PFO (61%) (11,12). It also has been associated with mitral valve (MV) prolapse and supraventricular arrhythmias.

An ASA is a putative risk factor for cardiac-derived emboli and cerebral ischemia. The incidence of ASA (using

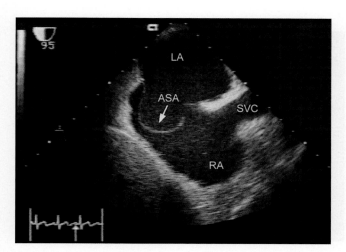

FIGURE 13.3. Two-dimensional modified mid-esophageal bicaval view demonstrating large aneurysmal atrial septum (*ASA, arrow*) bowing predominantly toward the right atrium (*RA*). *LA,* left atrium; *SVC,* superior vena cava.

15-mm dimensions) in patients evaluated with TEE following a cerebral ischemic event is 7.9% as compared with 2.2% in a comparable control group (11). Four mechanisms have been proposed to explain this increased risk: (a) thrombus formation on the LA side of the aneurysm; (b) paradoxic embolism via an associated PFO or ASD; (c) associated MV prolapse; and (d) associated supraventricular arrhythmias (11,13). Although current evidence strongly points to paradoxic embolism as the source for cerebral ischemia in ASA, the issue is not yet resolved.

ATRIAL SEPTAL DEFECTS

There are four morphologic types of ASDs: (a) ostium secundum defects; (b) ostium primum defects; (c) inferior and superior sinus venosus defects; and (d) CS defects. The pathophysiology of ASD is the result of anatomic and physiologic shunting at the atrial level. Physiologic left-to-right shunting refers to recirculation of oxygenated pulmonary venous blood into the pulmonary artery (PA) and back into the LA. Anatomically this involves flow of blood from the higher-pressure chamber (LA) to the lower-pressure chamber (RA). Normally mean RAP is lower than mean LAP because RV compliance is greater than LV compliance. This in turn is due to the fact that RV pressure is lower than LV pressure, and pulmonary vascular resistance is less than systemic vascular resistance. Blood flow from the LA to the RA can be evaluated echocardiographically with CFD and is often associated with volume overload of the LA, RA, and RV. Right ventricle volume overload can be qualitatively evaluated by TEE. A more quantitative measurement of RV volume overload relies on M-mode detection of intraventricular septal (IVS) shift toward the LV during diastole. A large left-to-right shunt at the atrial level is often associated with dilatation of the main PA and torrential pulmonary venous blood flow. The detection of bidirectional flow or right-to-left shunting at the atrial level is indicative of an elevated RAP. Elevated RAP is most likely the result of RV hypertension. Right ventricle hypertension results from pulmonary stenosis or RV outflow tract obstruction, primary pulmonary hypertension, and pulmonary vascular occlusive disease (PVOD). Pulmonary vascular occlusive disease should be considered in any patient with chronic exposure of the pulmonary circulation to excessive blood flow from a large ASD [pulmonary-to-systemic flow ratio (QP:QS) of >2:1].

Ostium Secundum Atrial Septal Defect

Ostium secundum defects are the most common type of ASD. The normal intact IAS consists of a central membranous portion and a thicker inferior and superior fatty limbus (14). The central membranous portion is formed by tissue of the septum primum and fossa ovalis. This membrane lies posterior to the superior aspect of the fatty limbus. Although a PFO results from incomplete fusion of an intact fossa ovalis membrane with the superior aspect of the fatty limbus, an ostium secundum ASD is the result of actual deficiencies in the membrane of the fossa ovalis. There are four morphologic types of ostium secundum ASDs:

- Virtual absence of the septum primum: the ASD is the entire fossa ovalis.
- Deficiency of the septum primum: the ASD is only a portion of the entire fossa ovalis.
- Completely fenestrated: the entire septum primum is fenestrated, creating multiple defects in the fossa ovalis.
- Partially fenestrated: a portion of the septum primum is absent and the remainder is fenestrated.

Ostium secundum ASDs are best visualized in a modified ME aortic valve SAX view with scanning between 30 and 60 degrees, or in the ME bicaval view. In both views the defect is limited to the area of the fossa ovalis. There is typically a rim of both anterior (retroaortic) and posterior tissue (Figs. 13.4 and 13.5). Ostium secundum ASDs are generally oval in shape, with a 2:1 ratio of the major to minor axis. The major axis is inferosuperior (IVC to SVC; ME bicaval view) ranging in size from 10 to 50 mm with a mean of 28 mm. The minor axis is anteroposterior (retro-aortic valve to posterior atrium; mid-esophagus aortic valve SAX with scanning between 30 and 60 degrees), ranging in size from 4 to 30 mm, with a mean of 15 mm (15). A fatty limbus tissue remnant frequently persists at both the anteroposterior and inferosuperior borders, but this rim of tissue may be small in the presence of a large defect.

Repair of ostium secundum ASDs generally requires patch closure with pericardium. Alternatively, homograft material or woven Dacron patch material can be used. A small ostium secundum ASD can be closed primarily. Caution must be exercised when a prominent EV exists because it

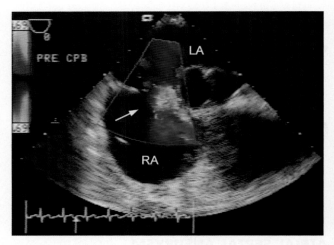

FIGURE 13.4. Modified mid-esophageal aortic valve short-axis view with color flow Doppler demonstrating ostium secundum atrial septal defect (*arrow*). The defect is confined to the area of the fossa ovalis with a rim of tissue posteriorly and anteriorly (retro-aortic).

can be mistaken for the inferior end of an ASD (16). Should this occur, postoperative TEE views of the closed ASD will readily demonstrate baffling of IVC blood into the LA.

Sinus Venous Atrial Septal Defect

Sinus venous defects are located either superiorly at the level of the RA and the SVC, or inferiorly at the level of the IVC. Superior defects comprise the majority of these lesions as inferior defects are rare. Both types are associated with partially anomalous pulmonary venous return (PAPVR). In the case of the superior defect, anomalous drainage of the right upper pulmonary vein into the SVC is the most common finding. Both defects are located posterior to the fossa ovalis.

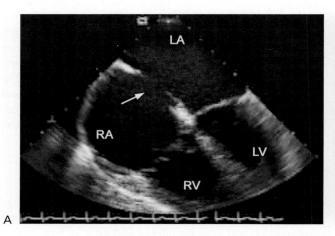
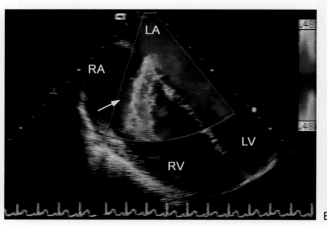

FIGURE 13.5. Ostium secundum atrial septal defect. **A:** Two-dimensional, mid-esophageal four-chamber view demonstrating that the defect (*arrow*) is confined to the region of the fossa ovalis. **B:** Color flow Doppler demonstrating predominant left-to-right shunting (*arrow*). *LA,* left atrium; *RA,* right atrium; *LV,* left ventricle; *RV,* right ventricle.

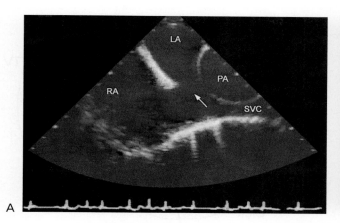
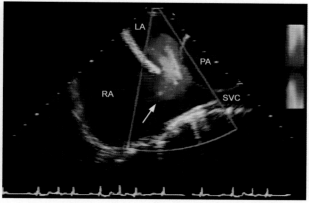

FIGURE 13.6. Sinus venous atrial septal defect. **A:** Two-dimensional, modified mid-esophageal bicaval view. Notice that the superior rim of the defect (*arrow*) is in the superior vena cava (*SVC*) at the level of the right pulmonary artery (*PA*). The fossa ovalis portion of the intraatrial septum is intact. **B:** Color flow Doppler demonstrating predominantly right-to-left shunting (*arrow*). *LA,* left atrium; *RA,* right atrium.

The defects are believed to result from a deficiency in the common wall that normally separates the right pulmonary veins from the RA and SVC, rather than a defect in the IAS or a change in the position of the pulmonary veins per se (17). Unroofing of the pulmonary veins (located posteriorly) permits drainage of the LA directly in the SVC and RA (located anteriorly). Intraatrial communication occurs at the level of the pulmonary veins rather than through an IAS defect.

Multiplane TEE is indispensable in imaging superior sinus venous ASDs and is superior to TTE in the diagnosis of this lesion (18). In an ME bicaval view, the superior aspect of the defect appears to be the right PA due to absence of the fatty limbus just below the SVC orifice (Fig. 13.6). The inferior aspect is the superior aspect of the IAS fatty limbus. In

this view, the SVC appears to override the RA and LA (19). Transverse plane imaging demonstrates the defect between the LA and the SVC–RA junction. The most common type of PAPVR can be detected with further withdrawal of the TEE probe. Transverse plane imaging will demonstrate the right upper pulmonary vein draining directly into the lateral wall of the SVC at the level of the right PA. This communication has a characteristic teardrop appearance (19) (Fig. 13.7).

In instances where the pulmonary veins are normally positioned, the defect is usually repaired with pericardium. Alternatively, the Warden procedure is performed when the pulmonary veins anomalously enter the SVC. The SVC is transected above the origin of the anomalous veins. The proximal end of the SVC is oversewn, and the SVC orifice is directed across the defect into the LA with a pericardial

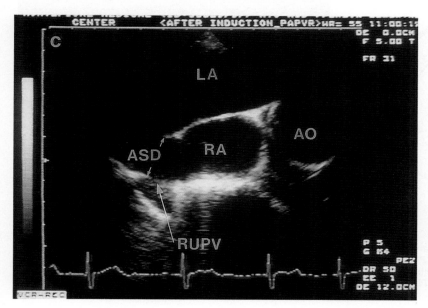

FIGURE 13.7. Sinus venous atrial septal defect (*ASD, arrow*) with partially anomalous pulmonary venous drainage. Transverse plane imaging at the level of the superior vena cava–right atrial (*RA*) junction. The superior vena cava–to–left atrial (*LA*) communication is visible, as is the drainage of the right upper pulmonary vein (*RUPV, arrow*). *AO,* aorta.

patch. The distal end of the SVC is then anastomosed end-to-end to the roof of the RA appendage.

Ostium Primum Atrial Septal Defect

Ostium primum ASDs occur most commonly in conjunction with defects of the inlet portion of the IVS and a common atrioventricular valve orifice, which together produce a complete atrioventricular canal defect. These defects occur as a result of failure of endocardial cushion fusion. This chapter focuses on isolated ostium primum ASDs, which develop when partial fusion of the endocardial cushions separate the two atrioventricular valves and close the ventricular septal communication, but fail to close the ostium primum. This defect occurs outside the confines of the fossa ovalis inferiorly at the level of the atrioventricular valves. The isolated ostium primum defect extends from the inferior IAS fatty limbus, to the crest of the IVS. A characteristic finding of this lesion is insertion of the septal portions of both atrioventricular valves on the IVS at the same level. Normally insertion of the TV to the IVS is inferior to the MV, producing the ventriculoatrial septum, which separates the RA from the LV. These defects are commonly associated with a cleft anterior MV leaflet and mitral regurgitation (MR), resulting from partial fusion of the anterosuperior and inferoposterior bridging leaflets, which normally fuse to form the anterior MV leaflet (Figs. 13.8 and 13.9).

In the ME four-chamber view, an ostium primum ASD appears as a defect extending from the inferior aspect of the IAS to the junction of the atrioventricular valves (Fig. 13.10). The MV cleft can be appreciated as discontinuity of the anterior MV leaflet in any of the short- and long-axis views that optimize imaging of this leaflet. CFD imaging can be used to assess the severity of the associated MR. Repair of

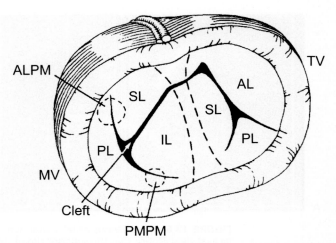

FIGURE 13.9. Separate atrioventricular valves as seen in an isolated ostium primum defect, viewed from above. A cleft is seen in the anterior leaflet of the mitral valve (*MV*) due to failure of fusion of the superior (*SL*) and inferior (*IL*) leaflets. *TV,* tricuspid valve; *ALPM,* anterior lateral papillary muscle; *PMPM,* posterior medial papillary muscle; *AL,* anterior leaflet; *PL,* posterior leaflet; *SL,* superior leaflet (mitral side), septal leaflet (tricuspid side); *VS,* ventricular septum.

his defect requires patch closure of the ASD. MV cleft repair is normally performed with interrupted sutures to create continuity of the anterior leaflet.

Coronary Sinus Atrial Septal Defect

Unroofing of the CS (posterior) allows direct communication with the LA (anterior). At its entry in the RA, the CS defect becomes the connection between the LA and RA.

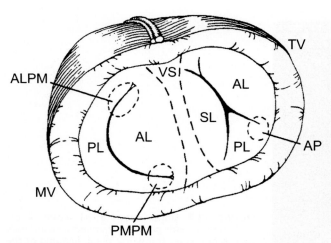

FIGURE 13.8. A pair of normal atrioventricular valves viewed from above. *MV,* mitral valve; *TV,* tricuspid valve; *ALPM,* anterior lateral papillary muscle; *PMPM,* posterior medial papillary muscle; *AP,* anterior papillary muscle; *AL,* anterior leaflet; *PL,* posterior leaflet; *SL,* septal leaflet; *VS,* ventricular septum.

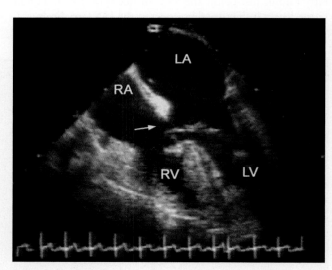

FIGURE 13.10. Ostium primum atrial septal defect. Two-dimensional mid-esophageal four-chamber view. The defect (*arrow*) is seen to extend from just below the inferior aspect of the fossa ovalis to the junction of the atrioventricular valves. The mitral and tricuspid valves are seen to insert at the same level. *RA,* right atrium; *LA,* left atrium; *RV,* right ventricle; *LV,* left ventricle.

CS ASDs are usually associated with a persistent LSVC and a large dilated CS. A persistent LSVC is easily detected in the ME four-chamber view. The vessel is seen in SAX as an echolucent circle in the ridge of tissue between the LA appendage and the left upper pulmonary vein. TEE probe advancement or slight retroflexion in this plane further demonstrates communication of the persistent LSVC with a dilated CS. The ME two-chamber view also provides a long-axis view of the persistent LSVC and a SAX view of the posterior CS communicating with the anterior LA.

Repair of CS ASDs requires patch closure of the CS roof, resulting in drainage of the CS and persistent LSVC blood flow to the RA. In the absence of an LSVC, the CS orifice can be oversewn, resulting in closure of the LA-to-RA communication while leaving a very small right-to-left shunt (CS to LA).

VENTRICULAR SEPTAL DEFECTS

A variety of nomenclature systems exist to describe congenital VSDs. Figure 13.11 illustrates a commonly used system. Conoventricular defects are also known as perimembranous or paramembranous defects, whereas conoseptal defects are also known as supracristal or subarterial defects. Most muscular and perimembranous VSD close spontaneously in infancy and childhood. Thus, an isolated VSD is a relatively rare occurrence in adults, yet most commonly present in the perimembranous or conoventricular location. These defects are located near or under the septal leaflet of the TV and communicate with the LV just below the aortic valve. These defects are commonly partially closed by a collection of TV and membranous septal tissue, giving an aneurysmal appearance to the IVS.

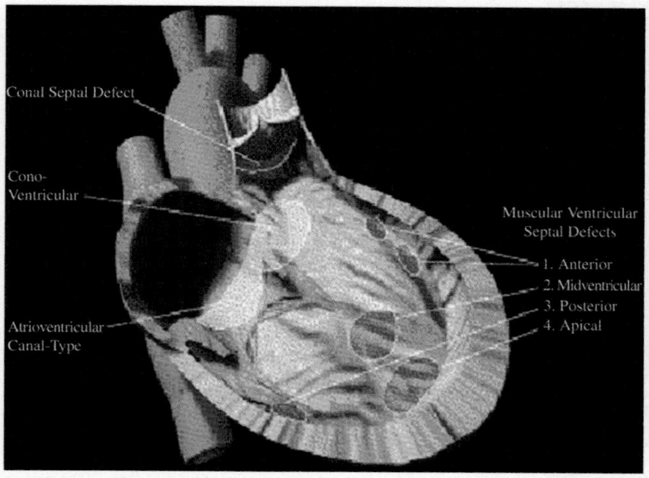

Perimembranous defects in adults are likely to be small and therefore restrictive. By definition, restrictive defects have a large pressure difference between the RV and LV. These small defects exhibit left-to-right shunting, with a QP:QS ratio of less than 1.5:1. Right ventricular systolic pressure (RVSP) can be estimated by using continuous-wave Doppler (CWD) to measure the peak velocity across the VSD. Using the modified Bernoulli equation: $RVSP = SBP - 4V^2$, where SBP is systolic blood pressure and V is the peak velocity across the VSD in meters per second. RVSP elevation in the presence of a small VSD should prompt a search for pulmonary stenosis, primary pulmonary hypertension, and PVOD. Further increases in RVSP produce bidirectional shunt flow across the VSD.

Congenital VSDs are best imaged in the ME long-axis and ME aortic valve SAX views. CFD is indispensable in identifying the defect, particularly if it is small (Fig. 13.12). In some instances of spontaneous closure, an aneurysmal septum with no evidence of trans-septal flow can be seen. In the ME aortic valve SAX view, the defect will be seen in close proximity to the TV, just beneath the right coronary cusp. It may be difficult to distinguish CFD flow associated with a perimembranous VSD from a TR jet. Spectral Doppler imaging, however, can be useful in this scenario. For example, let us assume that the systolic blood pressure = 120 mm Hg, RVSP = 39 mm Hg, and CVP = 14 mm Hg. If the peak velocity by CWD is 4.5 m/s, then the gradient is 81 mm Hg and thus more consistent with a VSD. However, if the peak velocity is 2.5 m/s, then the gradient is 25 mm Hg and the defect is more likely TR.

Congenital VSDs can usually be closed via a transatrial approach with retraction of the TV septal leaflet. The transatrial approach obviates the need for ventriculotomy and decreases

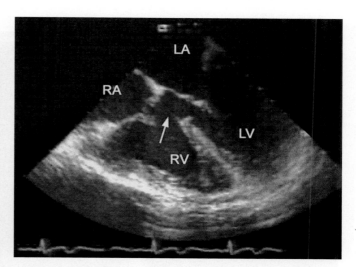

FIGURE 13.11. A view of the interventricular septum from the right ventricle demonstrating the position of various ventricular septal defects.

FIGURE 13.12. Perimembranous ventricular septal defect. Two-dimensional, mid-esophageal four-chamber view. The defect (*arrow*) is seen in proximity to the septal leaflet of the tricuspid valve. *RA*, right atrium; *LA*, left atrium; *RV*, right ventricle; *LV*, left ventricle.

the potential for ventricular dysfunction. In some instances, detachment and subsequent reattachment of the septal leaflet may be necessary to gain exposure.

Acquired VSDs in adults are usually associated with postinfarction rupture and have been diagnosed in 2% of patients following myocardial infarction. Postinfarction VSDs typically occur after an anterior myocardial infarction and involve the anterior middle or apical muscular portion of the IVS. Inferior septal defects can occur in the presence of an inferior wall myocardial infarction. These defects tend to involve the basal portion of the inferior septum. Survival after inferior septal rupture is poor, presumably due to the occurrence of concomitant extensive RV involvement following an inferior myocardial infarction.

Small acquired VSDs with serpiginous pathways may require CFD for detection. Other defects are large and easily identified. A large defect may have a QP:QS ratio of more than 2:1. The volume load associated with such lesions produces LV and RV dilatation when a large volume of blood is recirculated from the LV to the RV to the PA to the LA and back to the LV. Obviously, this has the potential to severely compromise systemic cardiac output, particularly when LV systolic function has been seriously compromised following a large myocardial infarction. Acquired VSDs are most optimally imaged in the ME four-chamber view, although it may be difficult to visualize the most anterior portion of the IVS given its greater distance from the transducer. Transgastric SAX views may be helpful to further delineate the VSD location (Figs. 13.13 and 13.14).

Acquired muscular VSDs require patch closure and are usually approached via a ventriculotomy in the infarcted area. These defects are a surgical challenge due to the friability of the surrounding tissue and the propensity for suture dehiscence. Postrepair TEE examination is essential to rule

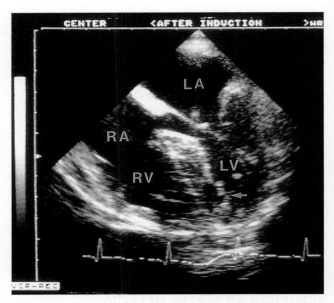

FIGURE 13.13. Ventricular septal rupture. Mid-esophageal four-chamber view. A large defect is seen in the apical region of the muscular septum. *RA,* right atrium; *LA,* left atrium; *RV,* right ventricle; *LV,* left ventricle.

out residual leaks, and to delineate any remaining serpiginous communications.

TUMORS

Cardiac tumors may be primary or secondary (metastatic). Primary cardiac tumors are rare, with an autopsy incidence of 0.05%. Secondary tumors are 20 times more common and are seen in 1% of autopsy examinations, almost always

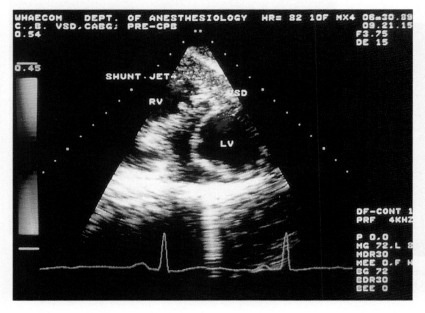

FIGURE 13.14. Ventricular septal rupture. Transgastric mid short-axis view. Color flow Doppler demonstrating a defect in the inferior portion of the muscular septum. *RV,* right ventricle; *LV,* left ventricle.

TABLE 13.1. PRIMARY CARDIAC TUMORS

Cardiac Tumor	Incidence (%)
Myxoma	45
Lipoma	20
Papillary fibroelastoma	15
Angioma	5
Hemangioma	5
Fibroma	3
Rhabdomyoma	1

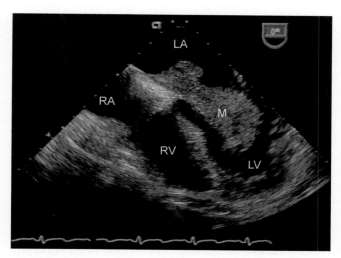

FIGURE 13.15. Atrial myxoma. A large tumor mass (*M*) is seen prolapsing across the mitral valve in diastole. The tumor is polypoid with multiple echolucent areas within the mass. *RA,* right atrium; *RV,* right ventricle; *LA,* left atrium; *LV,* left ventricle.

in the setting of widely disseminated disease. The clinical features most commonly associated with cardiac tumors include embolization, obstruction, and arrhythmias (20,21).

Primary Cardiac Tumors

The majority (75%) of primary cardiac tumors are benign (Table 13.1) (20,21). In adults, the myxoma is the most common benign primary tumor, whereas in children it is the rhabdomyoma. The majority of malignant primary cardiac tumors are angiosarcomas or rhabdomyosarcomas.

Atrial Myxoma

Atrial myxomas are intracavitary and can occur in any chamber, although most are found in the LA (90%), with the vast majority of the remaining portion being found in the RA. In addition, 90% of myxomas are solitary and 90% are attached to the IAS by a stalk or pedicle in the region of the fossa ovalis. The heterogenous and polypoid consistency of these tumors appears as small cystic echolucencies within the tumor mass. Tumors that have a fibrous composition are more likely to be obstructive. The tumor mass may compromise MV function by prolapsing back and forth across the MV producing a characteristic tumor "plop" heard on physical examination. Large myxomas may obstruct the MV inlet and produce functional mitral stenosis (Fig. 13.15). Systemic embolization also is a significant risk, occurring in 30% to 40% of patients. Tumors that have a polypoid or myxoid composition are more likely to embolize. In addition, these lesions are more likely to promote thrombus formation on their surface, which also can embolize. Once identified, atrial myomas are resected to prevent obstructive and embolic sequelae. Complete resection may require resection of part of the IAS, in which case patch closure of the resulting ASD may be necessary.

Lipoma

These encapsulated lesions generally originate in pericardial or epicardial fat and can grow to be enormous. They are less commonly found in the subendocardium and cardiac chambers. Lipomas involving the atrioventricular valves have been described as well. They tend to be solitary and asymptomatic. Symptoms are usually caused by growth and compression of adjacent structures. Resection is indicated unless the tumor encases the coronary arteries or is deeply infiltrative. The unique appearance of fat on magnetic resonance imaging makes this modality particularly useful for the diagnosis of lipoma.

Papillary Fibroelastoma

Papillary fibroelastoma is the most common tumor of cardiac valves. Prior to the use of TEE, the diagnosis of this tumor was made at surgery or autopsy. As a result, the incidence was underestimated (22). More than 90% are solitary, and the majority is small (<1–1.5 cm). The lesions, which are attached by a short pedicle, tend to be circular with multiple filiform projections off the surface. They are said to resemble a sea anemone. Most papillary fibroelastomas are located on cardiac valves (84%), with the majority of these located on the aortic valve and MV (54%). Involvement of the MV and TV is typically on the mid-portion of the atrial side, whereas involvement of the aortic valve and pulmonic valves can be anywhere, with equal frequency on the ventricular and arterial sides. The nonvalvular lesions are known to involve all intracardiac locations, including papillary muscles and chordae.

Papillary fibroelastomas are distinct from Lambl excrescences, which are found on 70% to 80% of adult valves (21). Lambl excrescences are small filamentous lesions that occur along the valve closure lines on the ventricular side of the valve. They are rarely found on the arterial side of semilunar valves.

Secondary Cardiac Tumors

Metastases to the heart generally affect the pericardium and are therefore frequently associated with an effusion. Intracavitary metastases are usually the result of hematogenous spread and consequently are much more common in right sided chambers. Renal cell carcinoma, hepatoma, Wilms tumor, and uterine leiomyoma can all spread to the right heart via the IVC.

THROMBUS

Thrombus is generally homogenous in appearance, tends to be more echogenic than the underlying myocardium, and typically exhibits a thin border of echolucency between itself and the underlying myocardium. This thin rim of echolucency helps to distinguish thrombus from infiltrative masses. Thrombi tend to laminate along endocardial surfaces without the discreet areas of attachment typical of myxomas. Thrombi usually appear in multiple imaging planes and move in concert with underlying myocardium.

Atrial Thrombus

Transesophageal echocardiography is clearly superior to TTE in detection and delineation of atrial thrombi (Fig. 13.16). Thrombus in the LA is relatively common and usually associated with stasis of blood, especially in the presence of LA dilatation and hypokinesis, atrial fibrillation (AF), native or prosthetic mitral stenosis, and LV dysfunction. Thrombus

in the setting of MR is less common despite LA dilatation because the high-velocity regurgitant jet prevents stasis (23). A large proportion of LA thrombi involve the left atrial appendage (LAA). Thus, careful examination of the appendage in multiple planes is necessary to rule out thrombi. The LAA has a narrow base and sharply terminates in a discreet, crenated apex. Often the comblike appearance of pectinate muscles is apparent. Blunting of the LAA apex is highly suggestive of thrombus. However, because more than 50% of patients have two or more small additional lobes of the LAA, it is important not to confuse the tissues separating these lobes with thrombus. In addition, care must be taken not to confuse thrombus with the ridge of tissue that separates the LAA from the left upper pulmonary vein (i.e., coumadin ridge).

Thrombus in the RA is unusual but may occur following embolization of a deep venous thrombosis (DVT) or thrombus that has formed on indwelling catheters or pacemaker leads. As discussed previously, the EV and Chiari network are commonly mistaken for RA thrombi. Similarly, the crista terminalis should not be confused with an RA mass. This muscular ridge runs from the anterior portion of the SVC orifice to the anterior portion of the IVC orifice and divides the anterior trabeculated portion of the RA from the posterior smooth portion. The RA appendage, which is broad based, short, and blunt, often contains prominent pectinate muscles.

Left atrial spontaneous echo contrast (SEC) has clearly been associated with thrombus formation and subsequent risk of thromboembolism for both patients in sinus rhythm and AF (24,25). SEC is defined as slowly swirling intracavitary echodensities (smoke) resulting from protein-mediated

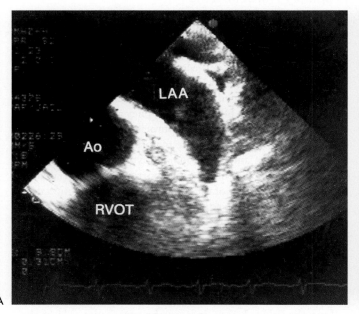
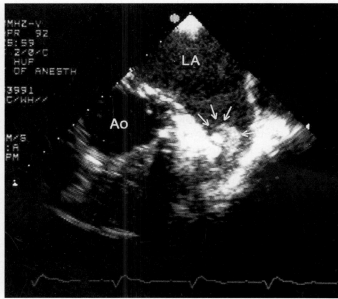

FIGURE 13.16. Left atrial appendage thrombus and spontaneous echo contrast. **A:** Normal left atrial appendage (*LAA*). **B:** A thrombus (*arrows*) is seen in the LAA apex of a patient with mitral stenosis. *Ao,* aorta; *RVOT,* right ventricular outflow tract; *LA,* left atrium.

red cell aggregation (26). Dense echo contrast can be seen easily at standard gain settings, whereas faint contrast requires enhanced gain settings for detection. LAA antegrade (emptying) velocity measured with pulsed-wave Doppler, has been identified as a method of stratifying the risk of thrombus and thromboembolism (27). In patients with nonvalvular AF and those in sinus rhythm, the incidence of SEC is related to peak antegrade LAA velocity. In the presence of AF, the incidence of SEC is 75% when peak antegrade LAA velocity is less than 20 cm/s as compared with 58% in patients with a peak velocity greater than 20 cm/s (28,29). In patients with sinus rhythm, the incidence of SEC is 87% with a peak antegrade LAA velocity of less than 40 cm/s compared with 19% in patients with a peak velocity of greater than 40 cm/s (29). The incidence of LAA thrombus is 89% in patients with AF and SEC as compared with 13% in patients with sinus rhythm and SEC. As expected, the incidence of LAA thrombus is higher in patients with dense echo contrast than in those with faint echo contrast (27). Alternatively, only 14% of patients with AF have RA SEC and less than 1% have an RA thrombus (30).

Ventricular Thrombus

Left ventricular thrombi are invariably associated with areas of stasis, most commonly associated with severely hypokinetic, akinetic, or aneurysmal wall segments. Consequently, LV thrombi are seen in up to 50% of patients following a large, transmural anterior myocardial infarction, and in 50% of patients with dilated cardiomyopathies. The overwhelming majority of LV thrombi are apical (Fig. 13.17).

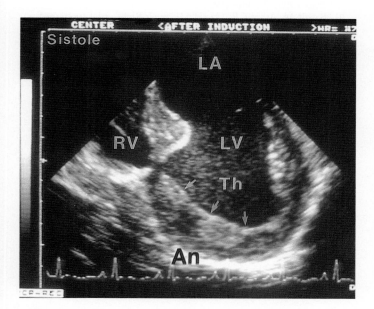

FIGURE 13.17. Left ventricular (*LV*) thrombus (*Th*). Midesophageal four-chamber view demonstrating a large apical ventricular thrombus. The underlying myocardium is akinetic and aneurysmal. *LA,* left atrium; *RV,* right ventricle; *An,* aneurysm.

Differentiation of thrombus from papillary muscles in the transgastric middle SAX view can be difficult, and often requires multiplane imaging.

Right ventricular thrombi are also associated with areas of stasis and systolic dysfunction occurring with myocardial infarction, dilated cardiomyopathy, myocardial contusion, and cor pulmonale. RV thrombi are almost always apical as well. Detection of RV thrombus is made more difficult by the trabeculated surface of the RV endocardium and the moderator band, which traverses the RV from the free wall to the septum near the ventricular apex.

KEY POINTS

- Four types of ASDs exist: ostium secundum (most common), ostium primum (associated with cleft MV), sinus venous (associated with PAPVR usually involving the right upper pulmonary vein and the SVC), coronary sinus (uncommon, associated with persistent LSVC drainage to the CS).
- Perimembranous VSDs tend to be small (restrictive) and are located close to the TV.
- Postinfarction ventricular septal rupture typically involves the anterior portion of the middle or apical IVS.
- Cardiac tumors are rare. Metastatic tumors are 20 times more common than primary tumors.
- Seventy-five percent of primary cardiac tumors are benign. The majority are myxomas, usually located in the LA.
- The presence of SEC and reduced antegrade LAA emptying velocity increases the likelihood that LA thrombus will be present.
- Right atrial thrombi occur following embolization of a DVT or thrombus that has formed on indwelling catheters or pacemaker leads.
- Ventricular thrombi are usually located in the apex and are invariably associated with underlying regions of impaired systolic function.

REFERENCES

1. Schmidt KG, Silverman NH, Rudolph AM. Assessment of flow events at the ductus venosus–inferior vena cava junction and at the foramen ovale in fetal sheep by use of multimodal ultrasound. *Circulation* 1996;93:826–833.
2. Schneider B, Hofmann T, Justen MH, et al. Chiari's network: normal anatomic variant or risk factor for arterial embolic events? *J Am Coll Cardiol* 1995;26:203–210.
3. Kerut EK, Norfleet WT, Plotnick GD, et al. Patent foramen ovale: a review of associated conditions and the impact of physiological size. *J Am Coll Cardiol* 2001;38:613–623.
4. Carson W, Chiu SS. Image in cardiovascular medicine. Eustachian valve mimicking intracardiac mass. *Circulation* 1998;97:2188.
5. Hamann GF, Schatzer-Klotz D, Frohlig G, et al. Femoral injection of echo contrast medium may increase the sensitivity of testing for a patent foramen ovale. *Neurology* 1998;50:1423–1428.

6. Konstadt SN, Louie EK, Black S, et al. Intraoperative detection of patent foramen ovale by transesophageal echocardiography. *Anesthesiology* 1991;74:212–216.

7. Schneider B, Zienkiewicz T, Jansen V, et al. Diagnosis of patent foramen ovale by transesophageal echocardiography and correlation with autopsy findings. *Am J Cardiol* 1996;77:1202–1209.

8. Fisher DC, Fisher EA, Budd JH, et al. The incidence of patent foramen ovale in 1,000 consecutive patients. A contrast transesophageal echocardiography study. *Chest* 1995;107:1504–1509.

9. Rao PS, Palacios IF, Bach RG, et al. Platypnea-orthodeoxia: management by transcatheter buttoned device implantation. *Catheter Cardiovasc Interv* 2001;54:77–82.

10. Shapiro GC, Leibowitz DW, Oz MC, et al. Diagnosis of patent foramen ovale with transesophageal echocardiography in a patient supported with a left ventricular assist device. *J Heart Lung Transplant* 1995;14:594–597.

11. Agmon Y, Khandheria BK, Meissner I, et al. Frequency of atrial septal aneurysms in patients with cerebral ischemic events. *Circulation* 1999;99:1942–1944.

12. Mugge A, Daniel WG, Angermann C, et al. Atrial septal aneurysm in adult patients. A multicenter study using transthoracic and transesophageal echocardiography. *Circulation* 1995;91:2785–2792.

13. Autore C, Cartoni D, Piccininno M. Multiplane transesophageal echocardiography and stroke. *Am J Cardiol* 1998;81:79G–81G.

14. Schwinger ME, Gindea AJ, Freedberg RS, et al. The anatomy of the interatrial septum: a transesophageal echocardiographic study. *Am Heart J* 1990;119:1401–1405.

15. Chan KC, Godman MJ. Morphological variations of fossa ovalis atrial septal defects (secundum): feasibility for transcutaneous closure with the clam-shell device. *Br Heart J* 1993;69:52–55.

16. Sapin PM, Salley RK. Arterial desaturation and orthodeoxia after atrial septal defect repair: demonstration of the mechanism by transesophageal and contrast echocardiography. *J Am Soc Echocardiogr* 1997;10:588–592.

17. Van Praagh S, Carrera ME, Sanders SP, et al. Sinus venosus defects: unroofing of the right pulmonary veins—anatomic and echocardiographic findings and surgical treatment. *Am Heart J* 1994;128:365–379.

18. Kronzon I, Tunick PA, Freedberg RS, et al. Transesophageal echocardiography is superior to transthoracic echocardiography in the diagnosis of sinus venosus atrial septal defect. *J Am Coll Cardiol* 1991;17:537–542.

19. Pascoe RD, Oh JK, Warnes CA, et al. Diagnosis of sinus venosus atrial septal defect with transesophageal echocardiography. *Circulation* 1996;94:1049–1055.

20. Vander Salm TJ. Unusual primary tumors of the heart. *Semin Thorac Cardiovasc Surg* 2000;12:89–100.

21. Grebenc ML, Rosado de Christenson ML, Burke AP, et al. Primary cardiac and pericardial neoplasms: radiologic-pathologic correlation. *Radiographics* 2000;20:1073–1103; quiz 1110–1111, 1112.

22. Shahian DM. Papillary fibroelastomas. *Semin Thorac Cardiovasc Surg* 2000;12:101–110.

23. Fatkin D, Kelly RP, Feneley MP. Relations between left atrial appendage blood flow velocity, spontaneous echocardiographic contrast and thromboembolic risk *in vivo. J Am Coll Cardiol* 1994;23:961–969.

24. Black IW. Spontaneous echo contrast: where there's smoke there's fire. *Echocardiography* 2000;17:373–382.

25. Sadanandan S, Sherrid MV. Clinical and echocardiographic characteristics of left atrial spontaneous echo contrast in sinus rhythm. *J Am Coll Cardiol* 2000;35:1932–1938.

26. Fatkin D, Loupas T, Low J, et al. Inhibition of red cell aggregation prevents spontaneous echocardiographic contrast formation in human blood. *Circulation* 1997;96:889–896.

27. Transesophageal echocardiographic correlates of thromboembolism in high-risk patients with nonvalvular atrial fibrillation. The Stroke Prevention in Atrial Fibrillation Investigators Committee on Echocardiography. *Ann Intern Med* 1998;128:639–647.

28. Zabalgoitia M, Halperin JL, Pearce LA, et al. Transesophageal echocardiographic correlates of clinical risk of thromboembolism in nonvalvular atrial fibrillation. Stroke Prevention in Atrial Fibrillation III Investigators. *J Am Coll Cardiol* 1998;31:1622–1626.

29. Goldman ME, Pearce LA, Hart RG, et al. Pathophysiologic correlates of thromboembolism in nonvalvular atrial fibrillation. I. Reduced flow velocity in the left atrial appendage (The Stroke Prevention in Atrial Fibrillation [SPAF-III] study). *J Am Soc Echocardiogr* 1999;12:1080–1087.

30. Bashir M, Asher CR, Garcia MJ, et al. Right atrial spontaneous echo contrast and thrombi in atrial fibrillation: a transesophageal echocardiography study. *J Am Soc Echocardiogr* 2001;14:122–127.

ECHOCARDIOGRAPHIC EVALUATION OF PERICARDIAL DISEASE

STANTON K. SHERNAN

Despite recent advances in medical imaging, echocardiography remains an essential technique for the diagnosis of pericardial disease. For example, echocardiography is an invaluable tool for quantifying the volume of pericardial effusions and diagnosing diastolic dysfunction associated with cardiac tamponade. In addition, the concurrent echocardiographic identification of a highly reflective thickened pericardium, associated with marked respiratory variation of intracardiac and systemic venous Doppler flow velocities, is often sufficient to make the diagnosis of constrictive pericarditis in a symptomatic patient. Two-dimensional (2D) echocardiography is also a relatively safe, noninvasive technique for identifying cysts, tumors, and other structural abnormalities of the pericardium. Following echocardiographic diagnosis, surgical intervention is frequently required for patients with pericardial disease who become symptomatic due to pericardial restraint associated with constrictive pericarditis, or cardiac chamber compression due to pericardial effusions or localized masses. This chapter will focus on the perioperative applications of transesophageal echocardiography (TEE) in the evaluation of pericardial disease.

PERICARDIAL ANATOMY AND PHYSIOLOGY

The pericardial cavity is a potential space between the visceral pericardium overlying the epicardial surface, and the parietal lining of the fibrous pericardium that separates the heart from other intrathoracic structures. The pericardium is restrained by posterior attachments to the pulmonary veins and venae cavae at the atrial level, and superior attachments to the great arteries. These posterior and superior attachments create the respective oblique pericardial and transverse sinuses. Complete congenital absence of the pericardium (CAP) is a rare, often asymptomatic disorder. Partial CAP, usually involving

the left side, potentially permits cardiac chamber herniation or entrapment. Echocardiographic findings in patients with congenital absence of the pericardium include exaggerated posterior left ventricle (LV) wall and paradoxic ventricular septal motion, the appearance of right ventricle (RV) dilatation from the transthoracic parasternal window due to a leftward shift of the entire heart, and the identification of other congenital cardiac anomalies (e.g., atrial septal defects, bicuspid aortic valve) (1). Although its definitive function remains to be delineated, the normal pericardium mechanically restrains the cardiac chambers from dilatation, limits ventricular filling, and may protect against excessive incompetence of atrioventricular valves (2).

PERICARDIAL EFFUSIONS

The visceral and parietal pericardium is normally separated by less than 20 to 30 mL of serous fluid in the pericardial cavity. They therefore appear echocardiographically as a single highly reflective linear interface that surrounds the external surface of the heart (2). Two-dimensional echocardiographic visualization of the pericardial cavity as an "echo-free space" depends on the volume and pattern of fluid distribution around the heart. Three-dimensional echocardiography also has shown promise for enhanced localization and quantification of pericardial effusions (3). Small pericardial effusions (<100 mL; <10 mm in width) tend to be localized behind the posterior LV wall (Fig. 14.1). The posterior pericardial cul-de-sac and lateral walls are relatively compliant, thus permitting initial fluid accumulation (4). Moderate-sized effusions (100–500 mL, 10–15 mm in width) expand laterally, apically, and anteriorly and can be seen throughout the entire cardiac cycle. Large pericardial effusions (>500 mL, >15 mm in width) tend to be more evenly distributed around the heart, although preferential posterior accumulation is still common (5). Large, chronically accumulating pericardial fluid effusions are often associated with excessive anteroposterior heart motion and counterclockwise rotation in the horizontal plane. Cardiac translation within the pericardial

S. K. Shernan: Department of Anesthesiology, Perioperative, and Pain Medicine, Brigham & Women's Hospital, Harvard Medical School, Boston, Massachusetts.

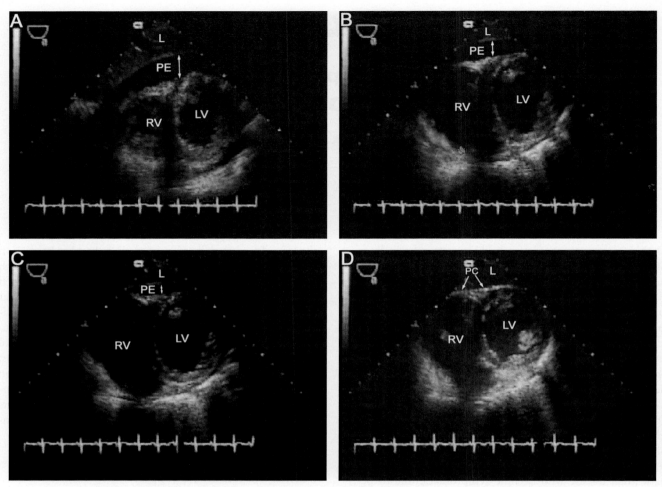

FIGURE 14.1. Intraoperative transesophageal echocardiographic transgastric middle short-axis images demonstrating decreasing pericardial effusion (*PE*) volume during surgical pericardiocentesis. **A:** Large pericardial effusion (900 mL, 16 mm in width) prior to pericardiocentesis (*arrows*). **B:** Moderate-sized pericardial effusion (600 mL, 11 mm in width) after removing 300 mL of fluid (*arrows*). **C:** Small pericardial effusion (300 mL, 8 mm in width) after removal of 600 mL of fluid (*arrows*). **D:** Minimal residual pericardial effusion following completed 900 mL pericardiocentesis (*arrows*). *LV,* left ventricle; *RV,* right ventricle; *PC,* pericardium; *L,* liver.

space accounts for electrocardiographic electrical alternans (6), the appearance of abnormal septal regional wall motion abnormalities and motion abnormalities of the cardiac valves (e.g., mitral and tricuspid valve prolapse, mitral valve systolic anterior motion, early systolic closure of the aortic valve, and mid-systolic notching of either the aortic valve or pulmonic valve) (7).

Pericardial effusions can be identified postoperatively in approximately 85% of cardiac surgical patients, although their size may vary, usually peaking by the 10th postoperative day (8). The clinical presentation of postoperative effusions also may vary from a spurious finding in an asymptomatic patient, to hemodynamic instability associated with local or circumferential cardiac chamber compression. The absolute size of the effusion, however, does not necessarily correlate with clinical signs because even relatively small, rapidly

accumulating effusions may produce symptoms. Although postoperative effusions may present as an isolated anterior effusion, they are often located posteriorly and loculated by restraint from adhesions within the pericardial space (9). Postoperative hemopericardium can present with thrombus, usually along the anterolateral right atrial (RA) free wall, and also may cause compression and hemodynamic compromise (10) (Fig. 14.2). Moderate or large pericardial effusions requiring surgical intervention also develop in patients with renal failure and following pericardial infiltration from lung and breast carcinoma (11). Primary pericardial neoplasms (e.g., mesothelioma, sarcoma, teratoma), however, are relatively uncommon (12).

A thorough TEE examination may be required to differentiate a pericardial effusion from similar appearing intrathoracic structures. The location of a large posterior pericardial

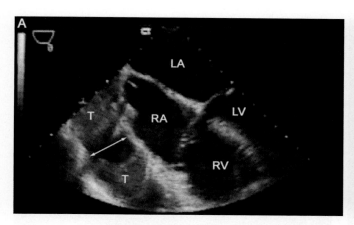

FIGURE 14.2. Intraoperative transesophageal echocardiographic mid-esophageal four-chamber **(A)** and bicaval **(B)** images of a large hemopericardium. A large pericardial effusion (↔) can be seen along with loculated, intrapericardial thrombus (*T*) adjacent to the right atrium (*RA*) in each view. *LA*, left atrium; *LV*, left ventricle; *RV*, right ventricle; *SVC*, superior vena cava.

fluid collection can be difficult to distinguish echocardiographically from a left pleural effusion, especially in a transgastric basal short-axis TEE view. However, a large left pleural effusion is usually easily identified in a long- or short-axis view of the descending thoracic aorta (Fig. 14.3). Benign

pericardial cysts may appear similar to echolucent pericardial effusions due to the presence of encapsulated clear fluid; however, they are most commonly round, sharply demarcated, and located in the right costophrenic angle (13). Pericardial cysts are usually asymptomatic; however, they can

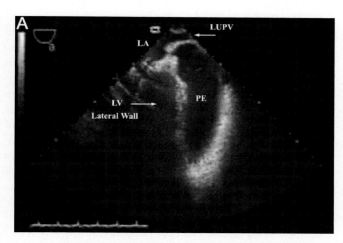

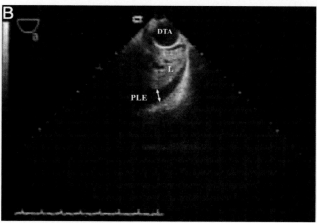

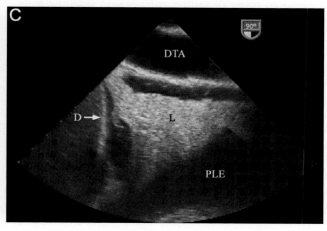

FIGURE 14.3. Intraoperative transesophageal echocardiographic (TEE) images demonstrating a large pericardial effusion (*PE*) and left pleural effusion (*PLE*). **A:** The PE can be seen adjacent to the lateral wall of the left ventricle (*LV, arrow*) and beneath the left upper pulmonary vein (*LUPV, arrow*) by advancing the probe to the transgastric depth while maintaining 0 degrees of rotation and turning the probe slightly leftward. *B:* A concurrent left PLE and collapsed left lung (*L, arrows*), can usually be seen beneath the descending thoracic aorta (*DTA*) by slightly withdrawing the TEE probe from the transgastric depth and turning further leftward while maintaining 0 degrees of rotation. **C:** Rotating to 90 degrees provides a long-axis view of the left PLE and DTA. *LA*, left atrium; *D*, diaphragm.

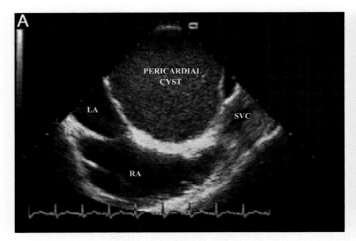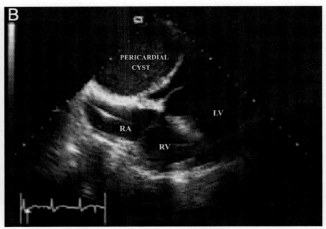

FIGURE 14.4. Intraoperative transesophageal echocardiographic mid-esophageal bicaval **(A)** and four-chamber **(B)** images of a large pericardial cyst (6 × 7 cm) compressing the left atrium (LA). *RA,* right atrium; *SVC,* superior vena cava; *RV,* right ventricle; *LV,* left ventricle.

be associated with chest pain, dyspnea, cough, significant arrhythmias, or even compression of the pulmonary artery, left atrium (LA), or pulmonary vein (Fig. 14.4) (14). Finally, isolated anterior pericardial effusions can develop following cardiac surgery, but they are relatively uncommon in the absence of posterior pericardial fluid. Loculated anterior echo-free spaces more commonly represent epicardial fat, especially in older, obese, diabetic, female patients (5,15). Thus, the differential diagnosis of an echolucent area should take into consideration its location and size, along with the patient's history and symptoms. The performance of at least a complete echocardiographic examination and even the use of contrast echocardiography have been suggested for further identifying an extracardiac echo-free space (16).

PERICARDIAL TAMPONADE

Cardiac tamponade is a clinical syndrome defined as the decompensated phase of cardiac compression resulting from increased intrapericardial compression. Cardiac tamponade is often characterized by an exaggerated decrease in systemic arterial pressure during spontaneous inspiration (i.e., pulsus paradoxus) associated with reduced LV stroke volume and the transmission of negative intrathoracic pressure to the aorta. Severe cardiac tamponade causing significant impairment of ventricular filling often requires surgical intervention to prevent circulatory collapse. Patients with severe cardiac tamponade usually become symptomatic when an excessively large or rapidly accumulating pericardial effusion develops (e.g., perioperative coagulopathy, vascular incisional or anastomotic dehiscence, ascending aortic dissection, coronary artery dissection following angioplasty, cardiac trauma, etc.). Postoperative pericardial tamponade has been reported in up to 2% of cardiac surgical patients (17).

Two-Dimensional Echocardiography

A variety of 2D echocardiographic signs have been reported in patients with symptomatic pericardial tamponade (Table 14.1). The echocardiographic signs of tamponade may actually precede clinical manifestations. Invagination of the anterior RV free wall and outflow tract often persists throughout diastole in severe tamponade but is usually terminated by atrial systole (Fig. 14.5) (18). Diastolic RA inversion associated with pericardial tamponade tends to occur later in diastole (4), even persisting into early systole after RV invagination has resolved (Fig. 14.6) (9,19). RA inversion becomes more specific for hemodynamically significant pericardial tamponade once its duration lasts longer than one third of the cardiac cycle (19). Elevated right heart pressures (e.g., RV hypertrophy/dilatation, RV infarction, pulmonic/tricuspid regurgitation) may prevent RA or RV diastolic collapse despite concurrent tamponade pathophysiology (20,21). Loculated left pericardial effusions that develop postoperatively, can cause LA or LV diastolic collapse, especially when adjacent left-sided cardiac chamber pressures are low (Fig. 14.7) (21).

Two-dimensional or M-mode echocardiographic examination of a patient with pericardial tamponade often reveals decreased LV dimensions during spontaneous inspiration

TABLE 14.1. ECHOCARDIOGRAPHIC FINDINGS ASSOCIATED WITH CARDIAC TAMPONADE

Early diastolic collapse of the right ventricle
Late diastolic to early systolic right or left atrial inversion
Decreased right atrial or ventricular size
Abnormal ventricular septal motion
Respiratory variation in ventricular chamber size
Inferior vena cava plethora with blunted respiratory changes
Respiratory variation in atrial-ventricular valve, pulmonary venous and hepatic vein Doppler flow velocity profiles

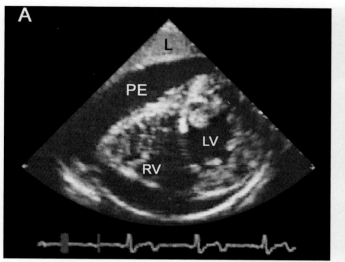
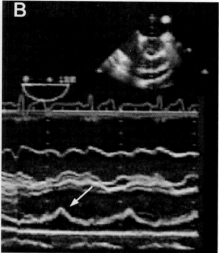

FIGURE 14.5. Intraoperative transesophageal echocardiographic (TEE) images demonstrating a large pericardial effusion (*PE*) and right ventricular (*RV*) diastolic collapse in a patient who became hemodynamically unstable following a left anterior descending coronary artery dissection during an attempt at angioplasty. The patient was brought to the operating room for emergent coronary artery bypass grafting. At the time of the initial TEE following general anesthesia induction, the presence of the hemopericardium was unknown. **A:** Transgastric short-axis view of large PE completely encompassing the RV and left ventricle (*LV*). *L,* liver. **B:** Two-dimensional and M-mode mid-esophageal four-chamber TEE images demonstrating RV diastolic collapse (*arrow*).

compared with expiration, and reciprocal changes in the RV size. The ventricular septum also tends to shift leftward during spontaneous inspiration and rightward during expiration (13). Inferior vena cava (IVC) dilatation and blunted respiratory variation also can occur in the presence of elevated right-sided pericardial pressure. Many of the described classic echocardiographic features of cardiac tamponade may not be present when small increases in intrapericardial volume are associated with rapid increases in pericardial pressure (e.g., cardiac trauma) or when effusions are loculated

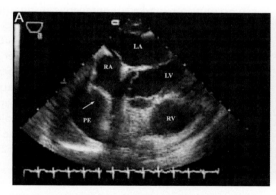
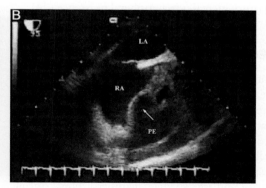
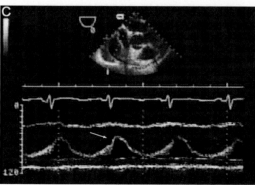

FIGURE 14.6. Intraoperative transesophageal echocardiographic (TEE) images demonstrating a large pericardial effusion (*PE*) and right atrial (*RA*) diastolic collapse. Mid-esophageal four-chamber image (*arrow*) **(A)** and bicaval two-dimensional TEE image **(B)** demonstrating large PE and RA collapse (*arrow*). **C:** Mid-esophageal four-chamber, M-mode images demonstrating right atrial (*RA*) collapse (*arrow*). *RV,* right ventricle; *LA,* left atrium; *LV,* left ventricle.

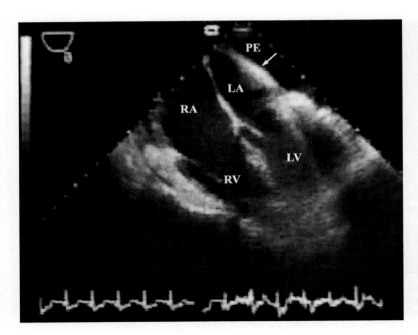

FIGURE 14.7. Intraoperative transesophageal echocardiographic mid-esophageal four-chamber images demonstrating left atrial (*LA*) diastolic collapse (*arrow*) associated with a loculated pericardial effusion (*PE*). *LV,* left ventricle; *RA,* right atrium; *RV,* right ventricle.

(22,23). Following pericardiocentesis, cardiac pressure and volume corrections are more likely to reflect the presence and degree of cardiac compression rather than the amount of fluid removed. After drainage, the more compliant RV may dilate significantly and develop abnormal septal motion consistent with volume overload and congestive heart failure (24). Left ventricle dilatation (pericardial shock) and pulmonary edema also may develop following pericardiocentesis in patients with underlying myocardial disease, due to the acute increase in venous return in the presence of persistent compensatory increases in peripheral resistance (24).

Doppler Echocardiography

In comparison with 2D echocardiography, Doppler echocardiographic features of pericardial tamponade are more sensitive measures of clinical severity (25). Doppler findings of pericardial tamponade are based on alterations of intrathoracic and intracardiac pressures that occur during respiration. Normally during spontaneous respiration, changes in intrathoracic pressures are almost equally transmitted to the pericardial space and intracardiac chambers. Thus, during spontaneous inspiration, both intrathoracic and intracardiac pressures decrease by approximately the same degree. As expected, compared with Doppler flow velocities measured during spontaneous expiration, normal differences in transmitral (10% decrease) and transtricuspid velocities (20% increase) during inspiration are relatively small (26). However, in patients with cardiac tamponade, significant pericardial effusions often blunt the transmission of intrathoracic pressure. Consequently, LA and LV filling pressure gradients are decreased during spontaneous inspiration, resulting in diminished pulmonary venous forward diastolic velocities,

delayed mitral valve opening, prolonged isovolumic relaxation time and decreased mitral E-wave velocity (27) (Fig. 14.8). Similarly, relative increases in LA and LV filling pressure gradients during spontaneous expiration are responsible for corresponding increases in LA and LV Doppler inflow velocities. Exaggeration of ventricular interdependence with pericardial tamponade is responsible for reciprocal changes in right-sided intracardiac flows, resulting in increased tricuspid E-wave velocities during spontaneous inspiration. Increased respiratory variations in patients with cardiac tamponade can account for marked spontaneous inspiratory decreases in transmitral velocities (>40%) and increases in transtricuspid velocities (>80%) compared with values measured during expiration. These transvalvular Doppler flow velocities tend to normalize following therapeutic pericardiocentesis (26). Alterations in the respiratory variation of right atrial inflow velocities (i.e., vena cavae and hepatic veins) are also altered by cardiac tamponade pathophysiology. For example, hepatic vein forward velocities decrease and reverse flows increase during spontaneous expiration (25).

CONSTRICTIVE PERICARDITIS

Constrictive pericarditis (CP) is characterized by a fibrotic, inflamed, or even calcified thickening of the pericardial sac that prevents normal diastolic filling. Hemodynamic features of CP include a narrow RV pulse pressure with normal systolic pressure and increased diastolic pressure, prominent RV early diastolic pressure dip and later plateau, and an additional prominent RA systolic pressure dip presenting as a "W" waveform (28). Pericardial constriction is associated with a variety of pathologic disorders, including infectious

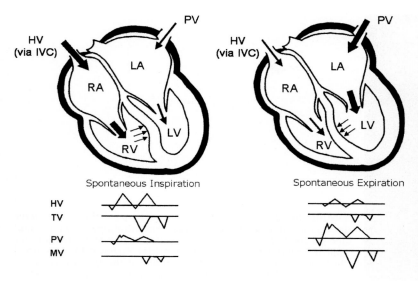

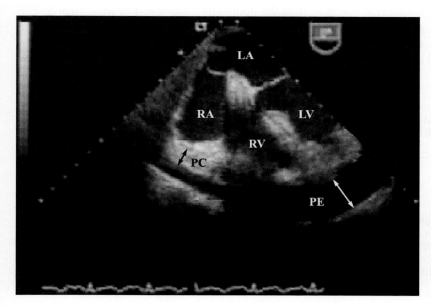

FIGURE 14.8. Effects of cardiac tamponade on right and left-sided intracardiac Doppler flow velocities during spontaneous respiration. Discordance between pressure changes in the thoracic vessels compared with intrapericardial and intracardiac pressure during spontaneous inspiration results in diminished pulmonary venous (*PV*) and transmitral valve (*MV*) Doppler flow velocities. Exaggeration of ventricular interdependence results in a consequential leftward shift of the ventricular septum, thus facilitating right ventricular (*RV*) filling. Consequently, hepatic venous Doppler flow velocities toward the inferior vena cava (*IVC*) and right atrium (*RA*), as well as transtricuspid valve (*TV*) flow, are increased. Reciprocal changes in intracardiac flow velocities occur during spontaneous expiration. *LA,* left atrium; *LV,* left ventricle.

diseases, metabolic disorders, radiation therapy, connective tissue disorders, and neoplastic disease (29). CP also has been reported in approximately 0.2% to 0.3% of cardiac surgical patients despite leaving the pericardium open prior to sternal closure (30). Hemopericardium, serosal injury, and post-pericardiectomy syndrome have all been proposed as possible causes of postoperative CP in the cardiac surgical population (31).

Two-Dimensional Echocardiography

The diagnosis of CP relies on the identification of a thickened, highly reflective echogenic interface surrounding the epicardial surface. Although determination of pericardial thickening is perhaps most accurate when measured using computed tomography or magnetic resonance imaging (32),

TEE may provide a reasonable, more practical and cost-effective alternative (Fig. 14.9). However, excessive gain, diminished lateral resolution, reverberation, and side lobe artifacts can sometimes interfere with echocardiographic imaging and identification of the actual pericardial thickness (Fig. 14.10). Furthermore, "thickening" of the pericardium may actually represent a pericardial effusion with thrombus and fibrinous, echodense adhesions. Several additional, nonspecific 2D and M-mode echocardiographic findings associated with CP also have been identified (Table 14.2).

Doppler Echocardiography

Although the etiology and pathology of CP differ from those of pericardial tamponade, both disorders share some common hemodynamic aberrations in restraining ventricular

FIGURE 14.9. Intraoperative transesophageal echocardiographic transgastric mid-esophageal four-chamber image in a patient with chronic effusive-constrictive pericarditis. Note the thickened pericardium (*PC, black arrow*) along the right atrium (RA) and right ventricle (RV) and the concurrent large pericardial effusion (*PE, white arrow*). *LA,* left atrium; *LV,* left ventricle.

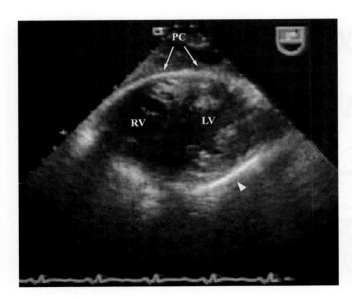

FIGURE 14.10. Intraoperative transesophageal echocardiographic transgastric middle short-axis image demonstrating mildly thickened and calcified echogenic pericardium (*PC, arrow*) along the inferior wall of the left (*LV*) and right (*RV*) ventricles. However, the pericardial thickness along the anterolateral border of the LV (*arrowhead*) is exaggerated due to diminished lateral resolution in the far field.

filling. During respiration, the thickened pericardium permits a profound dissociation between intrathoracic and intracardiac pressures and promotes hemodynamic changes associated with exaggerated ventricular interdependence. Consequently, reciprocal changes during spontaneous respiration in transmitral and pulmonary venous versus transtricuspid and hepatic vein Doppler flow velocities are similar to those observed in patients with pericardial tamponade (33). Frequently a respiratory variation of 25% in the transmitral peak early (E) velocity and an increased diastolic hepatic flow reversal is observed in patients with CP (13). However, up to 20% of patients with CP may not meet these criteria because the exponential shape of the LV pressure decay dictates that respiratory changes in the early diastolic transmitral pressure gradient are decreased at higher filling pressures. Consequently, when respiratory variation in the transmitral peak E-wave Doppler flow velocity is blunted or absent during the evaluation of suspected CP, repeat Doppler examination following preload reduction maneuvers (sitting or reverse Trendelenberg position) may be useful to unmask the characteristic respiratory variation (34).

TABLE 14.2. TWO-DIMENSIONAL AND M-MODE ECHOCARDIOGRAPHIC FINDINGS ASSOCIATED WITH CONSTRICTIVE PERICARDITIS

Paradoxical ventricular septal motion
Ventricular septal "bounce"
Diastolic flattening of the posterior left ventricle
Premature mid-diastolic pulmonary valve opening
Spontaneous inspiratory leftward shift of the atrial and
   ventricular septum
Enlarged hepatic veins; dilated inferior vena cava without
   variation in size during respiration
Normal ventricular size; normal or enlarged atria with reduced
   wall excursion

Because intrathoracic pressure changes associated with positive pressure ventilation are opposite in direction from those seen with spontaneous breathing (35), mechanical ventilation would be expected to reverse the respiratory variation pattern of LA and LV inflow velocities seen with CP (36,37). In a perioperative study of patients with CP undergoing pericardiectomy, the mean respiratory variation in transmitral peak E wave, as well as both pulmonary venous D wave and S wave, decreased significantly following pericardiectomy. In addition, patients who became asymptomatic after surgery had significantly less respiratory variation in mean mitral and pulmonary vein Doppler flow velocity compared with patients who remained symptomatic (38). In another clinical echocardiographic study of a similar patient population, all of the patients demonstrated evidence of LV dilatation following pericardiectomy (39). In addition, diastolic dysfunction was noted in more than half of the patients in the early postoperative period, yet resolved in the majority within 2 months. However, patients in this study in whom diastolic dysfunction persisted beyond the 2-month postoperative observation period remained symptomatic. Thus, the demonstration of respiratory variation in atrial and ventricular Doppler inflow profiles can be a useful technique to establish the diagnosis of hemodynamically significant pericardial pathology and to evaluate outcome following pericardiectomy. In general, pericardiectomy is most successful in patients who present with limited pericardial fibrosis/calcification and hepatic congestion. Interestingly, although atrioventricular valve incompetence is commonly associated with constrictive pericarditis (especially tricuspid valve regurgitation) (40), increased severity of mitral regurgitation has been reported postoperatively (41).

The distinction between CP and restrictive cardiomyopathy (RCM) may be difficult to determine from LV and LA Doppler inflow velocities alone. Both disorders can present with similar clinical manifestations related to decreased LV compliance. Consequently, either pathologic process may be associated with Doppler profiles resembling restrictive LV diastolic filling, including an elevated transmitral peak E-wave velocity and E/Atrial (A) ratio, shortened transmitral E-wave deceleration time, and a pulmonary venous systolic/diastolic ratio of less than 1 (34). The mechanism associated with an increase in chamber stiffness, however, is different for each of these pathologic disorders. In patients with CP, decreased ventricular compliance is directly related to pericardial constraint, whereas RCM usually involves an inherent myocardial disease or infiltrative process. Even more importantly, patients with CP tend to demonstrate an increase in ventricular interdependence and a greater dissociation of intrathoracic-intracardiac pressure changes during respiration, in comparison to patients with RCM. Consequently, CP can be differentiated from RCM echocardiographically by demonstrating respiratory variation in transmitral and pulmonary venous flows (27). In addition, patients with CP and preserved systolic function have more rapid transmitral color M-mode propagation velocities (Vp) compared to patients with RCM (42). Furthermore, a peak early velocity of longitudinal expansion (peak Ea) of 8.0 cm/s obtained by using Doppler tissue imaging (DTI) at the level of the lateral mitral annulus has been shown to be more sensitive (89%) and specific (100%) for differentiating patients with CP from RCM in comparison with Vp, or respiratory variation of either transmitral peak E-wave or pulmonary venous D-wave velocity (43,44). Interestingly, when constriction is more pronounced at the cardiac base as opposed to being evenly distributed, mitral annular velocities obtained by DTI may no longer differentiate constriction from restriction (45). In this scenario, echocardiographic evaluation should include color DTI, which facilitates the detection of an apical retraction phenomena, and regional strain rate imaging, which can provide less motion-dependent information about regional myocardial deformation. Finally, Doppler myocardial velocity gradients (MVGs), an index of myocardial contraction and relaxation that quantifies the spatial distribution of intramural velocities across the myocardium, also have been shown to be useful in differentiating CP from RCM. In comparison with CP, patients with RCM tend to have lower MVG values during ventricular ejection and rapid ventricular filling, and a positive rather than negative value during isovolumic relaxation (46). Thus, both conventional (respiratory variation of intracardiac Doppler flow velocities) and newer echocardiographic modalities (Ea, Vp, MVG) have been shown to be useful in discrimination RCM from CP.

SUMMARY

Echocardiography is a practical medical imaging technique that has several advantages for the evaluation of patients with pericardial disease. Conventional and newer echocar-

diographic techniques can be used to differentiate pericardial disorders with similar clinical presentations (CP vs. RCM) by understanding the differences in the underlying pathophysiologic processes, thus facilitating the determination of the most appropriate therapy. In addition, the identification of a significant pericardial effusion or pericardial constriction in a hemodynamically unstable, symptomatic patient can provide sufficient evidence to warrant prompt surgical intervention, thus avoiding a delay in diagnosis and further morbidity or mortality. Finally, in patients with pericardial disease who require surgical intervention, perioperative echocardiography including 2D and Doppler can provide important information related to the determination of postoperative functional status. Understanding the utility of echocardiography in evaluating patients with pericardial disease is therefore an important component of the ultrasonographer's knowledge base.

KEY POINTS
Pericardial Effusions

- Small pericardial effusions (<100 mL, <10 mm in width) tend to be localized behind the posterior LV wall. Moderate-sized effusions (100–500 mL, 10–15 mm in width) expand laterally, apically, and anteriorly and can be visualized throughout the entire cardiac cycle. Large pericardial effusions (>500 mL, >15 mm in width) tend to be more evenly distributed around the heart, although preferential posterior accumulation is still common.
- Pericardial effusions can be identified postoperatively in approximately 85% of cardiac surgical patients, although their size may vary, usually peaking by the 10th postoperative day. The absolute size of the effusion, however, does not necessarily correlate with clinical signs because even relatively small, rapidly accumulating effusions may produce symptoms.

Pericardial Tamponade

- Postoperative pericardial tamponade has been reported in up to 2% of cardiac surgical patients.
- Invagination of the anterior RV free wall and outflow tract often persists throughout diastole in severe tamponade but is usually terminated by atrial systole. Diastolic RA inversion associated with pericardial tamponade tends to occur later in diastole, even persisting into early systole after RV invagination has resolved.
- Spontaneous inspiration in patients with cardiac tamponade results in diminished pulmonary venous forward diastolic velocities, delayed MV opening, prolonged isovolumic relaxation time and decreased mitral E-wave velocity. During spontaneous expiration, LA and LV Doppler inflow velocities increase. Exaggeration of ventricular interdependence with pericardial tamponade is

responsible for reciprocal changes in right-sided intracardiac flows, resulting in increased tricuspid E-wave velocities during spontaneous inspiration.

Constrictive Pericarditis

- Constrictive pericarditis has been reported in approximately 0.2% to 0.3% of cardiac surgical patients.

- In patients with CP, reciprocal changes during spontaneous respiration in transmitral and pulmonary venous versus transtricuspid and hepatic vein Doppler flow velocities are similar to those observed in patients with pericardial tamponade. Mechanical, positive pressure ventilation reverses the respiratory variation pattern of LA and LV inflow velocities.

- Constrictive pericarditis can be differentiated from RCM echocardiographically by demonstrating respiratory variation in transmitral and pulmonary venous flows, more rapid transmitral color M-mode Vp, a peak Ea of 8.0 cm/s, and higher MVG values during ventricular ejection and rapid ventricular filling.

REFERENCES

1. Connolly H, Click R, Schattenberg T, et al. Congenital absence of the pericardium: echocardiography as a diagnostic tool. *J Am Soc Echocardiogr* 1995;8:87–92.
2. Sanfillippo A, Weyman A. Pericardial disease. In: Weyman A, ed. *Principles and practice of echocardiography,* 2nd ed. Philadelphia: Lea & Febiger, 1994:1102–1134.
3. Vasquez de Prada JA, Jiang L, Handschumacher MD, et al. Quantification of pericardial effusions by three-dimensional echocardiography. *J Am Coll Cardiol* 1994;24:254–259.
4. Feigenbaum H. Pericardial disease. In: Feigenbaum H, ed. *Echocardiography,* 5th ed. Baltimore: Williams & Wilkins, 1994:556–588.
5. Martin R, Rakowski H, French J, Popp R. Localization of pericardial effusion with wide-angle phased array echocardiography. *Am J Cardiol* 1978;42:904.
6. Yuste P, Torres-Carballada M, Miguel-Alonso J. Mechanism of electrical alternans in pericardial effusion: study with ultrasonics. *Arch Intern Cardiol Med* 1975;45:197.
7. Nanda N, Gramiak R, Gross C. Echocardiography of cardiac valves in pericardial effusion. *Circulation* 1976;54(3):500–504.
8. Weitzman L. The incidence and natural history of pericardial effusion after cardiac surgery: an echocardiographic study. *Circulation* 1984;69:506.
9. Douglas P. Pericardial disease. In: Sutton M, Oldershaw P, eds. *Textbook of adult and pediatric echocardiography and Doppler.* Boston: Blackwell Scientific, 1989:381–402.
10. Fyke F III. Detection of intrapericardial hematoma after open-heart surgery: the role of echocardiography and computer tomography. *J Am Coll Cardiol* 1985;5:1496.
11. Friedberg C. *Diseases of the heart.* Philadelphia: WB Saunders, 1966.
12. Cohen J. Neoplastic pericarditis. In Spodick D, ed. *Pericardial disease.* Philadelphia: FA Davis, 1976:257.
13. Oh J. Pericardial disease. In: Oh J, Seward J, Tajik A, eds. *The echo manual,* 2nd ed. Philadelphia: Lippincott Williams& Wilkins, 1999:181–194.
14. Antonini-Canterin F, Piazza R, Ascione L, et al. Value of transesophageal echocardiography in the diagnosis of compressive atypically located pericardial cysts. *J Am Soc Echocardiogr* 2002;15:192–194.
15. Spodick D. *Pericardial disease.* Philadelphia: FA Davis, 1976:814.
16. Nootens M, Ford K, Devries S. Utility of contrast echocardiography in the evaluation of a suspected right atrial mass. *Am J Cardiol* 1992;69:83.
17. **Pepi M, Muratori M, Barbieri P, et al. Pericardial effusion after cardiac surgery: incidence, site, size and hemodynamic consequences. *Br Heart J* 1994;72:327–331.**
18. **Leimgruber PP, Klopfenstein S, Wann SL, et al. The hemodynamic derangement associated with right ventricular diastolic collapse in cardiac tamponade: an experimental echocardiographic study. *Circulation* 1983;68:612.**
19. **Gillam L, Guyer D, Gibson T, et al. Hemodynamic compression of the right atrium: a new echocardiographic sign of cardiac tamponade. *Circulation* 1983;68(2):294–301.**
20. Hoit B, Fowler N. Influence of acute right ventricular dysfunction on cardiac tamponade. *J Am Col Cardiol* 1991;18:1787.
21. Brodyn N, Rose M, Prior F, et al. Left atrial diastolic compression in a patient with a large pericardial effusion and pulmonary hypertension. *Am J Med* 1990;88:1.
22. Russo A, O'Connor W, Waxman H. Atypical presentation and echocardiographic findings in patients with cardiac tamponade occurring early and late after cardiac surgery. *Chest* 1993;104:71–78.
23. **Ionescu A, Wilde P, Karsch K. Localized pericardial tamponade: difficult echocardiographic diagnosis of a rare complication after cardiac surgery. *J Am Soc Echocardiogr* 2001;14:1220–1223.**
24. Spodick D. Pericardial diseases. In: Braunwald E, Zipes D, Libby P, eds. *Heart disease,* 6th ed. Philadelphia: WB Saunders, 2001:1823–1876.
25. Burstow D, Oh J, Bailey K, et al. Cardiac tamponade: characteristic Doppler observations. *Mayo Clin Proc* 1989;64:312–324.
26. **Appleton C, Hatle L, Pop R. Cardiac tamponade and pericardial effusion: respiratory variation in transvalvular flow velocities studied by Doppler echocardiography. *J Am Coll Cardiol* 1988;11:1020.**
27. **Klein A, Cohen G, Petrolungo J, et al. Differentiation of constrictive pericarditis from restrictive cardiomyopathy by Doppler transesophageal echocardiographic measurements of respiratory variations in pulmonary venous flow. *J Am Coll Cardiol* 1993;2:1935–1943.**
28. Hancock W. Differential diagnosis of restrictive cardiomyopathy and constrictive pericarditis. *Heart* 2001;86(3):343–349.
29. Hirschmann JV. Fundamentals of clinical cardiology. *Am Heart J* 1978;96:110.
30. **Cimino J, Kogan A. Constrictive pericarditis following cardiac surgery—Cleveland Clinic experience: report of 12 cases and review. *Am J Cardiol* 1979;44:177–183.**
31. Lorell B. Pericardial diseases. In: Braunwald E, ed. *Heart disease: a textbook of cardiovascular medicine,* 5th ed. Philadelphia: WB Saunders, 1997:1478–1534.
32. Armstrong W, Feigenbaum H. Echocardiography. In: Braunwald E, Zipes D, Libby P, eds. *Heart disease,* 6th ed. Philadelphia: WB Saunders, 2001:160–236.
33. Hatle L, Appleton C, Popp R. Differentiation of constrictive pericarditis and restrictive cardiomyopathy by Doppler echocardiography. *Circulation* 1989;79:357.

34. Oh J, Tajik J, Appleton C, Hatle L, et al. Preload reduction to unmask the characteristic Doppler features of constrictive pericarditis: a new observation. *Circulation* 1997;95(4):796–799.

35. Hillman D. Physiological aspects of intermittent positive pressure ventilation. *Anaesth Intens Care* 1986;14:226–235.

36. **Abdalla I, Murray D, Awad H, et al. Reversal of the pattern of respiratory variation of Doppler inflow velocities in constrictive pericarditis during mechanical ventilation. *J Am Soc Echocardiogr* 2000;13:827–831.**

37. Skubas N, Beardslee M, Barzilai B, et al. Constrictive pericarditis: intraoperative hemodynamic and echocardiographic evaluation of cardiac filling dynamics. *Anesth Analg* 2001;92:1424–1426.

38. **Sun J, Abdalla I, Yang X, et al. Respiratory variation of mitral and pulmonary venous Doppler flow velocities in constrictive pericarditis before and after pericardiectomy. *J Am Soc Echocardiogr* 2000;14:1119–1126.**

39. Senni M, Redfield M, Ling H, et al. Left ventricular systolic and diastolic function after pericardiectomy in patients with constrictive pericarditis: postoperative and serial Doppler echocardiographic findings. *Circulation* 1997;96(Suppl I): 30.

40. Spodick D. Constrictive pericarditis. In: Spodick D, ed. *The pericardium: a comprehensive textbook.* New York: Marcel Dekker, 1997:214–259.

41. Buckingham R, Furnary A, Weaver M, et al. Mitral insufficiency after pericardiectomy for constrictive pericarditis. *Ann Thorac Surg* 1994;58(4):1171–1174.

42. Rodriguez, Ares MA, Vandervoot PM, et al. Does color M-mode flow propagation differentiate between patients with restrictive vs. constrictive physiology? [Abstract]. *J Am Coll Cardiol* 1996;27:268A.

43. Garcia MJ, Rodriguez L, Ares MA, et al. Differentiation of constrictive pericarditis from restrictive cardiomyopathy: assessment of left ventricular diastolic velocities in the longitudinal axis by Doppler tissue imaging. *J Am Coll Cardiol* 1996;27:108–114.

44. **Rajagopalan N, Garcia M, Rodriguez L, et al. Comparison of new Doppler echocardiographic methods to differentiate constrictive pericardial heart disease and restrictive cardiomyopathy. *Am J Cardiol* 2001;87:86–94.**

45. Arnold M, Voigt J, Kukulski T, et al. Does atrioventricular ring motion always distinguish constriction form restriction? A Doppler myocardial imaging study. *J Am Soc Echocardiogr* 2001;14:391–395.

46. Palka P, Lange A, Donnelly E, et al. Differentiation between restrictive cardiomyopathy and constrictive pericarditis by early diastolic Doppler myocardial velocity gradient at the posterior wall. *Circulation* 2000;102:655–662.

TRANSESOPHAGEAL ECHOCARDIOGRAPHIC EVALUATION OF THE AORTA AND PULMONARY ARTERY

ENRIQUE J. PANTIN
ALBERT T. CHEUNG

The thoracic aorta, its major branches and the pulmonary artery (PA) can be evaluated by transesophageal echocardiography (TEE) using two dimensional (2D) imaging and Doppler echocardiography. The majority of pathologic conditions affecting the thoracic and upper abdominal aorta produce structural lesions that can be detected by 2D imaging. The close proximity between the thoracic aorta and the esophagus enables TEE to provide high-resolution images of almost the entire aorta except for a distal segment of the ascending aorta and the proximal portion of the aortic arch that is shielded by the trachea. Transcervical, epicardial, or epiaortic ultrasound imaging can be used in addition to or as a substitute for TEE to evaluate the neck vessels, ascending aorta, and aortic arch during open-heart surgery (1).

Transesophageal echocardiography has many advantages over other imaging modalities to assess the thoracic aorta (Table 15.1) (2–4). For these reasons, TEE is considered the diagnostic procedure of choice for the emergency evaluation of patients with suspected aortic dissection, aortic aneurysms, or traumatic injury to the aorta, especially if the patient is clinically unstable. TEE is also useful for detecting complications associated with surgical emergencies involving the aorta, such as cardiac tamponade, aortic regurgitation, hypovolemia, myocardial ischemia, or malperfusion syndromes. Finally, intraoperative TEE is useful for assessing the success of the operative repair.

Transesophageal echocardiography can be performed in awake patients, but adequate topical anesthesia and intravenous sedation is essential for preventing hypertensive episodes in response to probe insertion performed to decrease the risk of acute aortic rupture in unstable patients with aortic dissection or traumatic aortic injury. Oversedation may cause hypotension in the hypovolemic patient or increase the risk for aspiration pneumonia (5). Transesophageal echocardiography is generally safe in anesthetized and intubated patients, but certain aortic diseases may make TEE hazardous. Patients with large descending thoracic aortic aneurysms causing compression of the esophagus may be at increased risk for esophageal perforation or aortic rupture as a consequence of TEE. Passage of the TEE probe into the esophagus can cause hypoxemia or airway compromise by extrinsic compression of the right PA or left main-stem bronchus in patients with large aneurysms of the ascending aorta (6,7). Routine use of TEE in cardiac surgical patients is useful for assessing the size, location, and severity of atherosclerotic lesions in the aorta to help identify patients at risk for stroke. Transesophageal echocardiography is also sensitive for diagnosing penetrating aortic ulcers that can develop into intramural hematoma or dissection (8).

ANATOMY OF THE AORTA

The aortic wall consists of three layers that are normally indistinguishable by TEE. Diseases or traumatic injury of the aortic wall can disrupt individual layers or cause the layers to separate, making them visible by TEE examination. The intima is a thin inner layer lined by endothelium in direct contact with blood that is most susceptible to injury and is also the site of atherosclerosis. The media is a thick layer consisting of intertwining sheets of elastic tissue that comprises 80% of the arterial wall thickness and provides tensile strength to the vessel. The adventitia is a thin outermost layer composed mainly of collagen and houses the vasa vasorum and aortic lymphatics.

The thoracic aorta can be divided into four regions: the aortic root, ascending aorta, aortic arch, and descending

E. J. Pantin: Department of Anesthesiology, University of Medicine and Dentistry of New Jersey; and Department of Anesthesiology, Robert Wood Johnson University Hospital, New Brunswick, New Jersey.

A. T. Cheung: Department of Anesthesiology, University of Pennsylvania; and Division of Cardiothoracic Anesthesia and Critical Care, Hospital of the University of Pennsylvania, Philadelphia, Pennsylvania.

TABLE 15.1. ADVANTAGES AND DISADVANTAGES OF TEE FOR THE DIAGNOSIS OF SURGICAL EMERGENCIES OF THE AORTA

Advantages of TEE
   Rapid diagnosis
   Generally less time consuming
   Portable and can be performed at the bedside
   Does not interfere with resuscitation efforts
   Provides information useful for resuscitation
   No instrumentation of aorta
   Ability to diagnose associated cardiac injuries
   Avoids radiographic contrast agents
   Readily available
   Relatively inexpensive
   Minimally invasive
   Low rate of complications

Disadvantages of TEE
   Operator dependent
   Interpretation requires experience
   Limited view of distal ascending aorta
   Limited view of aortic arch
   Requires sedation and topical anesthesia in awake patients
   Contraindicated in severe facial trauma or unstable cervical
     spine injury
   Contraindicated in esophageal injuries and
     pneumoperitoneum

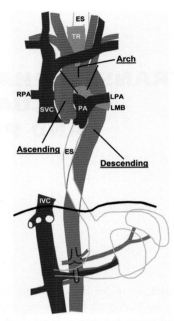

FIGURE 15.1. Anatomy of the aorta in relation to the esophagus. The aorta and branches are represented in red; the pulmonary artery (*PA*), superior vena cava (*SVC*), and inferior vena cava (*IVC*) in blue; the trachea (*TR*) and left main bronchus (*LMB*) in gray; and the esophagus (*ES*), stomach, spleen, and left kidney in yellow.

thoracic aorta (Fig. 15.1). The aortic root begins at the aortic valve annulus and includes the sinuses of Valsalva, and ends at the sinotubular junction where it joins the ascending aorta. The ascending aorta extends from the sinotubular junction to the origin of the innominate artery. The aortic arch that gives rise to the innominate, left carotid, and left subclavian arteries lies between the ascending and descending aorta. The descending aorta begins at the distal end of the origin of the left subclavian artery and extends caudally past the diaphragm (Fig. 15.2).

The combined length of the aortic root and ascending aorta measures 8.9 cm (range 7.6–10.2 cm). Transesophageal echocardiography typically can be used to image the proxi-

mal 7.4 cm (range 6.3–8.5 cm) of the aorta before the air-filled trachea or left main-stem bronchus intervenes between the esophagus and aorta, obscuring the acoustic window (9). The aortic root and ascending aorta are initially anterior and somewhat to the right of the esophagus. The descending aorta lies to the left of the spine just distal to the origin of the left subclavian artery but then moves toward the midline, directly in front of the spine as it crosses the diaphragm and continues into the abdomen, ending at the aortic bifurcation near the body of the fourth lumbar vertebra. In relation to the esophagus, the distal aortic arch is anterior to the esophagus. The descending thoracic aorta then winds around the

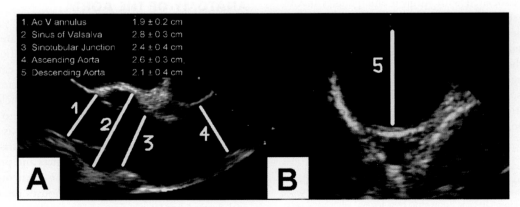

1. Ao V annulus	1.9 ± 0.2 cm
2. Sinus of Valsalva	2.8 ± 0.3 cm
3. Sinotubular Junction	2.4 ± 0.4 cm
4. Ascending Aorta	2.6 ± 0.3 cm,
5. Descending Aorta	2.1 ± 0.4 cm

FIGURE 15.2. A: Transesophageal echocardiographic (TEE) mid-esophageal long-axis view of the aortic root showing the standard anatomic landmarks for measuring aortic root and ascending aortic vessel diameters. **B:** TEE short-axis view of the descending thoracic aorta and vessel diameter.

TABLE 15.2. NORMAL RANGES FOR AORTIC AND PULMONARY ARTERY DIMENSIONS MEASURED BY TEE

Structure Diameter	Nonindexed (cm)	Range	Indexed[a] (cm/m²)	Range
Aortic valve annulus	1.9 ± 0.2	1.8–2.5		
Sinus of Valsalva	2.8 ± 0.3	2.1–3.4	1.6 ± 0.2	1.2–2.3
Sinotubular junction	2.4 ± 0.4			
Ascending aorta	2.6 ± 0.3			
Descending aorta (proximal)[b]	2.1 ± 0.4	1.4–3.0	1.2 ± 0.2	0.9–1.7
Descending aorta (distal)[c]	2.0 ± 0.4	1.3–2.8	1.1 ± 0.2	0.8–1.5
Main pulmonary artery	3.0			
(length)	5.0			
Right pulmonary artery	1.7 ± 0.3	1.2–2.2	1.0 ± 0.1	0.7–1.2
(length)[d]	5.5			
Left pulmonary artery	1.9			
(length)	3.0			
Right ventricular outflow tract	2.7 ± 0.4	1.3–3.6	1.5 ± 0.2	1.0–2.0

[a]Indexed relative to body surface area.
[b]Measured just below the aortic arch.
[c]Measured at the level of the diaphragm.
[d]Measured just beyond the main pulmonary artery during systole.
Data from references 7, 10–18, and 129–146.

esophagus in the left chest, becoming lateral to the esophagus in the mid-chest, then posterior to the esophagus at the diaphragmatic hiatus (Fig. 15.1, Table 15.2) (10).

The aortic root and the first several centimeters of the ascending aorta lie within the pericardial sac. The weakest area of the aortic wall is at the level of the sinus of Valsalva. Rupture of the aortic root or proximal ascending aorta can cause cardiac tamponade. The ascending aorta and arch are mobile, whereas the descending aorta is fixed to the thorax by the ligamentum arteriosum, just distal to the origin of the left subclavian artery, and by the paired intercostal arteries along the thoracic spine. The aortic isthmus is the region of aorta between the origin of the left subclavian artery and the ligamentum arteriosum and is the most common location for aortic coarctation, patent ductus arteriosus (PDA), and intimal disruptions caused by deceleration injuries or blunt chest trauma.

TRANSESOPHAGEAL ECHOCARDIOGRAPHY EVALUATION OF THE AORTA

The Society of Cardiovascular Anesthesiologists and American Society of Echocardiography TEE examination guidelines describe seven standard TEE cross-sectional views of the thoracic aorta (11). At the level of the left atrium (LA), at a multiplane angle between 120 and 160 degrees, the mid-esophageal aortic valve long-axis view (Fig. 15.3) provides a cross section through the aortic valve and aortic root. At the level of the right PA, at a multiplane angle of 0 degrees, the mid-esophageal ascending aortic short-axis view is obtained (Fig. 15.4). Multiplane rotation to 90 degrees produces mid-esophageal ascending aortic long-axis view at the level of the right PA (Fig. 15.5). The mid-esophageal ascending aorta

long- and short-axis views are useful for measuring the diameter of the ascending aorta. The air-filled trachea and left main-stem bronchus lie between the esophagus and the aortic arch and obscure the acoustic window for imaging the distal ascending aorta, the origin of the innominate artery, and proximal aortic arch, although they can sometimes be imaged by further manipulations of the TEE probe (9,12). At the level of the right PA, turning the probe to the left brings into view the descending aorta. Withdrawal of the TEE probe then generates the upper esophageal aortic arch long-axis view (Fig. 15.6). From this position, further withdrawal of the probe usually allows visualization of the left subclavian and carotid arteries as they branch off the aortic arch. Multiplane rotation to 90 degrees produces the upper esophageal aortic arch short-axis view (Fig. 15.7). The upper esophageal aortic arch short-axis view also images the left subclavian artery as it branches off the distal aortic arch and the main PA in long axis below the aortic arch. Advancing the TEE probe while keeping the aorta in the center of the image at a multiplane angle of 0 degrees allows the length of the descending aorta to be imaged in short axis (Fig. 15.8). The TEE descending aortic short-axis views also permit the detection of left pleural effusions that layer adjacent to the aorta in a supine patient. In a similar fashion, the length of the descending aorta can be imaged in long axis by advancing and withdrawing the TEE probe alongside the descending aorta at a multiplane angle of 90 degrees (Fig. 15.9). As the aorta is tracked distally, it becomes less pulsatile because it is less compliant and has a smaller diameter (13).

Precise localization of defects identified in the aortic root and ascending aorta by TEE is possible using anatomic references. The aortic valve, coronary ostia, sinuses of Valsalva, sinotubular junction, and right PA are easily identified anatomic landmarks useful for orientation of the

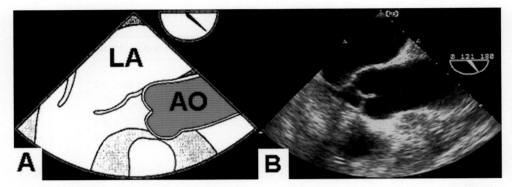

FIGURE 15.3. Transesophageal echocardiographic mid-esophageal aortic valve long-axis view at a multiplane angle of 121 degrees. *LA,* left atrium; *AO,* aortic root.

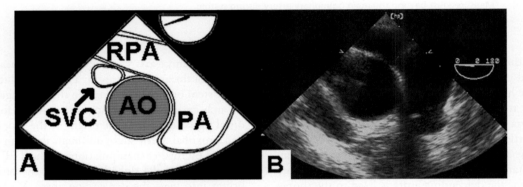

FIGURE 15.4. Transesophageal echocardiographic mid-esophageal ascending aortic (*AO*) short-axis view at a multiplane angle of 0 degrees. *RPA,* right pulmonary artery; *SVC,* superior vena cava; *PA,* main pulmonary artery.

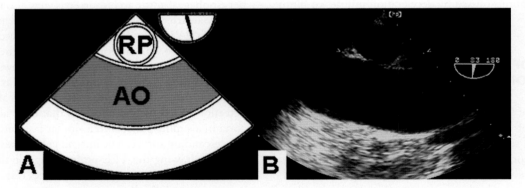

FIGURE 15.5. Transesophageal echocardiographic mid-esophageal ascending aorta (*AO*) long-axis view at a multiplane angle of 83 degrees. This cross section also provides a short-axis view through the right pulmonary artery (*RP*).

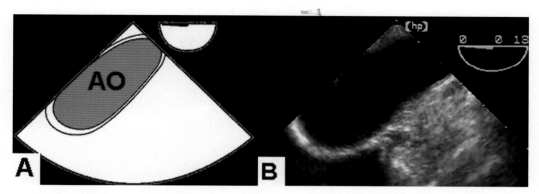

FIGURE 15.6. Transesophageal echocardiographic upper esophageal aortic arch long-axis view of the distal aortic arch (*AO*).

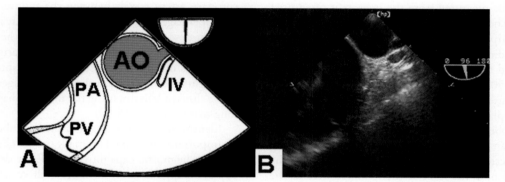

FIGURE 15.7. Transesophageal echocardiographic upper esophageal aortic arch (*AO*) short-axis view at a multiplane angle of 96 degrees. The origin of one of the arch vessels is seen at the 3 o'clock position. This cross section also provides a view of the pulmonic valve (*PV*) in long axis, the main pulmonary artery (*PA*) in long axis, and the innominate vein (*IV*) in short axis.

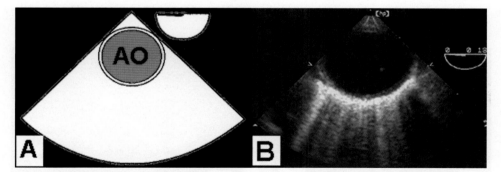

FIGURE 15.8. Transesophageal echocardiographic descending aorta (*AO*) short-axis view at a multiplane angle of 0 degrees.

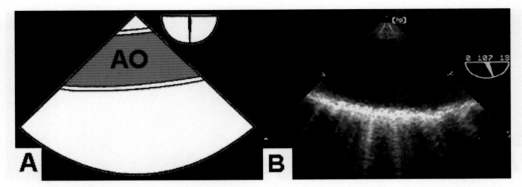

FIGURE 15.9. Transesophageal echocardiographic descending aorta (*AO*) long-axis view at a multiplane angle of 107 degrees.

cross-sectional imaging plane. Because there are few anatomic landmarks that can be used to identify the precise level of the imaging plane in the descending aorta, the depth of the TEE probe measured from the incisors is often used as a reference. The distal aortic arch is usually imaged with the TEE probe tip 20 to 25 cm from the incisors. The midthoracic descending aorta is usually imaged at a depth of 30 to 35 cm and the aorta at the diaphragmatic hiatus at a depth of 40 to 50 cm (14). Alternatively, the origin of the left subclavian artery can be used as a reference. The depth of the imaging plane is then determined by measuring the distance the probe has been advanced beyond the origin of the left subclavian artery (7). Another method for describing the depth of a lesion on the descending aorta is to turn the TEE probe and note the level of the lesion relative to the level of adjacent structures such as the LA or left ventricle. The location of defects on the aortic wall can be further described relative to the position of the esophagus as being adjacent, lateral, or on the opposite wall. Precise localization of defects in the descending thoracic aorta by TEE is often difficult when the aorta is tortuous or curves within the thorax.

It is possible to image many of the aortic branch vessels by TEE. The first branches off the aorta are the right and left main coronary arteries. The left main coronary artery is best imaged in the mid-esophageal aortic valve short-axis view as it branches off the left sinus of Valsalva. The left main coronary artery travels between the pulmonary trunk and LA appendage for 1 to 2 cm before it bifurcates into the left anterior descending coronary artery and the left circumflex coronary artery. The right coronary artery originates from the right sinus of Valsalva and travels in an anterior direction. The right coronary ostium also can be imaged in the far wall of the sinus of Valsalva using the mid-esophageal aortic valve long-axis view (Fig. 15.10).

Identification of the origin of the left subclavian artery is an important anatomic landmark in the TEE examination, but the diagnostic capability of TEE for detecting pathology or malperfusion of aortic branch vessels has not been established. The branch vessels are imaged using a combination of 2D imaging to identify the vessel lumen followed by color Doppler flow imaging to confirm that the structure is a vessel by detecting blood flow within the lumen. It is often necessary to decrease the Nyquist limit to 15 to 35 cm/s while using color Doppler flow imaging in order to visualize flow in a branch vessel, especially if flow is laminar and in a direction perpendicular to the ultrasound beam (Fig. 15.11). Using color Doppler flow imaging, it is

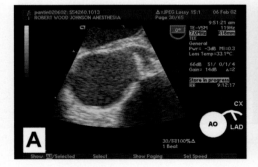 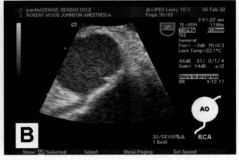

FIGURE 15.10. A: Transesophageal echocardiographic mid-esophageal short-axis views of the aortic root (*AO*) showing the left main coronary artery at the 1 o'clock position and its bifurcation into the left circumflex coronary artery (*CX*) and left anterior descending coronary artery (*LAD*). **B:** The right coronary artery (*RCA*) branches off the anterior wall of the aorta at the 6 o'clock position.

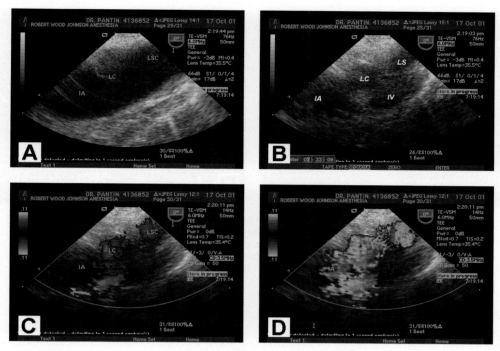

FIGURE 15.11. **A and B:** Transesophageal echocardiographic upper esophageal short-axis images of the innominate artery (*IA*), left carotid artery (*LC*), and left subclavian artery (*LS* and *LSC*). The innominate vein (*IV*) is anterior to the left carotid (*LC*) and left subclavian arteries (*LC*). **C and D:** Color Doppler flow imaging is useful for identifying the vessel lumens.

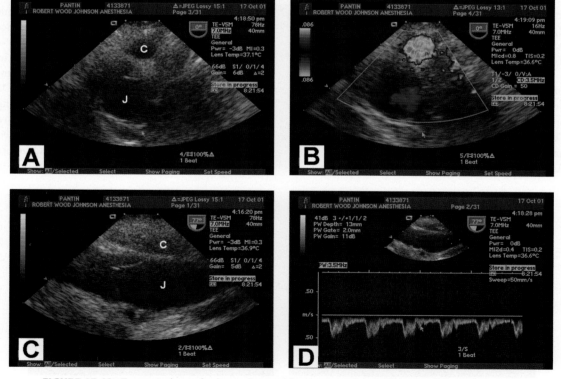

FIGURE 15.12. Transesophageal echocardiographic upper esophageal images of the right carotid artery (*C*), and the right internal jugular vein (*J*) in short axis at a multiplane angle of 0 degrees **(A and B)** and long axis at a multiplane angle of 77 degrees **(C)**. A valve in the internal jugular vein (*J*) was detected. Pulsed-wave Doppler demonstrated pulsatile blood flow in the right carotid artery **(D)**.

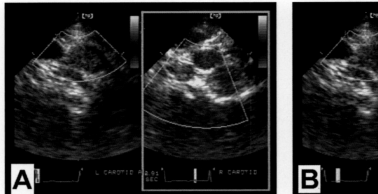

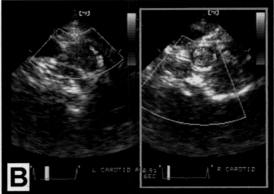

FIGURE 15.13. Transcervical surface two-dimensional ultrasound imaging of the left (*L*) and right (*R*) carotid arteries in a short-axis view in a patient with a type A aortic dissection who presented with a left hemispheric stroke. An intimal flap extended into the left carotid artery **(A)**. Color Doppler flow imaging of the carotid arteries showed a narrowed true lumen in the left carotid artery compressed by a thrombosed false lumen **(B)**.

sometimes possible to identify even small intercostal artery branches off the descending thoracic aorta.

The aortic arch branch vessel that is most consistently imaged by TEE is the left subclavian artery. Once the left subclavian artery is identified in short axis, the adjacent left carotid and innominate arteries can sometimes be visualized by turning the TEE probe toward the right. If the arch vessels are followed into the upper esophagus and pharynx, the carotid arteries and jugular veins can sometimes be imaged (Fig. 15.12). The aortic arch vessels in the neck can be imaged more consistently, even during surgery, by transcervical vascular ultrasound using a surface transducer. Transcervical ultrasound imaging is a useful supplement to TEE for the detection of dissection extending into the carotid arteries in patients with type A aortic dissection (Fig. 15.13).

Some branches off the abdominal aorta can sometimes be imaged by TEE using the transgastric views because the stomach may extend down to the level of the second lumbar vertebra. As the TEE probe enters the stomach, its posi-tion relative to the abdominal aorta will initially be anterior, then anterolateral, and finally left. To image the abdominal aorta, the TEE probe should be kept close to the gastric wall alongside the aorta. The first abdominal aortic branch vessel is the celiac trunk (Fig. 15.14), which branches off the anterior wall of the aorta just below the diaphragm. The celiac trunk is approximately 12 mm long and 6 mm in diameter. The superior mesenteric artery also branches off the anterior wall of the aorta 2 cm below the celiac trunk. Further down, the left and right renal arteries can be occasionally imaged (15).

It is difficult to quantify blood flow velocity in the thoracic aorta using TEE-derived Doppler echocardiography because of poor alignment with the blood flow. Doppler examination of the aorta is more useful for identifying flow disturbances caused by aortic dissection, intimal disruption, or stenosis. The Doppler examination also can be used to detect blood flow within a pseudoaneurysm, contained rupture, or false lumen of a dissection. In addition, color Doppler flow

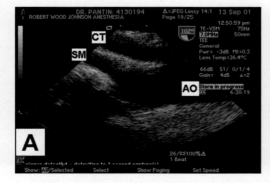

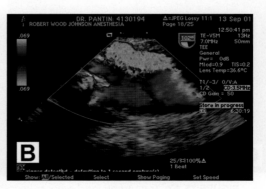

FIGURE 15.14. Transesophageal echocardiographic transgastric long-axis view of the abdominal aorta at a multiplane angle of 102 degrees **(A)** demonstrating the celiac trunk (*CT*) and superior mesenteric artery (*SM*). Color Doppler examination demonstrated blood flow in the vessels branching off the aorta **(B)**. *AO*, aortic arch.

imaging can be used to help locate aortic branch vessels or the sites of intimal tears in aortic dissection.

TRANSESOPHAGEAL ECHOCARDIOGRAPHY EVALUATION OF AORTIC DISEASE

Aortic diseases can be broadly classified as congenital or acquired. Congenital anomalies that affect the aorta that can be diagnosed by TEE in adults include aortic coarctation, PDA, bicuspid aortic valve with or without aortic aneurysm, and collagen vascular diseases causing aortic aneurysm or dissection. Acquired conditions of the aorta that can be diagnosed or evaluated using TEE include aortic rupture, aortic dissection, aortic aneurysm, pseudoaneurysm, atherosclerosis, traumatic aortic injury, tumors, and aortitis. The clinical application of TEE is also useful for endovascular aortic aneurysm stenting, aortic cannulation, and the positioning of intraaortic balloon pump (IABP) counterpulsation catheters or an endoaortic clamp.

CONGENITAL AORTIC DISEASES
Supravalvular Aortic Stenosis

Supravalvular aortic stenosis is a localized or diffuse narrowing of the ascending aorta distal to the coronary ostia at the superior border of the sinuses of Valsalva. Stenosis is caused by a discrete membrane in 10% of cases, a thickened and narrowed segment of the ascending aorta in 20%, and uniform hypoplasia of the ascending aorta in the majority of cases (7,16).

Coarctation of the Aorta

Coarctation of the aorta is caused by a localized deformity of the aortic wall that causes an eccentric narrowing of the lumen or even interruption of the aorta. In adults, the lesion is typically postductal, with the narrowing just beyond the origin of the left subclavian artery or distal to the insertion of the ligamentum arteriosum. Adults with coarctation of the aorta may require operation for revision of an earlier repair, restenosis after balloon aortoplasty, or repair of associated lesions. The accuracy of TEE for the diagnosis and evaluation of coarctation is limited because the region of aorta at the site of coarctation is typically difficult to image. In addition, TEE does not provide the ability to image the entire region of narrowing in a single cross-sectional imaging plane. Estimating the pressure gradient across the coarctation using the Bernoulli equation by TEE is also difficult because the ultrasound beam cannot usually be lined up with the direction of blood flow in the region of the coarctation. Transesophageal echocardiography can be used to detect enlargement and increased pulsation in the aorta and its branch vessels proximal to the stenosis. Color Doppler flow imaging typically demonstrates increased flow velocity and turbulence at the site of narrowing. In patients with coarctation, TEE is more useful for the detection and evaluation of anomalies and diseases associated with this condition. Up to 80% of patients with coarctation have associated bicuspid aortic valves that may require operation for aortic stenosis, aortic regurgitation, or aortic aneurysm. Other associated complications of coarctation that can be detected by TEE include endocarditis, aortic dissection, aortic aneurysm, aortic rupture, left ventricular hypertrophy, left ventricular dysfunction, or premature coronary artery disease (7,16).

Patent Ductus Arteriosus

A PDA is the persistence of the ductus arteriosus that provides a connection between the PA and the descending aorta in the fetus. TEE can be used for detecting PDA in adolescents and adults by demonstrating a shunt between the aorta and PA with color Doppler flow imaging. If there is flow from the PA into the aorta, the injection of echo contrast into a central vein can show contrast traversing through the right ventricle, PA, and into the descending aorta below the ductal area without the appearance of contrast in the ascending aorta. The PA pressure can be estimated by subtracting the Doppler-derived pressure gradient across the shunt from the arterial pressure (17,18). In adults, the ductus and its attachment to the descending aorta may be calcified. Longstanding left-to-right shunting through a PDA will cause pulmonary hypertension and associated right ventricular hypertrophy detectable by TEE. In one report, TEE correctly diagnosed the presence of a PDA masquerading as traumatic aortic rupture by aortography in a 17-year-old involved in a motor vehicle accident (19).

ACQUIRED AORTIC DISEASES
Aortic Dissection

Aortic dissection is caused by blood exiting the lumen of the aorta through one or several tears in the intimal wall of the aorta into a potential space created by cleavage within the intimal and medial layers of the vessel wall. The dissected aorta consists of a true and false lumen contained within the adventitia, separated by the dissecting or intimal flap that consists of aortic intima and media. The intimal tears create entry and reentry sites for blood flow between the true and false lumens. The most common site for aortic dissection is the proximal third of the ascending aorta or the descending thoracic aorta just beyond the left subclavian artery, but it can occur anywhere in the aorta (Fig. 15.15).

Aortic dissection is the most common surgical emergency of the aorta. Patients typically present with the sudden onset of severe chest or back pain. Limb ischemia, mesenteric ischemia, or renal failure indicates occlusion of the distal or mesenteric aortic branches by the dissection flap. Acute

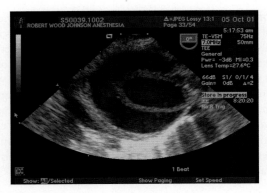

FIGURE 15.15. Transesophageal echocardiographic short-axis view of the mid-descending thoracic aorta in a patient with a type A aortic dissection that extended into the descending aorta with almost complete circumferential detachment of the intima.

respiratory failure or pulmonary edema indicates aortic regurgitation caused by extension of the dissection into the aortic root. Syncope or focal neurologic deficits indicate aortic arch involvement with malperfusion of the innominate or carotid arteries (Fig. 15.13). Refractory hypotension may indicate hypovolemia from rupture of the aorta or cardiac tamponade caused by hemopericardium from rupture of the proximal ascending aorta into the pericardial sac. Myocardial ischemia or infarction may be the consequence of dissection extension into the sinuses of Valsalva, causing malperfusion of the coronary ostia. Surviving patients with chronic aortic dissection will develop progressive aneurysmal dilatation as a consequence of the weakened aortic wall.

The most commonly used classification for aortic dissection is the Stanford classification, which divides dissections into two types (Fig. 15.16) (20). Stanford type A dissections involve the ascending aorta regardless of the distal extent and the site of intimal tear (Fig. 15.17). Stanford type B dissections are limited to the descending aorta distal to the origin of the left subclavian artery. The classification scheme described by DeBakey categorized dissections into those that involve the ascending aorta and extend through the arch into the descending aorta (type I), those confined to the ascending aorta (type II), and those that involve only the descending aorta (type III). Debakey type III dissections can be further subdivided into those that are confined to the descending thoracic aorta (type IIIa) and those that extend distally into the abdominal aorta (type IIIb) (Fig. 15.18) (20).

Aortic dissection is caused by degenerative or destructive diseases of the aortic media, usually in association with systemic hypertension, aging, or atherosclerosis. Aortic dissection can arise from cystic medial necrosis, rupture of the vasa vasorum, primary tear in the intima, rupture of an ulcerated atheromatous plaque, or trauma. Disorders associated with abnormal elastic tissue, such as Marfan syndrome, Ehlers-Danlos syndrome, osteogenesis imperfecta, idiopathic kyphoscoliosis, Turner syndrome, Noonan syndrome, coarctation of the aorta, bicuspid aortic valve, Takayasu disease, polycystic kidney disease, chronic corticosteroid treatment, or a family history of aortic dissection, predispose to aortic dissection. Aortic dissection also has occurred in young women in the third trimester of pregnancy, as an iatrogenic complication of coronary angiography, from injury at the aortic cannulation site after cardiac operations, or from retrograde arterial perfusion of the aorta via a femoral artery cannulation during cardiopulmonary bypass (7,20–27).

The identification of an intimal flap within the aortic lumen by TEE is diagnostic for aortic dissection (Table 15.3).

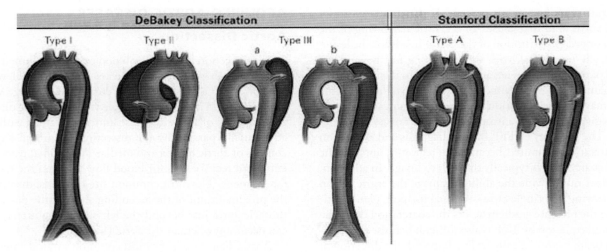

FIGURE 15.16. Illustration showing the DeBakey and Stanford classifications for aortic dissection. Acute Stanford type A aortic dissections involve the ascending aorta or aortic arch regardless of the number or location of entry sites and is considered a surgical emergency. (Reprinted from Kouchoukos NT, Dougenis D. Surgery of the thoracic aorta. *N Engl J Med* 1997;336:1876–1888, with permission.)

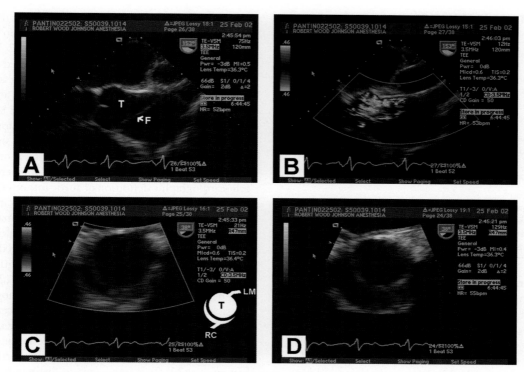

FIGURE 15.17. Transesophageal echocardiographic (TEE) mid-esophageal long-axis view of the aortic root **(A and B)** demonstrating an aortic dissection in a 43-year-old man with acute chest pain and myocardial ischemia in the right coronary artery distribution. An intimal flap (*F*) was imaged beginning at the anterior wall of the aortic root extending into the ascending aorta. TEE short-axis views of the aortic root **(C and D)** demonstrated the left main (*LM*) coronary ostium branching off the true lumen (*T*) and the right coronary artery (*RC*) branching off the false lumen.

The intimal flap should be imaged in more than one view, should exhibit a defined motion that is not parallel to the motion of any other cardiac or aortic root structure, and should not be confused with a reverberation or side lobe imaging artifact from intravascular catheters or another cardiac structure. The flap typically moves back and forth in synchrony with the cardiac cycle in a characteristic undulating motion as the true lumen fills with blood during systole (Fig. 15.19) (28). Central displacement of atherosclerotic intimal calcifications can sometimes be used to identify the endothelial surface of the intimal flap (29). On the TEE short-axis images of the aorta, the intimal flap can be seen separating the aorta into the true and false lumen. Although it is sometimes difficult to distinguish the true lumen from the false lumen of

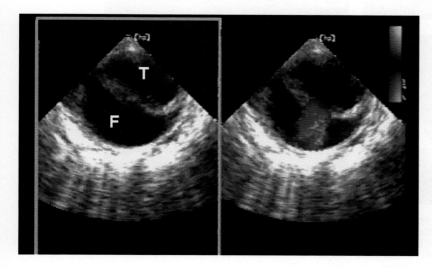

FIGURE 15.18. Transesophageal echocardiographic short axis view of the descending aorta in a patient with an aortic dissection. An intimal tear was identified. Color Doppler flow imaging demonstrated blood flow across the intimal flap through the tear exiting the true lumen (*T*) and entering the false lumen (*F*) during systole.

TABLE 15.3. TEE EXAMINATION IN AORTIC DISSECTION

Two-dimensional imaging
  Intimal flap
  Undulating motion of intimal flap
  True and false lumen separated by an intimal flap
  Aortic dilatation
  Central displacement of intimal calcification

Doppler examination
  Communication between true and false lumens at site of
    intimal tear
  Different blood flow patterns in true and false lumens

Atypical dissection
  Intramural hematoma
  Aortic intussusception
  Dissecting aneurysm
  Localized dissection

the aorta, the true lumen is typically smaller in diameter that the false lumen in diastole and expands during systole (29). Sometimes the true lumen can be identified within the aortic root and then tracked distally into the descending aorta. Color Doppler examination may detect blood flow from one lumen into the other across the intimal flap at the sites where there are intimal tears (21,22). Sometimes decreased blood flow within the false lumen may produce spontaneous echo contrast or thrombosis (21,22).

Aortic intramural hematoma is a variant of the classic aortic dissection. It is a life-threatening condition with a prognosis similar to that for aortic dissection (22,30–32). Aortic intramural hematoma also can be classified according to whether there is involvement of the ascending aorta and arch (type A) or if it is confined to the descending aorta (type B). Aortic intramural hematoma is characterized by hematoma tracking between the layers of the vessel wall along the length of the aorta. Aortic intramural hematoma is sometimes described as a dissection without an intimal tear or intimal flap. There is no intimal flap or flow within the hematoma. The echocardiographic definition of aortic intramural hematoma by TEE examination is a greater than 7 mm circumferential or crescentic thickening of the aortic wall imaged in short axis with central displacement of intimal calcification and a layered appearance of the aortic wall imaged in long axis extending for greater than 1 cm along the length of the vessel in the absence of an intimal flap (Fig. 15.20) (22,31,33,34). The density within the aortic wall has an echogenic pattern consistent with hematoma, often with echolucent spaces that may represent fresh blood. Partial or complete thrombosis of the false lumen of a classic aortic dissection may exhibit an echocardiographic pattern very similar to aortic intramural hematoma (22). It is important to distinguish aortic intramural hematoma from mural thrombus within the lumen of the aorta.

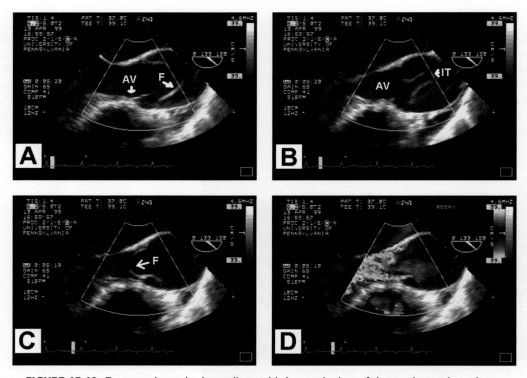

FIGURE 15.19. Transesophageal echocardiographic long-axis view of the aortic root in early systole **(A)** demonstrating a type A dissection with an intimal flap (*F, arrow*) originating at the sinotubular junction. An intimal tear (*IT, arrow*) can be identified in the late systolic image **(B)**. In diastole **(C)**, the intimal flap (*arrow*) prolapsed through the aortic valve (*AV*), causing severe aortic regurgitation diagnosed by color Doppler flow imaging **(D)**.

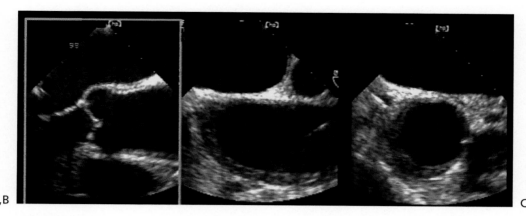

A,B   C

FIGURE 15.20. Emergent transesophageal echocardiography performed in a 63-year-old patient admitted with severe chest pain demonstrated an aortic intramural hematoma in the aortic root long-axis image that started at the level of the sinotubular junction **(A)**. The intramural hematoma produced a crescent-shaped density within the anterior wall of the aorta seen in the long-axis **(A and B)** and short-axis **(C)** views of the ascending aorta.

Other variants of the classic aortic dissection include a complete circumferential intimal tear and intussusception of the intimal flap distally into the vessel lumen, limited intimal tear with a bulge at the site of intimal disruption, penetrating atherosclerotic ulcer with surrounding hematoma, and traumatic dissection caused by instrumentation of the vessel during cardiac catheterization or surgery (Fig. 15.21) (21,135–137).

Upon the introduction of TEE, its clinical application for the diagnosis of aortic dissection became evident (35). Aortic dissection can be diagnosed by magnetic resonance imag-

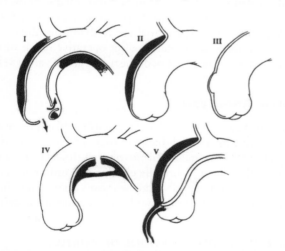

FIGURE 15.21. Illustrations showing the classification of aortic dissection variants. Type I, separation of intima producing a true and false lumen (classic); type II, intramural hematoma with separation of intima and no intraluminal tear or flap; type III, intimal tear without hematoma (limited dissection) and eccentric bulge; type IV, atherosclerotic penetrating ulcer with localized hematoma; type V, iatrogenic aortic dissection. (Reprinted from Svensson LG, Labib SB, Eisenhauer AC, et al. Intimal tear without hematoma. An important variant of aortic dissection that can elude current imaging techniques. *Circulation* 1999;99:1331–1336, with permission.)

ing (MRI), TEE, computed tomography (CT), aortography, or transthoracic echocardiography. Transesophageal echocardiography has many advantages for the evaluation of patients with suspected aortic dissection (Table 15.1) (2,20,28,36–39). The sensitivity and specificity of TEE for the diagnosis of aortic dissection is surpassed only marginally by MRI (Table 15.4) (40,41). In addition, TEE can be used to diagnose cardiac tamponade (Fig. 15.22), aortic regurgitation (Fig. 15.19), or myocardial ischemia associated with aortic dissection (Table 15.5). In a study of 65 patients with aortic dissection confirmed by surgery, the sensitivity of TEE was 97%; the sensitivity of aortography was 77% (40). The diagnosis of aortic dissection was missed by TEE in two patients who had small DeBakey type II aortic dissections, localized to the inner margin of the distal ascending aorta. Aortic dissection was missed by aortography in patients with intramural hematoma or completely thrombosed false lumens that were not enhanced by radiographic contrast. The inability to image the distal ascending aorta and aortic arch may explain the less than perfect ability of TEE to diagnose aortic dissection. Fortunately, it is rare that immediately life-threatening aortic dissections are confined to those regions of the aorta. The sensitivity of transthoracic echocardiography for the diagnosis of aortic dissection is low because of its limited ability to image the aorta (42). MRI has the greatest sensitivity and specificity for the diagnosis of aortic dissection, but the test is time consuming and difficult to perform in unstable patients (42). For this reason, a commonly used diagnostic strategy for patients with suspected aortic dissection is to perform MRI only if the patient is hemodynamically and neurologically stable. MRI is also useful for verifying a negative TEE examination or for evaluating patients where the TEE examination is inconclusive. Transesophageal echocardiography should be performed if the patient is unstable or if accompanying studies suggest a high likelihood of type A aortic dissection (29,42–44).

TABLE 15.4. SENSITIVITY AND SPECIFICITY OF TEE FOR DIAGNOSIS OF AORTIC DISSECTION

Study	N	Sensitivity	Specificity
Hashimoto et al., 1989 (131)	22	100%	100%
Ballal et al., 1991 (39)	34	97%	100%
Adachi et al., 1991 (35)	45	98%	NA
Simon et al., 1992 (44)	32	100%	100%
Erbel et al., 1993 (41)	168	99%	NA
Nienaber et al., 1993 (42)	110	98%	77%
Laissy et al., 1995 (43)	41	86%	90%
Bansal et al., 1995 (40)	65	97%	NA

NA, not available.

It is important to recognize several potential sources of imaging artifacts that can interfere with the TEE diagnosis of aortic dissection. False-positive diagnosis may occur owing to reverberation or side lobe artifacts appearing within the aortic lumen that are mistaken for an intimal flap. These ultrasound imaging artifacts may be generated by atherosclerotic plaques, sclerotic or ectatic regions of adjacent vessel walls, or intravascular catheters. In the mid-esophageal TEE images of the ascending aorta, the interface between the anterior LA or the posterior aortic wall and the anterior right PA or the posterior aortic wall may produce reverberation artifacts within the aortic lumen (45). Image artifacts can sometimes be eliminated by changing the transducer frequency. Artifacts caused by intravascular catheters can be eliminated by removing or repositioning the catheter. Artifacts also can be distinguished from actual defects by demonstrating that they cross anatomic boundaries or fail to alter blood flow patterns on the color Doppler examination (36,46,47). Marked tortuosity of the descending thoracic aorta folding back on itself may simulate an aortic dissection on the TEE examination (48). The false intimal flap generated by a tortuous aorta is thick, nonmobile, and present only in a localized segment of aorta. Periaortic fat may mimic an aortic intramural hematoma. Assessing the motion of periaortic masses relative to the aorta during respiration can sometimes be helpful for distinguishing whether the mass is part of the vessel wall. Misinterpretation of the TEE examination, poor-quality images, or incomplete examination as a consequence of inexperience is also a source of false-negative and false-positive diagnosis (Fig. 15.23) (7,32,36,48–50).

Intraoperative TEE combined with transcervical imaging of the carotid arteries can be used to detect extension of the dissection flap into the neck vessels. Transesophageal echocardiography with color Doppler flow imaging can detect cerebral malperfusion during aortic dissection repair by verifying aortic arch and carotid artery blood flow during the initiation of cardiopulmonary bypass, upon aortic cross-clamping, and after repair of the dissection (38). Intraoperative TEE also may assist in the detection of inadvertent femoral artery cannulation of the false lumen by detecting sudden expansion of the false lumen and collapse of the true lumen upon initiation of cardiopulmonary bypass (38,44). Intraoperative TEE is essential for verifying the absence of significant aortic regurgitation after operative repair of the aortic root with preservation of the native aortic valve (51).

Aortic Aneurysm

Aortic aneurysm is defined as an abnormal dilatation of the aorta producing a vessel diameter that is 50% greater than normal (52). True aneurysms involve all three layers of the aortic wall and can be broadly classified according to shape as saccular or fusiform. Pseudoaneurysms do not contain all or any layers of the aortic wall and develop from defects

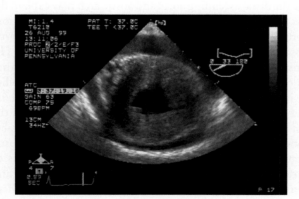

FIGURE 15.22. Transesophageal echocardiographic transgastric short-axis view of the left ventricle demonstrating fluid in the pericardial space surrounding the left ventricle, which was diagnostic for cardiac tamponade from hemopericardium caused by rupture of the proximal ascending aorta in a patient with a type A aortic dissection.

TABLE 15.5. COMPLICATIONS OF AORTIC DISSECTION DIAGNOSED BY TEE

Hemopericardium
Cardiac tamponade
Aortic regurgitation
Myocardial ischemia or infarction
Coronary involvement
Extension of dissection into aortic branch vessels
Hemothorax
Misplacement of the aortic cannula for cardiopulmonary bypass

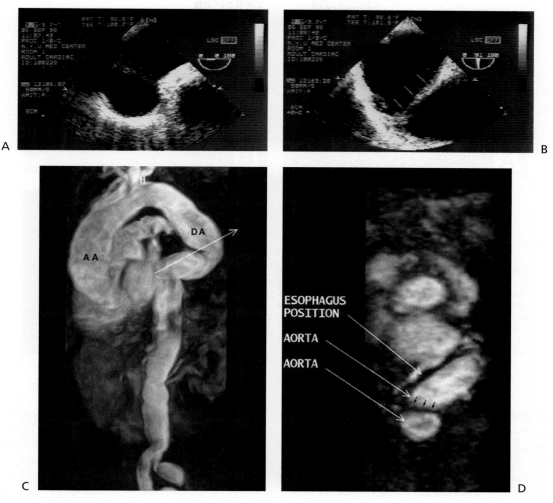

FIGURE 15.23. Transesophageal echocardiographic (TEE) short-axis **(A)** and long-axis **(B)** images of the descending aorta in a patient with severe tortuosity of a descending thoracic aortic aneurysm. The fold in the wall of the vessel (*arrows*) was mistaken for an intimal flap in the TEE images. Magnetic resonance imaging of the entire aorta **(C)** (*arrow*) and its relationship to the esophagus **(D)** explained the appearance of the TEE images. *AA*, ascending aorta; *DA*, descending aorta. (From: O'Connor CJ, Starck T, Goldin MD. Saccular outpouchings of an ascending aortic aneurysm: transesophageal echocardiographic appearance. *J Am Soc Echocardiogr* 1997;10:745–749, with permission.)

in the aortic wall such as the aortic cannulation site or suture lines (20,53). Pseudoaneurysms also may be caused by trauma, ruptured atherosclerotic plaque, or infection. The most common cause of an aortic aneurysm is atherosclerosis, often in combination with hypertension and aging. Chronic aortic dissections typically evolve into aneurysms. Less common causes include Marfan syndrome, Ehlers-Danlos syndrome, aortitis, and syphilis (54). Aortic aneurysm can be associated with bicuspid aortic valve and aortic coarctation. Annuloaortic ectasia is a term sometimes used to describe dilatation of the ascending aorta or aortic root not associated with any specific disease.

Transesophageal echocardiography can be used to characterize the size, location, and extent of thoracic aortic aneurysms. The TEE report should include measurements of the diameters of the aortic valve annulus, sinus of

Valsalva, and sinotubular junction from the mid-esophageal aortic valve long-axis image. Transesophageal echocardiography short-axis aortic diameters of the ascending aorta at the level of the right PA, distal aortic arch, descending aorta, and the site of maximum aneurysm size also should be reported. The diameter of the aneurysm measured by TEE does not always correlate exactly with dimensions measured by CT scan or MRI because of minor differences in the cross-sectional imaging plane and the ability to identify the endothelial wall of the vessel lumen.

Describing the location and extent of the aortic aneurysm using TEE is important for surgical management. Aortic aneurysms that involve the aortic root often cause central aortic regurgitation as a consequence of outward tethering of the aortic valve cusps and may require aortic valve replacement or resuspension (Fig. 15.24) (55).

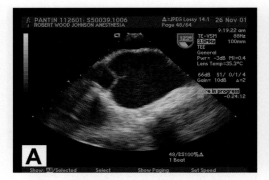
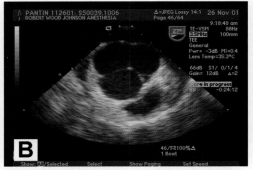
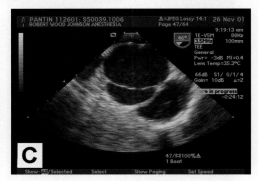

FIGURE 15.24. Transesophageal echocardiographic mid-esophageal aortic valve long-axis **(A)** and short-axis **(B and C)** images from a 32-year-old patient with Marfan syndrome demonstrating aneurysmal enlargement of the aortic root. There was dilatation of the sinuses of Valsalva **(B)** and elongation of the leading edge of the aortic valve cusps **(C)**.

Transesophageal echocardiography also can be used to detect dissection within the aneurysm or mural thrombus lining the wall of the aneurysm. The appearance of a new dissection flap within an aortic aneurysm may indicate a contained rupture. In dissecting aneurysms, the true lumen is usually much larger than the false lumen, and the false lumen is often thrombosed. Atherosclerotic aneurysms often have asymmetric mural thrombus and diffuse swirling echoes or spontaneous echo contrast within the lumen suggestive of low flow within the aneurysm (Fig. 15.25).

The TEE examination must be performed with care in patients with suspected aortic aneurysm. Large aortic aneurysms may cause external compression of the esophagus, making TEE hazardous. Symptoms of dysphagia may indicate esophageal involvement. Large aortic aneurysms also may compress the right PA, the right ventricular outflow tract, the trachea, or main-stem bronchus. The volume occupied by insertion of the TEE probe into the esophagus may be enough to provoke sudden severe cardiovascular collapse, airway obstruction, or aortic rupture. The TEE probe should not be advanced in the esophagus if resistance is encountered.

Aortic Atherosclerosis

Detecting and grading the severity of aortic atherosclerosis using TEE is important for estimating the risk of embolic stroke and peripheral embolization (56–64). The risk of stroke is greater than 10% in patients with atherosclerotic

disease in the ascending aorta or transverse arch (56). Transesophageal echocardiography diagnosis of significant atheromatous disease in the aorta has been shown to be an independent predictor of stroke and death in coronary artery bypass surgery patients (60,65). Other clinical studies also support that atheromatous disease detected by TEE at the time of operation in patients undergoing heart surgery predicted the risk of both intraoperative stroke and future cerebrovascular or peripheral embolic events when the patients were followed over time (38,60,66–69). The incidence of aortic atherosclerosis is greatest in male patients over 70 years of age who have a history of smoking, diabetes, peripheral vascular disease, hypertension, or hypercholesterolemia (70,71).

Atheromatous disease of the thoracic aorta appears on the TEE examination as irregularities and regions of thickening along the intimal surface of the vessel wall. In contrast, the normal thoracic aorta has a smooth intimal surface and uniform wall thickness. Intraluminal irregularities are the direct consequence of the atherosclerotic process, mural thrombus, or ulcerated lesions with attached thrombus (14). Atherosclerotic plaques often appear brighter by ultrasound imaging because of the specular echoes generated by the increased tissue density of the plaque. Calcified plaques or plaques containing calcium produce ultrasound shadowing. Transesophageal echocardiography assessment of aortic atherosclerotic disease should describe plaque thickness, location, and mobility. Plaque thickness is measured as the distance between the intimal surface of the atherosclerotic plaque and the outer edge of the aortic wall perpendicular to

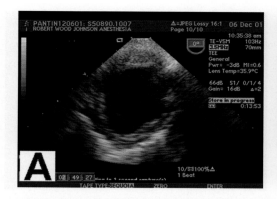
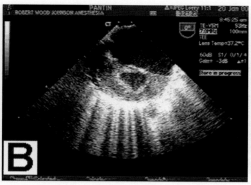
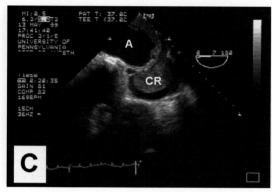

FIGURE 15.25. A and B: Transesophageal echocardiographic (TEE) short-axis views of the mid-descending thoracic aorta of atherosclerotic aneurysms and mural thrombus within the vessel lumen. **C:** TEE short-axis image of the mid-descending thoracic aorta (*A*) demonstrating a contained rupture with thrombus within the pseudoaneurysm cavity (*CR*).

the vessel wall. The most commonly used echocardiographic scale to describe the severity of atheromatous disease classifies disease into five grades (Table 15.6, Fig. 15.26) (60). The use of this scale has been demonstrated to yield reproducible interpretations with clinical value (72). Cardiac surgical patients with grade IV or V atheromatous disease have been demonstrated to have a significantly higher risk for perioperative stroke (73,74).

Detection of atherosclerotic disease in the ascending aorta and aortic arch is important during heart surgery to minimize the risk of embolization during aortic cannulation or aortic cross clamping. Ultrasound imaging is superior to digital palpation for the detection of all except hard calcific plaques (56,58,60,64,75). Although the distal ascending aorta and aortic arch cannot be imaged well by TEE, the detection of significant atherosclerotic plaques in the aortic root, proxi-

mal ascending aorta, or descending thoracic aorta by TEE suggests the presence of disease throughout the thoracic aorta (57). For examination of the ascending aorta and arch, intraoperative epiaortic ultrasound is more sensitive than TEE for the detection and grading of atheromatous disease (Fig. 15.27) (9,20,70,76). The intraoperative epiaortic ultrasound examination is performed directly in the surgical field by placing the transducer in a sterile sleeve. A standoff improves the ability to image the wall of the vessel nearest to the transducer (70).

Traumatic Aortic Injury

Transesophageal echocardiography has an important role in the emergency diagnosis of aortic injury caused by trauma (Table 15.7). Transesophageal echocardiography is typically

TABLE 15.6. GRADING OF AORTIC ATHEROSCLEROSIS USING TEE

Grade	Severity	Description
1	Normal	No intimal thickening
2	Mild	Intimal thickening =3 mm without irregularities
3	Moderate	Sessile atheroma >3 mm with intimal irregularities
4	Severe	Sessile atheroma =5 mm
5	Severe	Atheroma protruding =5 mm with mobile components

From Katz ES, Tunick PA, Rusinek H, et al. Protruding aortic atheromas predict stroke in elderly patients undergoing cardiopulmonary bypass: experience with intraoperative transesophageal echocardiography. *J Am Coll Cardiol* 1992; 20:70–77, with permission.

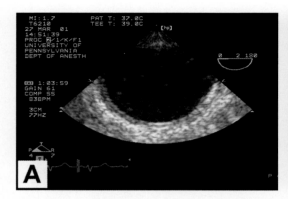
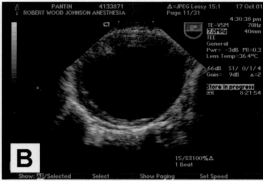
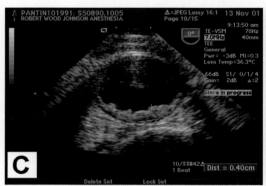
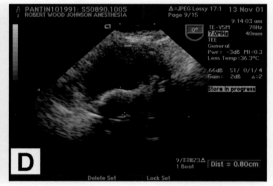
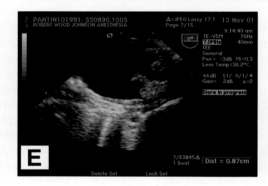

FIGURE 15.26. Echocardiographic grading of atherosclerotic disease of the thoracic aorta. **A:** Grade I, normal to mild intimal thickening. **B:** Grade II, uniform intimal thickening of less than 3 mm without protruding atheroma. **C:** Grade III, irregular atheroma protruding less than 5 mm. **D:** Grade IV, atheroma protruding at least 5 mm into the lumen. **E:** Grade V, atheroma with mobile components.

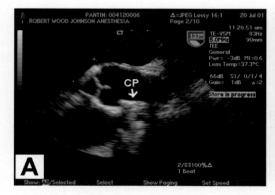
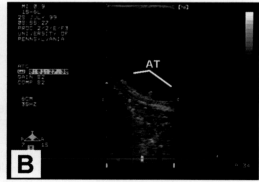

FIGURE 15.27. **A:** Transesophageal echocardiographic mid-esophageal long-axis view of the aortic root showing a calcified plaque (*CP, arrow*) in the anterior wall of the aortic root. **B:** Intraoperative epiaortic ultrasound image demonstrating mobile atheroma (*AT*) on the posterior wall of the ascending aorta **(B)**.

TABLE 15.7. SENSITIVITY AND SPECIFICITY OF TEE FOR DIAGNOSIS OF TRAUMATIC AORTIC INJURY

Study	n	Sensitivity	Specificity
Chirillo et al., 1996 (4)	131	93%	98%
Minard et al., 1996 (5)	29	57%	91%
Vignon et al., 1995 (86)	32	91%	100%
Smith et al., 1995 (81)	121	100%	98%
Saletta et al., 1995 (132)	114	63%	84%
Buckmaster et al., 1994 (77)	121	100%	98%
Karalis et al., 1994 (133)	25	100%	100%
Kearney et al., 1993 (134)	69	100%	100%
Brooks et al., 1991 (82)	21	100%	88%
Sparks 1991 (138)	11	100%	100%
Shapiro 1991 (139)	19	67%	100%

more accurate that aortography for the diagnosis of aortic injury and can be performed more rapidly without the risks associated with instrumentation of the vessel or radiographic contrast injection (77). In one series, the elapsed time between emergency department admission and operation when TEE was used for the diagnosis of aortic injury was as short as 30 minutes (4). In addition to aortic injury, TEE can be used to detect cardiac tamponade, left pleural effusion, hypovolemia, ventricular dysfunction caused by contusion, or injuries to the heart as a consequence of penetrating chest wounds.

The most common aortic injuries are caused by blunt chest trauma or rapid deceleration. The majority of aortic injuries are a consequence of high-speed motor vehicle accidents. Other causes include falls, crush, or blast injuries. In these types of accidents, it has been estimated that 4% to 17% of patients will have an injury to the aorta (78). Sudden deceleration generates the greatest shear forces in the region of the aortic isthmus because it is the region that separates the mobile aortic arch from the fixed descending aorta. Ninety percent of aortic injuries are in the region of the aortic isthmus, followed by injuries to the ascending aorta, the origin of the innominate artery, the descending thoracic aorta, and the arch vessels in decreasing order of frequency (78).

Rapid deceleration or blunt chest trauma typically causes a localized transverse laceration of the aortic wall that involves the intima, media, or entire vessel. It is estimated that 85% of patients with traumatic aortic rupture die at the scene. In survivors, the rupture or transection is contained within the remnants of the adventitial layer or by adjacent mediastinal structures. Among survivors, the estimated mortality rate is approximately 30% within the first 24 hours and 50% within the first week if the injury is not repaired.

The characteristic features of aortic injury by TEE examination is the presence of a mural flap at the site of injury and regional deformities in the vessel caused by the contained rupture (Table 15.8). The flap is commonly confined to only a 1- to 2-cm segment of the aorta. The flap is often described as a "thick flap" because it is made up of several layers of the vessel wall. The mural flap is typically less mobile than the intimal flap associated with aortic dissection. Sometimes intimal disruption produces a small defect in the lumen wall without a discrete flap, and other TEE features indicating aortic injury must be used to confirm the diagnosis (79,80). Intramural hematoma indicating a contained rupture appears as a thickening of the aortic wall at the site of injury (Fig. 15.28). A pseudoaneurysm also may form at the site of rupture. Hematoma surrounding the vessel at the site of rupture appears as a tissue density surrounding the aorta. The presence of a traumatic hemomediastinum is another sign of aortic injury and is defined by a separation exceeding 3 mm between the TEE probe within the esophagus and the anteromedial wall of the aortic isthmus or by blood detected between the posterolateral aortic wall and the left visceral pleura (79). Rupture of the aorta into the left pleural space can often be identified by TEE as a crescent-shaped effusion adjacent to the descending aorta. Doppler examination may demonstrate turbulent or nonlaminar blood flow at the site of injury caused by flow disturbance across the defect (79,81–86).

Problems encountered with the use of TEE to diagnose aortic trauma include the inability to image the entire aorta, failing to examine the short segment of aorta at the site of injury, or difficulty distinguishing between intimal disruption

TABLE 15.8. TEE FINDINGS IN TRAUMATIC AORTIC INJURY

Two-dimensional imaging
  Mural flap
  Intimal disruption
  Intramural hematoma
  Distortion of the vessel lumen
  Left pleural effusion
  Perivascular hematoma
  Pseudoaneurysm

Doppler imaging
  Nonlaminar flow across defect
  Blood flow in pseudoaneurysm cavity

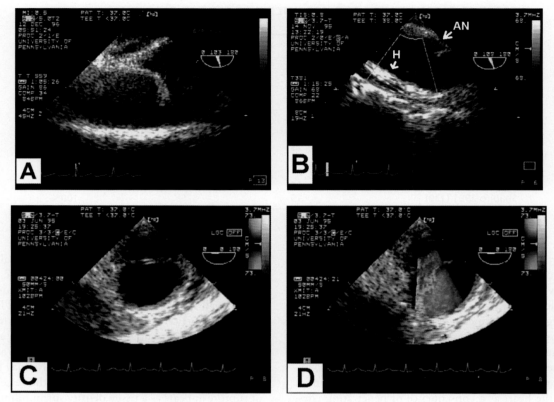

FIGURE 15.28. A: Transesophageal echocardiographic (TEE) long-axis view of the aortic isthmus in the region just distal to the origin of the left subclavian artery demonstrating a thick poorly mobile mural flap (*F, arrow*) diagnostic for traumatic intimal disruption caused by trauma in a patient involved in a high-speed motor vehicle accident. **B:** TEE long-axis view of the descending thoracic aorta just distal to the origin of the left subclavian artery demonstrated intramural hematoma (*H, arrow*) in the anterior wall of the aorta developing a pseudoaneurysm (*AN, arrow*), also diagnostic for aortic trauma. **C and D:** TEE short-axis view of the aortic isthmus demonstrates aortic transection and contained rupture with perivascular hematoma. Color Doppler flow imaging demonstrates nonlaminar flow disturbance at the site of the intimal disruption (**D**).

caused by injury and atherosclerotic disease (81). Fortunately, the vast majority of aortic injuries occur in segments of the aorta that can be imaged by TEE. The most common sites of injury should be examined carefully because the defect may be small and is typically confined to only a short segment of the vessel. Sometimes central venous or PA catheters can produce image artifacts within the aortic lumen that can be mistaken for a mural flap. Diverticula at the origin of the ductus arteriosus have been described and must not be confused with aortic injury (7). Aortography, contrast-enhanced CT, or MRI should be considered if the TEE examination is nondiagnostic or cannot be performed safely (79).

Masses and Tumors within the Aorta

Thrombus and atherosclerotic plaques are the most common abnormal masses detectable by TEE within the aorta. Aneurysms of the aorta are often lined by mural thrombus that appears as an eccentric, crescent-shaped density against the aneurysm wall (Fig. 15.25). Free-floating thrombus can sometimes be detected within a pseudoaneurysm, false lumen of a dissection, or within a contained rupture of the aorta (Fig. 15.25). Complete thrombosis of the aorta causing cardiovascular collapse also has been diagnosed by TEE (Fig. 15.29). Isolated vegetations within the thoracic aorta caused by bacterial endarteritis have been described where TEE was used to establish the diagnosis (87). Fibroelastoma, leiomyosarcoma of vascular origin, and malignant endothelioma are primary tumors of the aorta that may appear as polypoid masses in the lumen, but are extremely rare (88). The descending aorta may be invaded by tumor from the adjacent lung in patients with lung cancer. Sometimes TEE can be used to detect tumor invasion of the thoracic aorta or PA in patients undergoing lung resection for cancer.

Abnormalities of the Coronary Arteries

Transesophageal echocardiography also can help diagnose anatomic anomalies involving the origin of the coronary

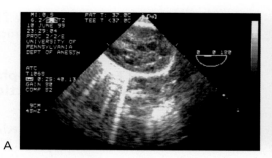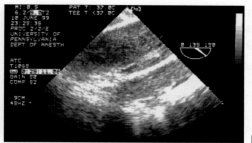

A   B

FIGURE 15.29. Transesophageal echocardiographic short-axis **(A)** and long-axis **(B)** views of the descending thoracic aorta in a patient with acute complete thrombosis of the descending thoracic aorta after repair of a thoracic aortic aneurysm. Tissue density consistent with thrombus occupied the entire lumen of the aorta.

arteries such as a coronary artery arising from the PA (89–93) or the right coronary artery arising from the left sinus of Valsalva (94). Multiplane TEE can be used to define the origin, course, and drainage site of a coronary artery fistula (95). Traumatic injury to the coronary arteries, severe proximal coronary artery stenosis, and embolization to the proximal coronary artery also have been detected by TEE (90,96,97).

Arteritis and Aortitis

Arteritis and aortitis are inflammatory processes that affect the aorta. Inflammation causes thickening and fibrosis of the involved vessel wall. Aortitis caused by bacterial infection may cause vegetations on the endothelial wall or mycotic aneurysms. Endarteritis and mycotic aortic aneurysms may develop from septic emboli, bacteremia, or contiguous spread. Endothelial defects in the aorta such as atherosclerotic plaques or mechanical injury from instrumentation may predispose to infection. The natural history of infected mycotic aneurysms is progressive enlargement and eventual rupture (98,99). Transesophageal echocardiography findings in aortitis are thickening of the aortic wall and periaortic fibrosis (100). Transesophageal echocardiography is often useful for distinguishing inflammation or mycotic aneurysms from intramural hematoma and dissection (101). Serial examination by TEE can be used to demonstrate the progression of endarteritis. The lesion usually begins as a focal thickening in the aortic wall that forms into an abscess with an echolucent cavity. Communication between the abscess cavity and the aortic lumen creates an enlarging mycotic aneurysm. Mycotic aneurysms appear on the TEE examination as focal saccular aneurysms or pseudoaneurysms of the aortic wall. Doppler examination can be used to demonstrate blood flow within the aneurysm or abscess cavity. Other forms of aortitis include Takayasu arteritis that often involves the aortic arch and its major branches. Takayasu arteritis causes vessel stenosis, calcification, or aneurysms and aortic regurgitation (Fig. 15.30). Luetic aneurysms are caused by spirochetal infection of the aortic media. The most common

location for syphilitic aortitis is the ascending aorta. The infection causes thickening of the aortic wall and aneurysmal dilatation that can lead to the development of aortic regurgitation, obliterative endarteritis, or coronary ostial obstruction (102).

Endovascular Stent Repair of Aortic Aneurysm

Endovascular stent repair has become an established treatment for abdominal aortic aneurysms but is still investigational for the repair of thoracic aortic aneurysms (103). Transesophageal echocardiography can potentially provide useful information on the size and luminal characteristics of the proximal and distal stent landing zones in the aorta to determine the feasibility of endovascular stent graft repair, to facilitate sizing of the graft, and to verify the patency of branch vessels after graft deployment (104,105). Results of some studies suggest that TEE may be used to detect the potential for endovascular leak and that TEE detection of spontaneous echo contrast or thrombosis within the excluded aortic lumen after stent graft deployment may predict successful exclusion of the aneurysm (106).

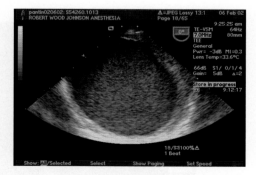

FIGURE 15.30. Transesophageal echocardiographic short-axis view of the descending thoracic aorta in a 23-year-old woman with Takayasu arteritis and a 6-cm diameter aortic aneurysm. Spontaneous echo contrast within the aneurysm lumen indicated decreased blood flow velocity.

Transesophageal Echocardiography to Guide Intraaortic Balloon Pump Positioning and Aortic Cannulation

Transesophageal echocardiography is useful for positioning IABP catheters inserted during surgery to ensure that they function with maximum effectiveness. The catheter tip and balloon can be imaged in the TEE descending aorta short-axis view. Once the distal tip of the catheter is identified, it should be positioned 2 cm distal to the origin of the left subclavian artery. If the left subclavian artery cannot be imaged by TEE, the tip of the balloon catheter can be positioned several centimeters below the point where the descending aorta becomes the distal aortic arch. Another approach is to adjust the TEE probe depth by imaging the aortic valve, then turn the TEE probe to the left without advancing or withdrawing until the descending aorta comes into view, then position the catheter so that its tip is in the same the plane as the aortic valve leaflets. TEE also can image inflation and deflation of the IABP (Fig. 15.31).

Transesophageal echocardiography can be used to detect complications or verify the absence of complications as a consequence of aortic cannulation for cardiopulmonary bypass. When TEE is used in cardiac surgery, the aorta should be examined after separation from cardiopulmonary bypass and after decannulation of the aorta to verify the absence of aortic dissection. When the use of aortic instrumentation has caused a dissection, vessel dilatation may not always be present. Inadvertent cannulation of the false lumen in a patient with an aortic dissection may cause obliteration of the true lumen and malperfusion of the aortic branch vessels upon initiation of cardiopulmonary bypass that can be detected by TEE. Minimally invasive cardiac surgery performed using cardiopulmonary bypass requires TEE for positioning the endoaortic balloon clamp in the ascending aorta (Fig. 15.32). TEE is necessary to detect proximal migration of the endoaortic balloon against the aortic valve or distal migration into the aortic arch. New investigational aortic cannulas designed to provide differential perfusion to the upper and lower body require intraoperative TEE for sizing and positioning of the cannula within the aortic arch (107).

Transesophageal Echocardiography Evaluation of Aortic Reconstruction with Prosthetic Graft

Aortic prosthetic tube grafts appear as an echogenic thin-walled circular structure in short axis by TEE. The TEE long-axis images display the corrugations in the wall of the graft (Fig. 15.33). The remaining native aortic wall is typically left behind after reconstruction and appears on the TEE examination as a tissue density surrounding the prosthetic graft. The free end of the prosthetic aortic arch graft within the lumen of the proximal descending thoracic aorta is a normal finding after the first stage of the "elephant trunk" reconstruction of the thoracic aorta. The proximal and distal anastomosis in patients who have undergone previous aortic grafting are often the sites of aneurysm, leaking, or rupture of the aorta.

TRANSESOPHAGEAL ECHOCARDIOGRAPHY EVALUATION OF THE PULMONARY ARTERY

Pulmonary Artery Anatomy

The main PA is the continuation of the infundibulum of the right ventricle. Its initial portion is intrapericardial and its distal portion is extrapericardial. The main PA is an anterior structure with a course directed superiorly, from right to left and from anterior to posterior. The posterior surface of the main PA rests on top of the LA, separated by the transverse sinus. At its base, the main PA is in front of the ascending aorta, but as it ascends, it courses under the aortic arch and divides into the right and left pulmonary arteries (10). The right PA travels in a horizontal direction from left to right behind the ascending aorta and the superior vena cava. It is just anterior and below the tracheal bifurcation. The left

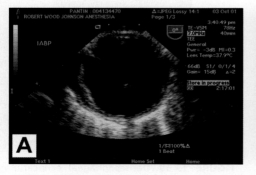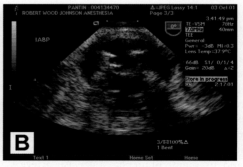

FIGURE 15.31. A: Transesophageal echocardiographic short-axis view of the aorta just distal to the origin of the left subclavian artery demonstrating the tip of an intraaortic balloon catheter properly positioned within the lumen of the descending thoracic aorta. **B:** shows the appearance of the catheter during balloon inflation.

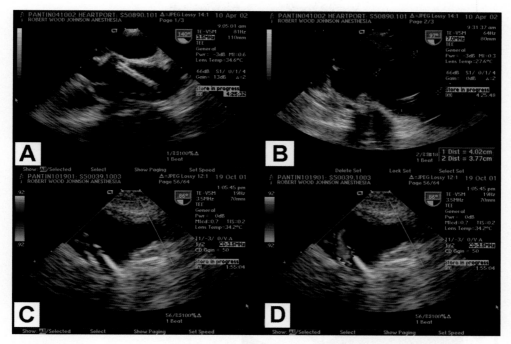

FIGURE 15.32. A: Transesophageal echocardiographic (TEE) mid-esophageal long-axis view of the aortic root demonstrating the tip of a deflated endoaortic balloon catheter in the proximal aorta. **B:** The endoaortic balloon was positioned just above the sinotubular junction and inflated with saline to occlude the proximal ascending aorta for cardiopulmonary bypass via the femoral artery and vein. **C and D:** TEE upper esophageal long-axis images of the ascending aorta showing the tip of an aortic cannula inserted through the anterior wall of the ascending aorta for standard cardiopulmonary bypass.

PA travels in an oblique direction laterally and posteriorly in front of the left main-stem bronchus.

Transesophageal Echocardiography Examination of the Pulmonary Artery

The PA and its branches appear in five of the standard multiplane TEE cross sections (11). The base of the main PA and pulmonic valve can be imaged in front and just to the left of the aorta in the TEE mid-esophageal right ventricular inflow and outflow view. The TEE upper esophageal aortic arch short-axis view also provides a long-axis image of the pulmonic valve and main PA below and behind the distal aortic arch. The distal main PA and its bifurcation can be imaged to the left of the ascending aorta in the TEE mid-esophageal ascending aorta short-axis view. The right PA is imaged in long axis behind the aorta in the TEE mid-esophageal ascending aorta short-axis view and in short axis behind the ascending aorta in the TEE mid-esophageal ascending aorta long-axis view. Only the proximal end of the left PA can be

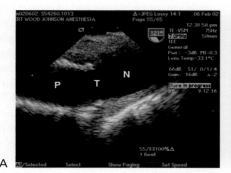

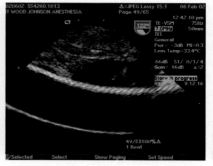

FIGURE 15.33. Transesophageal echocardiographic (TEE) long-axis view of the proximal descending thoracic aorta in a patient after graft repair of a descending thoracic aortic aneurysm. **A:** The transition zone (*T*) between the native aorta (*N*) and the prosthetic graft (*P*). **B:** TEE long-axis view of the prosthetic aortic graft surrounded by the native aortic wall that was left behind.

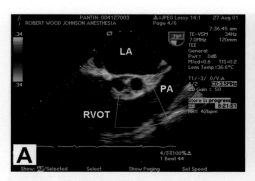
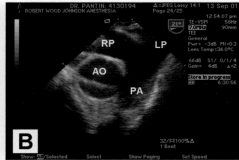

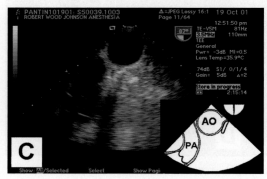

FIGURE 15.34. Transesophageal echocardiographic (TEE) views of the pulmonary artery. **A:** Mid-esophageal right ventricular inflow–outflow view at a multiplane angle of 79 degrees showing the main pulmonary artery (*PA*), right ventricular outflow tract (*RVOT*), and left atrium (*LA*). **B:** Mid-esophageal ascending aorta (*AO*) short-axis view at a multiplane angle of 21 degrees showing the bifurcation of the main pulmonary artery (*PA*) into the right pulmonary artery (*RP*) and left pulmonary artery (*LP*). **C:** Upper esophageal aortic arch short-axis view at a multiplane angle of 87 degrees showing the main pulmonary artery (*PA*) in long axis anterior to the distal aortic arch (*AO*).

imaged before it is obscured by the left main-stem bronchus (Fig. 15.34).

Doppler quantification of blood flow velocity in the main PA has been used to estimate cardiac output that correlates reasonably well with cardiac output measured by thermodilution, but the technique is cumbersome (108).

Transesophageal Echocardiography Evaluation of Diseases Involving the Pulmonary Artery

Transesophageal echocardiography can be useful in the evaluation of patients with pulmonary hypertension. In a study of 48 patients with pulmonary hypertension awaiting lung transplantation, preoperative TEE provided information that affected the conduct of the operation in 12 of the patients (25%). The TEE findings included proximal PA thrombi, patent foramen ovale with significant right-to-left shunting, atrial septal defect, double-outlet right ventricle, and ventricular septal defect (109). Pulmonary hypertension can cause dilatation of the PA. Color Doppler imaging of the main PA may exhibit reversal of systolic flow along the medial wall of the vessel in patients with pulmonary hypertension (110,111). Lesions in the wall of the PA can be

detected in patients with primary pulmonary hypertension and in approximately 48% of patients with chronic obstructive pulmonary disease (112). These lesions detected by TEE have been attributed to *in situ* thrombosis or atherosclerosis of the PA.

Transesophageal echocardiography is often useful for the evaluation of patients with suspected massive pulmonary thromboembolism (2,113–116). TEE can detect acute right ventricular dilatation and dysfunction as a consequence of pulmonary embolism and may even detect thrombus within the lumen of the PA (Fig. 15.35) (2,117). In a series of 24 consecutive medical intensive care unit patients with unexplained shock and jugular venous distension, TEE findings of right ventricular dilatation led to the diagnosis of massive pulmonary embolism with a sensitivity of 92% and specificity of 100% (118). In that series, TEE examination imaged central pulmonary thromboembolism in 12 patients. The combined accuracy of TEE and transthoracic echocardiography for the diagnosis of pulmonary embolism was lower in another study with a sensitivity of 59% and specificity of 77% (119).

Transesophageal echocardiographic assessment of PA flow characteristics predicted outcome after Fontan or hemi-Fontan procedures in a report of 10 patients no more than

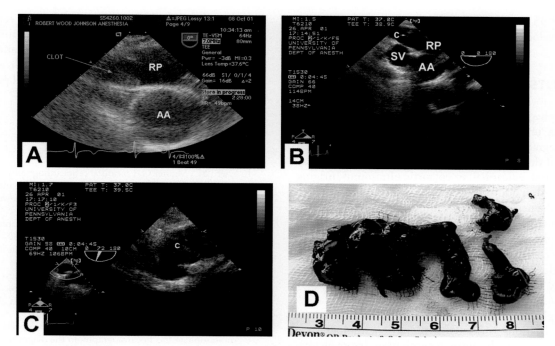

FIGURE 15.35. A: Transesophageal echocardiographic (TEE) mid-esophageal short-axis image of the ascending aorta (*AA*) demonstrating pulmonary embolus in the proximal right pulmonary artery (*RP*). **B and C:** TEE mid-esophageal short-axis images from another patient with recurrent pulmonary embolism also demonstrating thrombus (*c*) in the right pulmonary artery (*RP*). **D:** The pulmonary artery thrombus that was removed by pulmonary thromboembolectomy. *RP*, right pulmonary artery; *SV,* superior vena.

3 years of age who underwent direct anastomosis of the right atrium to the PA (120). Two distinct flow patterns across the atriopulmonary anastomosis were identified by TEE immediately after cardiopulmonary bypass. The normal flow pattern was biphasic forward flow with velocity peaks in systole and diastole. An abnormal flow pattern with flow reversal in diastole was observed in 4 patients who did poorly postoperatively. Reversal of diastolic PA flow after a Fontan operation predicted poor outcome and was attributed to elevated pulmonary vascular resistance or decreased left ventricular function (120).

Pulmonary artery stenosis can be caused by external compression from an anterior mediastinal tumor such as Hodgkin lymphoma or teratoma (121). An intraluminal PA fibroma is a rare tumor that can present as supravalvular PA stenosis (121). Primary sarcomas of the PA and right ventricle are also rare and may resemble acute or chronic pulmonary thromboembolism (113,122).

Transesophageal echocardiography can be used in the diagnosis of various other lesions involving the PA and branches, including fistulous communication between heart chambers and the great vessels caused by endocarditis, pulmonary arteriovenous malformation, idiopathic dilatation of the PA, aneurysm of the proximal right PA, and proximal interruption of the right PA (123–126). Pulmonary arteriovenous malformation can be detected by the transit of echo contrast injected into a central vein traversing the pulmonary vasculature and exiting from a pulmonary vein (127). Traumatic injury to the PA has been described presenting as cardiac tamponade caused by a PA laceration from a stab wound to the left chest (128).

NORMAL REFERENCE VALUES FOR THE AORTIC AND PULMONARY ARTERY

Transesophageal echocardiography can be used to quantify the size of the aorta and PA. Ideally, measurements should be performed with the ultrasound beam perpendicular to the acoustic interfaces and the calipers positioned from the inner edge to the inner edge of the structure being imaged. Image resolution should be optimized with the lowest possible gain setting. The electrocardiogram should be recorded to time the measurement in relation to the cardiac cycle.

Distinguishing normal from abnormal vascular and cardiac dimensions can be based not only in reference to "normal" values (Table 15.2), but also in comparison to other structures in a given individual. For example, aortic and pulmonic valve annular dimensions are similar within the same individual. Similarly, the aortic root and right ventricular outflow tract should be similar in size within an individual patient (129,130). It is also important to recognize that the size of the aorta, right PA, and superior vena cava increases with age (129). Finally, the normal aortic root blood flow velocity is 1.35 m/s (range 1–1.7 m/s) and the normal PA blood flow velocity is 0.75 m/s (range 0.6–0.9 m/s) (46).

KEY POINTS

- Transesophageal echocardiography can provide high-resolution images of almost the entire aorta except for a distal segment of the ascending aorta and the proximal portion of the aortic arch that is shielded by the trachea.
- Transcervical, epicardial, or epiaortic ultrasound imaging can be used in addition to or as a substitute for TEE to evaluate the neck vessels, ascending aorta, and aortic arch during open-heart surgery.
- Transesophageal echocardiography is the diagnostic procedure of choice for emergency evaluation of patients with suspected aortic dissection, aortic aneurysms, or suspected traumatic injury to the aorta if the patient is clinically unstable.
- Transesophageal echocardiography is useful for detecting complications associated with aortic pathology such as cardiac tamponade, aortic regurgitation, hypovolemia, myocardial ischemia, malperfusion syndromes, left pleural effusion, ventricular dysfunction caused by contusion, or injuries as a consequence of penetrating chest wounds.
- Insertion of the TEE probe into the esophagus can cause acute hypoxemia or airway compromise by extrinsic compression of the right PA or left main-stem bronchus in patients with large aneurysms of the ascending aorta.
- The most common site for aortic dissection is the initial third of the ascending aorta or the descending thoracic aorta just beyond the left subclavian artery.
- Aortic dissection is commonly classified using the Stanford classification that divides dissections into type A (involving the ascending aorta or aortic arch) or B (confined to the descending aorta).
- Identification of a mobile intimal flap separating the aorta into a true and false lumen seen in more than one view on TEE examination is diagnostic for aortic dissection.
- Aortic intramural hematoma is a variant of aortic dissection with similar prognosis.
- Aortic aneurysms that involve the aortic root often cause central aortic regurgitation as a consequence of outward tethering of the aortic valve cusps and may require aortic valve replacement or resuspension.
- Transesophageal echocardiography diagnosis of significant atheromatous disease in the aorta (>5 mm or mobile atheroma) is an independent predictor of stroke and death in coronary artery bypass surgery patients.
- Ultrasound imaging is superior to digital palpation for the detection of atherosclerotic plaques in the aorta.
- The detection of significant root, proximal ascending aorta, or descending thoracic aorta atherosclerosis by TEE suggests the presence of disease throughout the thoracic aorta.

- Ninety percent of traumatic aortic injuries occur in the region of the aortic isthmus, followed by injuries to the ascending aorta, at the origin of the innominate artery, the descending thoracic aorta and the arch vessels and are characterized by a "thick" mural flap and perivascular hematoma.

REFERENCES

1. Czer LSC, Maurer G. Epicardial echocardiography and Doppler color-flow mapping in the adult patient. In: deBruijn NP, Clements FM, ed. *Intraoperative use of echocardiography.* Philadelphia: JB Lippincott, 1991:157–161.
2. Heidenreich PA. Transesophageal echocardiography (TEE) in the critical care patient. *Cardiol Clin* 2000;18:789–805.
3. Vlahakes GJ, Warren RL. Traumatic rupture of the aorta. *N Engl J Med* 1995;332:389–390.
4. Chirillo F, Totis O, Cavarzerani A, et al. Usefulness of transthoracic and transoesophageal echocardiography in recognition and management of cardiovascular injuries after blunt chest trauma. *Heart* 1996;75:301–306.
5. Minard G, Schurr MJ, Croce MA, et al. A prospective analysis of transesophageal echocardiography in the diagnosis of traumatic disruption of the aorta. *J Trauma* 1996;40:225–230.
6. **Lefant F, Cittanova ML, Goarin JP, et al. Severe hypercapnia induced by acute dissecting aortic aneurysm. *Anesthesiology* 1998;89:780–782.**
7. Weyman AE, Griffin BP. Left ventricular outflow tract: the aortic valve, aorta, and subvalvular outflow tract In:. Weyman AE, ed. *Principles and practice of echocardiography,* 2nd ed Philadelphia: Lea & Febiger, 1994:498–574.
8. Lopez-Candales A. Assessing the aorta with transesophageal echocardiography. Update on imaging capabilities with today's technology. *Postgrad Med* 1999;106:157–158,161–166, 169.
9. **Konstadt SN, Reich DL, Quintana C, et al. The ascending aorta: how much does transesophageal echocardiography see? *Anesth Analg* 1994;78:240–244.**
10. Testut L, Jacob O. Cavidad torácica y su contenido. In: Testut L, Jacob O, ed. Anatomía topográfica, 8th ed Vol. I. Barcelona: Salvat, 1983:859–860,876–878.
11. **Shanewise JS, Cheung AT, Aronson S, et al. ASE/SCA guidelines for performing a comprehensive intraoperative multiplane transesophageal echocardiography examination: recommendations of the American Society of Echocardiography Council for Intraoperative Echocardiography and the Society of Cardiovascular Anesthesiologists Task Force for Certification in Perioperative Transesophageal Echocardiography. *Anesth Analg* 1999;89:870–884.**
12. Orihashi K, Matsuura Y, Sueda T, et al. Aortic arch branches are no longer a blind zone for transesophageal echocardiography: a new eye for aortic surgeons. *J Thorac Cardiovasc Surg* 2000;120:466–472.
13. Cholley BP, Shroff SG, Korcarz C, et al. Aortic elastic properties with transesophageal echocardiography with automated border detection: validation according to regional differences between proximal and distal descending thoracic aorta. *J Am Soc Echocardiogr* 1996;9:539–548.
14. Nakao T, Frymus M. Aortic plaque. In: Oka Y, Konstadt SA, eds. *Clinical transesophageal echocardiography: a problem oriented approach.* Philadelphia: Lippincott-Raven, 1996:113–123.
15. Orihashi K, Matsuura Y, Sueda T, et al. Abdominal aorta and visceral arteries visualized with transesophageal echocardiogra-

phy during operations on the aorta. *J Thorac Cardiovasc Surg* 1998;115:945–947.

16. Vicente T, Pinar E, Garcia A, et al. Utilidad de la ecocardiografia transesofagica en el diagnostico de coartacion de aorta atipica. [The usefulness of transesophageal echocardiography in the diagnosis of atypical aortic coarctation.] *Rev Esp Cardiol* 1997;50:802–805.

17. Andrade A, Vargas-Barron J, Rijlaarsdam M, et al. Utility of transesophageal echocardiography in the examination of adult patients with patent ductus arteriosus. *Am Heart J* 1995;130:543–546.

18. Shyu KG, Lai LP, Lin SC, et al. Diagnostic accuracy of transesophageal echocardiography for detecting patent ductus arteriosus in adolescents and adults. *Chest* 1995;108:1201–1205.

19. Smith JC, Smith DC, Ahrar K, et al. Patent ductus arteriosus masquerading as traumatic aortic rupture at aortography: the complementary role of transesophageal echocardiography. *J Vasc Interv Radiol* 1999;10:169–171.

20. **Kouchoukos NT, Dougenis D. Surgery of the thoracic aorta. *N Engl J Med* 1997;336:1876–188.**

21. **Svensson LG, Labib SB, Eisenhauer AC, et al. Intimal tear without hematoma. An important variant of aortic dissection that can elude current imaging techniques. *Circulation* 1999;99:1331–1336.**

22. Mohr-Kahaly S, Erbel R, Kearney P, et al. Aortic intramural hemorrhage visualized by transesophageal echocardiography: findings and prognostic implications. *J Am Coll Cardiol* 1994;23:658–664.

23. Vilacosta I, San Román JA, Aragoncillo P, et al. Atherosclerotic aortic rupture: documentation by transesophageal echocardiography. *J Am Soc Echocardiogr* 2001;14:152–154.

24. Sakakibara Y, Matsuda K, Sato F, et al. Aortic dissection complicating cardiac surgery in a patient with calcified ascending aorta. *Jpn J Thorac Cardiovasc Surg* 1999;47:625–628.

25. Andersen C, Joyce FS, Tingleff J, et al. Aortic dissection after cardiopulmonary bypass detected by intraoperative transesophageal echocardiography. *Acta Anaesthesiol Scand* 1997;41:1227–1228.

26. Katz ES, Tunick PA, Colvin SB, et al. Aortic dissection complicating cardiac surgery: diagnosis by intraoperative biplane transesophageal echocardiography. *J Am Soc Echocardiogr* 1993;6:217–222.

27. Chavanon O, Carrier M, Cartier R, et al. Increased incidence of acute ascending aortic dissection with off-pump aortocoronary bypass surgery? *Ann Thorac Surg* 2001;71:117–121.

28. Cigarroa JE, Isselbacher EM, DeSanctis RW, et al. Diagnostic imaging in the evaluation of suspected aortic dissection. Old standards and new directions. *N Engl J Med* 1993;328:35–43.

29. Deutsch HJ, Sechtem U, Meyer H, et al. Chronic aortic dissection: comparison of MR imaging and transesophagal echocardiography. *Radiology* 1994;192:645–650.

30. Lopez-Minguez JR, Merchan A, Arrobas J, et al. Hematoma intramural aortico. Un patron atipico equivalente a la diseccion aortica. [Aortic intramural hematoma. An atypical pattern equivalent to aortic dissection.] *Rev Esp Cardiol* 1995;48:634–637.

31. **Nienaber CA, Kodolitsch Y, Petresen B, et al. Intramural hemorrhage of the thoracic aorta: diagnostic and therapeutic implications. *Circulation* 1995;92:1465–1472.**

32. Ionescu AA, Vinereanu D, Wood A, et al. Periaortic fat pad mimicking an intramural hematoma of the thoracic aorta: lessons for transesophageal echocardiography. *J Am Soc Echocardiogr* 1998;11:487–490.

33. Flachskampf FA, Banbury M, Smedira N, et al. Transesophageal echocardiography diagnosis of intramural hematoma of the ascending aorta: a word of caution. *J Am Soc Echocardiogr* 1999;12:866–870.

34. Harris KM, Braverman AC, Gutierrez FR, et al. Transesophageal echocardiographic and clinical features of aortic intramural hematoma. *J Thorac Cardiovasc Surg* 1997;114:619–626.

35. Adachi H, Omoto R, Kyo S, et al. Emergency surgical intervention of acute aortic dissection with the rapid diagnosis by transesophageal echocardiography. *Circulation* 1991;84(suppl III):14–19.

36. Chu VF, Chow CM, Stewart J, et al. Transesophageal echocardiography for ascending aortic dissection: is it enough for surgical intervention? *J Card Surg* 1998;13:260–265.

37. Khandheria BK. Aortic dissection. The last frontier. *Circulation* 1993;87:1765–1768.

38. **Coletti G, Torracca L, La Canna G, et al. Diagnosis and management of cerebral malperfusion phenomena during aortic dissection repair by transesophageal Doppler echocardiographic monitoring. *J Card Surg* 1996;11:355–358.**

39. Ballal RS, Nanda NC, Gatewood R, et al. Usefulness of transesophageal echocardiography in assessment of aortic dissection. *Circulation* 1991;84:1903–1914.

40. Bansal RC, Chandrasekaran K, Ayala K, et al. Frequency and explanation of false negative diagnosis of aortic dissection by aortography and transesophageal echocardiography. *J Am Coll Cardiol* 1995;25:1393–1401.

41. Erbel R, Engberding R, Daniel W, et al. Echocardiography in diagnosis of aortic dissection. *Lancet* 1989;1:457–461.

42. Nienaber CA, Kodolitsch Y, Nicolas V, et al. The diagnosis of thoracic aortic dissection by noninvasive imaging procedures. *N Engl J Med* 1993;328:1–9.

43. Laissy JP, Blanc F, Soyer P, et al. Thoracic aortic dissection: diagnosis with transesophageal echocardiography versus MR imaging. *Radiology* 1995;194:331–336.

44. Simon P, Owen AN, Havel M, et al. Transesophageal echocardiography in the emergency surgical management of patients with aortic dissection. *J Thorac Cardiovasc Surg* 1992;103:1113–1118.

45. Losi MA, Betocchi S, Briguori C, et al. Determinants of aortic artifacts during transesophageal echocardiography of the ascending aorta. *Am Heart J* 1999;137:967–972.

46. Feigenbaum H. Diseases of the aorta. In: Feigenbaum H, ed. *Echocardiography*, 5th ed. Baltimore: Williams & Wilkins, 1994:652.

47. Kimura BJ, Phan JN, Housman LB. Utility of contrast echocardiography in the diagnosis of aortic dissection. *J Am Soc Echocardiogr* 1999;12:155–159.

48. O'Connor CJ, Starck T, Goldin MD. Saccular outpouchings of an ascending aortic aneurysm: transesophageal echocardiographic appearance. *J Am Soc Echocardiogr* 1997;10:745–749.

49. Katz ES, Applebaum RM, Earls JP, et al. Tortuosity of the descending thoracic aorta simulating dissection on transesophageal echocardiography. *J Am Soc Echocardiogr* 1997;10:83–87.

50. Patel S, Alam M, Rosman H. Pitfalls in the echocardiographic diagnosis of aortic dissection. *Angiology* 1997;48:939–946.

51. Keane MG, Wiegers SE, Yang E, et al. Structural determinants of aortic regurgitation in type A dissection and the role of valvular resuspension as determined by intraoperative transesophageal echocardiography. *Am J Cardiol* 2000;85:604–10.

52. Johnston KW, Rutherford RB, Tilson MD, et al. Suggested standards for reporting on arterial aneurysms. *J Vasc Surg* 1991;13:452–458.

53. Spencer KT, Kaji E, Drucker D. Transesophageal echocardiographic diagnosis of a mycotic ascending aortic pseudoaneurysm as a source of embolism. *J Am Soc Echocardiogr* 1998;11:1155–1157.

54. Meier JH, Seward JB, Miller FA Jr, et al. Aneurysms in the left ventricular outflow tract: clinical presentation, causes, and echocardiographic features. *J Am Soc Echocardiogr* 1998;11:729–745.

55. Tiller GE, Cassidy SB, Wensel C, et al. Aortic root dilatation in Ehlers-Danlos syndrome types I, II and III. A report of five cases. *Clin Genet* 1998;53:460–465.

56. Gardner TJ, Horneffer PJ, Manolio TA, et al. Stroke following coronary artery bypass grafting: a ten year study. *Ann Thorac Surg* 1985;40:574.

57. **Konstadt SN, Reich DL, Kahn R, et al. Transesophageal echocardiography can be used to screen for ascending aortic atherosclerosis. *Anesth Analg* 1995;81:225–228.**

58. Karalis DG, Chandrasekaran K, Victor MF, et al. Recognition and embolic potential of intra-aortic atherosclerotic debris. *J Am Coll Cardiol* 1991;17:73.

59. Ribakove GH, Katz ES, Galloway AC, et al. Surgical implications of transesophageal echocardiography to grade the atheromatous aortic arch. *Ann Thorac Surg* 1992;53:758.

60. Katz ES, Tunick PA, Rusinek H, et al. Protruding aortic atheromas predict stroke in elderly patients undergoing cardiopulmonary bypass: experience with intraoperative transesophageal echocardiography. *J Am Coll Cardiol* 1992;20:70–77.

61. Mitchell MM, Frankville DD, Weinger MB, et al. Detection of thoracic aortic atheroma with transesophageal echocardiography in patients without symptoms of embolism. *Am Heart J* 1991;122:1768.

62. Lanza GM, Zabalgoitia-Reyes M, Franzin L, et al. Plaque and structural characteristics of the descending thoracic aorta using transesophageal echocardiography. *J Am Soc Echocardiogr* 1991;4:19.

63. Tunick PA, Kronzon I. Protruding atherosclerotic plaque in the aortic arch of patients with systemic embolization: a new finding seen by transesophageal echocardiography. *Am Heart J* 1990;120:658.

64. Machleder HI, Takiff H, Lois JF, et al. Aortic mural thrombus: an occult source of arterial thromboembolism. *J Vasc Surg* 1986;4:473.

65. **Hartman GS, Yao FF, Bruefach M III, et al. Severity of aortic atheromatous disease diagnosed by transesophageal echocardiography predicts stroke and other outcomes associated with coronary artery surgery: a prospective study. *Anesth Analg* 1996;83:701–708.**

66. Jones EF, Kalman JM, Calafiore P, et al. Proximal aortic atheroma: an independent risk factor for cerebral ischemia. *Stroke* 1995;26:218–224.

67. Amarenco P, Cohen A, Tzourio C, et al. Atherosclerotic disease of the aortic arch and the risk of ischemic stroke. *N Engl J Med* 1994;331:1474–1479.

68. Tunick PA, Rosenzweig BP, Katz ES, et al. High risk for vascular events in patients with protruding aortic atheromas: a prospective study. *J Am Coll Cardiol* 1994;23:1085–1090.

69. The French Study of aortic Plaques in Stroke Group. Atherosclerotic disease of the aortic arch as a risk factor for recurrent ischemic stroke. *N Engl J Med* 1996;334:1216–1221.

70. Sylivris S, Calafiore P, Matalanis P, et al. The intraoperative assessment of ascending aortic atheroma: epiaortic imaging is superior to both transesophageal echocardiography and direct palpation. *J Cardiothorac Vasc Anesth* 1997;11:704–707.

71. Tribouilloy C, Peltier M, Andrejak M, et al. Correlation of thoracic aortic atherosclerotic plaque detected by multiplane transesophageal echocardiography and cardiovascular risk factors. *Am J Cardiol* 1998;82:1552–1555, A8.

72. Hartman GS, Peterson J, Konstadt SN, et al. High reproducibility in the interpretation of intraoperative transesophageal echocardiographic evaluation of aortic atheromatous disease. *Anesth Analg* 1996;82:539–543.

73. Mizuno T, Toyama M, Tabuchi N, et al. Thickened intima of the aortic arch is a risk factor for stroke with coronary artery bypass grafting. *Ann Thorac Surg* 2000;70:1565–1570.

74. Kutz SM, Lee VS, Tunick PA, et al. Atheromas of the thoracic aorta: a comparison of transesophageal echocardiography and breath-hold gadolinium-enhanced 3-dimensional magnetic resonance angiography. *J Am Soc Echocardiogr* 1999;12:853–858.

75. Marshall WG Jr, Barzilai B, Kouchoukos NT, et al. Intraoperative ultrasonic imaging of the ascending aorta. *Ann Thorac Surg* 1989;48:339.

76. Davila-Roman VG, Phillips KJ, Daily BB, et al. Intraoperative transesophageal echocardiography and epiaortic ultrasound for assessment of atherosclerosis of the thoracic aorta. *J Am Coll Cardiol* 1996;28:942–947.

77. Buckmaster MJ, Kearney PA, Johnson SB, et al. Further experience with transesophageal echocardiography in the evaluation of thoracic aortic injury. *J Trauma* 1994;37:989–995.

78. Pretre R, Chilcott M. Blunt trauma to the heart great vessels. *N Engl J Med* 1997;336:626–632.

79. Vignon P, Boncoeur MP, Francois B, et al. Comparison of multiplane transesophageal echocardiography and contrast-enhanced helical CT in the diagnosis of blunt traumatic cardiovascular injuries. *Anesthesiology* 2001;94:615–622.

80. Goarin JP, Cluzel P, Gosgnach M, et al. Evaluation of transesophageal echocardiography for diagnosis of traumatic aortic injury. *Anesthesiology* 2000;93(6):1373–1377.

81. **Smith MD, Cassidy JM, Souther S, et al. Transesophageal echocardiography in the diagnosis of traumatic rupture of the aorta. *N Engl J Med* 1995;332(6):356–362.**

82. Brooks SW, Cmolik BL, Young JC, et al. Transesophageal echocardiographic examination or a patient with traumatic aortic transection from blunt chest trauma. *J Trauma* 1991;31:841–845.

83. Galvin IF, Black IW, Lee CL, et al. Transesophageal echocardiography in acute aortic transection. *Ann Thorac Surg* 1991;51:310–311.

84. Locke TJ, Reeder GS, Khandheria BK, et al. Diagnosis of traumatic aortic rupture by transesophageal echocardiography. *J Thorac Cardiovasc Surg* 1991;101:555–556.

85. **Goarin JP, Catoire P, Jacquens Y, et al. Use of transesophageal echocardiography for diagnosis of traumatic aortic injury. *Chest* 1997;112:71–80.**

86. Vignon P, Gueret P, Vedrinne JM, et al. Role of transesophageal echocardiography in the diagnosis and management of traumatic aortic disruption. *Circulation* 1995;92:2959–2968.

87. Bansal RC, Ashmeik K, Razzouk AJ. An unusual case of vegetative aortitis diagnosed by transesophageal echocardiography. *J Am Soc Echocardiogr* 2001;14:237–239.

88. Navarra G, Occhionorelli S, Mascoli F, et al. Primary leiomyosarcoma of the aorta: report of a case and review of the literature. *J Cardiovasc Surg* 1994;35:333–336.

89. Kasprzak JD, Kratochwil D, Peruga JZ, et al. Coronary anomalies diagnosed with transesophageal echocardiography: complementary clinical value in adults. *Int J Card Imaging* 1998;14:89–95.

90. O'Rourke DJ, Flanagan M, Berman N, et al. Stenosis at the origin of an anomalous left main coronary artery arising from the pulmonary artery in a symptom-free adolescent girl: transesophageal echocardiographic findings. *J Am Soc Echocardiogr* 1996;9:724–726.

91. Sbraggia P, Habib G, Garcia M, et al. Naissance anormale de la coronaire gauche a partir de l'artere pulmonaire. Apport diagnostique des techniques echographiques. [Abnormal origin of the left coronary artery from the pulmonary artery. Diagnostic contribution of ultrasonographic technique.] *Ann Cardiol Angeiol (Paris)* 1996;45:507–511.

92. Rychik J, Jacobs ML. Intraoperative transesophageal echocardiographic imaging of intrapulmonary tunnel repair for anomalous left coronary artery originating from the pulmonary artery. *Echocardiography* 1997;14:33–38.

93. Hsu SY, Lin FC, Chang HJ, et al. Multiplane transesophageal echocardiography in diagnosis of anomalous origin of the left coronary artery from the pulmonary artery: a case report. *J Am Soc Echocardiogr* 1998;11:668–672.

94. Sasson Z, Grande P, Lorette I, et al. Proximal narrowing of anomalous right coronary artery from the left coronary sinus: delineation by omniplane transesophageal echocardiogram. *Can J Cardiol* 1996;12:529–531.

95. Lin FC, Chang HJ, Chern MS, et al. Multiplane transesophageal echocardiography in the diagnosis of congenital coronary artery fistula. *Am Heart J* 1995;130:1236–1244.

96. Bliss DW, Newth CJ, Stein JE. Blunt traumatic injury to the coronary arteries and pulmonary artery in a child. *J Trauma* 2000;49:550–552.

97. Thakur AC, Voros S, Nanda NC, et al. Transesophageal echocardiographic diagnosis of proximal coronary artery stenosis in patients with ischemic stroke. *Echocardiography* 1999;16:159–166.

98. Vilacosta I, Bustos D, Cigüenza R, et al. Primary mycotic aneurysm of the ascending aorta diagnosed by transesophageal echocardiography. *J Am Soc Echocardiogr* 1998;11:216–218.

99. Joffe II, Emmi RP, Oline J, et al. Mycotic aneurysm of the descending thoracic aorta: the role of transesophageal echocardiography. *J Am Soc Echocardiogr* 1996;9:663–667.

100. Harris KM, Malenka DJ, Plehn JF. Transesophageal echocardiographic evaluation of aortitis. *Clin Cardiol* 1997;20:813–815.

101. Kunzli A, von Segesser LK, Vogt PR, et al. Inflammatory aneurysm of the ascending aorta. *Ann Thorac Surg* 1998;65:1132–1133.

102. Frank MW, Mehlman DJ, Tsai F, et al. Syphilitic aortitis. *Circulation* 1999;100:1582–1583.

103. Mitchell RS, Dake MD, Sembre CP, et al. Endovascular stent-graft repair of thoracic aortic aneurysms. *J Thorac Cardiovasc Surg* 1996;111:1054–1062.

104. Dake MD, Kato N, Mitchell S, et al. Endovascular stent-graft placement for the treatment of acute aortic dissection. *N Engl J Med* 1999;340:1546–1552.

105. Nienaber CA, Fattori R, Lund G, et al. Nonsurgical reconstruction of thoracic aortic dissection by stent-graft placement. *N Engl J Med* 1999;340:1539–1545.

106. Fattori R, Caldarera I, Rapezzi C, et al. Primary endoleakage in endovascular treatment of the thoracic aorta: importance of intraoperative transesophageal echocardiography. *J Thorac Cardiovasc Surg* 2000;120:490–495.

107. Rehfeldt KH, Cook DJ. Transesophageal echocardiographic imaging of a new aortic cannula for differential perfusion during cardiopulmonary bypass. *Anesth Analg* 2001;92:338–340.

108. Kawahito S, Kitahata H, Tanaka K, et al. Pulmonary arterial pressure can be estimated by transesophageal pulsed Doppler echocardiography. *Anesth Analg* 2001;92:1364–1369.

109. Gorcsan J 3rd, Edwards TD, Ziady GM, et al. Transesophageal echocardiography to evaluate patients with severe pulmonary hypertension for lung transplantation. *Ann Thorac Surg* 1995;59:717–722.

110. Sloth E, Kruse M, Houlind KC, et al. The impact of ischemic heart disease on main pulmonary artery blood flow patterns: a comparison between magnetic resonance phase velocity mapping and transesophageal color Doppler. *Cardiovasc Res* 1997;36:377–385.

111. Murata I, Sonoda M, Morita T, et al. The clinical significance of reversed flow in the main pulmonary artery detected by Doppler color flow imaging. *Chest* 2000;118:336–341.

112. Russo A, De Luca M, Vigna C, et al. Central pulmonary artery lesions in chronic obstructive pulmonary disease: a transesophageal echocardiography study. *Circulation* 1999;100:1808–1815.

113. Amuchastegui LM, Marani LP, Caeiro A. Right ventricular outflow tract tumor mimicking a thrombus in the main pulmonary artery. *Echocardiography* 1997;14:611–614.

114. Parish JM, Rosenow EC 3rd, Swensen SJ, et al. Pulmonary artery sarcoma. Clinical features. *Chest* 1996;110:1480–1488.

115. Edasery B, Arunabh, Singh B, et al. Diagnosis of right pulmonary artery embolism by transesophageal echocardiography. A case report. *Angiology* 1995;46:341–344.

116. Abreu A, Branco L, Bento MJ, et al. Diagnostico de tromboembolismo paradoxal e pulmonar concomitante por ecocardiografia transesofagica: um caso clinico. [Diagnosis of paradoxal and concomitant pulmonary thromboembolism with transesophageal echocardiography: a clinical case.] *Rev Port Cardiol* 2000;19:823–828.

117. Caralps i Riera JM, Montiel Serrano J, Ruyra Baliarda X, et al. Trombosis arterial pulmonar en una paciente con valvulopatia mitro-tricuspidea. Valor anadido del ecocardiograma transesofagico peroperatorio. [Pulmonary artery thrombosis in a patient with mitral-tricuspid valve disease. Added value of perioperative transesophageal echocardiogram.] *Rev Esp Cardiol* 1996;49:621–622.

118. Krivec B, Voga G, Zuran I, et al. Diagnosis and treatment of shock due to massive pulmonary embolism: approach with transesophageal echocardiography and intrapulmonary thrombolysis. *Chest* 1997;112:1310–1316.

119. Steiner P, Lund GK, Debatin JF, et al. Acute pulmonary embolism: value of transthoracic and transesophageal echocardiography in comparison with helical CT. *AJR* 1996;167:931–936.

120. Kawahito S, Kitahata H, Tanaka K, et al. Intraoperative evaluation of pulmonary artery flow during the Fontan procedure by transesophageal Doppler echocardiography. *Anesth Analg* 2000;91:1375–1380.

121. Schroeder JK, Srinivasan V. Intraluminal pulmonary artery fibroma in a 7-year-old boy. *Pediatr Cardiol* 2000;21:480–482.

122. Pereira J, Oliver JM, Duran P, et al. Sarcoma primario de arteria pulmonar: diagnostico mediante ecocardiograma transtoracico y transesofagico. [Pulmonary artery primary sarcoma: diagnosis with transthoracic and transesophageal echocardiogram.] *Rev Esp Cardiol* 2000;53:142–144.

123. Almeida AA, Thomson HL, Burstow DJ, et al. Transesophageal echocardiography in an operation for pulmonary arteriovenous malformation. *Ann Thorac Surg* 1998;65:267–268.

124. Chang RY, Tsai CH, Chou YS, et al. Idiopathic dilatation of the pulmonary artery. A case presentation. *Angiology* 1996;47:87–92.

125. Barbier GH, Shettigar UR. Echocardiographic diagnosis of pulmonary artery aneurysm. *J Fla Med Assoc* 1995;82:470–472.

126. Thomas JM, Rajagopal S, George S, et al. Diagnosis of proximal interruption of right pulmonary artery by transoesophageal echocardiography. *Ind Heart J* 1998;50:83–84.

127. Brian CA, Payne RM, Link KM, et al. Pulmonary arteriovenous malformation. *Circulation* 1999;100:e29–e30.

128. Mechem CC, Alam GA. Delayed cardiac tamponade in a patient with penetrating chest trauma. *J Emerg Med* 1997;15:31–33.

129. Cohen GI, White M, Sochowski RA, et al. Reference values for normal adult transesophageal echocardiographic measurements. *J Am Soc Echocardiogr* 1995;8:221–230.

130. Kitzman DW, Scholz DG, Hagen PT, et al. Age-related changes in human hearts during the first 10 decades of life, part II (maturity): a quantitative anatomic study of 765 specimens from subjects 20 to 99 years old. *Mayo Clin Proc* 1988;63:137–146.

131. Hashimoto S, Kumada T, Osakada G, et al. Assessment of transesophageal Doppler echocardiography in dissecting aortic aneurysm. *J Am Coll Cardiol* 1989;14:1253–1262.

132. Saletta S, Lederman E, Fein S, et al. Transesophageal echocardiography for the initial evaluation of the widened mediastinum in trauma patients. *J Trauma* 1995;39:137–141.

133. Karalis DG, Victor MF, Davis GA, et al. The role of echocardiography in blunt chest trauma: a transthoracic and transesophageal echocardiographic study. *J Trauma* 1994;36:53–58.

134. Kearney PA, Smith DW, Johnson SB, et al. Use of transesophageal echocardiography in the evaluation of traumatic aortic injury. *J Trauma* 1993;34:696–701.

135. Ruvolo G, Voci P, Greco E, et al. Aortic intussusception: a rare presentation of type A aortic dissection evidenced by transesophageal echocardiography. *J Cardiovasc Surg* 1993;34385–34387.

136. Symbas PN, Kelly TF, Vlasis SE, et al. Intimo-intimal intussusception and other unusual manifestations of aortic dissection. *J Thorac Cardiovasc Surg* 1980;79:926–932.

137. Goldberg SP, Sanders C, Nanda NC, et al. Aortic dissection with intimal intussusception: diagnosis and management. *J Cardiovasc Surg* 2000;41:613–615.

138. Sparks MB, Burchard KW, Marrin CA, et al. Transesophageal Echocardiography–Preliminary results in patients with traumatic aortic rupture. *Arch Surg* 1991;711–713.

139. Shapiro MJ, Yanofsky SD, Trapp J, et al. Cardiovascular evaluation in blunt thoracic trauma using transesophageal echocardiography (TEE). *J Trauma* 1991;31:835–839.

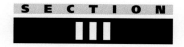

SECTION

III

PROBLEM-ORIENTED CASE DISCUSSIONS: APPLICATION OF THE FUNDAMENTAL CONCEPTS TO CLINICAL SCENARIOS

16

TRANSESOPHAGEAL ECHOCARDIOGRAPHY AND SURGICAL DEVICES: CANNULAS, CATHETERS, INTRAAORTIC BALLOON PUMPS, VENTRICULAR ASSIST DEVICES, AND OCCLUDERS

MARC E. STONE

GENERAL CONCEPTS

The echocardiographic appearance of intracardiac cannulas and catheters depends entirely on the orientation of the ultrasound beam with respect to the device. A perpendicular angle of beam intercept always results in the best image quality because a maximum amount of ultrasound energy is reflected back to the transducer. As depicted in Fig. 16.1, if the beam cuts perpendicularly through a cannula in short axis, that section is displayed as a circular "donut" (Fig. 16.1A). If the beam cuts perpendicularly through a cannula in long axis, a longitudinal "pipe" consisting of two parallel lines is displayed (Fig. 16.1B). An oblique angle of intercept results in deflection of the beam at an oblique angle, away from the transducer, which makes a poor image resolution. For this reason, if the beam intersects a cannula at an oblique angle, an oblique section with a variable appearance is displayed (Fig. 16.1C).

Cannulas are typically composed of high-density plastic. Some have metal tips or are reinforced circumferentially with metal wire. These materials are highly echogenic and tend to create artifacts, which can be mistaken for abnormalities of the cardiac chambers, valves, or great vessels. The echocardiographer must be aware of this possibility to avoid pitfalls in diagnosis and unnecessary interventions. Although cannulas and catheters themselves often cannot be well visualized, shadows and side-lobe artifacts are usually created. On occasion, it is only the presence of such artifacts, which suggests that something is present in that location (Fig. 16.2).

Shadowing results when the ultrasound beam fails to penetrate the dense plastic or metal components of a cannula, catheter, or other prosthetic device, casting a dark zone, or "shadow" behind the cannula or catheter. The shadow will always be cast toward the far field of the image sector, away from the source of the ultrasound beam (Fig. 16.1). Because there is no ultrasound beam in the zone of the shadow, neither two-dimensional (2D) imaging nor Doppler analyses can be performed there. Large shadows can obscure valve leaflets, ventricular walls, or entire cardiac chambers of interest, sometimes requiring the echocardiographer to use alternative imaging angles.

Side-lobe artifacts are the result of extraneous ultrasound beams generated diagonally from the edges of the ultrasound crystals but, when reflected back to the transducer, are interpreted as if they were part of the main central lobe. Such artifacts typically appear as a curved line across the display located at the same depth as the structure creating them. In a sense, side-lobe artifacts are a type of beam-width artifact.

CANNULAS FOR CARDIOPULMONARY BYPASS

Cardiopulmonary bypass (CPB) requires that venous blood returning to the heart be diverted to the bypass pump and then returned to the body, usually to an arterial vessel.

Routinely Used Venous Cannulas

In the case of full CPB, blood is typically collected at the level of the right atrium (RA) by a cannula introduced through the RA appendage. Venous cannulation is performed with either

M.E. Stone: Department of Anesthesiology, The Mount Sinai Medical Center, New York, New York.

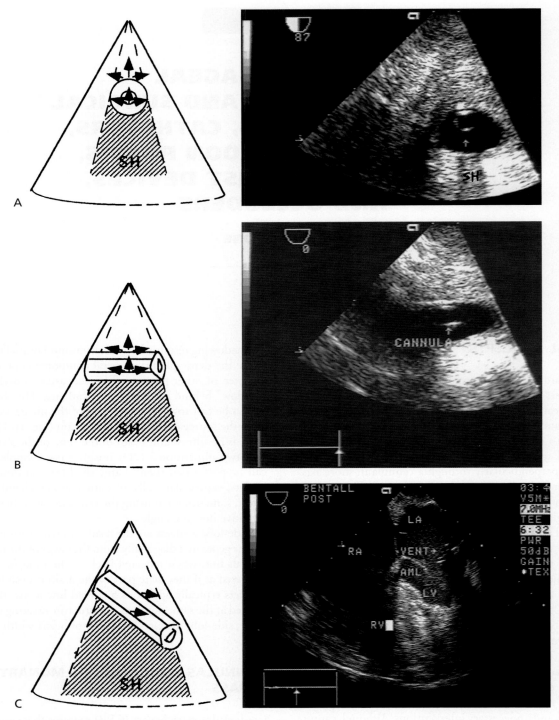

FIGURE 16.1. Transesophageal echocardiographic (TEE) appearance of cannulas based on their orientation within the ultrasound beam. The ultrasound beam is projected from the apex of the sector; *arrowheads* indicate potential directions of reflection of the ultrasound beam. *SH,* acoustic shadow. **A:** Short-axis view of a cannula perpendicular to the ultrasound beam. The *small arrow* in the photograph indicates the cannula within the lumen of the transverse aorta. As discussed in the text, it is rare to see an aortic cannula in this position. **B:** Long-axis view of the cannula perpendicular to the ultrasound beam. **C:** TEE appearance of a catheter at an oblique angle to the ultrasound beam. The photograph shows an oblique section of an intended left ventricular vent introduced through a left pulmonary vein. The catheter tip can be seen as two small parallel lines just to the right of the *small arrow*. The position of the acoustic shadow cast by the catheter suggests that the tip is in the left atrium. *RA,* right atrium; *RV,* right ventricle; *LA,* left atrium; *AML,* anterior mitral leaflet; *LV,* left ventricle.

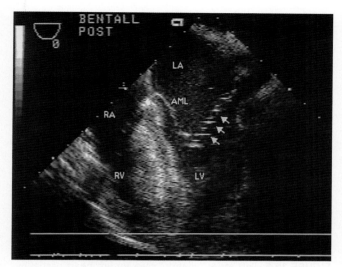

FIGURE 16.2. Imaging artifacts reveal the presence of a catheter. Oblique view of the same left ventricular vent as in Fig. 16.1C, now passed across the mitral valve into the left ventricle. Unlike Fig. 16.1C, the catheter itself cannot be clearly seen. Only the reverberations (*arrows*) and small beam-width artifacts reveal the location of the catheter. *RA,* right atrium; *RV,* right ventricle; *LA,* left atrium; *AML,* anterior mitral leaflet; *LV,* left ventricle.

a "double-staged" cannula [one port is positioned in the RA and a second, distal port positioned in the inferior vena cava (IVC)] or two separate cannulas [one in the superior vena cava (SVC) and one in the IVC].

One can usually see the venous cannula in the RA in the mid-esophageal four-chamber view at 0 degrees (Fig. 16.3) and in the mid-esophageal bicaval view at 90 degrees. Occasionally, one can see individual cannulas in the IVC and the SVC.

Routinely Used Arterial Cannulas

Once blood is diverted to the CPB machine, it is oxygenated, ventilated of carbon dioxide, and then returned, most often to the ascending aorta. Although the ascending aorta is reliably imaged in the ascending aorta long-axis view at 120 degrees, it is rare to see the routine arterial cannula in the ascending aorta because it is inserted at a point obscured from transesophageal echocardiography (TEE) by the trachea. The high acoustic impedance of the air-containing trachea obscures portions of the distal ascending aorta and proximal arch. Enough of the ascending aorta can usually be seen, however, to suggest the presence of significant calcification and atherosclerotic disease that will greatly increase the risk of stroke or distal embolization were routine "blind" aortic cannulation to be used (1–3). If significant disease is thought to be present, either from preoperative chest radiography, perioperative echocardiography, or direct surgical palpation, an aortic surface (or "epiaortic") ultrasonic examination can help to define potential cannulation sites away from calcifications and plaques (Fig. 16.4). Typically, a 7-MHz surface transducer is lubricated, placed into a sterile sheath (or laparoscopic camera drape), and passed to the surgeon in a sterile fashion for direct scanning of the aorta in the surgical field.

Occasionally, severe calcification, atherosclerotic plaques, or the surgical procedure itself (e.g., replacement of the ascending aorta or aortic arch) mandates that an alternative site (e.g., the right axillary artery) be used for the arterial cannulation. In this case, TEE 2D imaging with color flow mapping and continuous-wave Doppler analysis are useful to document that there is adequate flow in the aortic arch, to the head vessels, and distally during bypass. Useful TEE views include the upper esophageal aortic arch long-axis view

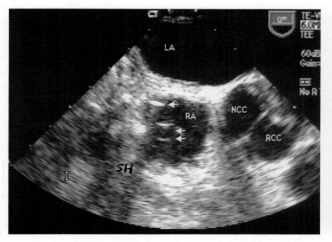
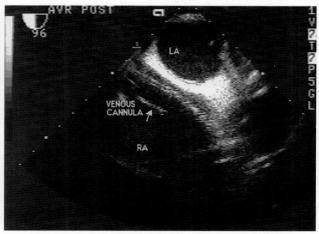

A   B

FIGURE 16.3. Venous cannula in the right atrium. **A:** Long-axis view of the tip of a venous cannula in the right atrium (*double arrows*). The *single arrow* indicates the pulmonary artery catheter. *RA,* right atrium; *LA,* left atrium; *SH,* acoustic shadow; *NCC,* noncoronary cusp of the aortic valve; *RCC,* right coronary cusp of the aortic valve. **B:** Long-axis view of a venous cannula in the right atrium. *RA,* right atrium; *LA,* left atrium.

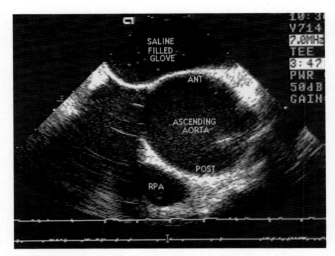

FIGURE 16.4. Epiaortic scanning. Seven-megahertz scan of the ascending aorta directly in the surgical field to assess the extent of atherosclerotic disease of the anterior ascending aortic wall prior to cannulation. Scanning through a saline-filled glove enhances visualization of the anterior aortic wall. The photograph depicts a site with no apparent plaque on the anterior wall. *ANT,* anterior aortic wall; *POST,* posterior aortic wall; *RPA,* right pulmonary artery.

at 0 degrees as well as the short- and long-axis views of the descending aorta. Additionally, TEE can detect a developing aortic dissection due to inadvertent cannulation of, or injury to, the intima of the axillary artery. Undetected, such an event might lead to malperfusion during bypass with catastrophic outcome. One could potentially detect a developing aortic dissection in the aortic arch long-axis view at 0 degrees, the ascending aorta short-axis view at 30 degrees, and the ascending aorta long-axis view at 120 degrees.

Cannulas for Partial Cardiopulmonary Bypass

Certain procedures (e.g., repair/replacement of the descending aorta) can be performed using partial left heart bypass, often with a centrifugal pump. In this case, only some of the patient's blood is diverted to the bypass pump; the native lungs continue to provide oxygenation and ventilation, and the heart continues to beat. Blood is diverted to the pump by a cannula placed in the left atrium (LA) through a left pulmonary vein and returned to an artery below the level of the repair (e.g., the femoral artery) to perfuse the viscera (retrograde perfusion) and lower extremities (antegrade perfusion). A mid-esophageal four-chamber view at 0 degrees and a mid-esophageal two-chamber view at 90 degrees are used to confirm the position of the venous cannula in the middle of the LA (Fig. 16.5) because poor venous return to the centrifugal pump may result if the cannula is passed into one of the right pulmonary veins. In addition, it is undesirable to have the cannula pass across the mitral valve into the left ventricle (LV), where it may cause mitral regurgitation and possibly induce arrhythmias.

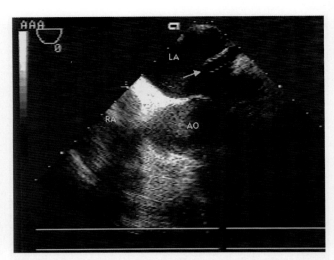

FIGURE 16.5. Left atrial "venous" cava for left heart partial bypass. Long-axis view of a left atrial venous cannula properly positioned in the left atrium for partial bypass. *LA,* left atrium; *AO,* ascending aorta.

In situations where femoral venous–femoral arterial bypass is used, TEE can be used to ensure the desired position of the venous cannula in the IVC near the entrance to the RA. One would start with a bicaval view at 90 degrees, and develop the image, following the IVC retrograde to visualize the cannula and to ensure that there is no dilatation of the hepatic veins with the commencement of pump flow.

CANNULAS FOR CARDIOPLEGIA

Antegrade cardioplegia solutions are often infused into the aortic root or selectively down the right and left main coronary arteries. When administration to the aortic root is planned, TEE is useful to exclude aortic insufficiency, which might otherwise result in LV distention and failure of the cardioplegia solution to go down the coronary arteries.

Retrograde cardioplegia is usually administered via a small balloon-tipped catheter inserted into the coronary sinus (CS). Once this cannula is introduced into the RA, and "blindly" advanced into the CS by the surgeon, a modified mid-esophageal four-chamber view is useful to confirm its position. On the rare occasion when blind introduction of the cannula fails, TEE can be used to guide the cannula toward the CS, as described by Aldea et al. (4). In their series, TEE imaging reportedly detected cannula misdirection into the IVC or right ventricle (RV), and assisted proper placement in patients with failed blind insertions.

The CS can usually be seen by attaining the mid-esophageal four-chamber view at 0 degrees and then developing the image by advancing the probe slightly. A small amount of retroflexion can often improve the image quality. The mouth of the CS can be seen opening into the RA just above the septal leaflet of the tricuspid valve (Fig. 16.6A),

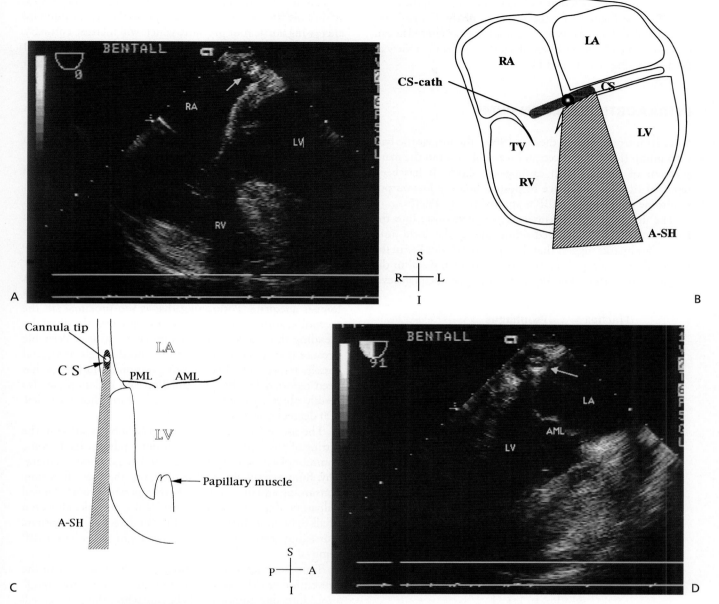

FIGURE 16.6. Retrograde cardioplegia cannula in the coronary sinus. **A:** The balloon of a cardioplegia cannula (*arrow*) can be seen in the mouth of the coronary sinus just above the septal leaflet of the tricuspid valve in this modified mid-esophageal four-chamber view. *RA,* right atrium; *RV,* right ventricle; *LV,* left ventricle. **B:** The path of the coronary sinus. *RA,* right atrium; *RV,* right ventricle; *LA,* left atrium; *LV,* left ventricle; *TV,* posterior tricuspid leaflet; *CS,* coronary sinus catheter; *A-SH,* acoustic shadow. **C and D:** Drawing and photograph of the cardioplegia catheter in the coronary sinus in the mid-esophageal two-chamber view. The catheter is seen as strongly echogenic (*arrow*), casting an acoustic shadow over the posterior left ventricular wall. *LA,* left atrium; *LV,* left ventricle; *AML,* anterior mitral leaflet; *PML,* posterior mitral leaflet; *CS,* coronary sinus; *A-SH,* acoustic shadow.

and the transverse path of the CS across the back of the heart can often be followed by the presence of the CS catheter (Fig. 16.6B). The retrograde cardioplegia catheter also can be seen in the CS in a mid-esophageal two-chamber view at 90 degrees (Fig. 16.6C and D).

INTRAAORTIC BALLOON PUMP

Since its introduction in the late 1960s, the intraaortic balloon pump (IABP) has been an invaluable asset in the management of patients with cardiogenic shock. It has been reported that the incidence of postcardiotomy low-output syndrome requiring an IABP is approximately 4% (5).

The device is typically inserted percutaneously into the femoral artery and advanced retrograde up the aorta until bodily landmarks suggest that the tip of the device lies in the proximal descending thoracic aorta, 2 to 3 cm distal to the left subclavian artery (Fig. 16.7). Assuming an adequate level

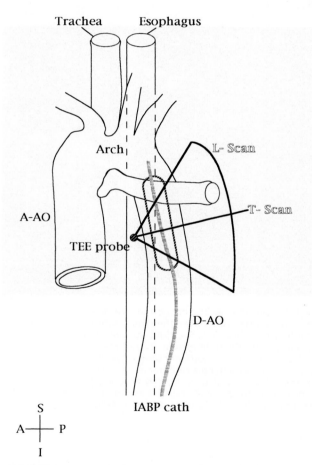

FIGURE 16.7. Drawing of the proper position of an intraaortic balloon pump in the descending thoracic aorta. Orientation of transverse and longitudinal transesophageal echocardiographic scanning planes are indicated (see Fig. 16.8). *A-AO,* ascending aorta; *D-AO,* descending aorta.

of saturated hemoglobin, balloon inflation at the beginning of diastole will increase oxygen supply to the myocardium by increasing aortic root pressure, which will increase coronary perfusion. Deflation just before the next systolic ejection will abruptly decrease aortic root pressure and facilitate forward ejection by decreasing impedance to opening of the aortic valve. This results in increased stroke volume with less myocardial work. In the absence of aortic insufficiency (which contraindicates IABP use and is easily detected by TEE) an optimally functioning IABP can increase cardiac output up to 20%.

Although the timing of balloon inflation and deflation are crucial for proper device function, the position of the balloon is also important to ensure optimal function of the device. Because the distal aortic arch and descending thoracic aorta are easily imaged in nearly all patients, TEE visualization of the device can ensure proper positioning. The descending aorta long-axis view at 90 degrees is the most useful for determining where the tip of the catheter lies (Fig. 16.8A and B), and may help to determine if the size of the balloon is adequate. Positioning that is too proximal (in the ascending aorta or aortic arch) or too distal (in the distal descending thoracic aorta or abdominal aorta) is undesirable because it may obstruct flow to the head vessels or visceral vessels, respectively. Inadvertent positioning in the LV has been reported (6). Balloon inflation and deflation are also readily observed from the descending aorta short-axis view at 0 degrees (Fig. 16.8C).

The use of TEE to assure correct balloon position in the setting of postcardiotomy low-output syndrome has become commonplace. Radiographic studies (e.g., chest radiography, fluoroscopy) also can be used, but they are often time consuming and inconvenient in the operating room. Digital palpation of the device in the aorta is also possible. However, of all these modalities, only TEE can detect and quantitate worsening aortic insufficiency that might necessitate IABP removal.

Transesophageal echocardiography also can assist in the prevention of IABP-related complications. As in any "blind" procedure, one cannot always be sure where the catheter will go, or what it has come in contact with when resistance is encountered. Prior to IABP placement, the aortic arch and descending thoracic aorta can be scanned in both short and long axis to detect atheromatous disease at risk of dislodgement and distal embolization during IABP placement. In the presence of a preexisting aortic dissection, TEE can assure that the device comes to rest in the "true lumen" (7). Shanewise et al. reported the TEE detection of an inadvertent passage of the IABP tip into the descending thoracic aortic intima, creating a dissection flap. The IABP was withdrawn from the aortic wall, and no extension of the dissection was observed during the remainder of the case (8). Coffin reported the accidental percutaneous placement of an IABP into the contralateral femoral artery. Continued

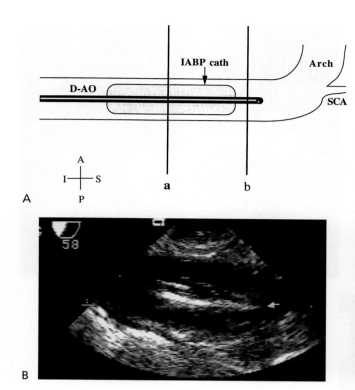

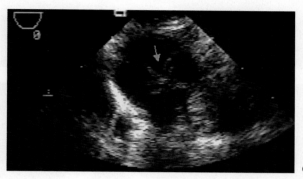

FIGURE 16.8. Intraaortic balloon pump (IABP) in the descending aorta. **A:** Drawing of an IABP in the descending aorta long-axis view. *D-AO*, descending aorta; *arch*, aortic arch; *SCA*, left subclavian artery; *a*, midportion of the device (see part **C**); *b*, IABP tip. **B:** Long-axis view of an IABP in the descending aorta. The *arrow* marks the tip of the device. **C:** Mid-portion of an IABP in the descending aorta short-axis view. The deflated balloon is seen as a stellate-shaped echodensity (*arrow*) in the aortic lumen, casting an acoustic shadow toward the far field of the scan sector.

unsatisfactory hemodynamics and failure to visualize the device in the proper position by TEE prompted further investigation as to its whereabouts (9).

PULMONARY ARTERY CATHETER

As TEE has become a standard of care in the operating room for most cardiac surgery requiring cardiopulmonary bypass, routine unquestioned use of the pulmonary artery catheter (PAC) is beginning to wane. However, the PAC remains a staple of cardiopulmonary monitoring in intensive care units and in those institutions where routine intraoperative TEE is not yet the standard.

The PAC is generally placed percutaneously via the internal jugular or subclavian veins, but in certain circumstances can be floated up from the femoral veins. Difficulties with placement are unusual, but there are times when passage across the tricuspid valve or pulmonic valve is problematic. Such situations might occur in patients with significant tricuspid or pulmonic regurgitation, severe tricuspid or pulmonic stenosis, or dilated cardiomyopathy with poor cardiac output, and possibly in those with anomalies of the RA, such as a Chiari network. In these circumstances, TEE 2D imaging can be helpful to accomplish safe flotation of the PAC. Several recent articles and letters to the editor of various journals describe the use of TEE to assist in the placement of a PAC under difficult situations (10,11).

One can see the entire intended course of the PAC from either the SVC or the IVC to either of the branch pulmonary arteries with the following sequence of TEE views:

- The bicaval view at 90 degrees allows visualization of the PAC as it enters the RA from either the SVC or the IVC and turns toward the tricuspid valve (Fig. 16.9A).
- An RV inflow–outflow view at 60 degrees allows visualization of the PAC as it enters the RV and floats out the pulmonic valve into the main PA (Fig. 16.9B). The standard mid-esophageal four-chamber view at 0 degrees also can be used to follow the PAC from the RA into the RV, but will not allow visualization of the passage into the main PA.
- The upper esophageal aortic short-axis view at 0 degrees allows visualization of the catheter tip as it floats into either the right or left branch PA (Fig. 16.9C). Use of this view may reduce the likelihood that the PAC is advanced so far as to increase the risk of PA rupture.

CENTRAL VENOUS CATHETERS

Ideally, the tip of a central venous catheter (CVC) should lie at the junction of the SVC and the RA. Correct positioning is rarely problematic in adults, but proper depth of insertion can be difficult to judge from surface landmarks alone in the pediatric population. In these small patients, a malpositioned CVC can increase the risk of serious

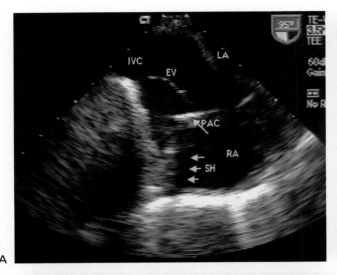

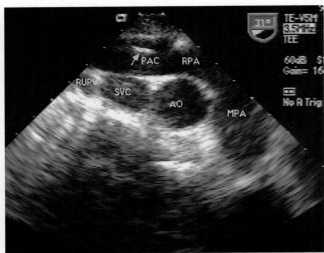

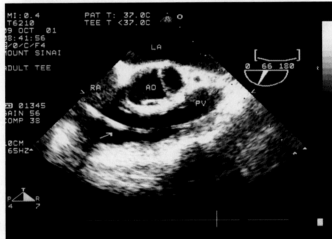

FIGURE 16.9. Passage of a pulmonary artery catheter. **A:** A pulmonary artery catheter (*PAC, single arrow*) is seen entering the right atrium in a modified bicaval view. An acoustic shadow (*three small arrows*) is cast from the catheter tip. *IVC,* inferior vena cava; *EV,* eustachian valve; *RA,* right atrium; *SH,* acoustic shadow; *LA,* left atrium. **B:** Appearance of a pulmonary artery catheter (*arrow*) in the right ventricular outflow tract. *RA,* right atrium; *LA,* left atrium; *AO,* aortic valve; *PV,* pulmonic valve. **C:** Final wedge position of the pulmonary artery catheter (*PAC, arrow*) in the right branch pulmonary artery. *RUPV,* right upper pulmonary vein; *SVC,* superior vena cava; *AO,* ascending aorta; *RPA,* right pulmonary artery; *MPA,* main pulmonary artery.

complications, most notably cardiac perforation resulting in tamponade (12). A recent study by Andropoulos et al. found that the use of perioperative TEE significantly improved the rate of proper CVC positioning in the pediatric population presenting for congenital heart surgery when compared with standard postoperative chest radiography (13). Useful views to assess CVC location include the bicaval view at 90 degrees and the mid-esophageal four-chamber view at 0 degrees.

VENTRICULAR ASSIST DEVICES

Ventricular assist devices (VADs) have become popular in the common management of intractable cardiogenic shock following cardiotomy, massive myocardial infarction, and in the patient with end-stage cardiomyopathy awaiting transplantation. "Destination therapy" is used in the occasional end-stage cardiomyopathy patient who undergoes intentionally permanent VAD placement in lieu of transplantation.

Several different devices are approved for clinical use, and an entirely new generation of devices is currently being developed; some are already in clinical trials.

Ventricular assist devices in common clinical use include the Abiomed BVS5000 (Abiomed, Danvers, MA, U.S.A.), the Novacor LVAS (World Heart, Ottawa, Canada), and the Thoratec VAD system and the HeartMate LVAS (Thoratec Corporation, Pleasanton, CA, U.S.A.). Centrifugal pumps (various manufacturers) are commonly used to provide temporary ventricular assistance and extracorporeal membrane oxygenation in the pediatric population.

In general, VADs are simply pumps that divert blood from the heart and return it downstream from the failing ventricle. A complete description of all such devices is beyond the scope of this chapter; however, currently approved devices all use the same cannulation strategies within the heart (Fig. 16.10).

Regardless of the specific device attached to these cannulas, TEE plays a critical role:

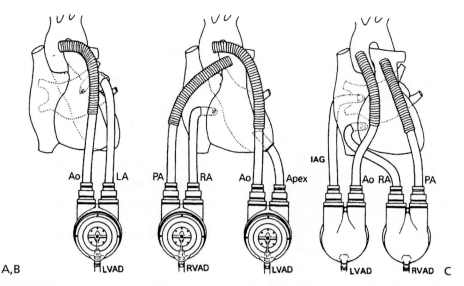

FIGURE 16.10. The various approaches used to cannulate the heart and great vessels for support by a ventricular assist device (VAD). The specific device depicted here is the Thoratec VAD, but the same cannulation strategies are used by all currently available VADs. **A:** Left ventricular assist device (*LVAD*). Blood is diverted to the LVAD from the left atrium and returned to the ascending aorta. **B:** Support of both the right (*RVAD*) and the left (*LVAD*) ventricle. This is also referred to as biventricular support (BiVAD). For RVAD support, blood is diverted from the right atrium and returned to the main pulmonary artery. For LVAD support, blood is diverted from the left ventricular apex and returned to the ascending aorta. **C:** BiVAD support, with a slightly different cannulation strategy. The LVAD diverts blood from the left atrium and returns it to the ascending aorta (as in **A**); however, the left atrium is cannulated via the interatrial groove behind the heart. The RVAD diverts blood from the right atrium and returns it to the main pulmonary artery as in the center panel. Notice, however, that in this configuration, the VADs are turned over and are on the opposite sides of the chest from those in the center panel. It is not depicted here, but an RVAD also use an inflow cannula from the right ventricular cavity. *AO*, aortic outflow cannula; *LA*, left atrial inflow cannula; *PA*, pulmonary artery outflow cannula; *RA*, right atrial inflow cannula; *APEX*, left ventricular apical inflow cannula; *IAG*, left atrial inflow cannula placed via the interatrial groove. (Reproduced with permission of the Thoratec Corporation, Pleasanton, CA, U.S.A.).

- In defining the need for a VAD through assessment of ventricular (dys)function
- In determining whether the right, left, or both ventricles require support [right ventricular assist devices (RVAD), left ventricular assist devices (LVAD), or bi-VAD, respectively]
- During VAD placement
- In the postoperative management of the patient supported by a VAD.

There are many reviews of the role of TEE in the perioperative period and in overall treatment of the VAD patient published in the literature (e.g., 14). A recent and particularly comprehensive review comes from the group at the Cleveland Clinic (15). The concepts described in this review specifically focus on the HeartMate LVAD, but are essentially applicable to all VADs, implantable or extracorporeal.

Before Ventricular Assist Device Placement

Transesophageal 2D imaging, Doppler analyses, and color-flow mapping are invaluable prior to VAD placement. Al-

though performing a complete TEE examination is always recommended, the echocardiographer must be aware of the intended cannulation strategy (Fig. 16.10), which will define the most important potential issues in a given patient and help direct the TEE examination. Specific considerations include:

1. Aortic atherosclerotic disease, calcifications, and mobile plaques. Thromboembolic events are a major source of morbidity and mortality in the VAD patient. Although the majority of these events occur as a result of inadequate anticoagulation while on VAD support, cannulation of a significantly diseased ascending aorta can increase the likelihood of a poor outcome. As discussed above, the ascending aorta long-axis view at 120 degrees and aortic surface scanning in the surgical field (epiaortic scanning) are useful views in which to detect such disease.
2. Valvular pathology must be identified and addressed prior to initiation of VAD support. The outflow from the VAD will be returned to either the ascending aorta or the main PA. Significant aortic or pulmonic valve regurgitation will prevent ventricular decompression by the device, and may

get worse over time. As the degree of insufficiency increases, VAD flows will increase, but at the expense of systemic perfusion, which will decrease. If the ventricular apex has been cannulated, stenotic mitral or tricuspid valves will impede VAD filling. In many cases where left apical cannulation is to be used, a stenotic mitral valve is simply excised.

3. Intracardiac shunts are crucial to identify prior to initiation of VAD support because worsened intracardiac shunting while on VAD support will greatly complicate patient management. While looking at Fig. 16.10, one may recall that the supported side of the heart will be nearly completely drained into a very low resistance pump. Patent foramen ovale (PFO) or septal defects [atrial (ASDs) or ventricular septal defects] will predispose to worsened intracardiac shunting while on VAD support. With an LVAD, right-to-left shunting can result in cyanosis. With an RVAD, left-to-right shunting will lead to excessive pulmonary blood flow at the expense of the systemic flow, potentially resulting in pulmonary edema and hypotension.

4. Is univentricular or biventricular assistance indicated? Often it is the LV that is failing; however, RV function must be carefully evaluated prior to instituting isolated LV support because there is an increased incidence of RV failure while on an isolated LVAD. Right ventricle failure is especially likely in patients with pulmonary hypertension, and in those requiring massive transfu-

sions. Even if it is the LV that is failing, patients with decreased RV function may benefit from biventricular support from the outset. Useful views to evaluate RV function include the mid-esophageal four chamber view at 0 degrees, the RV inflow–outflow view at 60 degrees, and transgastric views of the RV at 0 and 90 degrees. The TEE evaluation of RV function is discussed in detail elsewhere.

During Ventricular Assist Device Placement

Intraoperatively, TEE is useful to ensure:

1. Optimal cannula positioning. The LV apical cannula should be oriented away from the ventricular septum, pointing toward the mitral valve. This will ensure optimal cannula inflow. The tip of the cannula should be in the center of the ventricular chamber, away from the opposite ventricular free wall and papillary muscle, to decrease the chance of cannula obstruction once the ventricle is decompressed. Useful views for evaluating apical cannula position include the mid-esophageal four-chamber view at 0 degrees, the mid-esophageal two-chamber view at 90 degrees (Fig. 16.11A), and transgastric views of the LV at 0 degrees (Fig. 16.11B) and 90 degrees, including the deep transgastric view. If an interatrial approach from behind the heart is used for a LA cannulation, the bicaval

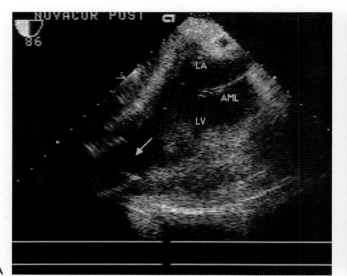
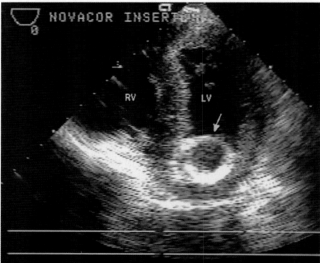

A   B

FIGURE 16.11. Left ventricular assist device (LVAD) apical inflow cannula position. **A:** Long-axis view of a left ventricular apical cannula (*arrow*) seen in the mid-esophageal two-chamber view. The *arrow* also shows the direction of blood flow into the cannula during VAD support. The position of this apical cannula is optimal, and the left ventricle is decompressed. *LA,* left atrium; *AML,* anterior mitral leaflet; *LV,* left ventricle. **B:** Short-axis view of a left ventricular apical cannula (*arrow*) in a transgastric view. Note the bulging of the interventricular septum to the left. This suggests either successful left ventricular decompression by the LVAD, right ventricular (*RV*) volume overload due to RV failure while on LVAD support, or possibly a combination of the two. *LV,* left ventricle.

view at 90 degrees and the mid-esophageal four-chamber view at 0 degrees are useful to assure that the cannula has not inadvertently been passed through the RA and across the interatrial septum into the LA. Such an occurrence would result in torrential intracardiac shunting if the patient were successfully weaned from the VAD and decannulated.

2. Complete de-airing of the device prior to engaging full VAD pumping.
3. Adequacy of ventricular decompression once support is engaged. Problems originating at the inflow and outflow cannulas often can be detected with TEE Doppler analyses and color flow mapping of VAD inflow and outflow.

The unusual angles involved in such Doppler analyses usually require a multiplane TEE probe, and imagination on the part of the echocardiographer in order to obtain a parallel angle for the ultrasound beam. Additionally, residual shunts or valvular pathology that may complicate postoperative management can be detected and addressed prior to leaving the operating room.

After Ventricular Assist Device Placement

Transesophageal echocardiography continues to play an important role in the postoperative period following VAD insertion. Most often, echocardiographic studies are requested

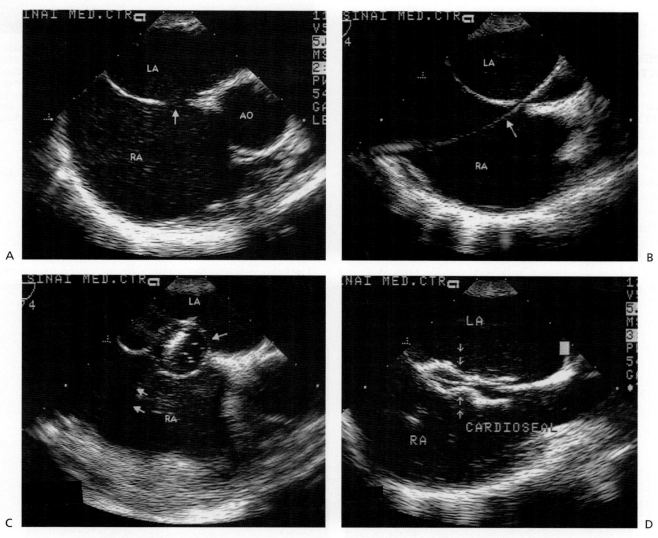

FIGURE 16.12. CardioSEAL closure of an atrial septal defect. **A:** A secundum-type atrial septal defect (*ASD*) is demonstrated (*arrow*). **B:** A balloon-tipped catheter (*arrow*) is passed over a guidewire through the ASD from the right atrium to the left atrium. **C:** Balloon (*single arrow*) used to size the ASD. The *double arrow* indicates an acoustic shadow cast by the unseen catheter. **D:** Final position of the CardioSEAL device. Note that the arms of the device straddle both sides of the interatrial septum. Ultimate occlusion of the ASD will occur over a period of days as the device is endothelialized. *LA,* left atrium; *RA,* right atrium; *AO,* aorta. (Images courtesy of S. Kamenir and R. Sommer, Division of Pediatric Cardiology, Mount Sinai School of Medicine, New York.)

to assist in the diagnosis of problems related to continued poor hemodynamics, or suspected poor device function. A comprehensive TEE examination at the bedside can rule out:

- Hypovolemia
- RV failure while on LVAD support
- Cannula problems
- Pericardial tamponade
- Conduit valve problems (e.g., regurgitation)
- Intracardiac thrombi

Additionally, TEE is routinely used in the assessment of ventricular recovery and potential device explantation (usually from the Abiomed; occasionally from the Thoratec; rarely from the HeartMate or the Novacor) (16).

DEVICES DEPLOYED TO CLOSE INTRACARDIAC DEFECTS

It is often possible to seal ASDs and other cardiac shunts (e.g., PFO, patent ductus arteriosus, atrial fenestration of a Fontan conduit, etc.) with devices deployed during cardiac catheterization. TEE 2D imaging, Doppler flow analyses, and color-flow mapping are routinely used during these procedures to assess the feasibility of defect closure by a percutaneously deployed device, to select the type and size of device, to guide and orient device placement, as well as to assess the success of device deployment in closing the shunt (17). Momenah et al. reported several echocardiographic predictors of residual leakage following transcatheter closure of interatrial defects using the CardioSEAL device (18). A typical sequence of events during CardioSEAL closure of a

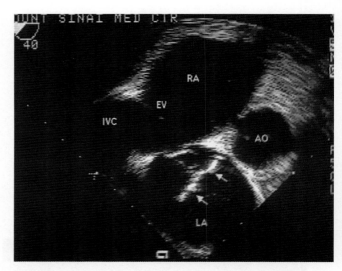

FIGURE 16.13. CardioSEAL closure of a patent foramen ovale. Following passage of a guidewire and catheter across the PFO, a CardioSEAL device is deployed. The *arrows* indicate the direction in which the device will be pulled to cover the PFO. *RA,* right atrium; *EV,* eustachian valve; *IVC,* inferior vena cava; *AO,* ascending aorta; *LA,* left atrium. (Images courtesy of S. Kamenir and R. Sommer, Division of Pediatric Cardiology, Mount Sinai School of Medicine, New York.)

secundum-type ASD is shown in Fig. 16.12 and of a PFO in Fig. 16.13.

UNEXPECTED DEVICES

The echocardiographer occasionally encounters unexpected surgical devices. The location, characteristic appearance

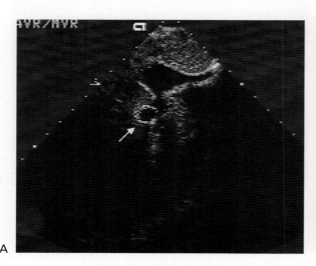

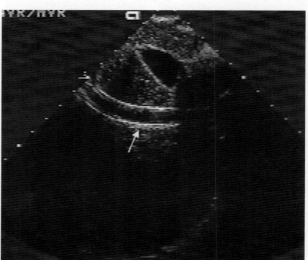

FIGURE 16.14. Short-axis **(A)** and long-axis **(B)** views of a transjugular intrahepatic portosystemic shunt unexpectedly found in the liver of a patient who presented for aortic and mitral valve replacement.

of the prosthetic material, and presence or absence of flow through the device can assist in device identification. Figure 16.14 depicts an unexpected finding of a transjugular intrahepatic portosystemic shunt in a patient who presented for aortic and mitral valve replacement. During the preanesthesia assessment, the patient had denied prior surgery or previous medical illnesses.

KEY POINTS

■ The conduct of cardiopulmonary bypass requires various cannulas, catheters, vents, and pressure lines. Due to the proximity of the esophagus to the mediastinum, transesophageal echocardiography (TEE) can provide high-quality images of the cardiac structures and intracardiac devices, and can assist in the placement and confirmation of the position of such devices. TEE 2D imaging, color-flow mapping, and Doppler analyses can:

Confirm the position of cannulas, catheters, vents, pressure lines, and conduits.

Detect and potentially diagnose problems with cannula and conduit flows.

Assure proper positioning of cannulas used for retrograde cardioplegia.

Assure adequate blood flow in the aortic arch during bypass when alternative arterial cannulation sites (e.g., the axillary artery) are used.

Identify significant aortic atherosclerotic disease, calcifications, and mobile plaques.

■ TEE is invaluable prior to, during, and following the placement of VADs to:

Assist in determining the need for VAD support through assessment of ventricular function.

Identify intracardiac shunts and valvular pathology that will complicate patient management once VAD support is engaged.

Assist with postoperative management and potential weaning from VAD support.

■ Additionally, TEE is routinely used in the operative setting to confirm the proper position of an intra-aortic balloon pump.

■ Furthermore, TEE can be used to:

Assist the flotation of a PAC when difficulties are encountered.

Assist with determination of central line positioning in the pediatric population.

Allow proper positioning of percutaneously introduced devices deployed to seal intra-cardiac shunts.

REFERENCES

1. Gardner TJ, Horneffer PJ, Manolio TA, et al. Stroke following coronary artery bypass grafting: a ten-year study. *Ann Thorac Surg* 1985;40:574–581.
2. **Blauth CI, Cosgrove DM, Webb BW, et al. Atheroembolism from the ascending aorta. An emerging problem in cardiac surgery.** *J Thorac Cardiovasc Surg* **1992;103:1104–1112.**
3. **Marschall K, Kanchuger M, Kessler K, et al. Superiority of transesophageal echocardiography in detecting aortic arch atheromatous disease: identification of patients at increased risk of stroke during cardiac surgery.** *J Cardiothorac Vasc Anesth* **1994;8:5–13.**
4. **Aldea GS, Connelly G, Fonger JD, et al. Directed atraumatic coronary sinus cannulation for retrograde cardioplegia administration.** *Ann Thorac Surg* **1992;54:789–790.**
5. **Smedira NG, Blackstone EH. Postcardiotomy mechanical support: risk factors and outcomes.** *Ann Thorac Surg* **2001;71(Suppl):60–66.**
6. **Kantrowitz A, Wasfie T, Freed PS, et al. Intraaortic balloon pumping 1967 through 1982: analysis of complications in 733 patients.** *Am J Cardiol* **1986;57:976–983.**
7. Nakatani S, Beppu S, Tanaka N, et al. Application of abdominal and transesophageal echocardiography as a guide for insertion of intraaortic balloon pump in aortic dissection. *Am J Cardiol* 1989;64:1082–1083.
8. **Shanewise JS, Sadel S. Intraoperative transesophageal echocardiography to assist the insertion and positioning of the intraaortic balloon pump.** *Anesth Analg* **1994;79:577–580.**
9. Coffin SA. The misplaced intraaortic balloon pump. *Anesth Analg* 1994;78:1182–1183.
10. **Safwat AM. Difficult floatation of a pulmonary artery catheter: echocardiographic diagnosis.** *J Clin Anesth* **2001; 13(May):239–240.**
11. **Zimmermann P, Steinhübel B, Greim CA. Facilitation of pulmonary artery catheter placement by transesophageal echocardiography after tricuspid valve surgery.** *Anesth Analg* **2001;93:242–243.**
12. Bar-Joseph G, Galvis AG. Perforation of the heart by central venous catheters in infants: guidelines to diagnosis and management. *J Pediatr Surg* 1983;18:284–287.
13. Andropoulos DB, Stayer SA, Bezold LI, et al. A controlled study of transesophageal echocardiography to guide central venous catheter placement in congenital heart surgery patients. *Anesth Analg* 1999;89:65–70.
14. **Hauptman PJ, Body S, Fox J, et al. Implantation of a pulsatile external left ventricular assist device: role of intraoperative transesophageal echocardiography.** *J Cardiothorac Anesth* **1994;8(3):340–341.**
15. **Scalia GM, McCarthy PM, Savage RM, et al. Clinical utility of echocardiography in the management of implantable ventricular assist devices.** *J Am Soc Echo* **2000;13(8):754–763.**
16. Barzilai B, Davila-Roman VG, Eaton MH, et al. Transesophageal echocardiography predicts successful withdrawal of ventricular assist devices. *J Thorac Cardiovasc Surg* 1992;104(5):1410–1416.
17. **Elzenga NJ. The role of echocardiography in transcatheter closure of atrial septal defects.** *Cardiol Young* **2000;10(5):474–483.**
18. Momenah TS, McElhinney DB, Brook MM, et al. Transesophageal echocardiography predictors for successful transcatheter closure of defects within the oval fossa using the CardioSEAL septal occlusion device. *Cardiol Young* 2000;10(5):510–518.

RHEUMATIC MITRAL STENOSIS

BONNIE MILAS
JOSEPH S. SAVINO
ALBERT T. CHEUNG

Rheumatic fever is the predominant cause of acquired calcific mitral stenosis in adults and accounts for 77% of cases of mitral stenosis in the United States and Western Europe (1). Although the prevalence of rheumatic fever has decreased in the United States, it remains an important health-care problem in underdeveloped areas and nonindustrialized countries (Fig. 17.1).

Rheumatic mitral disease is characterized by progressive deformation, thickening, calcification, and fusion of heart valves that can produce both valvular stenosis and regurgitation (2). Mitral stenosis is usually the predominant feature, and the clinical symptoms parallel the decrease in size of the mitral valve orifice (1).

Mitral stenosis has a bimodal age distribution (3). Disease in the younger age group (20–39 years) is characterized by a severe initial episode or recurrent episodes of rheumatic endocarditis that produce accelerated valve injury, with rapid scarring and contracture of leaflets. Mitral stenosis in the older age group (50–60 years) results from a milder or asymptomatic initial episode of rheumatic carditis, followed by a gradual progression of leaflet injury. After the initial injury, leaflet calcification, thickening, and deformation are accelerated by the chronic effects of abnormal transvalvular blood flow (3). The latency between acute rheumatic fever and clinical symptoms of mitral stenosis ranges from 11 to 21 years (Fig. 17.2). Valve obstruction progresses at a variable rate. Debilitating disease occurs at an average of 9 years (range 5–13 years) after the onset of symptoms. A decrease in valve area greater than 0.1 cm^2/year, an increased mean and peak transvalvular pressure gradient, severe valve immobility, calcification, and thickening of leaflets and subvalvular

apparatus are echocardiographic findings that suggest a more progressive course of disease (2). The estimated 5-year mortality rate in patients with severe mitral stenosis who do not undergo operation is approximately 60% (1). Heart failure is the most common cause of death, but pulmonary hypertension, pulmonary edema, dysrhythmia, and stroke are common causes of morbidity and mortality.

SCIENTIFIC PRINCIPLES

The normal mitral valve permits laminar diastolic blood flow from the left atrium (LA) to the ventricle, prevents regurgitant systolic flow via a valve and sphincter action, and contributes to ventricular contraction.

Anatomy

The normal mitral valve consists of a fibrous annulus, two leaflets, and subvalvular attachments to the ventricular wall. The mitral annulus is a funnel-shaped atrioventricular membrane incorporated in the free wall of the heart; it directs diastolic blood flow inferiorly, anteriorly, and toward the left side of the heart. The functional mitral valve is composed of a large triangular anterior mitral leaflet and a broad, crescent-shaped posterior leaflet. The anterior mitral leaflet is continuous at its attachment with the noncoronary and left coronary cusps of the aortic valve. When the mitral valve opens in diastole, the anterior leaflet forms the separation between the left ventricular inflow and outflow tracts. The posterior leaflet is composed of the posteromedial (P3), middle (P2), and anterolateral (P1) scallops. Although the surface areas of the anterior and posterior mitral leaflets are nearly equal, the broader attachment of the posterior leaflet to the mitral annulus renders it shorter and less mobile.

The subvalvular apparatus of the mitral valve is composed of the papillary muscles and chordae tendineae. The chordae are divided into first-, second-, and third-order chordae based on the location of their attachment to the valve leaflets. First-order chordae attach to the edges of the valve leaflets, giving

B. Milas: Department of Anesthesiology, University of Pennsylvania, Hospital of the University of Pennsylvania, Philadelphia, Pennsylvania.

J. S. Savino: Department of Anesthesia, University of Pennsylvania School of Medicine; and Department of Anesthesia, Hospital of the University of Pennsylvania, Philadelphia, Pennsylvania.

A. T. Cheung: Department of Anesthesiology, University of Pennsylvania; and Division of Cardiothoracic Anesthesia and Critical Care, Hospital of the University of Pennsylvania, Philadelphia, Pennsylvania.

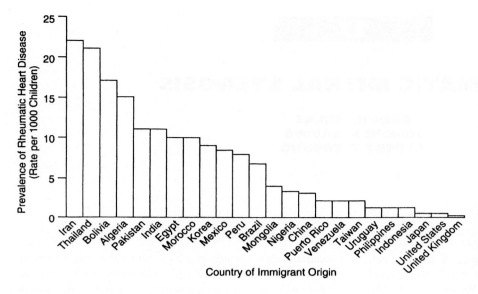

FIGURE 17.1. The prevalence of rheumatic heart disease in children plotted according to their country of origin. (From Carroll JD, Feldman T. Percutaneous mitral balloon valvotomy and the new demographics of mitral stenosis. *JAMA* 1993;270:1731, with permission.)

the mitral valve its typical serrated appearance in the transgastric basal short-axis view. Second-order chordae attach to the ventricular surface of the leaflets, and third-order chordae attach near the mitral annulus. Both the anterolateral and posteromedial papillary muscles have chordal attachments to both leaflets.

Physiology

The normal mitral valve opens to form an orifice with a cross-sectional area that ranges from 4 to 6 cm². A mitral valve area (MVA) of 1.6 to 2 cm² is considered mild mi-

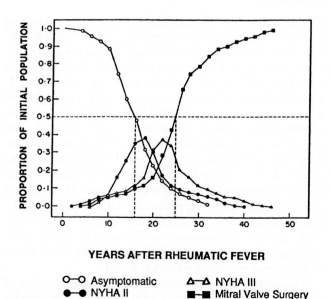

FIGURE 17.2. Progression of symptoms of rheumatic mitral stenosis. [From Horstkotte D, Niehues R, Strauer BE. Pathomorphological aspects, aetiology and natural history of acquired mitral valve stenosis. *Eur Heart J* 1991;12(suppl B)55, with permission.]

tral stenosis, 1.0 to 1.5 cm² is moderate mitral stenosis, and less than 1 cm² is severe mitral stenosis. The normal mitral valve has a negligible diastolic transvalvular pressure gradient. The diastolic transvalvular pressure gradient increases with progressive decrease in the MVA. Severe mitral stenosis can produce transvalvular gradients in diastole of greater than 20 mm Hg. For a given orifice size, however, the transvalvular pressure gradient is dependent on the transvalvular flow rate. When cardiac output is low, the diastolic transvalvular pressure gradient decreases and may underestimate the severity of stenosis.

The mitral valve is normally competent during ventricular systole and protects the pulmonary circulation against the systemic pressures generated by the left ventricle. Mitral regurgitation is prevented by the coaptation of the LA surfaces of the mitral valve leaflets along its commissure (Fig. 17.3). Because the leaflets oppose each other for several millimeters along their surfaces, valve competence is maintained despite small increases in annular size.

Blood flow across the mitral valve during diastole is biphasic (Fig. 17.4). Early diastolic filling (E phase) begins when the ventricular pressure decreases to less than the LA pressure, causing the mitral valve to open. Although early diastolic filling is primarily governed by the pressure gradient between the LA and ventricle, diastolic "suction" produced by ventricular relaxation can augment early diastolic filling when transvalvular pressures are low. Late diastolic filling (A phase) occurs with the onset of atrial contraction. Left atrial enlargement or loss of sinus rhythm decreases the atrial contribution to left ventricular filling (Fig. 17.5).

Blood flow velocities across the mitral valve are generally low because the normal transvalvular pressure gradient is small and the mitral valve orifice is large. The average value for the peak velocity of blood flow through the normal mitral valve is 0.9 m/s in the adult and can be measured by pulsed-wave Doppler echocardiography. Distortion of the mitral

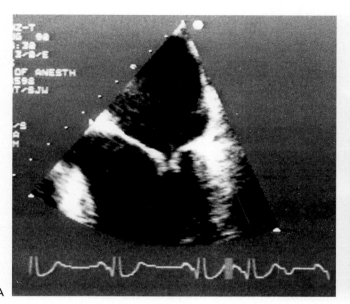
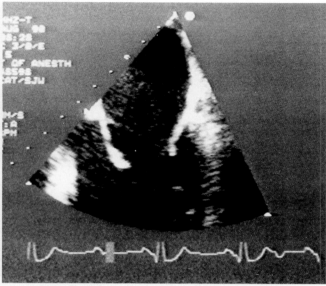

A   B

FIGURE 17.3. Two-dimensional transesophageal echocardiography of a normal mitral valve (**A,** systole; **B,** diastole) demonstrating that the site of coaptation is the left atrial surface (and not the edges) of the leaflets.

valve orifice and decreases in the effective mitral valve orifice size produce turbulent transvalvular flow that is characterized by high-velocity, multidirectional blood flow patterns.

The normal anatomy and function of the mitral valve permits a more effective left ventricular contraction. The nonrigid mitral annulus has a sphincter action with maximum circumferential fiber shortening at the base of the heart. In addition, chordae tendineae pull the mitral annulus and the base of the heart toward the ventricular apex and shorten the longitudinal axis of the left ventricle during systole. Disturbances in the normal mitral contribution to ventricular contraction contribute to the worsening of ventricular function after replacement of the mitral valve with a rigid prosthesis. Sparing the chordae and papillary muscles during mitral valve repair and replacement is associated with improved postoperative ventricular function (4).

Pathophysiology

Rheumatic carditis can be a sequela of upper respiratory infections caused by group A streptococci. The precise mechanism in the pathogenesis of rheumatic carditis is not fully understood, but autoimmune-mediated tissue injury is believed to be an important factor. Rheumatic carditis can produce exudative and proliferative inflammatory lesions in any part of the heart. A verrucous acute valvulitis, most commonly involving the mitral and aortic valves, causes valve edema and deformity. Rheumatic involvement of all four heart valves is unusual. Acute rheumatic myocarditis also can cause ventricular dysfunction and congestive heart failure.

Fibrous thickening of the valve leaflets, fusion of the posteromedial and anterolateral commissurae, shortening of chordae, and calcification of the valve apparatus are the

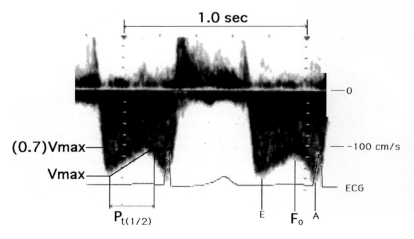

FIGURE 17.4. Intraoperative transesophageal echocardiography with continuous-wave Doppler across a mitral valve in a patient in sinus rhythm. Early diastolic (E phase) transmitral flow begins with a rapid acceleration of blood into the ventricle followed by a more gradual decay in transmitral velocity. The slope of the diastolic deceleration in the transmitral blood velocity is a function of valve orifice area and transvalvular pressure gradient. The deceleration of transmitral blood velocity during diastole was interrupted (F_0) by atrial contraction (A phase).

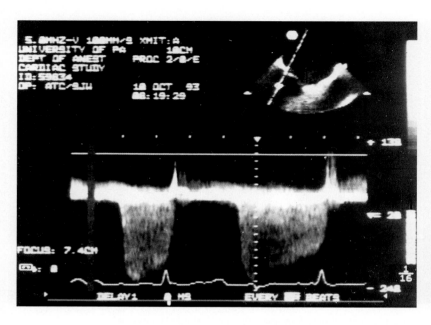

FIGURE 17.5. Intraoperative transesophageal echocardiography with continuous-wave Doppler across the mitral valve of a patient with mitral stenosis and atrial fibrillation. The absence of an atrial contraction and an irregular R-R interval produced beat-to-beat differences in the diastolic transmitral flow pattern and loss of the A wave.

morphologic features of rheumatic mitral stenosis. The extent of calcification varies and is inversely related to the size of the stenotic orifice. Calcium deposits begin in the commissure and extend to the leaflet bodies, subvalvular apparatus, and valve annulus. Inflammation and calcium deposits erupt through the leaflet endothelium, causing surface ulceration and thrombosis. Systemic embolization associated with rheumatic mitral stenosis has traditionally been attributed to LA thrombi, but also may be caused by valve surface thrombi and fragmentation.

The physiologic features of mitral stenosis are the direct result of impaired diastolic emptying of blood from the LA through a narrowed mitral valve orifice or subvalvular apparatus. In conditions that demand an increase in cardiac output, the limitation of diastolic blood flow through the stenotic mitral valve causes an acute increase in LA, pulmonary venous, and pulmonary artery pressures. Interstitial and alveolar pulmonary edema occurs when pulmonary venous hydrostatic pressure exceeds the pulmonary capillary oncotic pressure. Chronically increased pulmonary venous pressure leads to right ventricular hypertrophy and dilatation. Right ventricular pressure overload in combination with right ventricular dilatation may render the tricuspid valve incompetent (Fig. 17.6). Left atrial dilatation caused

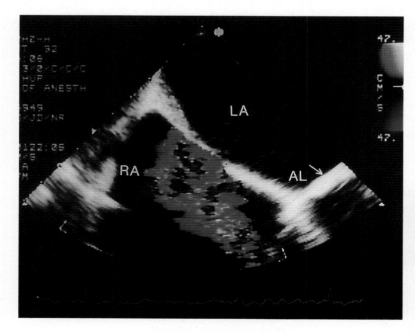

FIGURE 17.6. Intraoperative two-dimensional transesophageal echocardiography image in a patient with mitral stenosis and tricuspid regurgitation. The systolic jet within the right atrium (*RA*) produced an aliasing and high-variance color Doppler signal, suggesting severe tricuspid regurgitation. Other pertinent findings included a dilated left atrium (*LA*), thickened anterior mitral valve leaflet (*AL*), and rightward displacement of the interatrial septum (*IAS*). The tricuspid regurgitation resolved after mitral valve replacement.

by chronic increases in LA pressure produces a high-volume, low-flow chamber with a propensity for thrombosis formation. Left atrial mural thrombi are more common than free-ball thrombi, but the latter are more likely to cause acute mitral valve obstruction and sudden death. Dilatation of the LA decreases the effect of atrial systole to augment left ventricular filling and increases the risk of atrial flutter or fibrillation.

Left ventricular dysfunction is often associated with rheumatic mitral stenosis. Left ventricular regional wall motion abnormalities, a decreased ejection fraction, decreased left ventricular stroke work, and increased left ventricular end-diastolic pressure can be detected in as many as 50% of patients with significant mitral stenosis (5,6). Disease affecting the normal function of the mitral valve annulus, subvalvular apparatus, and papillary muscles impairs the ability of the mitral valve to augment ventricular contraction and relaxation. A potential cause of left ventricular dysfunction is rheumatic carditis, which may impair the systolic function of the ventricle, independent of valve disease. Chronic decreases in left ventricular preload produced by mitral stenosis may cause ventricular remodeling and an "atrophic" ventricle. Regional wall motion abnormalities of the posterobasal myocardium without coronary artery disease occur with severe rheumatic mitral stenosis and suggest a mechanical "tethering" of the myocardium caused by a scarred mitral valve and annulus.

Patients with mitral stenosis who are scheduled for mitral valve surgery have various clinical symptoms. The clinical evaluation is a factor in determining the need for operation, perioperative mortality, and postoperative function. The most common symptoms associated with mitral stenosis are limitations in physical activity, dyspnea, cough, orthopnea, and paroxysmal nocturnal dyspnea. Symptoms are exacerbated with conditions that demand an increase in cardiac output such as exercise, pregnancy, anemia, fever, or thyrotoxicosis. A subjective method of categorizing patients based on the severity of their symptoms uses the New York Heart Association (NYHA) classification. Palpitations are caused by paroxysmal supraventricular tachycardia, atrial flutter, or atrial fibrillation.

The murmur of mitral stenosis is a low frequency diastolic rumbling best heard at the apex, but is sometimes inaudible when the stenosis is severe. Systolic murmurs may indicate the presence of mitral or tricuspid regurgitation or concomitant aortic stenosis. A prominent pulmonic component of the S2, pulmonic systolic ejection click, and sternal heave suggest right ventricular enlargement and pulmonary hypertension. Jugular venous distention, hepatomegaly, pleural effusions, and dependent edema are signs of right ventricular failure. Pulmonary edema is manifested by tachypnea, wheezing, and rales. An irregular pulse indicates atrial fibrillation.

Laboratory studies are often useful for evaluating patients before operation. Wide, notched P waves in leads I and II in association with flat or inverted P waves in lead III of the electrocardiogram are indicative of right atrial (RA) hypertrophy and termed P-mitrale. Right axis deviation combined with atrial fibrillation or P-mitrale is an electrocardiographic pattern associated with mitral stenosis. Postoperative restoration of sinus rhythm is more likely when the duration of atrial fibrillation is less than 1 year (7). The chest roentgenogram may provide information useful for estimating pulmonary venous pressure, cardiac chamber size, and even calcification of the mitral valve in the occasional patient. Radiographic evidence of right ventricular dilatation includes a decrease in the space between the anterior border of the heart and the sternum on the lateral chest radiograph and a leftward deviation of the left heart border on the posteroanterior view. Extreme LA enlargement causes an elevation of the right main-stem bronchus, posterior displacement of the esophagus, and enlargement of the right heart border. Pulmonary venous hypertension increases the size of vessels in the upper lung fields and a loss of definition of vessel borders in the lower lung fields due to perivascular edema in the dependent regions. The presence of Kerley B lines suggests that pulmonary venous pressures exceed 20 mm Hg. Alveolar edema suggests that pulmonary venous pressures exceed 30 mm Hg. Cardiac catheterization is routinely performed in older patients with mitral stenosis because coronary artery disease is common in these patients.

The diagnosis and evaluation of mitral stenosis are based on the results of echocardiography and cardiac catheterization.

DIAGNOSIS

Gorlin Formula

The MVA can be estimated at cardiac catheterization by using the Gorlin equation:

$$\text{MVA (cm}^2) = \text{CO (mL/s)}/[38(\Delta P)^{1/2}]$$

where CO is cardiac output and ΔP is transvalvular pressure gradient.

An absolute or gold standard measurement of MVA has not been developed; however, the Gorlin formula is usually used as a standard for comparison. Accurate determination of MVA depends on the ability to measure antegrade blood flow through the mitral valve. Cardiac output, measured by the Fick equation or thermodilution, is the limiting factor determining the accuracy of the MVA measurement. LA-to-RA shunting, which is common after balloon valvuloplasty, decreases the ability to accurately measure cardiac output and MVA according to the Gorlin equation.

Treatment

Rheumatic mitral stenosis can be treated with medical therapy, percutaneous balloon valvulotomy, closed commissurotomy, open commissurotomy, mitral valve repair, mitral valve replacement with a prosthetic valve, or a combination of these techniques. Drug therapy does not change the size of the mitral valve orifice but is aimed at improving symptoms and preventing the complications associated with mitral stenosis. Anticoagulation decreases the risk of LA thrombus and complications related to systemic embolization. Digoxin decreases atrioventricular node conduction and is used to control the ventricular rate in patients with atrial fibrillation or flutter. Diuretics are used to manage pulmonary edema and congestive heart failure. Inotropic and vasoactive agents are used in end-stage disease, usually as a bridge to surgical operation. Although medical treatment may improve symptoms, only surgical treatment has improved survival.

Percutaneous Balloon Valvulotomy

Percutaneous balloon valvulotomy for the management of mitral stenosis was first reported in 1984 and is an alternative to surgery. The procedure is conducted in the cardiac catheterization laboratory with fluoroscopic and, on occasion, echocardiographic guidance. A balloon-tipped transvenous catheter is inserted into the LA by an interatrial septal puncture. The collapsed balloon is positioned across the mitral valve orifice and rapidly inflated and deflated (Fig. 17.7). Inflation of the balloon can be repeated with successively larger balloon diameters until a decrease in the pressure gradient across the mitral valve is detected. The procedure is often performed with two balloon-tipped catheters aligned side by side across the mitral valve orifice to achieve a greater balloon diameter during inflation. The balloon increases the effective MVA and decreases the mitral valve gradient by mechanically disrupting the rheumatic mitral valve. Balloon

valvulotomy splits the commissures, enlarges the orifice, and fractures the valve leaflets. Successful valvulotomy increases the estimated MVA by 1 to 2 cm². Successive increases in effective MVA during valvulotomy can be quantified using transesophageal echocardiography (TEE) in the cardiac catheterization laboratory. A successful procedure produces immediate increased cardiac output, decreased LA pressure, and decreased pulmonary artery pressure.

Echocardiography is useful to determine if patients are candidates for percutaneous balloon valvulotomy. Structural deformity of the mitral valve rather than MVA predicts whether percutaneous balloon dilation will be successful. An echocardiographic grading system based on structural deformity of the mitral valve apparatus can be used to predict the likelihood of successful balloon valvulotomy (Table 17.1) (8). Thickening of the valve leaflet, extensive calcification, restricted leaflet mobility, and subvalvular disease increase the echocardiographic grade of the valve and increase the likelihood of a suboptimal outcome (i.e., an increase in valve area of less than 25%). Small valve area was not associated with suboptimal outcome. Increased echocardiographic grades were also associated with increased mortality, restenosis after valvulotomy, NYHA class for heart failure, and increased need for mitral valve surgery. Echocardiographic evaluation prior to balloon valvulotomy is also performed to grade and detect the severity of mitral regurgitation. If mitral regurgitation is present, the severity typically increases after valvulotomy.

Echocardiography is useful for detecting complications of mitral valvulotomy that include worsening of mitral regurgitation, residual atrial septal defect (Fig. 17.8), cardiac tamponade from catheter perforation of the atria, systemic embolization of valve fragments or LA clot, aortic to RA

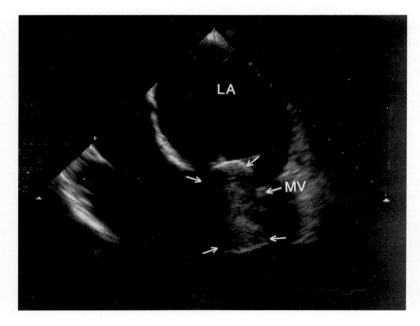

FIGURE 17.7. Transesophageal echocardiographic image of a rheumatic mitral valve during balloon mitral valvotomy. An Inoue balloon catheter was inserted into the patient's femoral vein, passed through the interatrial septum, and positioned in the mitral valve orifice (*MV*). Inflation of the balloon (*arrows*) caused commissural splitting and expansion of the mitral valve orifice. *LA*, left atrium.

TABLE 17.1. GRADING OF RHEUMATIC MITRAL VALVE BASED ON ECHOCARDIOGRAPHIC CHARACTERISTICS

Grade	Mobility	Subvalvular Thickening	Thickening	Calcification
1	Highly mobile valve with only leaflet tips restricted	Minimal thickening just below the mitral leaflets	Leaflets near normal in thickness (4–5 mm)	A single area of increased echo brightness
2	Leaflet middle and base portions have normal mobility	Thickening of chordal structures extending up to one third of the chordal length	Middle leaflets normal, considerable thickening of margins (5–8 mm)	Scattered areas of brightness confined to leaflet margins
3	Valve continues to move forward in diastole, mainly from the base	Thickening extending to the distal third of the chords	Thickening extending through the entire leaflet (5–8 mm)	Brightness extending into the middle portion of the leaflets
4	No or minimal forward movement of the leaflets in diastole	Extensive thickening and shortening of all chordal structures extending down to the papillary muscles	Considerable thickening of all leaflet tissue (>8–10 mm)	Extensive brightness throughout much of the leaflet tissue

Maximum score = 16 (score = sum of grade for each category, maximum = 16).
From Wilkins GT, Weyman AE, Abascal VM, et al. Percutaneous balloon dilatation of the mitral valve: an analysis of echocardiographic variables related to outcome and the mechanisms of dilation. *B Heart J* 1988;60:299, with permission.

fistula, and death. The echocardiographic appearance of the mitral valve, echocardiographic valve score, or total balloon inflation diameter has not been useful for predicting the likelihood of developing mitral regurgitation after valvulotomy. The severity of preexisting mitral regurgitation increases in 14% to 37% of patients after valvulotomy. Mitral regurgitation after valvulotomy may be caused by injury to chordae or papillary muscle, fracture of the valve leaflets, or poor leaflet coaptation from deformation of the valve orifice. The presences of active endocarditis or a LA thrombus are contraindications to percutaneous balloon valvulotomy. Transesophageal echocardiography is the most sensitive diagnostic test for detecting LA thrombus (Fig. 17.9). If a LA thrombus is detected, TEE can be repeated after 6 months of anticoagulation therapy to reassess the suitability of balloon valvulotomy.

Operative Treatment

Operative treatment for mitral stenosis includes closed commissurotomy, open commissurotomy with valve reconstruction, or mitral valve replacement. Closed commissurotomy is rarely performed anymore because of percutaneous balloon valvulotomy and refinements in cardiopulmonary bypass. In the past, closed commissurotomy was achieved by splitting the fused commissure and mitral leaflets, using either the surgeon's index finger or a valve dilator inserted through an atriotomy. The procedure is accomplished via a left thoracotomy

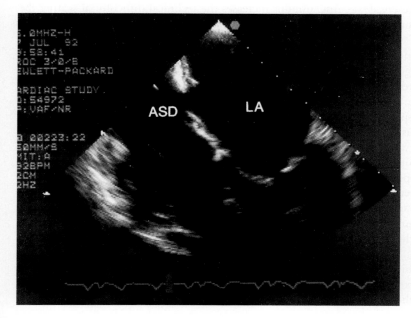

FIGURE 17.8. Transesophageal echocardiographic image of a patient with rheumatic mitral disease scheduled for mitral valve repair or replacement. A large atrial septal defect (*ASD*) was demonstrated due to prior attempt at balloon valvulotomy via a transseptal approach.

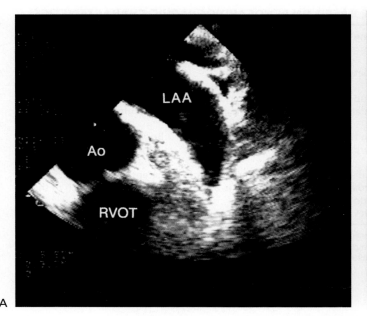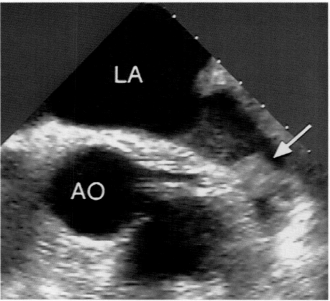

A

B

FIGURE 17.9. A: Intraoperative two-dimensional basal short-axis transesophageal echocardio-graphic image of a normal left atrial appendage (*LAA*). *Ao,* aorta; *RVOT,* right ventricular outflow tract. **B:** *Arrow* indicates a well-defined thrombus in the left atrial appendage with surrounding spontaneous echo contrast. Basal short-axis multiplane views at angles of approximately 30 to 45 degrees are useful for thrombus detection in the multilobed left atrial appendage.

and does not require systemic anticoagulation or cardiopul-monary bypass. The efficacy of digital commissurotomy is limited, and the use of a mechanical dilator is associated with mitral regurgitation. The ideal candidate for closed com-missurotomy has early rheumatic mitral stenosis limited to commissure fusion. The major limitation of closed commis-surotomy is that the increase in MVA is unpredictable and often produces mitral regurgitation. Major complications in-clude incomplete valvulotomy, bleeding, and embolization of clot or valve debris. Closed commissurotomy is reserved for emergency circumstances when alternatives are not avail-able.

Open commissurotomy can be performed in patients with mitral stenosis who do not have significant mitral regurgita-tion. Open commissurotomy is performed using cardiopul-monary bypass, and it permits direct visualization of the mitral valve to enable the debridement of calcium, splitting of fused chordae, removal of LA thrombi, or exclusion of the LA appendage. An open procedure permits the valve to be inspected after commissurotomy to assess valve opening and closure, and to test for valve competency. Intraoperative echocardiography is performed to assess the effectiveness of the commissurotomy and detect the presence and severity of mitral regurgitation immediately after the procedure (Fig. 17.10). Immediate valve replacement can proceed if the open commissurotomy fails to achieve a satisfactory result.

Mitral valve replacement with a prosthetic or biopros-thetic valve is usually performed in patients with extensive fibrosis and calcification of the valve apparatus or who have

significant mitral regurgitation. Unlike prosthetic valve re-placement for myxomatous degeneration or ischemic mi-tral regurgitation, the rheumatic mitral valve and portions of the subvalvular apparatus are frequently excised almost in their entirety. Division of subvalvular structures, how-ever, may predispose the patient to left ventricular rupture. Preservation of the chordae to the posterior annulus may prevent this rare but serious complication of mitral valve replacement. Severe calcification and deformity of the mi-tral annulus increases the technical difficulty of seating the valve prosthesis and increases the risk for paravalvular re-gurgitation. Most prosthetic valves have a functional MVA of 1.2 to 2.0 cm^2 (9). Bioprosthetic valves do not require long-term anticoagulation, but have the disadvantage of de-creased long-term durability, often failing 7 to 10 years after implantation. For this reason, they are reserved for elderly pa-tients or when anticoagulation is contraindicated. Mechan-ical bileaflet valves are the most commonly used prosthetic valves in the mitral position. Their two leaflets provide a low profile with a relatively large effective orifice area. Small jets of mitral regurgitation are normally detectable by TEE and must be distinguished from paravalvular regurgitation that typically produces larger and eccentric regurgitant jets (see Chapter 11). The bileaflet mechanical valves have a proven record of durability but require lifelong anticoagulation ther-apy and its associated risks.

Mitral valve reconstructive surgery, with ring an-nuloplasty as an alternative to mitral valve replace-ment in rheumatic mitral stenosis with associated mitral

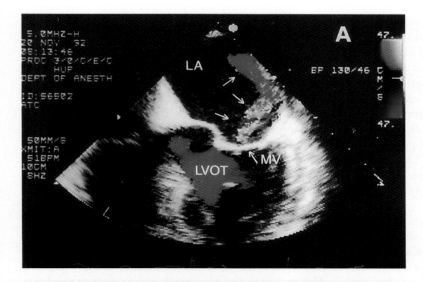

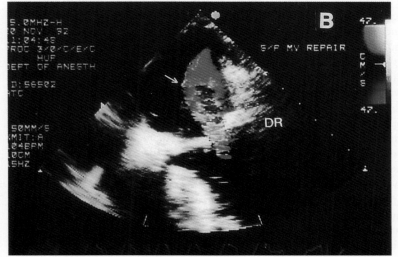

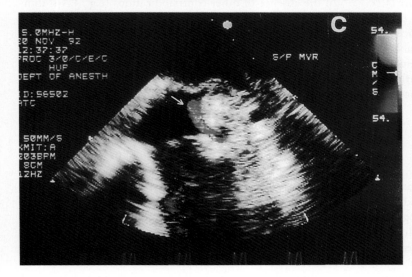

FIGURE 17.10. Intraoperative two-dimensional transesophageal echocardiogram (TEE) with Doppler color flow mapping. **A:** Precardiopulmonary bypass TEE showed a mitral regurgitant jet (*arrows*), a dilated left atrium (*LA*), and thickened mitral leaflets. *LVOT,* left ventricular outflow tract; *MV,* mitral valve. **B:** TEE images acquired immediately after commissurotomy, valve repair, and ring annuloplasty. Color Doppler flow mapping showed severe residual mitral regurgitation (*arrow*). The repair had failed. The Duran ring (*DR*) can be seen in cross section. **C:** TEE images in the same patient after mitral valve replacement with a Carpentier-Edwards bioprosthetic valve. Color Doppler flow mapping showed a perivalvular leak (*arrow*) in the posterolateral region of the mitral annulus. After reinstitution of cardiopulmonary bypass and left atriotomy, an avulsed annular suture was discovered and repaired at that location. The absence of the left ventricular outflow tract and aorta in the image plane indicated that the perivalvular leak was located in the posterior portion of the mitral annulus.

regurgitation, is possible in select patients. The routine surgical correction of the regurgitant rheumatic mitral valve is controversial. Unsuccessful repairs are common and are associated with a severalfold increase in hospital mortality rates. Patients with rheumatic mitral disease who undergo repair are more likely to return for reoperation than those who have had valve replacement. Advocates of rheumatic valve repair boast a decreased risk for long-term thromboembolism and late mortality in their patients when compared with patients who underwent prosthetic valve replacement (10). The routine use of TEE for reconstructive surgery permits the detection of early failures and prompt correction, usually at the time of operation (10).

Atrial fibulation remains to be one of the more prevalent arrhythmias that affect patients with mitral stenosis. Primary treatment of atrial fibulation is usually aimed at controlling ventricular rate and reducing the risk for thromboembolism, rather than correction of the underlying pathophysiology. The earliest attempts at correction of medically refractory atrial fibulation involved atrioventricular node ablation and pacemaker insertion. Although this method did address the issue of rate control, it did not correct the loss of atrial contraction or the continued susceptibility to thromboembolism. In 1991, Cox and associates (11) developed the Maze procedure, whereby both atrial appendages were excised and the pulmonary veins were isolated. Appropriately placed atrial incisions interrupt conduction roots of the reentrant currents and direct the sinus impulse from the sinoatrial node to the atrioventricular node along a specific path. The most current Maze III procedure is highly effective but has not been widely used due to concerns regarding increased bypass and cross-clamp times, bleeding from multiple suture lines, technical difficulty, and unfamiliarity with the procedure. Surgical radiofrequency ablation has been proposed as an alternative to the Maze procedure (12). Radiofrequency energy is delivered via a hand-held flexible probe to create lesions in the LA, with possible placement of additional RA lesions. Surgical radiofrequency ablation may simplify the procedure and make intraoperative correct of atrial fibrillation more feasible for patients presenting for concurrent mitral valve surgery. Early results are encouraging (2).

ECHOCARDIOGRAPHY

Mitral stenosis produces a characteristic pattern of anatomic and pathophysiologic features that can be detected and quantified by two-dimensional and Doppler echocardiography. The clinical experience with echocardiography for diagnosing and quantifying the severity of mitral stenosis is based primarily on transthoracic echocardiography. Although studies directly comparing TEE with transthoracic echocardiography in patients with mitral stenosis are lacking, the basic principles of the two techniques are the same. The standardized

multiplane TEE imaging planes for evaluation of the mitral valve described in the American Society of Echocardiography (ASE)/Society of Cardiovascular Anesthesiologists (SCA) guidelines correlate closely with the standard cross-sectional views obtained by transthoracic echocardiography. In some instances, such as for the detection of LA thrombus, TEE is superior to transthoracic echocardiography. The position of the transesophageal echocardiographic transducer directly behind the LA permits improved image resolution of structures near the mitral valve. The major disadvantage with TEE is that the probe is confined within the esophagus and only limited views of the heart can be obtained. Sometimes acquiring the standard transesophageal echocardiographic views may be more difficult in patients with mitral stenosis, because LA dilatation causes the esophagus to be deviated posteriorly. In addition, right ventricular hypertrophy causes a leftward displacement of the left ventricle in relation to the esophagus.

The anatomic and functional examination of the heart and mitral valve with two-dimensional and Doppler echocardiography provide information pertinent to the surgical care of the patient with mitral stenosis. A qualitative assessment of leaflet disease and the presence of mitral regurgitation or LA thrombus determine the appropriateness of commissurotomy, valve repair, or valve replacement. The echo score, developed by Wilkins, is an attempt to quantify the severity of the morphologic derangement of the rheumatic mitral valve to establish a predictor of outcome after percutaneous balloon valvotomy. Valve scores of less than 7 were associated with a "good" increase in MVA, defined as a postvalvotomy valve area of greater than 1.5 cm^2 and a greater than 25% increase in valve area. All patients with a valve score of less than 4 had an effective increase in valve area after balloon dilation. Valve scores of greater than 8 were associated with a greater than 58% chance of suboptimal outcome (13;14). In the absence of other contraindications (e.g., LA thrombus, severe mitral regurgitation), patients with relatively low valve scores tend to be good candidates for percutaneous mitral balloon valvotomy. Because the morbidity rate of the procedure is low, percutaneous balloon valvulotomy also can be tried in patients with high valve scores, but they are more likely to require surgical intervention.

Preoperative tricuspid regurgitation caused by pulmonary hypertension and right ventricular dilatation may improve after correction of the mitral stenosis. TEE can be used to help determine the need for tricuspid annuloplasty if tricuspid regurgitation is severe. In the absence of rheumatic involvement of the tricuspid valve, tricuspid valve replacement is rarely necessary. In patients who had a percutaneous balloon valvulotomy, echocardiographic examination of the intraatrial septum can usually detect a small atrial septal defect at the site of the transseptal puncture that can be surgically closed at the time of operation.

Although intraoperative TEE is rapidly being recognized as the standard of care for evaluating the success of mitral valve repair, it is important to recognize certain limitations.

Physiologic conditions, such as aortic insufficiency, affect the functional assessment of the mitral valve and the quantification of MVA. Measurements of mitral valve function obtained by intraoperative TEE may differ from those obtained in awake patients. Changes in cardiovascular function caused by the operation, the actions of general anesthetic agents, and the effects of vasoactive drugs may modify quantitative measures of mitral valve function. Provocative testing may be necessary when performing intraoperative TEE assessment of valve function. Provocative testing of valve function by changing heart rate, blood volume, or blood pressure may be necessary to simulate the transvalvular flow and loading conditions encountered in the awake state.

Two-Dimensional Echocardiography

The mitral valve leaflets can be examined in their entirety by multiplane TEE using the mid-esophageal four-chamber view, mid-esophageal commissural view, and mid-esophageal long-axis view. Alternatively, serial cross-sectional images of the valve beginning at the posteromedial commissure and extending to the anterolateral commissure can be acquired beginning from the four-chamber view by retroflexion and anteflexion of the probe tip. Complete assessment of mitral valve pathology from multiple echocardiographic imaging planes is particularly useful for the planning of mitral valve repair.

Rheumatic disease can cause a variety of lesions affecting the mitral valve, and a description of the extent of disease is useful for evaluating patients for valvuloplasty or valve replacement. Fibrosis and scarring produces a thickening of the mitral valve leaflets and restricts their mobility. In rheumatic disease, leaflet thickening typically is most severe at the leaflet edges, progressing toward the body of the leaflet, then to the annulus. Calcification appears as focal echogenic densities that cast far-field shadows. Leaflet calcification causes irregular leaflet surfaces that can ulcerate, cavitate, and generate thrombus. The motion and separation of thickened valve leaflets may be restricted. Fusion of the leaflet edges produces diastolic doming of the anterior leaflet, because the increased LA pressure pushes the usually more pliable body of the anterior leaflet toward the left ventricle. The diastolic displacement of the broad mid-portion of the anterior leaflet retracts the fused posterior leaflet in a paradoxic anterior direction. The transgastric basal short-axis image at the level of the mitral valve demonstrates loss or deformity of the typical open "fish mouth" appearance and can sometimes be used to estimate the valve orifice size. The normally serrated edges of the valve leaflets may be obscured by multiple areas of focal calcification (Figs. 17.11, 17.12, and 17.13).

Left atrial dilatation is caused by chronic increases in LA pressure, and the interatrial septum bows toward the RA. The normal atrial size is 38 ± 6 mm in the antero-posterior dimension and 39 ± 7 mm in the mediolateral

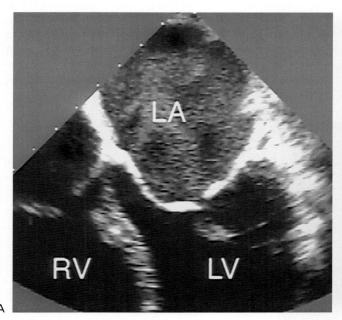

A

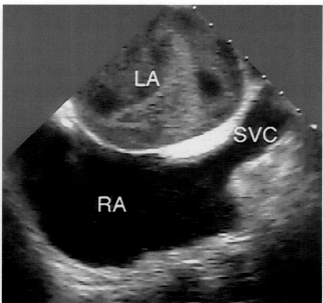

B

FIGURE 17.11. A: Intraoperative two-dimensional transesophageal echocardiographic image at end-diastole in a patient with rheumatic mitral stenosis. The dilated left atrium was filled with spontaneous echo contrast. The image also demonstrated poor leaflet separation and doming of the anterior mitral leaflet. **B:** Multiplane image of the atria and the interatrial septum obtained in a bicaval view, at an angle of approximately 90 degrees. This multiplane view is useful for thorough assessment of the atria and for detection of a patient foramen ovale. *LA,* left atrium; *LV,* left ventricle; *RV,* right ventricle; *SVC,* superior vena cava.

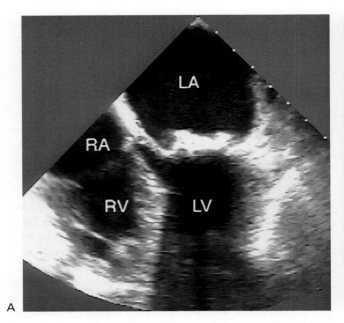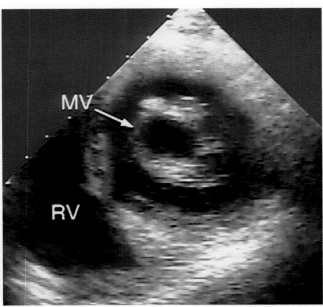

FIGURE 17.12. A: Intraoperative two-dimensional transesophageal image of a four-chamber view in a patient with rheumatic mitral stenosis. Extensive calcification with acoustic shadowing in the left ventricular cavity was demonstrated. **B:** Deep transgastric short-axis view of the stenotic mitral valve from the left ventricular aspect, during diastole (*arrow*). Calcification of the leaflets and extremely limited leaflet separation were noted. This view also can be used to perform planimetry measurements of the mitral valve orifice area and to detect the origin of mitral regurgitation during ventricular systole. *LA,* left atrium; *LV,* left ventricle; *RV,* right ventricle; *MV,* mitral valve.

dimension (15). Spontaneous echo contrast has the appearance of "smoke" in the LA and can be observed by TEE in greater than 50% of patients with mitral stenosis (Fig. 17.11). Spontaneous echo contrast suggests the presence of blood stasis and is associated with mitral stenosis, LA dilatation, and atrial fibrillation; the absence of significant mitral regurgitation; and an increased risk of thromboembolism.

Thrombus appears on TEE as an abnormal echogenic density within the LA, often residing in the LA appendage (Fig. 17.9). It is frequently difficult to distinguish mural thrombus in the atrial appendage from hypertrophied pectinate muscle or normal reflections in the wall of the atrium. Thrombus can be free, adherent to the LA wall (mural thrombus), or pedunculated. Thrombus may have irregular borders. A dark, less

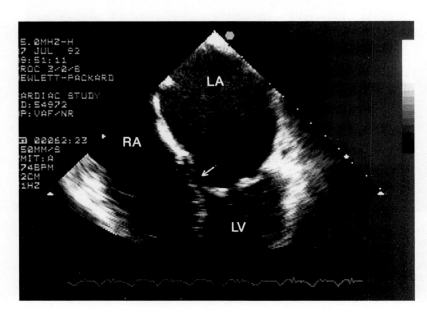

FIGURE 17.13. Intraoperative two-dimensional transesophageal echocardiographic image at end-diastole in a patient with rheumatic mitral stenosis. Diastolic doming (*arrow*) of the anterior mitral valve leaflet is characteristic of mitral stenosis. *LA,* left atrium; *LV,* left ventricle; *RA,* right atrium.

echogenic central region within the thrombus suggests central liquefaction. Pedunculated thrombi or free-ball thrombi are more likely to produce systemic embolization and mitral valve obstruction.

The left ventricle of patients with mitral stenosis is typically small and appears underfilled. Nonischemic posterobasal regional wall motion abnormalities are often present and attributable to rheumatic disease. Area ejection fraction is mildly decreased or normal. Severe left ventricular dysfunction is unusual but, if present, suggests coexisting disease, such as aortic valve disease, severe mitral regurgitation, or rheumatic carditis. In the presence of pulmonary hypertension, the crescent-shaped right ventricle increases in size and becomes more spherical. Wall thickness may exceed that of the left ventricle. Increased right ventricular systolic pressures may cause flattening or leftward deviation of the interventricular septum, or paradoxic interventricular septal motion.

Planimetry

Orifice area can be measured directly using two-dimensional echocardiography by manual planimetry of the cross-sectional view of the mitral orifice imaged from the transesophageal transgastric basal short-axis view. Studies have been performed demonstrating that transthoracic planimetric MVA measurements are reproducible and accurate compared with values derived from cardiac catheterization (16,17). The measurement is performed by acquiring short-axis tomographic images of the limiting mitral valve orifice. The valve area is measured by manually tracing the orifice. Measured orifice areas of less than 2.0, less than 1.5, and less than 1.0 cm^2 are graded as mild, moderate, and severe mitral stenosis, respectively. The ability to measure valve area accurately using this method depends on the technique and the extent of valve disease. A true tomographic image plane across the narrowest mitral valve opening is often difficult to obtain, especially when valve leaflets are severely deformed or when there is subvalvular stenosis (Fig. 17.14). The smallest mitral valve orifice may be missed if the tomographic plane is not directed through the apex of the funnel-shaped mitral valve, thereby underestimating the severity of mitral stenosis. Increased instrument gain settings increase the echogenicity of the borders of the mitral valve opening, especially if the valve is extensively calcified, and may lead to underestimation of the true MVA and overestimation of the severity of mitral stenosis (Fig. 17.15) (17). Commissurotomy usually renders the mitral valve orifice nonplanar, irregular, and difficult to quantify by planimetry. Using the width of the color Doppler jet across the mitral valve in two or more different long-axis planes may aid in identifying the borders of the mitral orifice and also has been used for direct estimation of the stenotic mitral valve orifice area.

$$MVA = (\pi/4)(a \times b)$$

where a is the jet width in a long-axis view (e.g., mid-esophageal four-chamber view) and b is the jet width in the corresponding orthogonal long-axis view (e.g., mid-esophageal two-chamber view).

Doppler Echocardiography

Doppler estimates of transmitral blood flow velocity permit quantification of the MVA and transvalvular pressure gradient. The sample volume is positioned between the tips of the open mitral leaflets. The mid-esophageal long-axis imaging planes through the mitral valve align transmitral blood flow along the same axis as the ultrasound transmission. The angle of incidence between the direction of blood flow and the Doppler signal is usually less than 20 degrees, negating the need to correct the incidence angle when calculating flow velocity.

Transmitral blood flow velocities are normally between 0.60 and 1.3 m/s and are within the bandwidth of pulsed-wave Doppler. A stenotic or distorted mitral orifice causes turbulent flow, an increased distribution of flow velocities, and an increase in the peak transmitral blood flow velocity (V_{max}). This blood flow pattern produces a widening of the spectral bandwidth on pulsed-wave Doppler and a mosaic of colors on the color Doppler variance flow map (Fig. 17.16). The increased peak velocities may exceed the Nyquist limit of pulsed-wave Doppler. Range-gated pulsed-wave Doppler with a high-pulse repetition frequency, upward shifting of the baseline velocity, or continuous-wave Doppler are frequently required for accurate estimation of the V_{max} across the stenotic valve (Fig. 17.5). A V_{max} of greater than 1.3 m/s is a sensitive but not specific indicator of mitral stenosis. The V_{max} may be increased in the absence of significant mitral stenosis by increased cardiac output, tachycardia, increased inotropic state, presence of a ventricular septal defect, or mitral regurgitation (18). An aortic regurgitant jet crossing the path of the continuous-wave ultrasound beam may be misinterpreted as an increase in the V_{max} and can falsely suggest mitral stenosis (18).

Transmitral Pressure Gradient

The diastolic pressure gradient across the mitral valve is estimated from the transmitral blood flow velocities using the simplified Bernoulli equation. The transvalvular pressure gradient calculated by Doppler correlates well with direct measurements obtained by cardiac catheterization (19). The instantaneous peak transmitral pressure (P_{max}) gradient is calculated as follows:

$$\Delta P_{max} = 4(V_{max})^2$$

where V_{max} is the peak transmitral blood flow velocity measured in m/second and the peak pressure gradient is measured in mm Hg.

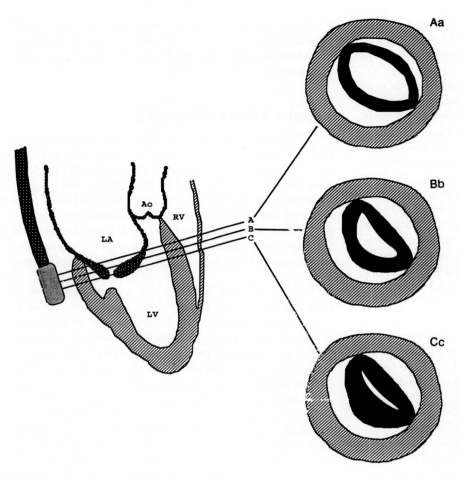

FIGURE 17.14. Schematic diagrams demonstrating the use of two-dimensional transesophageal echocardiographic basal short-axis views for measuring the stenotic mitral valve orifice size by planimetry. The imaging planes (*A, B,* and *C*), used to locate the mitral valve orifice, are acquired by adjusting probe depth or flexion and extension of the probe tip. The cross-sectional areas of the mitral valve inlet as they appear on the corresponding two-dimensional echocardiograms (*Aa, Bb,* and *Cc*) are dependent on the level of the imaging plane. An imaging plane that traverses the mitral valve inlet at the level of the limiting orifice (*C*) is necessary for accurate estimation of the mitral valve area using planimetry. *Ao,* aorta; *RV,* right ventricle; *LA,* left atrium; *LV,* left ventricle.

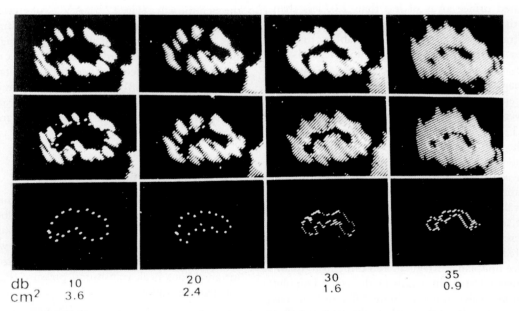

db	10	20	30	35
cm²	3.6	2.4	1.6	0.9

FIGURE 17.15. The mitral valve orifice size determined by manual planimetry is dependent on the receiver gain setting. The top row has two-dimensional phased-array ultrasound images of an excised stenotic mitral valve with increasing receiver gain levels (dB). The middle row displays the mitral valve orifice traced with a light pen. The bottom row shows light pen–traced mitral valve orifices with their corresponding areas (cm²) determined by planimetry. (From Martin RP, Rabowski H, Kleiman JH, et al. Reliability and reproducibility of two-dimensional echocardiographic measurement of the stenotic mitral valve orifice area. *Am J Cardiol* 1979;43:560, with permission.)

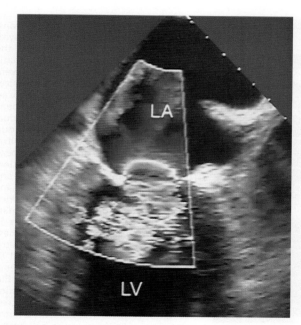

FIGURE 17.16. Intraoperative transesophageal echocardiographic color Doppler flow velocity map across a rheumatic mitral valve demonstrates a narrow diastolic orifice, producing flow convergence and high-velocity, high-variance transmitral flow velocities. *LV,* left ventricle, *LA,* left atrium.

Valve pressure gradients are usually expressed as peak or mean gradients. P_{max} is calculated by using the peak velocity. Therefore, a $V_{max} = 2$ m/s produces a $P_{max} = 16$ mm Hg. Calculation of a mean valve gradient requires integration of the spectral velocity and temporal averaging, a measurement that is simple to perform using modern echocardiography equipment. The mean diastolic pressure gradient across the mitral valve is calculated by integrating the spectral velocity over time throughout diastole and using the mean blood flow velocity to calculate the pressure gradient (Fig. 17.17). The major limitation of using the transvalvular pressure gradient to estimate the severity of mitral stenosis is that the pressure gradients are dependent on blood flow. At any given mitral valve orifice size, the transmitral pressure gradient is directly related to the cardiac output (Fig. 17.18).

Pressure Half-Time

The diastolic blood velocity profile across the mitral valve is altered in mitral stenosis. The rate of deceleration of diastolic blood flow velocity is a function of LA emptying and the instantaneous transvalvular pressure gradient over time. The normal transmitral blood flow velocity decays rapidly in diastole because the LA pressure decreases rapidly upon opening of the mitral valve. The impedance to LA emptying in patients with mitral stenosis causes an increased transvalvular pressure gradient throughout diastole and causes a more gradual decay in the transvalvular blood flow velocity. The rate of diastolic decay measured by Doppler echocardiography provides a functional estimation of the MVA. The

methodology is based on determining the pressure half-time ($P_{t1/2}$), or the time it takes for the peak diastolic pressure gradient to decrease by one half. The $P_{t1/2}$ is determined by measuring the time for V_{max} to decrease to 70% of its original value (Fig. 17.17) (18):

Definitions: $P_{t1/2} =$ time required for transmittal pressure gradient to equal $\dfrac{P_{max}}{2}$

$V_{t1/2} =$ blood velocity at pressure half-time

Given: $P = 4V^2$ (modified Bernouelli equation)

Derivation:

$$\text{at any time } t \; P_t = 4[V_t]^2$$
$$\text{at } t = P_{t1/2} \; P_t = \frac{P_{max}}{2} \text{ and } V_t = V_{t1/2},$$
$$\frac{P_{max}}{2} = 4[V_{t1/2}]^2$$
$$\text{by substituting } P_{max} = 4V_{max}^2$$
$$\frac{4V_{max}^2}{2} = 4[V_{t1/2}]^2$$
$$V_{t1/2} = \frac{V_{max}}{\sqrt{2}}$$
$$V_{t1/2} \approx 0.7\,V_{max}$$

The estimated MVA can then be calculated from the $P_{t1/2}$ with the following equation:

$$\text{MVA (cm}^2) = 220/P_{t1/2} \text{ (milliseconds)}$$

In patients with atrial fibrillation, the estimation of MVA is customarily based on the average of Doppler measurements obtained over 5 to 10 cardiac cycles.

The shape of the transvalvular blood flow velocity profile is determined not only by the mitral valve orifice size but also by LA and ventricular compliance, the transvalvular pressure gradient, and cardiac output. Variability in these factors can lead to inaccuracies when the $P_{t1/2}$ measurement is used to determine the MVA. After valvuloplasty, increased LA compliance or decreased left ventricular diastolic compliance slows the deceleration of blood flow through the mitral valve independent of changes in mitral valve orifice size. In aortic regurgitation, retrograde filling of the left ventricle acutely increases left ventricular diastolic pressures and decreases left ventricular diastolic compliance. These changes promote the deceleration of transmitral valve blood flow velocity in diastole, increase the rate of decay of diastolic transmitral blood flow velocity, decrease the $P_{t1/2}$ for any fixed mitral valve orifice size, and lead to an underestimation of the severity of mitral stenosis using the $P_{t1/2}$ method.

Pressure half-time and peak inflow velocity measurements are also affected by changes in the cardiovascular status of the patient. $P_{t1/2}$ measurements can overestimate the MVA by 50% to 100% during exercise (21,22). Exercise-induced increases in heart rate, inotropy, and cardiac output increase the

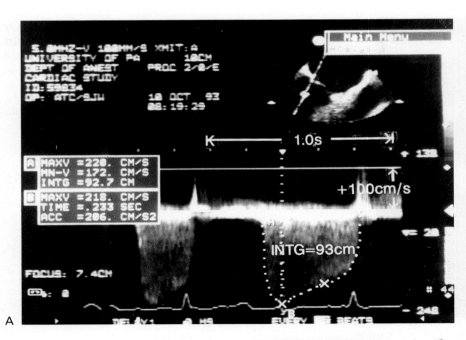

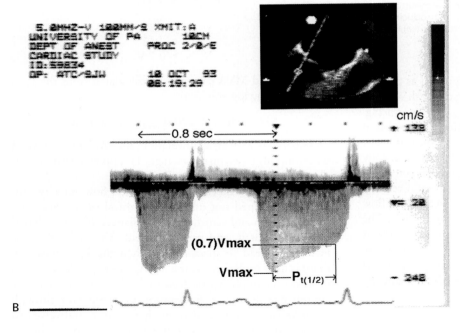

FIGURE 17.17. Intraoperative transesophageal echocardiogram with continuous-wave Doppler across the mitral valve in a patient with rheumatic mitral stenosis. Measurements were made with the vertical plane transducer using biplane transesophageal echocardiography **(inset)**. The increased peak velocity (V_{max} = 220 cm/s) and gradual deceleration of blood flow velocity during diastole was characteristic of mitral stenosis. The absence of the A-wave peak was consistent with atrial fibrillation. Functional estimates of the peak and mean transmitral pressure gradient and mitral valve orifice size were obtained from this echocardiogram. It is customary to use the average values of three to five cardiac cycles for calculating these parameters. **A:** The area of the spectral envelope (*Vdt* or *INTG*) is measured by manual planimetry of the outer border of the diastolic transmitral velocity profile. The diastolic time interval is the duration of antegrade diastolic blood flow across the mitral valve. **B:** The calculated mitral valve area using the pressure half-time is shown.

$$\text{Peak } \Delta P = 4 \times (V_{max})^2$$
$$= (4)\,(2.20 \text{ m/s})^2$$
$$= 19 \text{ mm Hg}$$
$$\text{Mean } \Delta P = 4 \times [\text{Vdt/diastolic time interval}]^2$$
$$= 4 \times [0.927 \text{ m/0.533 s}]^2$$
$$= 12.1 \text{ mm Hg}$$

Pressure half-time
$$V_{max} = 2.20 \text{ m/s}$$
$$0.7\,V_{max} = 1.58 \text{ m/s}$$
$$P_{t1/2} = \text{time interval from } V_{max}$$
$$\text{to } 0.7\,V_{max}$$
$$P_{t1/2} = 350 \text{ m/s}$$
$$MVA = 220/P_{t1/2}$$
$$= 220/350 \text{ m/s}$$
$$= 0.63 \text{ cm}^2$$

Continuity equation for mitral valve orifice area (MVA)
$$MVA = \text{stroke volume/Vdt}$$
$$= 50 \text{ cm}^3/93 \text{ cm}$$
$$= 0.54 \text{ cm}^2$$

where stroke volume = thermodilution CO/HR.

transmitral pressure gradient in early diastole and produce an increase in the peak inflow velocity. Exercise decreases the $P_{t1/2}$, regardless of the actual mitral valve orifice size, because the $P_{t1/2}$ is a function of the peak inflow velocity. The correlation between MVA estimated from the $P_{t1/2}$, two-dimensional echocardiography, and cardiac catheterization data are variable, ranging from $r = 0.70$ to $r = 0.90$.

Continuity Equation

The continuity equation, based on the conservation of mass, permits the calculation of MVA. The net antegrade blood flow through the mitral valve must be equal to the net antegrade blood flow through the left ventricular outflow tract or main pulmonary artery (Fig. 17.17).

Transmitral blood flow in diastole = cardiac stroke volume:

$$\int \text{Vdt}_{MV} \times MVA = \text{stroke volume (SV)}$$

$$MVA = SV/\int \text{Vdt}$$

The time-velocity integral is determined by measuring the area outlined by the outer border of the spectral display

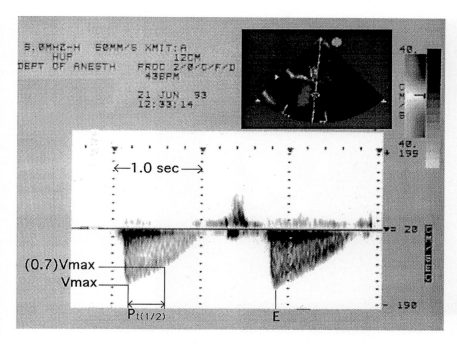

FIGURE 17.18. Determination of transmitral pressure gradients and mitral valve orifice area (*MVA*) using continuous-wave Doppler TEE across the rheumatic mitral valve in a patient with a low cardiac output. Measured values: diastolic time interval = 0.910 s, Vdt = 73.4 cm, V_{max} = 132 cm/s.

$$0.7\ V_{max} = 92\ cm/s$$
$$P_{t1/2} = 413\ m/s$$
$$Peak\ \Delta P = 4 \times (V_{max})^2$$
$$= 4 \times (1.32\ m/s)^2$$
$$= 7\ mm\ Hg$$
$$Mean\ \Delta P = 4 \times (V_{mean})^2$$
$$= 4 \times (Vdt/diastolic\ time\ interval)^2$$
$$= 4 \times (0.734\ m/0.910s)^2$$
$$= 2.6\ mm\ Hg$$
$$MVA = 220/P_{t1/2}$$
$$= 220/(413\ m/s)$$
$$= 0.5\ cm^2$$

The relatively low values of the transmitral pressure gradients in this patient with critical mitral stenosis can be explained by a low cardiac output.

of the transmitral Doppler signal. Stroke volume can be determined by thermodilution or Doppler echocardiography. Stroke volume (SV) also can be determined from the product of the annular cross-sectional area of the left ventricular outflow tract or pulmonary artery and the time-velocity integral through the respective structure is equal to the stroke volume. The continuity equation method of determining MVA is invalid in the presence of mitral or aortic regurgitation. A reasonable ($r = 0.7$–0.9) correlation exists between MVA determined by the continuity equation and other methods (23,24).

Flow Convergence

Blood flow proximal to a stenotic orifice converges in a concentric pattern and provides a method for functional determination of the stenotic orifice size (25). Color Doppler flow mapping produces a series of concentric isovelocity hemispheric surfaces on the LA side of the stenotic mitral valve (Fig. 17.19). If the LA is large relative to the mitral valve orifice size and if the isovelocity surface areas are hemispheric for a circular orifice, then the peak flow through the orifice can be calculated as follows: peak antegrade mitral flow = ($2\pi r^2$) ("aliasing" velocity), where r is the distance from the center of the mitral valve orifice to the first aliasing at a given Nyquist limit. The "funnel angle" restricts the region of proximal flow and is incorporated in the equation when examining antegrade flow through the mitral valve. Factoring in the inflow angle, peak antegrade mitral flow is calculated as ($2\pi r^2$) ($\alpha/180$) (aliasing velocity).

By assuming that flow through the isovelocity surface area is equal to the flow through the stenotic orifice, the conti-

nuity equation can then be applied to determine the mitral valve orifice area as follows: MVA = (peak antegrade mitral flow)/(V_{max}), where V_{max} is the peak inflow velocity through the mitral valve measured by continuous-wave Doppler. Preliminary studies suggest that the MVA determined from the proximal isovelocity surface area correlates ($r = 0.9$) with the MVA measured by planimetry, the Gorlin equation, and the $P_{t1/2}$ (Figs. 17.20 and 17.21) (26). The ability to estimate the inflow angle, the presence of subvalvular stenosis, determination of the exact center of the mitral valve orifice to measure the radius to the first aliasing boundary, and a nonhemispheric shape of the isovelocity surface contour can influence the accuracy of MVA calculations using the flow convergence method.

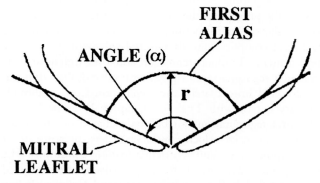

FIGURE 17.19. Schematic diagram of proximal flow convergence producing a series of concentric isovelocity hemispheric surfaces on the left atrial side of a stenotic mitral valve. (Adapted from Weyman AE. Left ventricular inflow tract I: the mitral valve. In: Weyman AE, ed. *Principles and practice of echocardiography,* 2nd ed. Philadelphia: Lea & Febiger, 1994:391, with permission.)

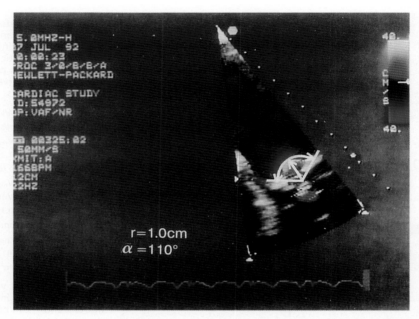

FIGURE 17.20. Transesophageal echocardiographic color Doppler flow map of transmitral blood velocity during diastole before balloon valvulotomy. As blood within the left atrium (*LA*) accelerates away from the ultrasound transducer, the color flow map changes from blue to yellow (*arrows*). This color interface represents the acceleration of blood flow velocity beyond the selected aliasing velocity (Nyquist limit = 40 cm/s). The mosaic of colors within the left ventricle (*LV*) downstream to the plane of the mitral valve suggests high-velocity turbulent blood flow though the stenotic orifice. When combined with the value for V_{max}, measured by continuous-wave Doppler, a functional estimation of the mitral valve orifice area (*MVA*) was determined using the proximal flow convergence method.

$$MVA = 2\pi r^2 \, (\alpha/180°) \times (V_{alias})/(V_{max})$$
$$= 2\pi \, (1.0 \text{ cm})^2 (110 \text{ degrees}/180 \text{ degrees})$$
$$\times (40 \text{ cm/s})/10 \text{ cm/s}$$
$$= 1.0 \text{ cm}^2$$

where r = the isovelocity radius of the proximal flow convergence region, α = the funnel angle of the flow convergence region, V_{alias} = the selected aliasing velocity, and V_{max} = the peak blood flow velocity measured by continuous-wave Doppler (not shown). The MVA simultaneously calculated from the pressure half-time was 1.0 cm^2 and from the cardiac catheterization data using the Gorlin formulas was 0.9 cm^2.

Immediately after mitral surgery, the transesophageal echocardiographic examination is repeated to assess the success of the procedure, the presence of intracavitary air, and ventricular size and function. TEE is sensitive for detecting technical complications after mitral valvuloplasty or valve replacement. Residual stenosis, residual regurgitation, paravalvular regurgitation, or prosthetic valve dysfunction can be detected immediately after separation from cardiopulmonary bypass with TEE (see Chapter 20). The severity of mitral regurgitation can be graded based on the maximum jet area, jet velocity, number of jets, presence of jet wall impingement, and ventricular loading conditions. The intraoperative assessment after mitral valve repair is targeted to detect flail leaflet segments, improved leaflet mobility, altered leaflet coaptation, mitral regurgitation, and to quantify the increase in the mitral valve orifice area. A successful mitral valvuloplasty increases leaflet excursion, decreases calcification, increases MVA, and does not result in signif-

icant mitral regurgitation. Recalculation of MVA and mitral valve pressure gradient permits quantitative estimates of treatment efficacy. Any open chamber cardiac procedure has the potential to introduce air into the left heart. Intracavitary air appears on the echocardiographic examination as specular, echogenic signals in the LA, pulmonary veins, or left ventricle.

Case Report

A 71-year-old man with aortic and mitral stenosis was scheduled for aortic valve replacement and mitral valvuloplasty. The history included rheumatic fever and mitral stenosis with closed commissurotomies at age 40 and 48 years. The patient developed increasing shortness of breath, orthopnea, and exercise intolerance. The medical history was notable for smoking, chronic obstructive pulmonary disease, chronic atrial fibrillation, an embolic stroke at age 53 years, and no

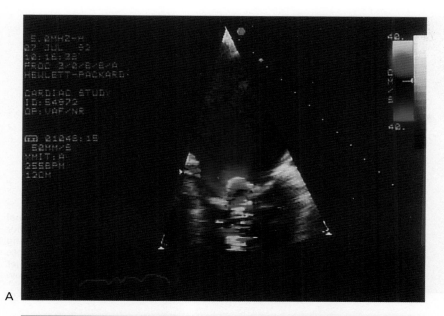

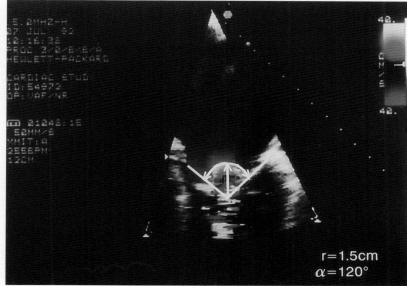

r=1.5cm
α=120°

FIGURE 17.21. A: Transesophageal echocardiographic color Doppler flow map of transmitral blood flow after balloon valvulotomy. **B:** The isovelocity radius (*r*) of the proximal flow convergence region has increased to 1.5 cm at the same aliasing velocity (V_{alias} = 40 cm/s) with a funnel angle (α) of 120 degrees. The peak transmitral blood flow velocity (V_{max}), measured by continuous-wave Doppler, decreased to 180 cm/s. The mitral valve area calculated by the proximal flow convergence method was 2.1 cm², by the pressure half-time was 1.8 cm², and by the Gorlin formula was 1.9 cm². These measurements suggested an increase in MVA after balloon valvulotomy.

angina. Cardiac catheterization revealed aortic stenosis with an aortic valve area of 0.75 cm² and a peak aortic valve gradient of 60 mm Hg, and mitral stenosis with an MVA of 1.4 cm² and a mean gradient of 12 mm Hg. No mitral regurgitation was detected. Coronary angiography showed 60% stenosis of the left anterior descending and right coronary arteries. Ventriculography showed a dilated and severely hypokinetic left ventricle with an ejection fraction of 25%, aortic regurgitation, and tricuspid regurgitation. The right ventricle was dilated with pulmonary artery pressures of 58/40 mm Hg.

After induction of general anesthesia and tracheal intubation, a TEE probe was inserted into the esophagus. The two-dimensional TEE examination performed before by-

pass revealed severely calcified mitral leaflets with restricted mobility, commissure fusion, and focal calcification in the mitral annulus and leaflet tips (Fig. 17.11). The aortic valve had poor leaflet mobility and numerous focal areas of calcification and thickening accompanied with post-stenotic dilatation of the aortic root. The left ventricle was hypertrophied, dilated, and severely hypokinetic. Spontaneous echo contrast filled the LA, and the LA appendage could not be detected. No intracardiac masses were appreciated. Doppler examination revealed severe aortic regurgitation (Fig. 17.22), 1+ mitral regurgitation, diastolic transmitral peak velocity that exceeded 200 cm/s (aortic regurgitation rendered the diastolic transmitral flow velocity difficult to interpret), and 1+ tricuspid regurgitation. Color flow Doppler across the

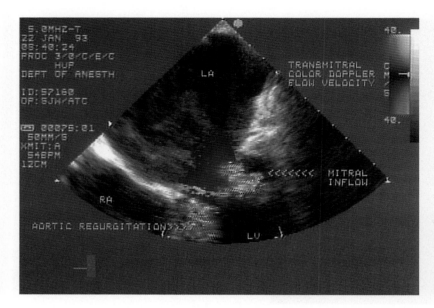

FIGURE 17.22. Intraoperative two-dimensional transesophageal echocardiography with color Doppler flow map across the mitral valve during diastole demonstrates high-velocity, high-variance transmitral blood flow. An aortic regurgitation jet was partially imaged in the left ventricular outflow tract. *LA,* left atrium; *RA,* right atrium.

mitral valve produced a high-variance, high-velocity diastolic flow map, suggesting turbulent blood flow.

During hypothermic cardiopulmonary bypass and retrograde cardioplegia of the heart, the aortic valve was replaced with a no. 27 Carpentier-Edwards bioprosthesis. An open mitral valve commissurotomy included commissure splitting and excision of calcified lesions near the edges of the anterior and posterior leaflets. Separation from cardiopulmonary bypass was achieved with dobutamine, epinephrine, and intraarterial blood pressure (IABP) counterpulsation. Postcardiopulmonary bypass TEE demonstrated improved separation and excursion of the mitral valve leaflets (Fig. 17.23), with a peak transmitral flow velocity of less than 1.0 m/s and

trace mitral regurgitation. Compared with the precardiopulmonary bypass examination, the left ventricular chamber was smaller with improved systolic function. The IABP was removed on postoperative day 2, and mechanical ventilation was discontinued on postoperative day 3. The patient was discharged from the intensive care unit on postoperative day 4 and discharged from the hospital on postoperative day 8.

CONCLUSION

Intraoperative TEE alters management of patients with rheumatic mitral stenosis. The ability to obtain precise

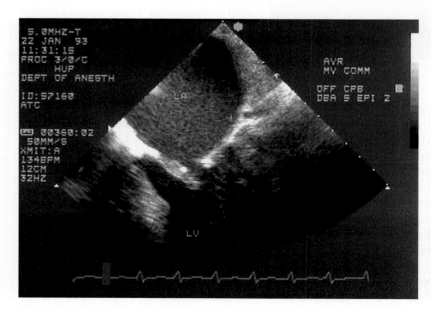

FIGURE 17.23. Intraoperative two-dimensional transesophageal echocardiographic image in a patient after mitral valvuloplasty demonstrates increased separation of the mitral leaflets during diastole compared with the images obtained before cardiopulmonary bypass. *LA,* left atrium.

anatomic and functional information about the mitral valve has enabled mitral valve repair in patients who would otherwise undergo valve replacement. The success of a valvuloplasty or valve replacement can be assessed immediately afterward.

Perioperative TEE of the stenotic rheumatic mitral valve can characterize and quantify:

1. Mitral valve anatomy and function, before and after valvuloplasty
2. Left atrial thrombus
3. Disease of the aortic and tricuspid valves
4. MVA (before and after valvuloplasty) and detection of residual stenosis
5. Mitral regurgitation (before and after valve surgery)
6. Right and left ventricular function
7. Prosthetic valve function and paravalvular regurgitation
8. Intracavitary air
9. ASD (after balloon valvuloplasty)
10. Left atrial size (for RF ablation)

KEY POINTS

■ Rheumatic carditis can be a sequela of upper respiratory infections caused by group A streptococci and results in an autoimmune-mediated tissue injury-leading to mitral stenosis.
■ Normal cross-sectional area ranges from 4 to 6 cm^2, and 1.6 to 2 cm^2 is considered mild mitral stenosis, 1.0 to 1.5 cm^2 is moderate mitral stenosis, and less than 1 cm^2 is severe mitral stenosis.
■ Left ventricular dysfunction is often associated with rheumatic mitral stenosis.
■ Orifice area can be measured by manual planimetry of the cross-sectional view of the mitral orifice imaged from the transesophageal transgastric basal short-axis view.
■ Mitral valve area can be calculated from the $P_{t1/2}$ with the following equation: MVA (cm^2) $= 220/P_{t1/2}$ (milliseconds).
■ Mitral valve area also can be calculated by proximal isovelocity surface area (PISA): MVA = peak antegrade mitral flow or $(2 \pi r^2)$ (aliasing velocity)/(V$_{max}$).
■ Additional diagnoses to consider with mitral stenosis include LA dilatation and thrombus, right ventricular failure, tricuspid regurgitation, and aortic valve disease.

REFERENCES

1. Horstkotte D, Niehues R, Strauer BE. Pathomorphological aspects, aetiology and natural history of acquired mitral valve stenosis. *Eur Heart J* 1991;12(suppl B):55.
2. Gordon SPF, Douglas PS, Come PC, et al. Two-dimensional and Doppler echocardiographic determinants of the natural history of mitral valve narrowing in patients with rheumatic mitral stenosis: implications for follow-up. *J Am Coll Cardiol* 1992;19:968.
3. **Carroll JD, Feldman T. Percutaneous mitral balloon valvotomy and the new demographics of mitral stenosis. *JAMA* 1993;270:1731.**
4. Okita Y, Miki S, Kusuhara K, et al. Analysis of left ventricular motion after mitral valve replacement with a technique of preservation of all chordae tendineae. *J Thorac Cardiovasc Surg* 1992;104:786.
5. Mohan JC, Khalilulla M, Arora R. Left ventricular intrinsic contractility in pure rheumatic mitral stenosis. *Am J Cardiol* 1989;64:240.
6. Liu CP, Ting CT, Yang TM, et al. Reduced left ventricular compliance in human mitral stenosis. *Circulation* 1992;85:1447.
7. Probst B, Goldschlager N, Seltzer A. Left atrial size and atrial fibrillation in mitral stenosis: factors influencing their relationship. *Circulation* 1973;48:1281.
8. Wilkins GT, Weyman AE, Abascal VM, et al. Percutaneous balloon dilatation of the mitral valve: an analysis of echocardiographic variables related to outcome and the mechanism of dilatation. *Br Heart J* 1988;60:299.
9. Khuri SF, Folland ED, Sethi GK, et al. Six-month post-operative hemodynamics of the Hancock heterograft and the Bork-Shiley prosthesis: results of a Veterans Administration Cooperative prospective randomized trial. *J Am Coll Cardiol* 1988;12:8.
10. Yau TM, El-Ghoneimi YA, Armstrong S, et al. Mitral valve repair and replacement for rheumatic disease. *J Thorac Cardiovasc Surg* 2000;119(1):53–60.
11. Sundt TM III, Camillo CJ, Cox JL. Advances in supraventricular tachycardia. *Cardiol Clin* 1997;15:1–11.
12. Williams MR, Stewart JR, Bolling SF, et al. Surgical treatment of atrial fibrillation using radiofrequency energy. *Ann Thorac Surg* 2001;71:1939–1944.
13. **Abascal VM, Wilkins GT, O'Shea JP, et al. Prediction of successful outcome in 130 patients undergoing percutaneous balloon mitral valvotomy. *Circulation* 1990;82:448.**
14. Weyman AE. Left ventricular inflow tract I: the mitral valve. In: Weyman AE, ed. *Principles and practice of echocardiography*, 2nd ed. Philadelphia: Lea & Febiger, 1994:391.
15. **Cohen GI, White M, Sochowski R, et al. Reference values for normal adult transesophageal echocardiographic measurements. *J Am Soc Echocardiogr* 1995;May–June:227.**
16. Nichol PM, Gilbert BW, Kisslo JA. Two-dimensional echocardiographic assessment of mitral stenosis. *Circulation* 1977;55:120.
17. Martin RP, Rabowski H, Kleiman JH, et al. Reliability and reproducibility of two-dimensional echocardiographic measurements of the stenotic mitral valve orifice area. *Am J Cardiol* 1979;43:560.
18. Kandath D, Nanda NC. Conventional and color Doppler assessment of mitral and tricuspid stenosis. In: Nanda NC, ed. *Textbook of color Doppler echocardiography*. Philadelphia: Lea & Febiger, 1989:168.
19. **Halbe D, Bryg RJ, Labovitz AJ. A simplified method for calculating mitral valve area using Doppler echocardiography. *Am Heart J* 1988;116:877.**
20. Thomas JD, Weyman AE. Doppler mitral pressure half-time: a clinical tool in search of theoretical justification. *J Am Coll Cardiol* 1987;10:923.
21. **Braverman AC, Thomas JD, Lee RT. Doppler echocardiographic estimation of mitral valve area during changing hemodynamic conditions. *Am J Cardiol* 1991;68:1485.**
22. Voelker W, Regel B, Dittmann H, et al. Effect of heart rate on transmitral flow velocity profile and Doppler measurements of

mitral valve area in patients with mitral stenosis. *Eur Heart J* 1992;13:152.

23. Nakatani S, Masuyama T, Kodama K, et al. Value and limitations of Doppler echocardiography in the quantification of stenotic mitral valve area: comparison of the pressure half-time and the continuity equation methods. *Circulation* 1988;77:78.

24. Derumeaux G, Bonnemain T, Remadt F, et al. Non-invasive assessment of mitral stenosis before and after percutaneous balloon mitral valvotomy by Doppler continuity equation. *Eur Heart J* 1992;13:1034.

25. Recusani F, Bargiggia GS, Yoganathan AP, et al. A new method for quantification of regurgitant flow rate using color Doppler flow imaging of the flow convergence region proximal to a discrete orifice. An *in vitro* study. *Circulation* 1991;83:594.

26. **Rodriguez L, Thomas JD, Monterroso V, et al. Validation of the proximal flow convergence method. Calculation of orifice area in patients with mitral stenosis.** *Circulation* **1993;88:1157.**

18

CONGESTIVE HEART FAILURE (HEMODYNAMIC INSTABILITY)

KAZUMASA ORIHASHI

APPLICATION OF TRANSESOPHAGEAL ECHOCARDIOGRAPHY IN MANAGING CONGESTIVE HEART FAILURE

Clinical appearance of congestive heart failure (CHF) varies much in severity among individual cases. The extreme form of heart failure appears as cardiogenic shock or cardiac arrest, which necessitates immediate cardiopulmonary resuscitation (CPR) or ventilatory/circulatory support. In addition, CHF is often complicated by other pathologies that cause or result from CHF. Prompt and accurate diagnosis and treatment for every pathology is needed. However, diagnostic examinations such as cardiac catheterization or coronary angiography are not practically feasible in patients with a critically ill condition such as cardiac arrest, but it is essential to obtain accurate and real-time information at bedside. Ultrasonography including echocardiography is most suitable for this purpose. However, the transthoracic approach often fails to show the heart under CPR or mechanical ventilation with positive airway pressure. Transesophageal echocardiography (TEE) is advantageous because it can clearly show the heart and vessels with least interference and minimal disturbance on therapeutic interventions.

In treating CHF patients with limited tolerance, it is important to make the correct diagnosis and proceed with "safe" and "secure" treatment without causing iatrogenic complications. This chapter focuses on the problems encountered in the clinical setting, and demonstrates how TEE can be used for this purpose.

ETIOLOGIES OF CONGESTIVE HEART FAILURE

Figure 18.1 illustrates mechanisms of circulatory derangement. The factors in italic letters indicate etiologies of CHF.

K. Orihashi: Department of Surgery, Graduate School of Biomedical Sciences, Hiroshima University; and Division of Thoracic and Cardiovascular Surgery, Hiroshima University Hospital, Hiroshima, Japan.

Mechanisms of CHF are summarized into four categories: (a) stenosis of the cardiovascular lumen, (b) valvular dysfunction, (c) myocardial dysfunction, and (d) shunt (Table 18.1). Transesophageal echocardiography is used for determining the cause of CHF and other circulatory derangement by examining each chamber, valve, and vessel, as well as blood flow.

When stenosis is present along the cardiac chamber, valve, or vessel, the chamber before stenosis is subjected to pressure overload. Figure 18.2 illustrates the changes seen in aortic stenosis. Hypertrophy of the left ventricle (LV) is apparent in B mode. Opening of the aortic valve is limited. Post-stenotic turbulent flow in color Doppler mode indicates the presence of a stenotic portion. The severity of the stenosis can be assessed by measuring the area in B mode or the pressure gradient in continuous-wave Doppler mode. Congestion in the left atrium (LA) and pulmonary vein (PV) occurs secondarily.

When valvular regurgitation is present, a fraction of blood returns to the previous chamber and causes volume overload. Figure 18.2B illustrates the changes caused by mitral regurgitation (MR). A dilated LA can be seen in B mode. Regurgitant flow is readily recognized with regurgitant jet flow in color Doppler mode. The severity of MR is assessed by measuring the area of the regurgitant jet, or by measuring the regurgitant volume by means of proximal isovelocity surface area method.

Myocardial dysfunction is recognized by reduced contraction or abnormal dilatation of the LV (Fig. 18.2C). Abnormal wall motion is recognized in B mode. The LA also may be dilated. MR is often present. When contraction is impaired, it is important to know whether it is diffuse or regional. LV aneurysm also reduces cardiac performance because a portion of LV work is wasted.

The presence of a shunt forms a loop circuit and causes volume overload along it. Dilatation of chambers and vessels is the result (Fig. 18.2D). In addition, pressure overload causes hypertrophy on the right heart. Dilatation with hypertrophy is recognized in B mode, while shunt flow is depicted in color Doppler mode.

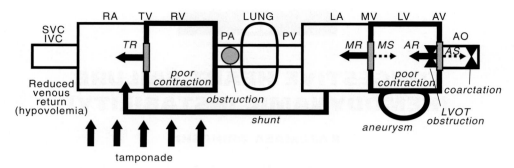

FIGURE 18.1. Mechanisms of circulatory derangement. *SVC,* superior vena cava; *IVC,* inferior vena cava; *RA,* right atrium; *TV,* tricuspid valve; *RV,* right ventricle; *PA,* pulmonary artery; *PV,* pulmonary vein; *LA,* left atrium; *MV,* mitral valve; *LV,* left ventricle; *AV,* aortic valve; *AO,* aorta; *TR,* tricuspid regurgitation; *MR,* mitral regurgitation; *MS,* mitral stenosis; *AR,* aortic regurgitation; *AS,* aortic stenosis; *LVOT,* left ventricular outflow tract.

Any of these pathologies leads to congestion of blood. Clinical manifestation of congestion in the left heart is pulmonary congestion (dyspnea), whereas that in the right heart is peripheral edema.

ASSOCIATED DISEASES RELATED TO CONGESTIVE HEART FAILURE

Congestive heart failure is often complicated by several other pathologies. One must be mindful of these pathologies as well as CHF because they can cause other troubles secondarily unless they are diagnosed and treated appropriately.

TABLE 18.1. ETIOLOGIES OF CONGESTIVE HEART FAILURE

Stenosis of cardiac or vascular lumen
    Congenital: aortic coarctation etc.
    Acquired: pulmonary artery spasmus, pulmonary embolism, etc.
    Hypertrophic obstructive cardiomyopathy
    Neoplasm inside cardiac lumen

Valvular dysfunction
    Stenosis: rheumatic, arteriosclerotic, congenital, etc.
    Regurgitation: rheumatic, degenerative, arteriosclerotic, infective endocarditis, etc.
    Prosthetic valve dysfunction: stuck valve, valve dehiscence

Myocardial dysfunction
    Impaired contraction: myocardial infarction, cardiomyopathy, cardiac contusion, etc.
    Impaired diastolic function: cardiomyopathy, etc.
    Rhythm and conduction disturbance: marked bradycardia or tachycardia, cardiac arrest, etc.
    Ineffective contraction: ventricular aneurysm

Shunt
    Congenital: atrial septal defeft, ventricular septal defect, patent ductus arteriosus, etc.
    Acquired: ventricular septal perforation, ruptured sinus of Valsalva, etc.

Mitral Regurgitation

Mitral regurgitation can be a cause, an accompanying disease, or a result of CHF. Mitral regurgitation can be caused by a number of mechanisms, which are schematically illustrated in Fig. 18.3. A deformed leaflet caused by sclerosis or fusion of leaflets can be responsible for inadequate coaptation. In cases of infective endocarditis, the leaflet can be perforated, and it is through this perforation that regurgitation occurs (1). Dysfunction of the subvalvular apparatus disturbs appropriate coaptation. Torn, shortened, or elongated chordae tendineae can cause MR. Torn papillary muscle (Fig. 18.4) occurs most commonly in acute myocardial infarction and causes severe MR. Dilatation of the mitral annulus, often associated with chronic LV dilatation, causes coaptation failure of the mitral leaflet (2). When the LV is acutely dilated, relative shortening of the subvalvular system occurs, and the subvalvular apparatus is pulled toward the apex. The coaptation point is deviated toward the ventricular apex, and inappropriate coaptation is the result. Transesophageal echocardiography is used to differentiate these mechanisms of MR in order to determine which surgical procedures or pharmacologic intervention are indicated.

Atrial Fibrillation and Mural Thrombus

When overload on the atrium is sustained, atrial fibrillation often occurs. It causes the following two problems: thrombus formation and reduced cardiac performance. As blood in the LA stagnates, thrombus often appears, especially in the LA appendage (3). It may cause a systemic arterial embolism, including cerebral infarction. On the other hand, impaired diastolic function of the LV can be responsible for overload on the LA. In these patients, atrial kick contributes to a large fraction of LV inflow. As atrial kick is lost in atrial fibrillation, cardiac output is significantly reduced. Transesophageal echocardiography clearly visualizes stagnated blood flow as spontaneous echo contrast as well as thrombus formation.

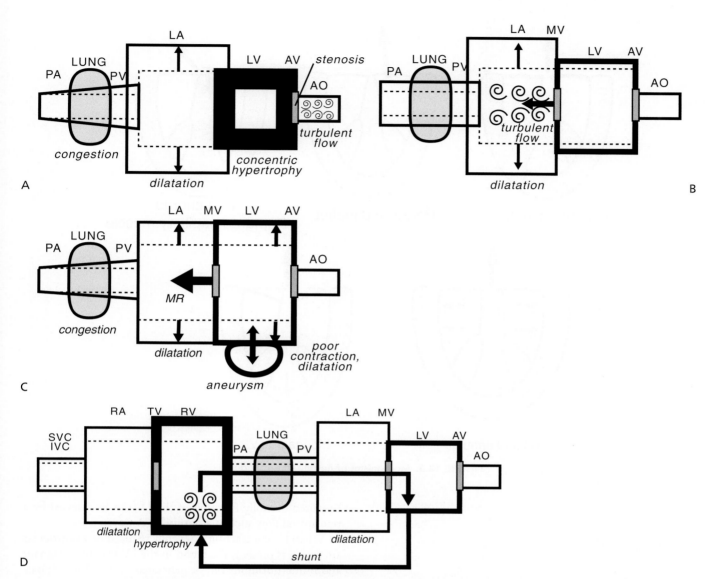

FIGURE 18.2. Etiology-oriented morphologic and hemodynamic changes. **A:** Aortic stenosis. **B:** Mitral regurgitation. **C:** Left ventricular dysfunction. **D:** Ventricular septal defect. *PA,* pulmonary artery; *PV,* pulmonary vein; *LA,* left atrium; *LV,* left ventricle; *AV,* aortic valve; *AO,* aorta; *MV,* mitral valve; *SVC,* superior vena cava; *IVC,* inferior vena cava; *RA,* right atrium; *TV,* tricuspid valve; *RV,* right ventricle.

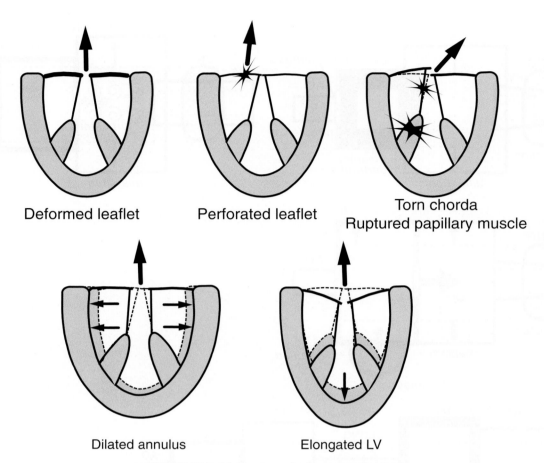

Deformed leaflet   Perforated leaflet   Torn chorda
                                                Ruptured papillary muscle

Dilated annulus   Elongated LV

FIGURE 18.3. Mechanisms of mitral regurgitation.

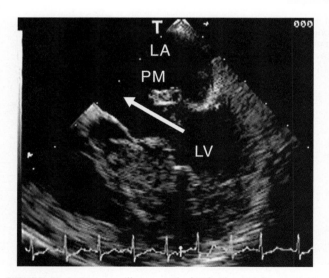

FIGURE 18.4. Torn papillary muscle (*PM*). The PM flips into the left atrium (*LA*). *LV,* left ventricle.

Impaired diastolic function of the LV can be assessed by a transmitral flow such as a dominant A wave.

When LV contraction is severely reduced or a ventricular aneurysm is present, the blood in the LV becomes stagnant and mural thrombus can be generated (4,5). This is apparent with TEE by spontaneous echo contrast and echogenic thrombus on the wall.

Pleural effusion and atelectasis are often found in CHF patients. Pleural effusion compresses the lung parenchyma from behind and causes atelectasis. Use of vasodilators disturbs hypoxic vasoconstriction and considerably increases A-aDO2. In addition, lung edema interferes with oxygenation. Transesophageal echocardiography clearly shows atelectasis and pleural fluid on the dorsal side (Fig. 18.5) and is helpful for immediately assessing the drainage and increase of air content in the alveoli, which is depicted by a marked increase in echogenicity in the lung parenchyma (6).

GUIDING PLACEMENT OF THE SWAN-GANZ CATHETER

Hemodynamic changes in patients with CHF are commonly monitored continuously by means of a pulmonary

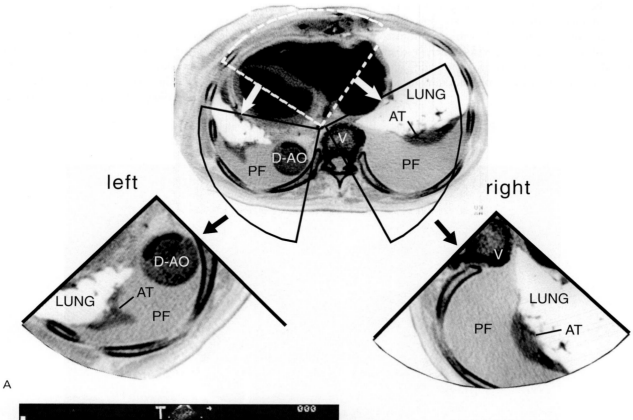

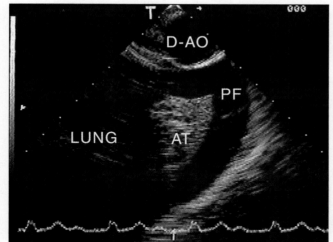

FIGURE 18.5. Pleural effusion and atelectasis. **A:** Computed tomography scan showing scanning planes possible with transesophageal echocardiography (TEE). **B:** TEE view. *AT,* atelectasis; *PF,* pleural fluid; *D-AO,* descending aorta; *V,* vertebra.

artery catheter. However, it is sometimes difficult to insert the catheter in the intensive care unit (ICU) under the guidance of pressure tracing without fluoroscopy. The presence of tricuspid regurgitation with a dilated right atrium (RA) also makes this procedure difficult. Ventricular arrhythmias often make one hesitant to advance the catheter.

Transesophageal echocardiography helps guide this procedure by showing the position of the catheter and advancement of the ballon without being stuck (Fig. 18.6) (7). The catheter tip may unintentionally enter the inferior vena cava or RA appendage, make a loop in the RA, or become trapped at the right ventricular apex (Fig. 18.7). Transesophageal echocardiography can be used to clearly

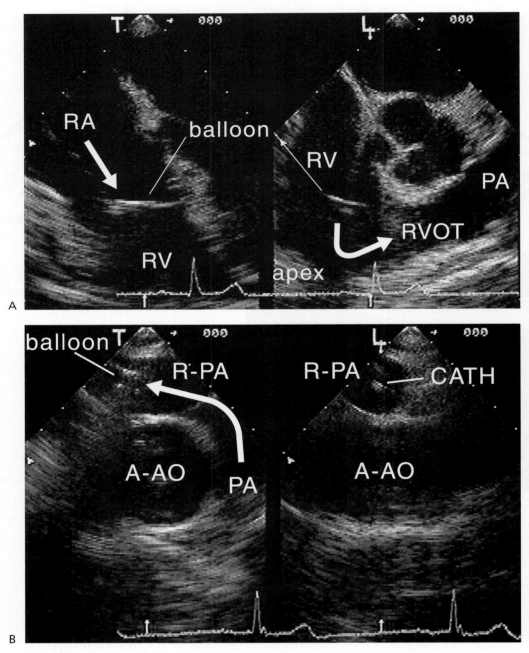

FIGURE 18.6. Guidance of Swan-Ganz catheter placement. **A:** From right atrium (*RA*) to right ventricular outflow tract (*RVOT*). **B:** From main pulmonary artery (*PA*) to the right pulmonary artery (*R-PA*). *RV,* right ventricle; *A-AO,* ascending aorta; *CATH,* catheter.

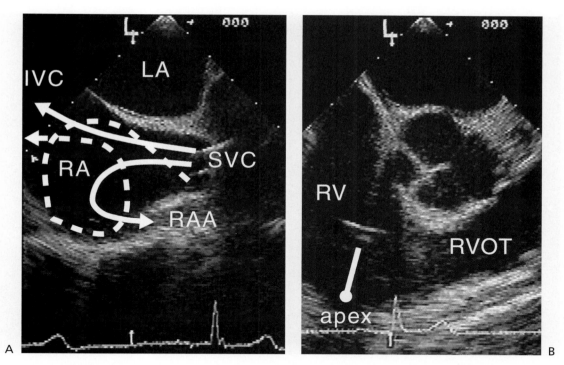

FIGURE 18.7. Pitfalls in placing a Swan-Ganz catheter. **A:** In the right atrium (*RA*). **B:** In the right ventricle (*RV*). *SVC,* superior vena cava; *IVC,* inferior vena cava; *RAA,* right atrial appendage; *RVOT,* right ventricular outflow tract; *LA,* left atrium.

monitor these events and to show when the catheter should be withdrawn. When a ventricular arrhythmia occurs with the catheter tip in the right ventricle, the movement of the balloon should be checked. If the balloon is immobilized at the ventricular apex, the catheter should be withdrawn with the balloon deflated and advanced again. If the balloon is not stuck, the catheter should be quickly advanced further into the pulmonary artery.

ROLE OF TRANSESOPHAGEAL ECHOCARDIOGRAPHY DURING SURGERY

When patients with CHF are undergoing surgery, it is important to achieve the best possible results without (iatrogenic) complications. To this end, one should use TEE to (a) provide as much information as possible for both anesthesiologists and surgeons regarding the causes and mechanisms of CHF as well as associated diseases; (b) avoid pitfalls; (c) guide procedures, which are otherwise invisible from the surgeon; (d) detect unexpected events during surgery and provide information for decision making; and (e) assess the results of surgical intervention immediately following it. This is especially important when a patient with severe hemodynamic instability needs emergency surgery and little information is available preoperatively.

In the following pages, several experiences of managing patients with circulatory derangement are presented.

CASE PRESENTATIONS

Case 1

A 42-year-old man who had undergone mitral valve replacement due to MR 6 years earlier experienced a sudden onset of severe back pain and was transferred to our hospital. Although he was conscious and hemodynamically stable on arrival, he suddenly had a cardiac arrest. Cardiopulmonary resuscitation was started without any diagnosis determined: the most probable diagnoses included aortic dissection, acute myocardial infarction, prosthetic valve dysfunction (stuck valve), and pulmonary embolism.

Computed tomography (CT) was not feasible in this situation. Transesophageal echocardiography under CPR ruled out cardiac tamponade, aortic dissection, and pulmonary embolism within a few minutes. One of two discs of mitral prosthesis appeared to be stuck in the closed position (Fig. 18.8A). Because spontaneous echo contrast was seen in the ascending aorta, I told the doctor to compress the chest more strongly. The disc soon started to open (Fig. 18.8B). A stuck valve was ruled out.

Because of cardiac arrest (standstill), the diagnosis of myocardial infarction could not be made from electrocardiographic (ECG) or echocardiographic findings. It was essential to resume cardiac function. After acidosis and oxygenation was corrected to a normal level under cardiac massage, TEE showed that only a small portion of the LV was fibrillating, although the ECG monitor showed a flat

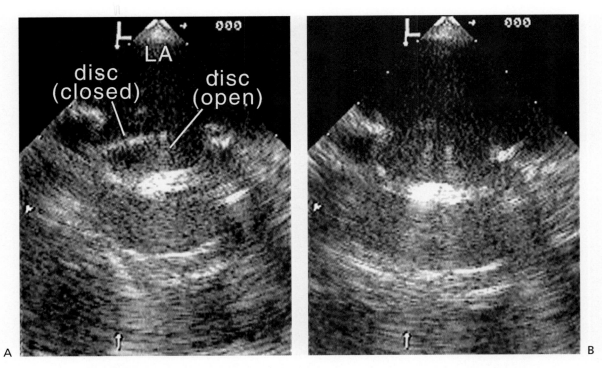

FIGURE 18.8. Pseudo-stuck valve during cardiopulmonary resuscitation. **A:** Under inadequate massage. **B:** With adequate massage, the valve opens. *LA,* left atrium.

line. Direct current (DC) shock successfully defibrillated the heart, and pacing from the body surface was captured. Transesophageal echocardiography demonstrated severe hypokinesis of the anterior wall, suggesting myocardial ischemia as the most probable cause.

Comments

In cardiac arrest, cardiac catheterization is not appropriate because it takes too much effort and time to check only one or two causes among the number of possible causative diseases. In CPR, one should rule out (a) severe hypovolemia, (b) pericardial tamponade, and (c) severe pulmonary embolism because cardiac massage is hardly effective in these situations. The first two can be solved only with rapid infusion and pericardial drainage, respectively. In patients with pulmonary embolisms, percutaneous cardiopulmonary support (PCPS) is the only way to restore an adequate cerebral perfusion. These three situations can be diagnosed or ruled out with TEE. Transesophageal echocardiography is also used for assessing the treatment (cardiac massage, infusion, drainage, etc.) in real time and for guiding placement of the PCPS cannula. When spontaneous echo contrast is seen in the ascending aorta with the cardiac valve closed, it indicates that the massage is inadequate.

Cardiac contraction must be resumed in order for the clinician to examine myocardial ischemia as a cause of cardiac arrest. Transesophageal echocardiography clearly shows whether the heart is fibrillating or in arrest, and it enables the clinician to make the decision to apply DC shock. The ECG

monitor can be misleading. When the heart remains in arrest despite correction of acidosis and hypoxemia, one may attempt pacing. I have experienced several cases in which ventricular pacing was easily instituted with excellent LV contraction despite a misleading ECG.

Case 2

A 64-year-old woman had syncope and fell on the 4th postoperative day after right upper lobectomy. Because she was cyanotic and the pulse was weak with poor oxygenation, she was intubated and transferred to the ICU, but soon had a cardiac arrest. Under CPR, PCPS was introduced with the cannulae inserted into the femoral vessels (Seldinger method) by an experienced physician. However, the systemic blood pressure was as low as 35 mm Hg and oxygenation remained poor.

The patient's condition was still too unstable for her to undergo CT. Despite possible misplacement of cannulae, we hesitated to replace the cannula under transient circulatory arrest without a definite diagnosis. Transesophageal echocardiography showed that (a) the right pulmonary artery was filled with thrombus (Fig. 18.9A) and (b) the right heart was not adequately drained and antegrade blood flow was present in the heart and in the descending aorta (Fig. 18.9B and C). She was diagnosed as having a pulmonary embolism, and the arterial cannula was shown to be misplaced into the femoral vein.

A guidewire was inserted into the contralateral femoral artery. The artery was cannulated after TEE showed the

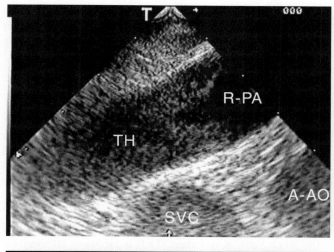

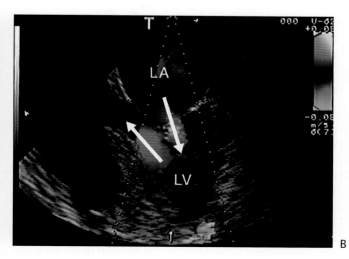

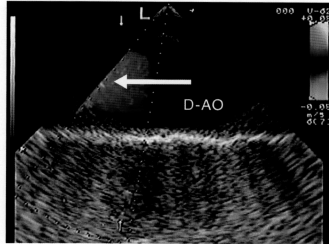

FIGURE 18.9. Transesophageal echocardiography views of case 2. **A:** Thrombus (*TH*) in the right pulmonary artery (*R-PA*). **B:** Unusual antegrade flow in the heart. **C:** Antegrade flow in the descending aorta (*D-AO*). **D:** Guidewire visualized in the D-AO. *A-AO,* ascending aorta; *SVC,* superior vena cava; *LA,* left atium; *LV,* left ventricle.

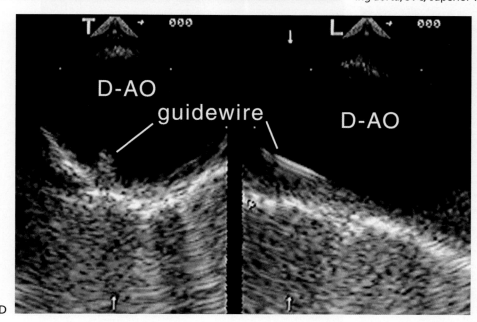

guidewire in the descending aorta (Fig. 18.9D). As soon as PCPS was resumed, cyanosis disappeared and systemic pressure recovered.

Comments

Under CPR, it is not easy to cannulate the femoral vessels correctly. Pulsation under cardiac massage is not reliable for identifying the artery, and the color of blood is misleading. The surgeon should find the guidewire in the descending aorta or inferior vena cava as soon as the vessel is entered. Locating the guidewire rules out both wrong cannulation and the accidental entry of the guidewire into the contralateral iliac vessel or a branch vessel. This process is important to avoid iatrogenic injury of a wrongly entered vessel. Once the venous cannula is advanced, the position of the cannula tip is adjusted to the RA level for the most effective drainage. After PCPS is started, new development of aortic dissection should be ruled out with TEE.

Case 3

A 61-year-old woman who had undergone aortic and mitral valve replacement 6 years before was referred to our hospital with subacute onset of CHF: blood pressure 90 mm Hg, pulse rate 120 beats/min, oxygen partial pressure (PaO_2) 88.7 mm Hg with 2 L/min of oxygen. Chest radiography showed bilateral pleural effusion. A stuck valve was strongly suggested, and TEE was undertaken in the awake state. One of two discs was stuck in the closed position, surrounded by

thrombus (Fig. 18.10). Because she had increasing dyspnea and shock, she was intubated and PCPS was instituted under TEE guidance before she was transferred to the operating room.

Comments

In cases of previous valve replacement, dysfunction of valve prosthesis should be considered as a possible cause of new onset of CHF. In this case, precordial echo showed a small LV and unusual motion of the prosthesis. A stuck valve mitral disc can be suspected by absence of half the mitral flow or an unusually small valve area assessed by continuous-wave Doppler (pressure half-time) by means of precordial echo. However, it cannot show the disc, and the cause of the stuck valve is not clear. TEE is far more effective for diagnosing stuck valve and its cause. When PCPS needs to be introduced before surgery because of hemodynamic instability, misplacement of cannulae can considerably exacerbate the condition. Secure institution under TEE guidance is preferable.

Case 4

A 69-year-old man was diagnosed with CHF caused by aortic stenosis with pressure gradient of 200 mm Hg associated with marked LV hypertrophy by means of precordial echocardiography. Clinicians were unable to advance the catheter into the LV. After induction of anesthesia, TEE revealed moderate aortic regurgitation but no stenosis, as well as LV

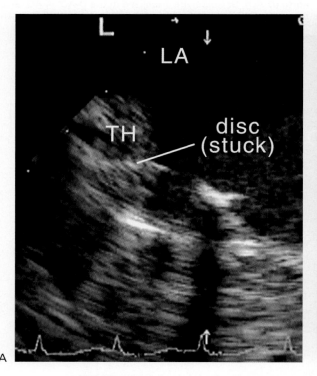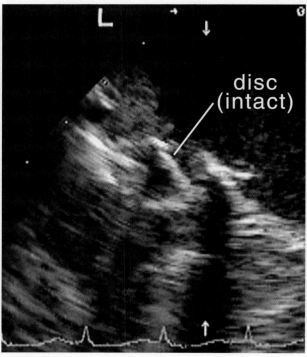

FIGURE 18.10. Stuck valve in case 3. **A:** Diastole. **B:** Systole. *LA,* left atrium; *TH,* thrombus.

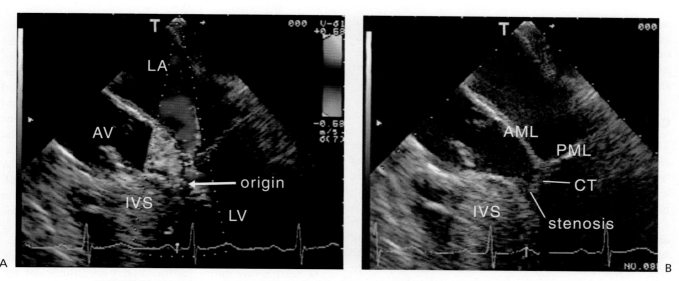

FIGURE 18.11. Left ventricular outflow tract at the chordal level. *AV,* aortic valve; *AML,* anterior mitral leaflet; *PML,* posterior mitral leaflet; *CT,* chorda tendinae; *IVS,* interventricular septum; *LA,* left atrium; *LV,* left ventricle. **A:** The color flow Doppler shows turbulence at the point of obstruction. **B:** The area of stenosis is seen.

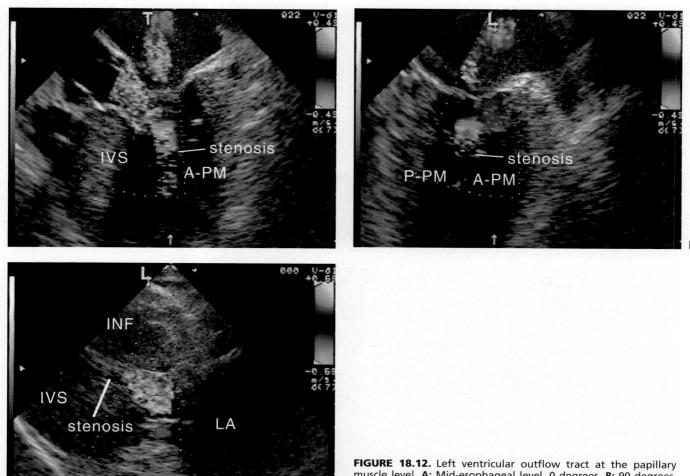

FIGURE 18.12. Left ventricular outflow tract at the papillary muscle level. **A:** Mid-esophageal level, 0 degrees. **B:** 90 degrees. **C:** Transgastric view, 90 degrees. *LA,* left atrium; *A-PM,* anterolateral papillary muscle; *IVS,* interventricular septum; *P-PM,* posteromedial papillary muscle; *INF,* inferior wall.

outflow obstruction. Systolic anterior motion of the mitral leaflet was recognized. Stenosis was localized at the chorda tendinea just below the leaflet where turbulent flow originated (Fig. 18.11). He underwent aortic valve replacement and myectomy of the interventricular septum.

Comment

The site of obstruction in the LV outflow tract varies among individuals. This patient had stenosis at the chordal level. Another patient had stenosis at the papillary muscle level (Fig. 18.12). The LV wall and papillary muscle were markedly hypertrophic and caused stenosis at systole. In such a case, mitral valve replacement may be indicated. TEE is useful for clarifying the exact level of stenosis and making surgical decisions. In case 4, TEE was helpful for guiding the surgeon as to how far the muscle should be resected, and to rule out a postintervention ventricular septal defect.

Case 5

A 40-year-old man underwent coronary artery bypass grafting (CABG) due to an old myocardial infarction. At weaning from bypass, TEE revealed pooled air at the LV apex (Fig. 18.13A). Bright dots appeared in the inferior wall at the basal level (Fig. 18.3B), then spread toward the apex (Fig. 18.13C). The inferior wall became dyskinetic. The myocardium remained brightly echogenic for longer than 1 hour. Weaning from bypass failed twice and an intraaortic balloon pump (IABP) was instituted. It worked, and LV function gradually improved after 2 hours, and the echogenic dots disappeared.

Comment

The period of weaning from cardiopulmonary bypass is risky because the heart is loaded with increasing preload within a short period. If LV reserve is inadequate, CHF will occur. Transesophageal echocardiography clearly shows a dilated LV with poor contraction, associated with MR and dilated LA. Based on the TEE findings as well as pressure data, one should consider putting the patient back on bypass. Because cardiopulmonary bypass reduces preload, the cardiac performance appears to improve. Similarly, when a left ventricular assist device (VAD) is applied to such cases, preexisting MR improves (8). Heart failure during this period is reversible in most cases. TEE is helpful for assessing recovery of cardiac function and making decisions to institute IABP, PCPS, or VAD.

Prevention is of primary importance. Two major causes of heart failure during cardiac surgery are insufficient cardioplegia and air embolism of the coronary artery.

Cardioplegia

For effective and secure myocardial protection, the cardioplegic solution needs to be perfused to the entire myocardium and remain there without being washed out.

In antegrade cardioplegia, one should check for aortic regurgitation because it allows the cardioplegic solution to escape into the LV. Not only is the amount of effective cardioplegic solution reduced, but also the LV is dilated and perfusion of cardioplegic solution is disturbed. Left ventricle venting is needed in such cases. Transesophageal

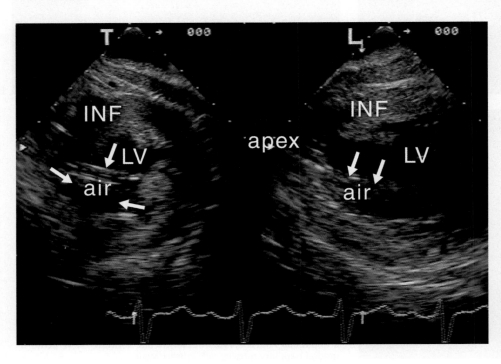

FIGURE 18.13. Coronary air embolism in case 7. Air (*arrow*) is depicted as bright dots in the myocardium. *LV,* left ventricle; *INF,* inferior wall.

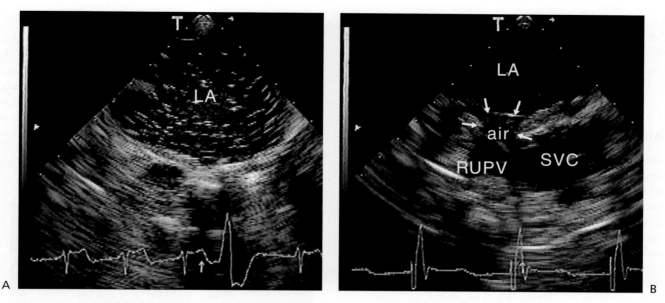

FIGURE 18.14. Retained air in two forms. **A:** The bubble is seen. Note the many echo-dense areas. **B:** The pooled form is seen. Note the concentrated dense area in the roof of the left atrium. *LA,* left atrium; *SVC,* superior vena cava; *RUPV,* right upper pulmonary vein.

echocardiography is helpful for examining both aortic regurgitation and expansion of the LV. In retrograde cardioplegia, one must assure that the coronary sinus cannula stays in place. It may slip back to the RA while the heart is manipulated. The cannula in the coronary sinus can be visualized with TEE.

When the heart resumes beating or fibrillating soon after cardioplegic solution is given, one should check inadequate aortic cross-clamping and poor venous drainage. In the former, blood leaks into the aortic root and washes out the cardioplegic solution. This leak is detected in color Doppler mode. When venous drainage is inadequate, the remaining

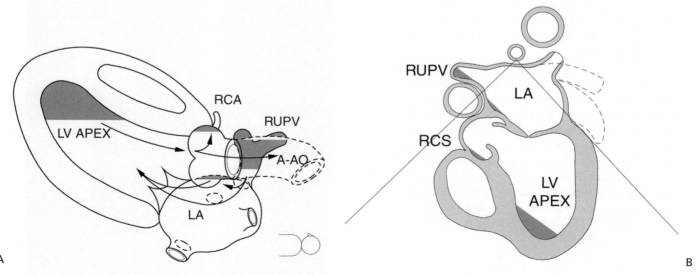

FIGURE 18.15. Common sites of air retention are shown by the shaded areas. **A:** Areas of air retention are shown in a long-axis transgastric diagram. **B:** Areas of air retention are shown in a mid-esophageal diagram. *LV,* left ventricle; *RCA,* right coronary artery; *RUPV,* right upper pulmonary vein; *A-AO,* ascending aorta; *LA,* left atrium; *RCS,* right coronary sinus of Valsalva.

blood enters pulmonary circulation and returns to the LA. Deoxygenated blood enters the coronary artery and cardioplegic solution is replaced. One should check whether the lumens of cardiac chambers have antegrade blood flow in them.

Air Embolism

Air embolism occurs not only in open heart surgery with cardiotomy, but also in CABG, as shown in case 5. Retained air can enter the coronary arteries, especially the right coronary artery, and cause myocardial ischemia. Multiple DC shocks are necessary to defibrillate the heart, heart block is commonly observed, and LV contraction is severely impaired and often associated with MR for longer than 30 minutes. Once coronary air embolism occurs with hemodynamic instability, the patient needs a second pump-run to unload the heart and wash out the air. When air emboli are numerous, they may cause myocardial infarction. In patients undergoing mitral valve repair, one should be careful in assessing severity of MR because it can be influenced by impaired cardiac function.

Transesophageal echocardiography is useful for detecting the presence and location (or even amount) of retained air (9,10). Air is visualized as bubbles or in the pooled form (Fig. 18.14). Figure 18.15 shows the common sites of air retention in the latter form: right upper PV, LV apex, and LA. It amounts to several milliliters. Air emboli are depicted as highly echogenic dots in the myocardium, mainly in the inferior wall, posteromedial papillary muscle, and inferior septum near the atrioventricular node, often associated with atrioventricular block or wall motion abnormalities of the corresponding region. Transesophageal echocardiography is also helpful for guiding elimination of the air by informing the surgeon of the exact site of retention and immediately assessing the results.

When heart failure is sustained and the patient requires institution of an IABP, TEE is helpful for secure placement of the catheter without iatrogenic complications (6,11). As a guidewire is inserted, TEE assures that it is in the descending aorta. This finding rules out (a) an unexpected entry of the guidewire (followed by catheter) into the contralateral iliac artery or other branch arteries and (b) development of a new aortic dissection. Thus, iatrogenic injury to the aorta and its branch artery is avoided. After the catheter is advanced along the guidewire, the position of the catheter tip is adjusted with the help of TEE. After the IABP is started, the cardiac function is monitored.

When heart failure does not improve with the IABP, placement of a VAD is indicated. Transesophageal echocardiography is helpful for monitoring cardiac performance under circulatory assistance, detecting complications such as thrombus formation, and decision making in weaning from the VAD (12–14).

Case 6

A 17-year-old boy underwent an implantable cardioverter defibrillator (ICD) implant due to Brugada syndrome. The endocardial lead was advanced under fluoroscopic guidance. Although the position of the lead tip appeared to be acceptable, the R-wave amplitude was low and pacing threshold was unusually high. It was not clear whether it was due to a myocardial lesion. However, TEE revealed that the lead was in the left hepatic vein, which was only 2 cm from the right ventricle (Fig.18.16A). The lead was withdrawn and

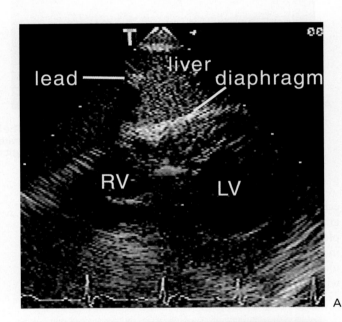

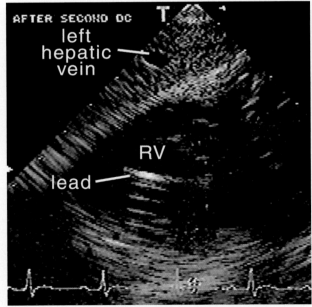

FIGURE 18.16. A: Accidental entry of an implantable cardioverter defibrillator lead into the left hepatic vein. *RV,* right ventricle; *LV,* left ventricle. **B:** Correct positioning of the lead in the RV.

advanced again with the stylet bent more acutely. Transesophageal echocardiography assured that the lead was in the right ventricle (Fig. 18.16B). Every parameter was acceptable.

Comments

An ICD implant is often indicated for patients with CHF, who may experience complications with thrombus formation in the LA or LV. Even a test shock can considerably deteriorate LV function or cause thromboembolism. In another patient, spontaneous echo contrast and small thrombus was found in the LA appendage. After test shock, TEE confirmed that the thrombus stayed there. Transesophageal echocardiography is helpful for monitoring reduced contraction after shock delivery or placement of a lead, which are hardly recognized with the conventional monitoring or imaging system. In the former case, immediate pharmacologic or mechanical intervention would have been needed if the cardiac performance remained low. In the latter case, the hepatic vein would have been injured with the screw or the rigid lead unless TEE detected misplacement of the lead.

Case 7

A 75-year-old woman underwent aortic root replacement due to aortic dissection that involved the right coronary artery, which was revascularized with a saphenous vein graft. At chest closure, systemic blood pressure suddenly decreased. Transesophageal echocardiography revealed reduced wall motion of the inferior wall. Compression of the saphenous vein graft by the drain tube was suspected, and the chest was opened immediately. After the position of the drain was changed, the sternum was closed again. This time, the patient was hemodynamically stable.

Comments

One should be careful at closure of the pericardium and sternum, especially in cases of CHF. When a long pump time is needed, the myocardium is often edematous at the time of chest closure. Even pericardial suture can compress the right ventricle, just as in pericardial tamponade. Sternal closure has a similar effect on the heart. When TEE demonstrates a compressed right heart with low cardiac output, it may be necessary to incise the pleura or leave the sternum open to avoid excessive compression on the right heart.

Accidental obstruction of the coronary graft is another risk at chest closure. It is caused by kinking of the saphenous vein graft or compression of the graft by the drain tube in the pericardial space. Graft trouble can be immediately detected by reduced wall motion of the corresponding region. Transesophageal echocardiography can verify improved wall motion after the cause is removed.

SUMMARY

The role of TEE in managing CHF patients is summarized in the Key Points. Each step of diagnosis, decision making, treatment, and assessment is proceeded with more reliability and safety. This is important especially in treating critically ill patients.

However, some effort is required to gain the needed information. The quality and quantity of information depends on how one considers the patient's condition and how effectively TEE is used. There is definitely a learning curve. *Echo* is a reference to *sound*. Echo information is a reflection of what and how one sounds.

KEY POINTS

- Transesophageal echocardiography can be used to help make a definite diagnosis and rule out the majority of possible diseases, especially when other diagnostic measures are not feasible due to the patient's condition, thus simplifying the tree of decision making.
- Transesophageal echocardiography can be used to detect other pathologies associated with or caused by CHF.
- Transesophageal echocardiography can guide many therapeutic interventions.
- Following therapy, TEE can verify that the clinical decision made was correct and efficacious.

REFERENCES

1. Horstkotte D. Endocarditis: epidemiology, diagnosis and treatment. *Z Kardiol* 2000;89(suppl 4):2–11.
2. Kranidis A, Koulouris S, Filippatos G, et al. Mitral regurgitation from papillary muscle rupture: role of transesophageal echocardiography. *J Heart Valve Dis* 1993;2:529–532.
3. Stoddard MF, Dawkins PR, Prince CR, et al. Left atrial appendage thrombus is not uncommon in patients with acute atrial fibrillation and a recent embolic event: a transesophageal echocardiographic study. *J Am Coll Cardiol* 1995;25:452–459.
4. Siostrzonek P, Koppensteiner R, Gossinger H, et al. Hemodynamic and hemorheologic determinants of left atrial spontaneous echo contrast and thrombus formation in patients with idiopathic dilated cardiomyopathy. *Am Heart J* 1993;125(2 Part 1):430–434.
5. Shen WF, Tribouilloy C, Rida Z, et al. Clinical significance of intracavitary spontaneous echo contrast in patients with dilated cardiomyopathy. *Cardiology* 1996;87:141–146.
6. Orihashi K, Hong YW, Chung G, et al. New applications of two-dimensional transesophageal echocardiography in cardiac surgery. *J Cardiothorac Vasc Anesth* 1991;5:33–39.
7. Orihashi K, Nakashima Y, Sueda T, et al. Usefulness of transesophageal echocardiography for guiding pulmonary artery catheter placement in the operating room. *Heart Vessels* 1994;9:315–321.
8. Holman WL, Bourge RC, Fan P, et al. Influence of left ventricular assist on valvular regurgitation. *Circulation* 1993;88(5 Part 2):309–318.

9. Orihashi K, Matsuura Y, Hamanaka Y, et al. Retained intracardiac air in open heart operation examined by transesophageal echocardiography. *Ann Thorac Surg* 1993;55:1467–1471.
10. Orihashi K, Matsuura Y, Sueda T, et al. Pooled air in open heart operations examined by transesophageal echocardiography. *Ann Thorac Surg* 1996;61:1377–1380.
11. Tatar H, Cicek S, Demirkilic U, et al. Exact positioning of intra-aortic balloon catheter. *Eur J Cardiothorac Surg* 1993;7:52–53.
12. Gruber EM, Seitelberger R, Mares P, et al. Ventricular thrombus and subarachnoid bleeding during support with ventricular assist devices. *Ann Thorac Surg* 1999;67:1778–1780.
13. Mets B. Anesthesia for left ventricular assist device placement. *J Cardiothorac Vasc Anesth* 2000;14:316–326.
14. Scalia GM, McCarthy PM, Savage RM, et al. Clinical utility of echocardiography in the management of implantable ventricular assist devices. *J Am Soc Echocardiogr* 2000;13:754–763.

MITRAL VALVE EVALUATION OF THE PATIENT WITH ISCHEMIC HEART DISEASE

ALEXANDER N. CHAPOCHNIKOV
SOLOMON ARONSON
DAVID JAYAKAR

Mitral regurgitation (MR) that accompanies acute myocardial ischemia or infarction is associated with an unfavorable prognosis for both medical and surgical treatment. It has been reported that up to 41% of coronary artery bypass-grafting (CABG) candidates may also have chronic ischemic mitral insufficiency (1). When the severity of ischemic mitral regurgitation (IMR) necessitates CABG and mitral valve repair or replacement, the combined procedure may lead to significantly increased in-hospital mortality compared with that for CABG alone. This risk is further enhanced in patients over 80 years of age (2). It has previously been demonstrated that CABG alone can lead to reduction of IMR severity (3). On the other hand, significant residual MR after revascularization is associated with increased immediate postoperative and long-term morbidity and mortality (4,5).

The intraoperative severity assessment of residual MR is further complicated by hemodynamic changes related to the effect of general anesthesia and is often underestimated (6). Intraoperative transesophageal echocardiography (TEE) in experienced hands enables precise assessment of the mechanism and may improve intraoperative decision making and patient outcome. This chapter discusses the anatomic and physiologic principles of IMR and reviews the use of TEE in the diagnosis of this condition (7,8).

SCIENTIFIC PRINCIPLES

Prevalence and Outcome

Ischemic MR is present in 7% to 31% of patients undergoing coronary angiography (4,9). In a series of 140 patients with

mitral insufficiency, 26% had IMR (10), with other reported causes of MR in that series being 41% myxomatous degeneration, 17% rheumatic valvular disease, 12% endocarditis, and 2% congenital pathology (Fig. 19.1). The same group reported that among 755 patients who had undergone a primary operation for MR (11), the total operative mortality rate was 4.0%, whereas the mortality rate in the group of patients with combined repair and CABG was 6.6%. Analysis of 150 consecutive patients with IMR undergoing either repair (63%) or replacement has been reported to result in different long-term outcome based on the underlying pathophysiology, rather than the type of procedure (12). It was found that the functional subset of IMR (annular dilatation or restrictive leaflet motion) had the worse long-term (5-year) survival rate (43%) compared with the structural IMR (ruptured chordae or papillary muscle) repair (76%) or structural/replacement groups (89%). The predictor of worse long-term survival (repair of functional IMR) indicates that pathophysiologic mechanisms may be the major determinants of survival, rather than the type of surgical intervention (12). Retrospective analysis of 1,292 patients at the Cleveland Clinic over a 5-year period revealed an overall incidence of IMR of 6.5%, of which 40% had valve prolapse and 60% had restrictive leaflet motion due to regional or global left ventricular (LV) dilatation (13). Forty-two percent of the patients had rheumatic valvular disease; 44% had degenerative valvular disease; and 6% had endocarditis or congenital valve malformation. A mean follow-up (3 ± 1.6 years) interval after repair revealed a superior survival in the patients with valve leaflet prolapse (96%) versus 48% for those with restricted valvular motion (13,14).

In a reported series by Seipelt and colleagues, 262 patients underwent mitral valve operations (replacement, 198; repair, 64) in combination with coronary revascularization. MR was determined to be secondary to coronary artery disease (CAD) in 31% patients (19.5% in-hospital mortality), whereas 53%

A. N. Chapochnikov: Rockford Anesthesiologists Associated; Swedish-American Hospital; and OSF St. Anthony Medical Center, Rockford, Illinois.
S. Aronson: Chicago, Illinois.
D. Jayakar: Department of Cardiac Surgery, University of Chicago, Chicago, Illinois.

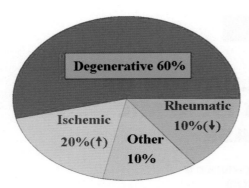

FIGURE 19.1. Prevalence of mitral valve disease. Ischemic etiology is increasing while rheumatic etiology is decreasing in the U.S. population.

of cases had a rheumatic etiology and 16% were attributed to degenerative changes, with a combined in-hospital mortality rate of 6.7% (15). Mitral valve repair was performed in 37% of the patients with IMR versus 19% with rheumatic or degenerative disease. The survival rates (valve-related event-free survival) in the 1st, 5th, and 10th years were 94%, 66%, and 53% in the IMR group, compared with 95%, 76%, and 41% in rheumatic or degenerative group.

The reported in-hospital mortality rate for isolated CABG is 3%, whereas isolated mitral valve procedures carry a reported in-hospital mortality rate of 3% to 7% (16,17).

Combined mitral valve surgery and CABG is associated with a reported in-hospital mortality rate of 7% to 20% (2,16–18), with advanced age of the patients (≥80 years) being described as an independent risk factor leading to increased in-hospital mortality (19.6% vs. 12.2% in younger patients) as well as congestive heart failure (CHF), acute onset of ischemia requiring intensive care, LV end-diastolic pressure greater than 15 Torr, and New York Heart Association class IV (2,8).

Investigators have reported that patients with grade 2 or less ischemic MR (group I) who underwent CABG alone had reduced angina pectoris and improved functional status equal to CABG patients without MR (group II) (19). In that series, IMR patients were older and had lower preoperative LV ejection fraction (42% vs. 58%). The 30-day mortality rates were similar (4.5% in both groups), as were the survival rates at 1 year (91% vs. 93%) and 3 years (84% vs. 88%). The severity grade of MR increased in 2% of the patients and was unchanged in 36% (19).

At the Society of Cardiovascular Anesthesiologists (SCA) Annual Meeting in April 2002, it was reported that isolated off-pump coronary artery bypass (OPCAB) may offer improvement and resolution of mild IMR (20). A total of 144 patients undergoing OPCAB were evaluated retrospectively. Sixteen of 144 required conversion to cardiopulmonary bypass (CPB), and 5 patients among them had moderate IMR. Of the remaining 128 patients who tolerated the OPCAB procedure, 109 were examined by preoperative, in-

traoperative, and postoperative echocardiography. Fourteen patients were excluded from the study because nonischemic mitral valve pathology was found. Forty-eight of 109 patients (44%) had varied degrees of IMR, 11 patients (10%) had moderate IMR, 37 patients (34%) had mild or trace IMR, and none had severe IMR. Three of five patients with moderate IMR who required conversion to CPB died postoperatively due to low output syndrome and respiratory failure. Postoperative transthoracic echocardiography (TTE) or TEE revealed no improvement in IMR degree in four of these five patients. The patients with moderate IMR who tolerated OPCAB had postoperative TTE at 1 to 35 weeks, which showed improvement in MR severity in 9 of 11. All had functional improvement. No deaths were reported in the moderate IMR OPCAB group. The researchers concluded that OPCAB patients with moderate IMR who required conversion to on-pump CABG represented a high-risk group, whereas patients with moderate or less IMR who tolerated OPCAB appeared to benefit from revascularization alone. This may be important in the subgroup of patients with IMR and perioperative risk, which strongly preclude aortic occlusion and initiation of CPB (20).

Anatomy

The mitral valve (MV) is a complex structure consisting of two leaflets (posterior and anterior), the chordal structures (primary, secondary, and tertiary), the papillary muscles [anterolateral (AL) and posteromedial (PM)], and the ventricular wall extending between the base of the PM papillary muscle insertion and the annulus of the MV. While the LV remains in systole, the leaflets come together, forming the coaptation point, which along with AL and PM commissures create a "line of coaptation."

The posterior leaflet consists of three scallops: medial, middle, and lateral. The corresponding portions of the anterior leaflet are medial, middle, and lateral thirds. The chordae, which consist of connective tissue (mainly collagen bundles), extend from the head of each papillary muscle to the nearest half of each leaflet.

The primary chordae attach to the tip of the leaflet, the secondary chordae attach to the mid-portion of the leaflet, and the tertiary chordae attach to the base of the leaflet or mitral annulus. These tertiary chordae (also referred to as "stay" chordae) form a posterior chordal structure that has a stabilizing function. Interruption of the tertiary chordae due to ischemic/necrotic rupture in the corresponding myocardial zone (including papillary muscle) will have a significant impact on the maintenance of normal LV geometry and ventricular function. The number of papillary muscle heads varies from one to five.

The blood supply to the PM papillary muscle was provided by one vessel (either right coronary artery or obtuse marginal artery) in 63% of the patients and two vessels in 37% (21). The AL papillary muscle had a double-vessel blood supply (obtuse marginal and diagonal) in 71% and single-vessel supply in 29%. In a study that included 20 patients monitored by TEE during coronary surgery, selective coronary graft injections of sonicated albumin microbubbles were performed to assess graft patency and papillary muscle perfusion. It was demonstrated that in the subgroup of 10 patients with an old inferior myocardial infarction (MI), MR was present only among those 6 with a single rather than a double blood supply.

Presently used nomenclature systems include both Carpentier classification, where the posterior MV leaflet is divided into P1, P2, and P3 (lateral, middle, and medial) scallops and the Duran classification (22). The latter uses a P1, PM, P2 for the same scallops, respectively, where the middle scallop is subdivided into the PM1 and PM2 with regard to the chordae that come from the corresponding AL papillary muscle (PM1) or the PM papillary muscle (PM2). The anterior leaflet (comprising 60%–70% of the mitral valve area and 30% of the annular circumference) is also divided differently. The Carpentier classification provides A1, A2, and A3 nomenclature (lateral, middle, medial) segments, respectively, versus a division into A1 and A2 portions (by Duran classification) with the corresponding papillary muscles attached via chordae. The specific approach to the anterior leaflet division may reflect different mitral regurgitant pathophysiology and a different approach from the surgical standpoint. The American Society of Echocardiography and the SCA incorporate the anatomic classification represented by the Carpentier scheme. Mitral valve regurgitation may be caused by malfunctioning of any component of the mitral valve apparatus. Chronic regurgitation leads to dilatation of the left atrium (LA) and the annulus, which loses its physiologic elliptoid shape during systole. The resulting circular annulus portends poor leaflet coaptation and MR. Increased LA dimension suggests an advanced degree of MR, although smaller dimensions do not exclude insufficiency.

Mechanism

Mitral regurgitation as a primary complication of ischemic heart disease was initially described by Burch and De Pasquale in 1963, when they recognized papillary muscle dysfunction as a primary consequence of ischemia (23).

There are many ways to classify IMR, for example, acute versus chronic, or by underlying pathology such as CAD with annular dilatation, CAD with ischemic or infarcted papillary muscles, or CAD with restrictive chordae or leaflet pathology with or without annular dilatation (24). The classification of mitral valve insufficiency proposed by Alain Carpentier included a description as follows: Type I: pure dilatation of the annulus, leaflet motion normal, leaflet perforation may be present; Type II: leaflet prolapse due to chordal rupture or elongation or papillary muscle rupture or elongation; and Type III: restricted leaflet motion due to posterior papillary muscle dysfunction in conjunction with LV dysfunction (25).

Acute transient MR during ischemic episode occurs primarily due to leaflet restriction as a result of ventricular dyskinesia, rather than of annular dilatation (26). Segmental asynergy of the LV wall was found in up to 96% of the patients with acute severe MR. The inferior wall was impaired in 86% (Fig. 19.2) (27).

It is important to distinguish IMR that is described in the context of other organic causes of MR from the IMR described among patients with CAD and no primary organic mitral valve disease. The latter type may be as high as 57%, with prevalence up to 90% represented by incomplete mitral leaflet closure in patients with acute MI and acute IMR (14).

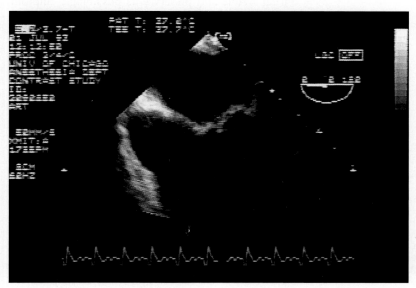

FIGURE 19.2. Prolapsed posterior leaflet of the mitral valve. Magnified view of left atrium and coapted mitral valve leaflets forming a chevron shape.

The current understanding about the mechanism of IMR after acute MI involves consideration of unbalanced ventricular forces, changes in papillary muscle geometry, asymmetric widening of the annulus, expansion of the border zone myocardium, and early systolic leaflet loitering.

The normal saddle shape of the valve promotes caudal opening, with less force required to open the valve than to close it (Fig. 19.3) (28). The diastolic LA pressure to LV pressure gradient determines the rate of mitral valve leaflet opening. The rate of change of the early systolic LV to LA pressure gradient affects (in part) the degree of mitral leaflet closure. If this gradient is low (as seen with LV dysfunction), then MR will occur. This principle was examined by Dent et al. (28) when global LV function was changed by altering the left main coronary artery flow while maintaining constant LA pressure. Left ventricular end-systolic dimension and peak positive LV rate of pressure development (dP/dt) correlated well with the degrees of mitral leaflet opening and closure. They concluded that LV systolic function determines the extent (both opening and closure) of mitral leaflet excursion (28).

Papillary muscle dynamics also play a significant role in proper mitral leaflet closure in normal hearts. In a diseased heart, even a preexisting single blood supply to the PM papillary muscle can uncommonly lead to its necrosis. On the other hand, the consequent LV systolic dysfunction of ischemia may significantly contribute to the geometry changes of the mitral valve apparatus. The tethering distance (Fig. 19.4) between an ischemic PM papillary muscle tip and the anterior annulus has been measured experimentally. Initial inferior ischemia alone produced papillary muscle tip retraction with restricted closure and mild to moderate MR

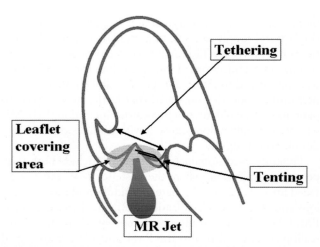

FIGURE 19.4. Echocardiography-derived indices to assess ischemic mitral regurgitation include tethering (the distance between the posteromedial papillary muscle and the anterior annulus), tenting height (the distance of the mitral valve leaflet from the tip to the hinge point of restrictive motion), leaflet covering area, and mitral valve regurgitant jet area. *MR,* mitral regurgitation.

(regurgitant fraction, 25%), whereas the addition of papillary muscle ischemia consistently decreased MR and tethering distance. It was concluded that papillary muscle contractile dysfunction paradoxically decreased MR because the inferobasal ischemia reduced leaflet tethering and improved coaptation (29).

The otherwise normal constant distance between the tip of the papillary muscle and the annulus may become variable in ischemic heart disease, whereas the papillary muscle tip to the leaflet edge distance (determined by the length of the primary chorda) remains constant despite the presence of ischemic changes. If the primary chorda is intact, tethering of the leaflet edges occur, which leads to restrictive leaflet closure and MR (Fig. 19.5). The annulus area normally decreases by 25% during systole and preserves its physiologic elliptoid shape. Most changes in annulus shape are posterior.

Komeda and associates used an acute ischemic dog model along with radiopaque markers and simultaneous biplane videofluoroscopy to evaluate annular dimensions during regional (posterolateral wall) LV ischemia (30). They demonstrated that end-systolic mitral annulus area increased (4.9 vs. 5.9 cm²) and IMR occurred in an asymmetric manner, with the most anterior annular segment lengths not changed. Markedly increased radial dislocation of PM papillary muscle at end-systole, dilatation (in the septal-lateral direction) of the mitral annulus, and AL apical motion (tethering) of the posterior mitral leaflet all led to MR. Based on these data, it might seem that an initial procedure of choice would be a ring annuloplasty provided that TEE assessment revealed no leaflet prolapse. The ring annuloplasty, although causing augmentation of leaflet coaptation, may in some circumstances not completely eliminate MR due to the fact that it does not normalize the radial displacement of the posterior

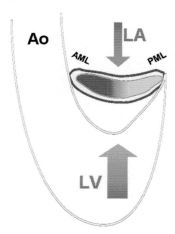

FIGURE 19.3. The saddle-shaped mitral valve requires greater force to move the leaflets cephalad than caudad. Ischemic mitral regurgitation also may occur when the pressure gradient between the left ventricle and the left atria during early systole is low due to increased left atrial end-diastolic pressure, or diminished left ventricular early systolic pressure. *AML,* anterior mitral leaflet; *PML,* posterior mitral leaflet; *LA,* left atrium; *LV,* left ventricle; *Ao,* aorta.

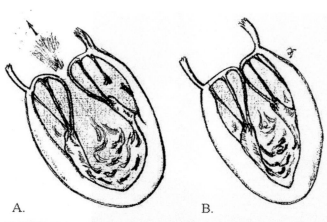

FIGURE 19.5. Mechanisms of ischemic mitral regurgitation are attributable to apical tethering of the left ventricle resulting in restricted mitral valve leaflet motion and poor leaflet coaptation. The annulus is apically displaced due to chordae tendineae retaining their length constant between the tips of the leaflets and the papillary muscles **(A)**. The normal mitral valve apparatus is demonstrated **(B)**.

mitral leaflet and the PM papillary tips in the radial direction. Thus, the tethering effect may not be eliminated, and an additional procedure such as chordal extension (or replacement with expanded synthetic chordae), posterior papillary muscle elongation, or even excision of the posterior LV wall between the PM bases may be necessary.

The Surgical Anterior Ventricular Endocardial Restoration (SAVER) trial has demonstrated that surgical anterior ventricular endocardial restoration can be used for remodeling the dysfunctional and dilated anterior portion of the LV after anterior MI (31). In this important series of 439 patients, concomitant CABG was performed in 89% and mitral repair in 22%. Mitral valve replacement was necessary in 4% of the patients.

Gorman and associates in an acute infarction sheep model demonstrated that circumflex coronary artery occlusion (which subtended 32% of the posterior LV) produced acute 2 to 3+ MR. Sonomicrometry transducers implanted around the mitral annulus and the tips and bases of papillary muscles revealed that the mitral annulus was dilated asymmetrically orthogonal to the line of leaflet coaptation. Although annular area increase was rather small (9.2%), when combined with tethering of the leaflet scallops, it was sufficient to produce moderate to severe MR (32).

Radiopaque markers sutured around the mitral annulus, to the central free mitral leaflet edges, and to both papillary muscle tips and bases again helped reveal changes in mitral annular dimensions and leaflet closing dynamics in pre- and postinduction of acute ischemia (33). During control (preischemic phase), leaflet coaptation occurred 23 msec after end-diastole, whereas during ischemia (with LV dysfunction) coaptation was delayed to 115 msec after end-diastole with MR occurring. Mitral annulus area was also 14% larger during ischemic conditions compared with control measure-

ments. In that experimental model, the posterior papillary muscle tip was displaced laterally and posteriorly, but no apical displacement was noted. "Loitering" of the leaflets associated with posterior mitral annulus enlargement and circularization led to incomplete mitral leaflet coaptation during early systole, not at end-systole (33). This early systolic mitral annular dilatation and shape change, as well as altered posterior papillary muscle motion, should be considered as one of the mechanisms by which incomplete mitral leaflet coaptation occurs during acute IMR.

Carpentier and associates showed that mitral valve incompetence could not be produced by infiltrating the papillary muscle with formaldehyde. In order to get MR, it was also necessary to infiltrate the myocardial wall that supports the papillary muscle. These experimental findings were revealed when Dr. Carpentier commented on a similar conclusion made by Llaneras et al. (34).

The role of an LV shape in the development of functional MR in heart failure was demonstrated by Sabbah and associates (35). Global LV shape changes were induced in dogs by multiple sequential intracoronary microembolizations. Sixty-one percent of animals developed 1+ to 3+ MR during heart failure. End-systolic sphericity index increased 72%. Animals without MR were found with only a 30% increase of the same index. These data support the concept of spherical LV shape as a determinant of functional MR (35–37). The same group of researchers (35) commented on the mechanism of functional MR with the emphasis on the LV chamber enlargement and LV reshaping along with papillary muscle dysfunction, regional LV wall motion abnormalities, and dilatation of the mitral valve annulus (38).

The concept of simultaneous ischemic impairment of the anterior papillary muscle and mitral annulus dilatation contributing to clinically significant MR remains controversial. In a sheep model it was shown that simultaneous mitral annular dilatation and anterior papillary muscle dislocation produced no MR (39). Implanted radiopaque markers with biplane videofluoroscopy revealed significantly increased (11%–13%) mitral valve area 1 week after chemical obliteration of the anterior annular and leaflet muscles. Exclusive intercommissural axis increase and AL displacement of the anterior papillary muscle tip were noted at end-systole with displacement toward the mitral annulus. The posterior papillary muscle geometry remained unchanged. The presence of biaxial annular enlargement resulted in MR, which suggested that septolateral axis elongation (as observed with proximal circumflex coronary artery occlusion) may play a role in development of clinically significant IMR. It was reported that ischemia delays leaflet coaptation and shifts it to the late end-diastole (40). Ischemia was also associated with a significant increase in end-diastolic annular area (8.0 vs. 6.7 cm^2) and septal-lateral annular diameter (2.9 vs. 2.5 cm, $p = 0.02$).

The importance of mitral annulus dynamics was described during rapid atrial pacing as a close link was shown to

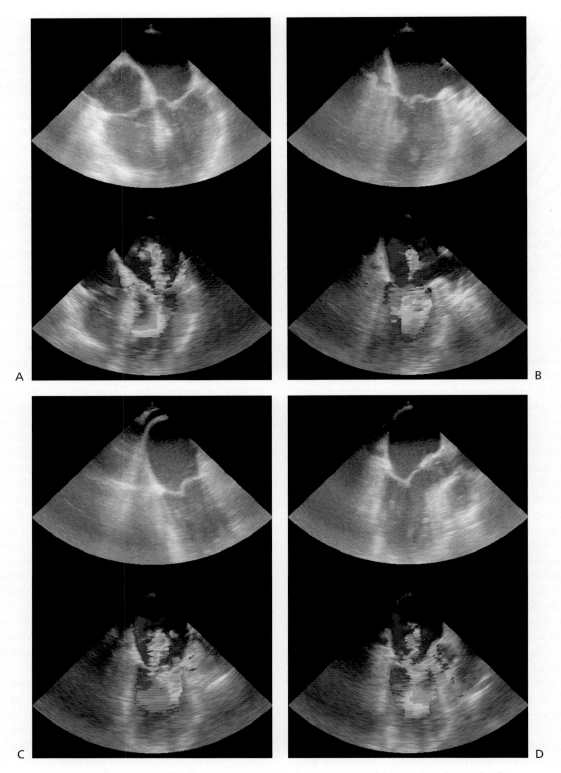

FIGURE 19.6. Tomographic planes of the mitral valve apparatus with corresponding color-flow Doppler (*CFD*) images are demonstrated. There are mid-esophageal (*ME*) four-chamber view **(A)**, ME commissural view **(B)**, ME two-chamber view **(C)**, ME long-axis view **(D)**, and transgastric short-axis view (*TG SAX*) **(E)**.   (*continued*)

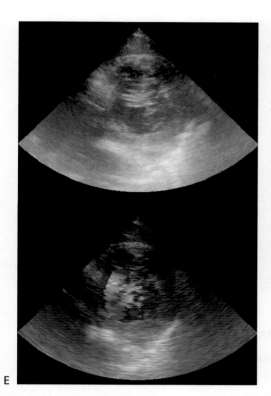

E

FIGURE 19.6. (*continued*) The central regurgitant jet is visualized in all views. The TG SAX CFD image may suggest the anatomic location of the jet regarding the posterior leaflet scallops. Of note, complete analysis of the severity of the regurgitant jet requires evaluation of the proximal isovelocity surface area and pulmonary vein flow pattern.

exist between mitral annulus area reduction and LA volume reduction during diastole. Rapid pacing at 140 per minute helped to reliably couple a minimum mitral annulus area and LA volume (41). Annuloplasty has been shown in animal models to decrease the distance from the papillary muscle tip to the annulus in control and ischemic conditions (42).

The chronic phase seen in postinfarcted myocardium is characterized by its dilatation and an increased distance from the tip of papillary muscles to the tip of the leaflets. Progression of MR parallels changes in LV geometry where increased leaflet tethering, leaflet tenting, and leaflet restriction take place. Restoring this tethering geometry toward normal, using ventricular remodeling procedures, has been demonstrated (43). During 8 weeks of observation following ligation of the circumflex coronary artery, LV dilatation was noted, as was a shift of the papillary muscles posteriorly and mediolaterally. The leaflet tethering distance increased with the progression of MR. By multiple regression analysis it was shown that the only independent predictor of MR was tethering distance.

The paradoxic decrease in IMR with papillary muscle dysfunction was reported in an animal model (29). Three-dimensional (3D) echocardiography was used to measure the tethering distance between the ischemic PM papillary

muscle tip and anterior annulus. Initial inferior ischemia alone produced papillary muscle tip retraction with restricted closure and mild to moderate MR (regurgitant fraction, 25%). However, adding papillary muscle ischemia consistently decreased MR and tethering distance. It was concluded that papillary muscle contractile dysfunction could paradoxically decrease MR from inferobasal ischemia by reducing leaflet tethering and improving coaptation.

The multiple mechanisms of IMR suggest that our understanding of this subject continue to evolve. Clinical decision making regarding the type of repair may be difficult. Annular ring implantation alone (rigid vs. flexible with the intention to preserve the elliptoid shape during mitral annular dynamics) or with the addition of leaflet or subvalvular procedures as well as possible LV wall remodeling all should be based on comprehensive understanding of the underlying mechanisms.

THE ECHOCARDIOGRAPHIC EXAMINATION

Two-dimensional (2D) TEE enables the mitral valve to be seen in several tomographic planes [mid-esophageal (ME) four-chamber, commissural, two-chamber, long-axis, and transgastric short-axis (TG SAX) views] (Fig. 19.6).

Pulsed-wave (PW) Doppler and color-flow Doppler imaging of the LA will delineate the regurgitant jet. Fine manipulation of the TEE probe allows inspection of the mitral valve in the aforementioned planes. Transgastric short-axis reveals the mitral valve and mitral annulus with the P3 scallop as the uppermost on the screen (the closest to the TEE probe). The ME images (two- and four-chamber views) allow focusing on the specific scallops of the posterior leaflet and the specific regions of the anterior leaflet. These views also survey the motion of the leaflets relative to the annulus. In these views the leaflet coaptation point below the annulus gives the classic appearance of the chevron (Fig. 19.7).

A systematic study of these views often reveals the mechanism of injury. Elongated chordae may lead to prolapse of one or both leaflets. Marked prolapse of the affected leaflet may have a "flail" appearance in the direction of the LA. Flail leaflets are commonly caused by ruptured chordae and less commonly by infarcted and ruptured papillary muscle. Ruptured primary or secondary chordae may be seen as a fluttering thin structure in the LA during systole. In contrast, shorter tertiary chordae or just elongated chordae do not prolapse into the LA during systole, but rather appear as an excessively mobile structure near the tip of the leaflets during diastole. The presence of a flail leaflet helps to distinguish isolated severe mitral leaflet prolapse with intact chordae from the ruptured subvalvular structures.

Infarcted papillary muscle in combination with infarction of the nearest LV myocardium also may lead to the regurgitation. This happens secondary to a lack of the tethering

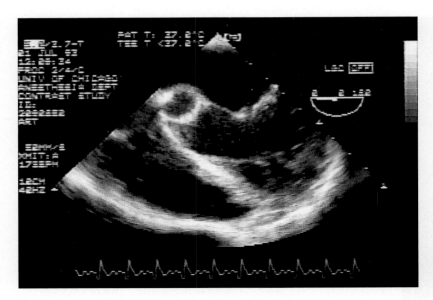

FIGURE 19.7. Classic chevron shape of coapted mitral valve leaflets in a long-axis view. The posterior leaflet prolapses into the left atrium.

function normally performed by this myocardial structures. On the other hand, when this dilated myocardial segment is moving dyskinetically, it prevents proper coaptation of the leaflets during systole. Echocardiographic findings such as papillary muscle atrophy with increased echogenicity on the SAX view, thinning of the adjacent myocardium, or akinetic or dyskinetic motion during systole indicate a previously infarcted state. Of note, postinfarction changes (connective tissue development) of papillary muscle with its subsequent shrinkage may lead to the retraction of chordal structure and regurgitation.

Severity of MR assessed with intraoperative TEE and postoperative TTE has been compared. Intraoperative TEE assessment tends to downgrade evaluation of MR severity (5). It has been observed that systolic blood pressure, mean arterial pressure, and LV end-diastolic and end-systolic dimensions become significantly lower during the intraoperative TEE examination compared with the preoperative TEE examination (5,6). Although preoperative assessment of severity may be preferable when deciding whether to perform mitral valve surgery (6), intraoperative TEE evaluation is critical in order to determine the mechanism of MR and guide a strategy for repair.

Phenylephrine may help increase the patient's blood pressures to preoperative values and provide an adequate hemodynamic environment for the intraoperative MR grading.

Three-dimensional echocardiography has been used to evaluate mechanism of disease (44). Real-time 3D echocardiography of LV function after infarct exclusion surgery for ischemic cardiomyopathy has been reported as an excellent quantitative assessment mode for changes in LV volume and function after complex LV reconstruction. Currently 3D echocardiography and real-time 3D echocardiography are labor-intensive and time-consuming manipulations and not yet available for widespread intraoperative application.

CLINICAL INFORMATION

Case 1

A 75-year-old man with hypertension, unstable angina, and diabetes mellitus had a history of inferior wall MI and a preoperative electrocardiogram (ECG) showing a Q wave in leads II, III, and aVF. Preoperative cardiac catheterization revealed 80% stenosis of the left ascending artery, total stenosis of the first marginal artery, and total stenosis of the proximal right coronary artery. Before \ c bypass, TEE revealed severely hypokinetic inferior septal, inferior, and inferoposterior segments in the SAX view and apical, middle, and inferobasal segments in the long-axis view. Color Doppler imaging showed mild to moderate MR originating from the site of the PM commissure shown in the two-chamber view (Fig. 19.8). The mitral annulus was slightly dilated (3.5-cm diameter in the three-chamber view). Pulmonary venous systolic flow was normal. The patient underwent CABG to the left anterior descending artery, the first marginal artery, and the posterior descending artery. The patient was weaned from bypass without inotropic therapy. After CABG, TEE showed improvement of all inferior segments and only trivial MR (Fig. 19.9). The postoperative course was uneventful.

Case 2

A 73-year-old woman had a history of inferior wall MI and a preoperative ECG showing a Q wave in leads II, III, and aVF. Preoperative cardiac catheterization revealed 80% stenosis of the left main trunk, 90% stenosis of the left circumflex artery, and 90% stenosis of the proximal right coronary artery. Ejection fraction was 50%. Before CPB, TEE revealed an akinetic inferior septal segment; hypokinetic inferior, inferoposterior, and posterolateral segments in the SAX view (Fig. 19.10);

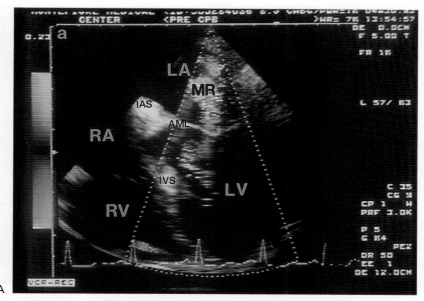

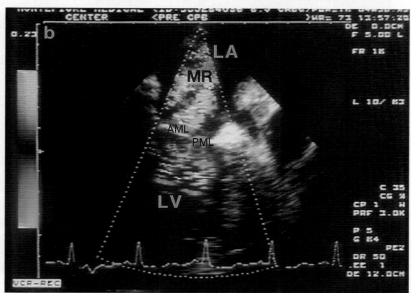

FIGURE 19.8. Color Doppler imaging shows mild to moderate mitral regurgitation in the three chamber view **(A)** originating from the site of the posteromedial commissure in the two-chamber view **(B)**. *MR,* mitral regurgitation; *LA,* left atrium; *RA,* right atrium; *LV,* left ventricle; *RV,* right ventricle; *IAS,* interatrial septum; *IVS,* interventricular septum; *AML,* anterior mitral leaflet; *PML,* posterior mitral leaflet.

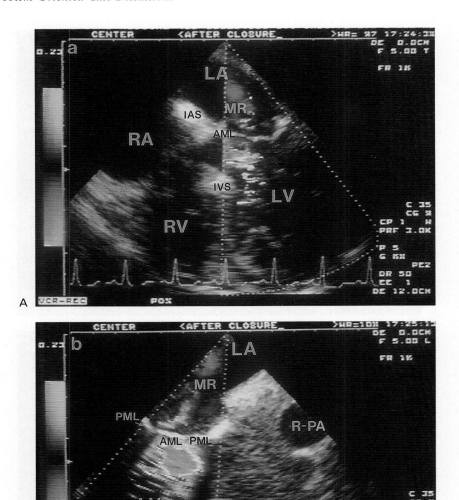

FIGURE 19.9. Color Doppler imaging shows trivial mitral regurgitation in the three-chamber view **(A)** originating from the site of the posteromedial commissure in the two-chamber view **(B)**. *MR,* mitral regurgitation; *LA,* left atrium; *RA,* right atrium; *RV,* right ventricle; *LV,* left ventricle; *IAS,* interatrial septum; *IVS,* interventricular septum; *AML,* anterior mitral leaflet; *PML,* posterior mitral leaflet; *R-PA,* right pulmonary artery.

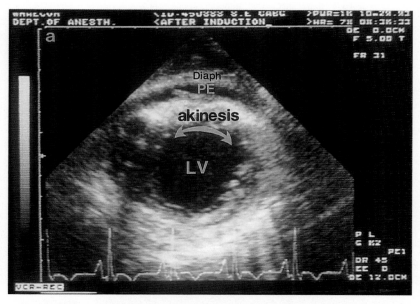

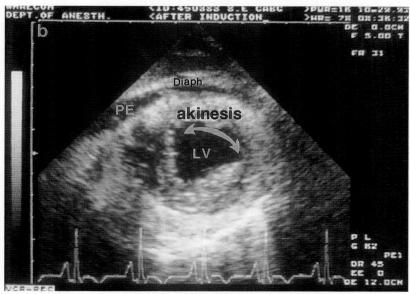

FIGURE 19.10. Short-axis view of the left ventricle (*LV*) in the transverse scan at end-diastole **(A)** and end-systole **(B)**. *Arrow* shows akinetic inferior septum (*IS*), inferior (*I*), inferoposterior (*IP*), and posterolateral segments of the LV. *Diaph,* diaphragm; *PE,* pericardial effusion.

and akinetic apical, middle, and inferobasal segments in the long-axis view (Fig. 19.11). Color Doppler imaging showed severe MR originating from the site of the PM commissure (Fig. 19.12), and decreased pulmonary venous systolic flow (systolic < diastolic) was noted in PW Doppler mode (Fig. 19.13). The mitral annulus was mildly dilated (3.7 cm diameter in the three-chamber view). An intraaortic balloon pump was placed before the CPB, but akinetic wall motion and severe MR did not improve. The patient underwent CABG using veins to the left anterior descending artery and the first marginal artery. After the patient was initially weaned from bypass, MR was still severe (Fig. 19.14) and wall motion of all inferior segments was still akinetic. The patient underwent

another bypass and annuloplasty was added. She was weaned from bypass with inotropic therapy (epinephrine, amrinone) and intraaortic balloon pump. After CABG, color Doppler imaging showed remarkably reduced MR (Fig. 19.15) associated with normalization (systolic > diastolic) of the pulmonary venous systolic flow (Fig. 19.16). Transesophageal echocardiography also revealed a little improvement of inferior septal and posterolateral segments in the SAX view and the inferobasal segment in the long-axis view, but other inferior segments were still akinetic. The diameter of the mitral annulus was shown as 3.1 cm in the three-chamber view. The postoperative course was uneventful without complications.

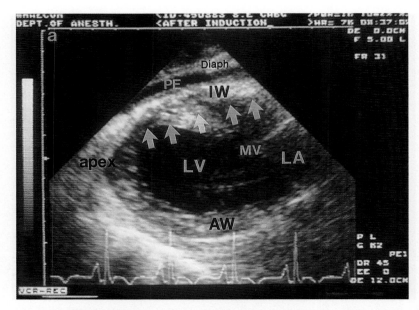

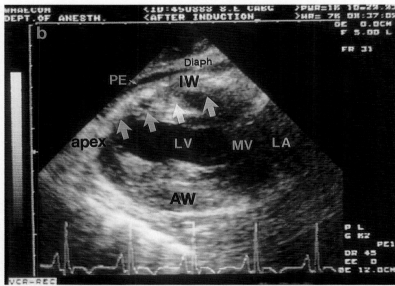

FIGURE 19.11. Long-axis view of the left ventricle (*LV*) in the longitudinal scan at end-diastole **(A)** and end-systole **(B)**. *Arrows* show akinetic apical, middle, and basal-inferior segments of the LV. *LA,* left atrium; *LV,* left ventricle; *MV,* mitral valve; *AW,* anterior wall; *IW,* inferior wall; *PE,* pericardial effusion; *Diaph,* diaphragm.

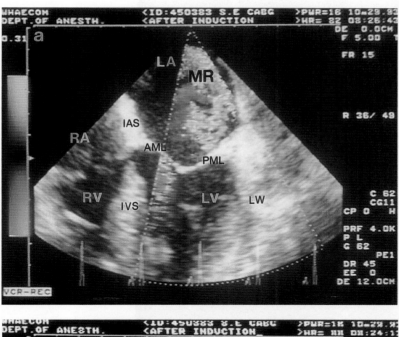

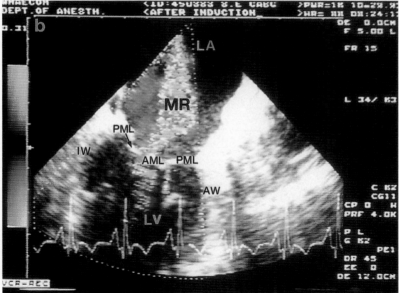

FIGURE 19.12. Color Doppler imaging shows severe mitral regurgitation originating from the posteromedial commissure in the three-chamber view **(A)** and the two-chamber view **(B)**. *MR,* mitral regurgitation; *LA,* left atrium; *RA,* right atrium; *RV,* right ventricle; *LV,* left ventricle; *IAS,* interatrial septum; *IVS,* interventricular septum; *AML,* anterior mitral leaflet; *PML,* posterior mitral leaflet; *LW,* lateral wall; *AW,* anterior wall; *IM,* inferior wall.

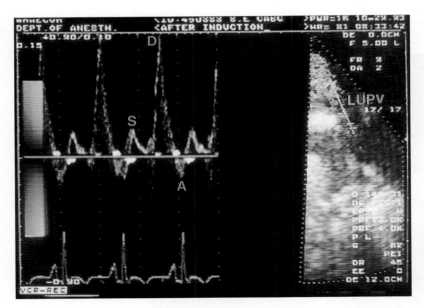

FIGURE 19.13. Decreased left pulmonary venous systolic flow compared with diastolic flow in the pulsed-wave mode. Negative velocity **(A)** is seen just after the D wave. *S*, peak pulmonary venous systolic filling; *D*, peak pulmonary venous diastolic filling; *LUPV*, left upper pulmonary vein.

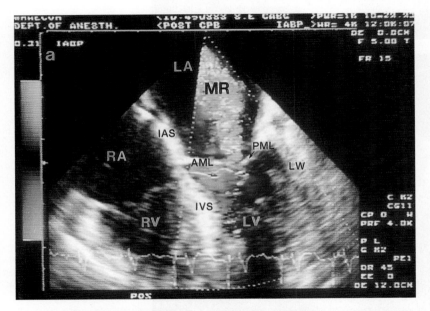

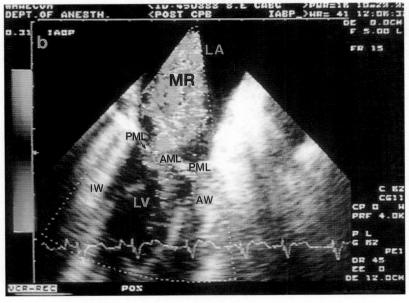

FIGURE 19.14. After revascularization, color Doppler imaging continues to show severe mitral regurgitation originating from the site of postero-medial commissure in the four-chamber view **(A)** and the two-chamber view **(B)** after initial weaning from the bypass. *MR*, mitral regurgitation; *LA*, left atrium; *RA*, right atrium, *RV*, right ventricle; *LV*, left ventricle; *IAS*, interatrial septum; *IVS*, interventricular septum; *AML*, anterior mitral leaflet; *PML*, posterior mitral leaflet; *LW*, lateral wall; *AW*, anterior wall; *IW*, inferior wall.

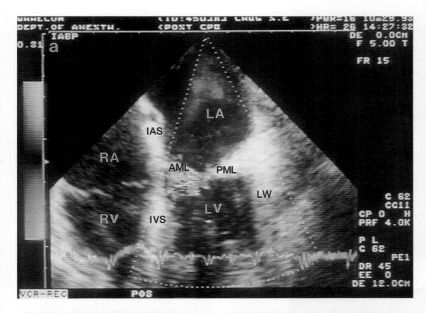

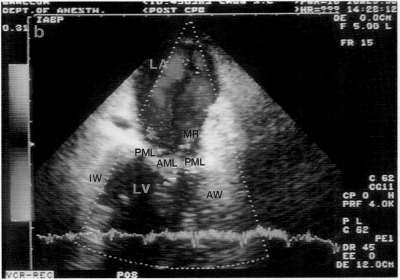

FIGURE 19.15. Color Doppler imaging shows trivial mitral regurgitation in the four-chamber view **(A)** and the two-chamber view **(B)** after annuloplasty. *MR,* mitral regurgitation; *LA,* left atrium; *RA,* right atrium; *RV,* right ventricle; *LV,* left ventricle; *AML,* anterior mitral leaflet; *PML,* posterior mitral leaflet; *IAS,* interatrial septum; *IVS,* interventricular septum; *LW,* lateral wall; *AW,* anterior wall; *IW,* inferior wall.

CLINICAL DECISION MAKING

Because of the increased risks associated with mitral valve surgery in ischemic heart disease, TEE has been used to assess the underlying mechanisms of injury of the mitral valve apparatus and to guide the formulation of a surgical plan (45–47). Before intraoperative TEE became routinely available, surgeons relied on the filling of the arrested LV with fluid to test the competency of the repaired mitral valve. The parallel line of leaflet closure to the posterior part of the ring also indicated a good apposition of the leaflets (25).

These techniques were less sensitive than using TEE during beating heart conditions, because testing an arrested heart may not accurately reflect physiologic changes.

Assessment of residual mitral incompetence (after unclamping the aorta) by digital palpation of the LA for a systolic thrill or by identification of a V wave of the LA pressure tracing are also unreliable due to variations in preload, LA size, and chamber compliance. Two-dimensional TEE with color-flow imaging allows evaluation of the function of the valve. The presence and severity of MR and the location of the regurgitant jet can be clearly ascertained.

The severity of regurgitation can be measured by the size of the jet relative to the atrium. Data obtained from this technique correlate well with angiographic data (4), but overestimation of the mitral regurgitant central jet is possible. The color Doppler flow method is not a quantitative approach. Entrained nonregurgitant blood flow within the LA may increase the overall color jet area, which may be important

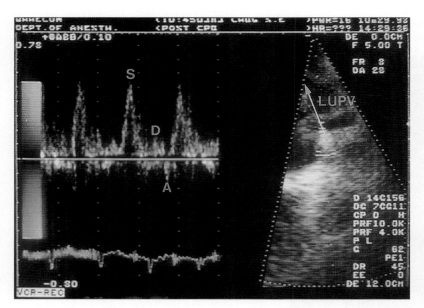

FIGURE 19.16. Normalization of left pulmonary venous systolic flow (*PVSF*) in pulsed-wave mode after annuloplasty. *LUPV,* left upper pulmonary vein; *S,* peak pulmonary venous systolic filling; *D,* peak pulmonary diastolic filling; *A,* negative velocity seen just before the S wave.

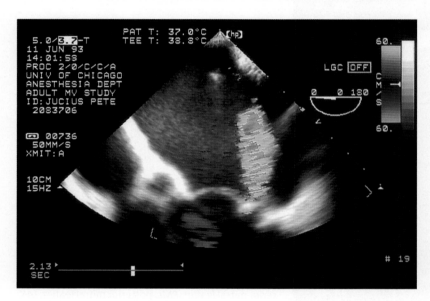

FIGURE 19.17. A posteriorly displaced regurgitant jet in a patient with a prolapsed anterior valve leaflet. Note the aliasing of the color hues, demonstrating high-velocity flow.

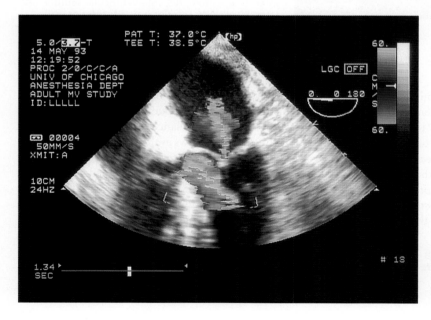

FIGURE 19.18. Central regurgitant jet in a patient with diffuse coronary disease. This type of jet is seen in patients with bileaflet restricted mobility or with either restricted or excessive mobility of both mitral valve leaflets.

in the estimation of ischemic/functional MR. In addition, an eccentric regurgitant jet may be attenuated by viscous forces within the wall of the LA, as well as increased heart rate. Other methods to assess the severity of MR include pulmonary venous flow velocity, vena contracta, regurgitant fraction, and proximal isovelocity surface area (PISA) analysis.

Anesthetic technique, hemodilution, temperature, and the use of vasoactive drugs influence the hemodynamic variables that determine the severity of MR during surgery. These factors can affect preload, afterload, heart rate, and rhythm, which significantly influence the degree of MR at a given time. Discordance between angiographic and echocardiographic evidence of mitral insufficiency may involve patients with unstable hemodynamics during angiography and those with high LV end-diastolic pressures whose disease has been palliated with thrombolytic therapy (4).

In a study comparing echocardiographic assessment with surgical inspection of the mitral valve, the direction of the regurgitant jet elucidated the mechanism of MR (14). In general, the jet is directed away from an excessively mobile leaflet and toward a leaflet with restricted mobility. For example, a posteriorly displaced jet can be seen in the presence of a flail or prolapsed (excessive mobility) anterior leaflet or a fibrotic or calcified (restricted mobility) posterior leaflet (Fig. 19.17). Mitral regurgitation with normal leaflet motion as manifested by a central Doppler jet is usually seen with annular dilatation associated with ischemic disease. Less commonly, a central jet is seen with bileaflet prolapse secondary to papillary muscle rupture or with restricted leaflet motion as in rheumatic heart disease (Fig. 19.18).

Interrogation of the mitral valve apparatus in multiple planes before using color Doppler is useful to visualize and diagnose the mechanism of injury causing insufficiency. Tomographic images of all components of the mitral valve apparatus should be obtained and recorded, recognizing that 2D and Doppler determination of leaflet dysfunction and jet direction correctly diagnoses the mechanism of disease in up to 85% of patients (14). A useful way to differentiate severe from moderate or mild mitral insufficiency is to examine flow patterns in the pulmonary vein during systole. At the ME level, the echocardiographic probe is positioned posterior to the LA. Rotation of the omniplane allows interrogation of the left upper pulmonary vein. Color Doppler helps locate the maximum flow for the subsequent use of the PW mode. The PW cursor positioned 1 cm into the vein will permit a high-quality signal. Left upper pulmonary vein flow is the easiest to image with TEE. Mitral regurgitation is graded on a scale of 1 to 4 depending on the direction and ratio of the systolic and diastolic components of pulmonary venous velocity tracings. The presence of systolic flow reversal in the pulmonary vein has been shown to be 93% sensitive and 100% specific for detecting mitral insufficiency graded at 4 or more. A problem of many noninvasive techniques is their inability to directly measure regurgitant flow rate at the lesion.

The power-velocity integral at the vena contracta was described as a method for direct quantification of regurgitant volume flow. Flow rate is a product of velocity and area, where the Doppler signal can produce backscattered acoustic power that can be used as an estimation of flow rate:

$$\text{Velocity} \times \text{Power} = \text{Flow Rate}$$

Backscattered power returning to the ultrasound transducer is a nonlinear function of hematocrit, and the backscattered power in the Doppler spectrum of flow velocities is linearly proportional to the cross-sectional area of flow within the beam. The power-velocity integral at the vena contracta provides an accurate direct measurement of regurgitant flow.

Regurgitant volume can be indirectly measured as a difference between SV through the MV (SVmv) and a nonregurgitant reference valve such as the aortic valve (AV) (SVav). Further calculation of the regurgitant fraction (RFmv = SVmv − SVav/SVmv) can grade MR severity, where 30% to 50% is considered moderate. Limitations of this method include assumption that the left ventricular outflow tract (LVOT) and AV orifice and mitral annulus are circular, aortic regurgitation is absent, and no ventricular septal defect is present. Furthermore, the calculation error is squared if the LVOT or MV annulus area is not measured accurately.

Proximal isovelocity surface area analysis was introduced as a quantitative Color Doppler flow measurement approach. Laminar flow stream narrows and accelerates proximal to a regurgitant valve orifice. This creates a hemispheric flow convergence region (FCR) where at each point the flow has the same velocity. Volume flow rate (mL/s) can be calculated as PISA (cm^2) multiplied by the isovelocity of the PISA (cm/s). The first PISA, with an isovelocity corresponding to the "aliasing" velocity (at one half the Nyquist sampling limit) is identified as blue and red color interface proximal to the orifice. The instantaneous flow rate (Q) at the FCR can be calculated as: $Q = 2\pi r^2 Vr$. The grading of MR by using FCR radius correlates with angiographic MR.

Measurements of effective mitral regurgitant orifice area (ROA) and regurgitant volume are derived from the PISA method. ROA is equal to Q/V, where Q is the maximum instantaneous regurgitant flow rate in mL/min and V is measured by CWD in cm/s. The ROA grade of MR is as follows: 1+ (mild) degree, ROA (cm^2) <0.1; 2+ (moderate), 0.1 to 0.25 cm^2 (with regurgitant volume of 25–40 mL); 3+ (moderate-severe), 0.25 to 0.5 cm^2 (40–55 mL); 4+ (severe), >0.5 cm^2 (or >55 mL).

Recent experimental findings suggest that a simplified formula can reliably estimate regurgitant volume and that blood viscosity does not affect the grade of regurgitation by the PISA method.

When evaluating mitral annuloplasty procedures, there are two primary complications: functional stenosis and dynamic obstruction of the LVOT. Ring annuloplasty, which uses a downsized ring, may result in functional stenosis. In patients requiring ring annuloplasty, the valve area can be assessed with planimetric measurements. PW or continuous-wave Doppler measurement of flow velocity can be used to obtain the pressure half-time (t½) or (PHT) of diastolic flow, which can be used to calculate the effective valve area as follows:

$$\text{Mitral valve area (cm}^2) = 220/t_{1/2}$$

The normal range of PHT is 50 to 70 msec. Tachycardia, prolonged PR interval, and aortic insufficiency may alter its measurement. Of note, the mitral valve area is approximately 1 cm² when the PHT is 220 msec, so mitral valve area is equal to $220/t_{1/2}$.

Echocardiographic evidence of systolic anterior motion (SAM) of the mitral leaflets in the presence of normal septal thickness is associated with the high-velocity flow disturbance seen in dynamic obstruction of the LVOT. With a rigid Carpentier-Edwards ring for annuloplasty, the risk of the LVOT obstruction is 4.5% to 17%. Freeman and colleagues reported that severe SAM of the anterior leaflet could cause moderate to severe MR in 9.1% of patients during separation from CPB after mitral valve repair.

Experimental research of ring annuloplasty in an animal model indicated that its implantation can reliably prevent delayed leaflet coaptation, which occurs after acute LV ischemia. Preischemic implantation of both the Duran and the Physio rings facilitated timely coaptation after induction of ischemia (40).

Preischemic implantation of either ring also preserved papillary–annular distances, which invariably tended to increase after the induction of ischemia in the control group (42). In a chronic ischemia animal model, reduction of MR was achieved by restoring tethering geometry toward normal by plication of the infarct region. Myocardial bulging was reduced without muscle excision or CPB. Immediately and up to 2 months after plication, mitral insufficiency was reduced (trace to mild) as tethering distance decreased (43).

In this experiment, implantation of a ring before induction of ischemia not only prevented delayed coaptation and preserved tethering distance as above, but also prevented disturbances in the geometry of both mitral valve leaflets (48).

Neither flexible nor semirigid mitral annuloplasty rings appear to affect global or basal regional LV systolic function (48). It has been shown that rigid fixation of the mitral annulus does not result in regional systolic dysfunction at the base of the LV (49).

A recent report of how mitral annular area and intercommissural and anteroseptal dimensions change throughout the cardiac cycle in a sheep model has demonstrated that a flexible Tailor partial ring preserves physiologic mitral annular folding dynamics (50).

A double-orifice technique in mitral valve repair (51) may represent a simple solution for complex problems associated with bileaflet prolapse, prolapse of either leaflet, lack of leaflet coaptation for restricted motion, or erosion of the free edge. In a series of 260 patients, a 5-year freedom from reoperation was achieved in 90% with this procedure. However, an ischemic cause of MR was only attributed to 2.3% of the patients, whereas degeneration was found in 81% of the

patients. The group of patients without annuloplasty (20%, when annulus was not dilated or it was severely calcified) showed an inferior rate of freedom from reoperation (70%). None of six patients with IMR required reoperation during the follow-up period. Although overall survival at 5 years was 94.4%, in this series outcome data for IMR were not as positive.

Dilated cardiomyopathy with functional mitral insufficiency required repair of MR in 59% in a reported series of 49 patients, with 75% of the patients having an ischemic etiology (52). The importance of mitral valve coaptation depth (MVCD), which is defined as the distance between the annulus and the coaptation point of the leaflets and is equivalent to the Mayo term *coaptation height*, was emphasized. As compared with healthy individuals with an average distance of 4.1 mm, the cardiomyopathic patients with an MVCD of less than 10 mm had postoperative functional MR of 1.2 degree. If preoperative MVCD was greater than 11 mm, it led to an average postrepaired MR degree of 2.5. In this series, late survival was similar in both repair and replacement groups, with functional class also similar in those who survived (73%) at a mean follow-up period of 24 months.

It has been suggested that surgeons be more aggressive and not ignore substantial degrees of IMR at the time of CABG (45). Whether to perform a simple ring annuloplasty or a more reliable chordal-preserving mitral valve replacement (MVR) remains a challenging question. In one recent report, patients who underwent mitral repair (although not as sick as those who required MVR) had survival rates similar to those of the MVR group (52).

Valve repair with a downsized annuloplasty ring, in order to enhance coaptation, works satisfactorily in most cases of functional IMR, but the surgeon must pay attention to the interpretation of the associated mechanism and direction of the regurgitation. Simple ring annuloplasty may be sufficient if a Carpentier type I pathology is present, but it is not a remedy in case of type III restricted systolic leaflet motion. Reduction of septal-lateral but not the intercommissural dimension should be performed. Both partial or complete and flexible or rigid rings perform well (46,47). Do all patients undergoing CABG who have more than mild MR need a concomitant mitral annuloplasty? This question remains to be answered, but preliminary data suggest that patients with moderate or less IMR who tolerated off-pump CABG appear to benefit from revascularization alone (20).

In summary, ischemic mitral insufficiency carries a worse prognosis than MR from other causes (4,9,13). The use of TEE enables the assessment of valvular function in real time so that surgical plans and techniques can be adopted.

KEY POINTS

- Up to 41% of CABG candidates also may have chronic ischemic mitral insufficiency.

- Coronary artery bypass grafting alone can lead to reduction of IMR severity.
- Significant residual MR after revascularization is associated with increased immediate postoperative and long-term morbidity and mortality.
- Combined mitral valve surgery and CABG is associated with a reported in-hospital mortality rate of 7% to 20%.
- The intraoperative severity assessment of residual MR is further complicated by hemodynamic changes related to the effect of general anesthesia and is often underestimated.
- Intraoperative TEE evaluation is critical in order to determine the mechanism of MR and guide a strategy for repair.
- Acute transient MR during an ischemic episode occurs primarily due to leaflet restriction as a result of ventricular dyskinesia, rather than of annular dilatation (type IIIb).
- Valve repair with a downsized annuloplasty ring, in order to enhance coaptation, works satisfactorily in most cases of functional IMR.
- Patients with moderate or less severe IMR who tolerated off-pump CABG appear to benefit from revascularization alone.

REFERENCES

1. Izhar U, Daly R, Dearani J, et al. Mitral valve replacement or repair after previous coronary artery bypass grafting. *Circulation* 1999;100(suppl II):84–89.
2. Alexander K, Anstrom K, Muhlbaier L, et al. Outcomes of cardiac surgery in patients age ≥80 years: results from the national cardiovascular network. *J Am Coll Cardiol* 2000;35:731–738.
3. **Duarte I, Shen Y, MacDonald M, et al. Treatment of moderate regurgitation and coronary disease by coronary bypass alone: late results. *Ann Thorac Surg* 1999;68:426–430.**
4. Sheikh KH, Bengtson JR, Rankin JS, et al. Intraoperative transesophageal Doppler color flow imaging used to guide patient selection and operative treatment of ischemic mitral regurgitation. *Circulation* 1991;84:594–604.
5. **Aklog L, Filsoufi F, Flores K, et al. Does coronary artery bypass grafting alone correct moderate ischemic mitral regurgitation? *Circulation* 2001;104(suppl I):68–75.**
6. **Grewal K, Malkowski M, Piracha A, et al. Effect of general anesthesia on the severity of mitral regurgitation by transesophageal echocardiography. *Am J Cardiol* 2000;85:199–203.**
7. **Shanewise J, Cheung A, Aronson S, et al. ASE/SCA guidelines for performing a comprehensive intraoperative multiplane transesophageal echocardiography examination: recommendations of the American Society of Echocardiography Council for intraoperative echocardiography and the Society of Cardiovascular Anesthesiologists Task Force for certification in perioperative transesophageal echocardiography. *J Am Soc Echocardiogr* 1999;12:884–900.**
8. Miller J, Lambert A, Shapiro W, et al. The adequacy of basic intraoperative transesophageal echocardiography performed by experienced anesthesiologists. *Anesth Analg* 2001;92:1103–1110.
9. Hickey M, Smith L, Muhlbaier L, et al. Current prognosis of ischemic mitral regurgitation. Implications for future management. *Circulation* 1988;78(suppl I):51–59.
10. Cohn L, Kowalker W, Bhatia S, et al. Comparative morbidity of mitral valve repair versus replacement for mitral regurgitation with and without coronary artery disease. *Ann Thorac Surg* 1988;45:284–290.
11. Cohn L, Kowalker W, Bhatia S, et al. Comparative morbidity of mitral valve repair versus replacement for mitral regurgitation with and without coronary artery disease. 1988. Updated in 1995. *Ann Thorac Surg* 1995;60:1452–1453.
12. Cohn L, Rizzo R, Adams D, et al. The effect of pathophysiology on the surgical treatment of ischemic mitral regurgitation: operative and late risks of repair versus replacement. *Eur J Cardiothorac Surg* 1995;9:568–574.
13. Hendren W, Nemec J, Lytle B, et al. Mitral valve repair for ischemic mitral insufficiency. *Ann Thorac Surg* 1991;52:1246–1251.
14. Stewart W, Currie P, Salcedo E, et al. Evaluation of mitral leaflet motion by echocardiography and jet direction by Doppler color flow mapping to determine the mechanism of mitral regurgitation. *J Am Coll Cardiol* 1992;20:1353–1361.
15. Seipelt R, Schoendube F, Vazquez-Jimenez J, et al. Combined mitral valve and coronary surgery: ischemic versus non-ischemic mitral valve disease. *Eur J Cardiothorac Surg* 2001;20(2):270–275.
16. Ferguson T, Dziuban F, Edwards F, et al. STS National Database: current changes and challenges for the new millennium. *Ann Thorac Surg* 2000;69:680–691.
17. Andrade I, Cartier R, Panisi P, et al. Factors influencing early and late survival in patients with combined mitral valve replacement and myocardial revascularization and in those with isolated replacement. *Ann Thorac Surg* 1987;44:607–613.
18. Lytle B, Cosgrove D, Gill C, et al. Mitral valve replacement combined with myocardial revascularization: early and late results for 300 patients, 1970 to 1983. *Circulation* 1987;44:1179–1190.
19. **Ryden T, Bech-Hanssen O, Brandrup-Wognsen G, et al. The importance of grade 2 ischemic mitral regurgitation in coronary artery bypass grafting. *Eur J Cardiothorac Surg* 2001;20:276–281.**
20. **Chapochnikov A, Jayakar D, Jeevanandam V, et al. Off-pump coronary artery bypass alone can remedy ischemic mitral regurgitation of moderate degree. 24th Annual Meeting of the Society of Cardiovascular Anesthesiologists, April 2002.**
21. Voci P, Bilotta F, Caretta Q, et al. Papillary muscle perfusion pattern. A hypothesis for ischemic papillary muscle dysfunction. *Circulation* 1995;91(6):1714–1718.
22. Bollen B, Luo H, Oury J, et al. A systematic approach to intraoperative transesophageal echocardiographic evaluation of the mitral valve apparatus with anatomic correlation. *J Cardiothorac Vasc Anesth* 2000;14(3):330–338.
23. Burch G, De Pasquale N, Phillips J. Clinical manifestations of papillary muscle dysfunction. *Arch Intern Med* 1963;59:508–520.
24. Grigioni F, Enriquez-Sarano M, Zehr K, et al. Ischemic mitral regurgitation. Long-term outcome and prognostic implications with quantitative Doppler assessment. *Circulation* 2001;103:1759–1764.
25. Carpentier A. Cardiac valve surgery—the "French correction." *J Thorac Cardiovasc Surg* 1983;86:323–337.
26. Fehrenbacher G, Schmidt D, Bommer W. Evaluation of transient mitral regurgitation in coronary artery disease. *Am J Cardiol* 1991;68:868–873.
27. Sharma S, Secker J, Israel D, et al. Clinical, angiographic and anatomic findings in acute severe ischemic mitral regurgitation. *Am J Cardiol* 1992;70:277–280.
28. **Dent J, Spotnitz W, Nolan S, et al. Mechanism of mitral leaflet excursion. *Am J Physiol* 1995;269:H2100–H2108.**

29. **Messas E, Guerrero J, Handschumacher M, et al. Paradoxic decrease in ischemic mitral regurgitation with papillary muscle dysfunction. Insights from three-dimensional and contrast echocardiography with strain rate measurement. *Circulation* 2001;104;1952–1960.**
30. Glasson J, Komeda M, Daughters G, et al. Three-dimensional dynamics of the canine mitral annulus during ischemic mitral regurgitation. *Ann Thorac Surg* 1996;62:1059–1068.
31. Athanasuleas C, Stanley A, Buckberg G, et al. Surgical anterior ventricular endocardial restoration (SAVER) in the dilated remodeled ventricle after anterior myocardial infarction. *J Am Coll Cardiol* 2001;37:1199–209.
32. Gorman J 3rd, Gorman R, Jackson B, et al. Distortions of the mitral valve in acute ischemic mitral regurgitation. *Ann Thorac Surg* 1997;64:1026–1031.
33. **Glasson J, Komeda M, Daughters G, et al. Early systolic mitral leaflet "loitering" during acute ischemic mitral regurgitation. *J Thorac Cardiovasc Surg* 1998;116:193–205.**
34. Llaneras M, Nance M, Streicher J, et al. Pathogenesis of ischemic mitral insufficiency. *J Thorac Cardiovasc Surg* 1993;105:439–443.
35. Sabbah H, Kono T, Rosman H, et al. Left ventricular shape: a factor in the etiology of functional mitral regurgitation in heart failure. *Am Heart J* 1992;123:961–966.
36. Lamas G, Mitchell G, Flaker G. Clinical significance of mitral regurgitation after acute myocardial infarction. *Circulation* 1997;96:827–833.
37. Di Donato M, Sabatier M, Dor V. Effects of the Dor procedure on left ventricular dimension and shape and geometric correlates of mitral regurgitation one year after surgery. *J Thorac Cardiovasc Surg* 2001;121:91–96.
38. Kono T, Sabbah H, Rosman H, et al. Mechanism of functional mitral regurgitation during acute myocardial ischemia. *J Am Coll Cardiol* 1992;19:1101–1105.
39. Green G, Dagum P, Glasson J, et al. Mitral annular dilatation and papillary muscle dislocation without mitral regurgitation in sheep. *Circulation* 1999;100(suppl II):95–102.
40. Timek T, Glasson JR, Dagum P, et al. Ring annuloplasty prevents delayed leaflet coaptation and mitral regurgitation during acute left ventricular ischemia. *J Thorac Cardiovasc Surg* 2000;119:774–783.
41. Timek T, Lai D, Dagum P, et al. Mitral annular dynamics during rapid atrial pacing. *Surgery* 2000;128:361–367.
42. Dagum P, Timek T, Green R, et al. Coordinate-free analysis of mitral valve dynamics in normal and ischemic hearts. *Circulation* 2000;102(suppl III):62–69.
43. Liel-Cohen N, Guerrero J, Otsuji Y, et al. Design of a new surgical approach for ventricular remodeling to relieve ischemic mitral regurgitation. *Circulation* 2000;101:2756–2763.
44. Otsuji Y, Handschumacher M, Schwammenthal E, et al. Insights from three-dimensional echocardiography into the mechanism of functional mitral regurgitation: direct *in vivo* demonstration of altered leaflet tethering geometry. *Circulation* 1997;96:1826–1834.
45. **Miller DC. Ischemic mitral regurgitation redux—to repair or to replace? *J Thorac Cardiovasc Surg* 2001;122:1059–1062.**
46. Gillinov A, Wierup P, Blackstone E, et al. Is repair preferable to replacement for ischemic mitral regurgitation? *J Thorac Cardiovasc Surg* 2001;122:1125–1141.
47. Grossi E, Goldberg J, LaPietra A, et al. Ischemic mitral valve reconstruction and replacement: comparison of long-term survival and complications. *J Thorac Cardiovasc Surg* 2001;122:1107–1124.
48. Lai D, Timek T, Dagum P. The effects of ring annuloplasty on mitral leaflet geometry during acute left ventricular ischemia. *J Thorac Cardiovasc Surg* 2000;120:966–975.
49. Green G, Dagum P, Glasson J. Semirigid or flexible mitral annuloplasty rings do not affect global or basal regional left ventricular systolic function. *Circulation* 1998;98(suppl II):128–136.
50. Dagum P, Timek T, Green G, et al. Three-dimensional geometric comparison of partial and complete flexible mitral annuloplasty rings. *J Thorac Cardiovasc Surg* 2001;122:665–673.
51. Alfieri O, Maisano F, De Bonis M. The double-orifice technique in mitral valve repair: a simple solution for a complex problem. *J Thorac Cardiovasc Surg* 2001;122:674–681.
52. Calafiore A, Gallina S, Di Mauro M. Mitral valve procedure in dilated cardiomyopathy: repair or replacement? *Ann Thorac Surg* 2001;71:1146–1153.

TRANSESOPHAGEAL ECHOCARDIOGRAPHIC EVALUATION OF PROSTHETIC VALVE DYSFUNCTION

SANDRA I. REYNERTSON
ERIC K. LOUIE

Transesophageal echocardiography (TEE) plays a major role in the diagnostic armamentarium of the clinician managing patients with suspected prosthetic valve dysfunction. In Chapter 11 the fundamental concepts involved in imaging and evaluating prosthetic valves is discussed in detail, and these principles will be applied to five clinical examples in this chapter.

Transesophageal echocardiography has several advantages over other imaging devices and procedures for the evaluation of prosthetic valves:

- Transesophageal echocardiography is a relatively unobtrusive technique, which can be quickly applied at the bedside, in the critical care environment, in the emergency room, and in the operating room (unlike computed tomography, magnetic resonance imaging, and contrast angiography).
- Transesophageal echocardiography can evaluate newly implanted mechanical prostheses without risk of displacing ferro-magnetic surgical clips or creation of distorting artifacts (unlike magnetic resonance imaging and computed tomography).
- Transesophageal echocardiography can conveniently evaluate upstream and downstream of mechanical prostheses without transprosthetic or trans-septal catheterization.
- Transesophageal echocardiography provides real-time dynamic integration of intracardiac flow events and cardiac valvular anatomy (and pathologic anatomy).
- Transesophageal echocardiography provides an alternative to transthoracic echocardiography (TTE) under condi-

tions where transthoracic acoustic windows are inadequate (due to body habitus, hyperinflated lungs, and subcutaneous emphysema).
- Transesophageal echocardiography complements TTE in the evaluation of the left atrial (LA) aspect of mechanical mitral prostheses (acoustically "hidden" from TTE), whereas TTE may provide complementary information about the left ventricular aspect of mechanical mitral prostheses.
- Depending on prosthesis orientation and cardiac positioning either, TEE or TTE may achieve superior alignment of the Doppler beam to measure transvalvular gradients.
- Transesophageal echocardiography is often superior to TTE with regards to spatial resolution and the interrogation of unique portions of cardiac anatomy (e.g., the pulmonary veins) due to the proximity of the TEE piezoelectric crystal to cardiac structures (just posterior to the LA). This proximity enables the use of higher carrier frequencies than are conventionally used in adult TTE studies, so higher image resolution is achieved.

As we shall explore in the rest of this chapter, these advantages of the TEE technique have been exploited to facilitate the diagnosis and treatment of a wide variety of prosthetic valve disorders in critically ill patients. The addition of TEE to the toolkit of the cardiovascular specialist has greatly shaped our diagnostic and therapeutic strategies applied in the management of prosthetic valve dysfunction.

PROSTHETIC MITRAL VALVE OBSTRUCTION

Case 1

Three months following mitral valve replacement with a St. Jude Medical prosthesis for endocarditis, a 45-year-old woman presented with slurred speech of sudden onset and generalized weakness, while inadequately anticoagulated (international normalized ratio = 1.7). Previously she had

S. I. Reynertson: Department of Medicine, Stritch School of Medicine, Loyola University, Maywood, Illinois; and Coronary Care Unit, Department of Medicine, Edward Hines, Jr. Veterans Affairs Hospital, Hines, Illinois.

E. K. Louie: Department of Medicine, Division of Cardiology, Stritch School of Medicine, Loyola University, Maywood, Illinois; and Medicine and Neurology Service Line, Edward Hines, Jr. Veterans Affairs Hospital, Hines, Illinois.

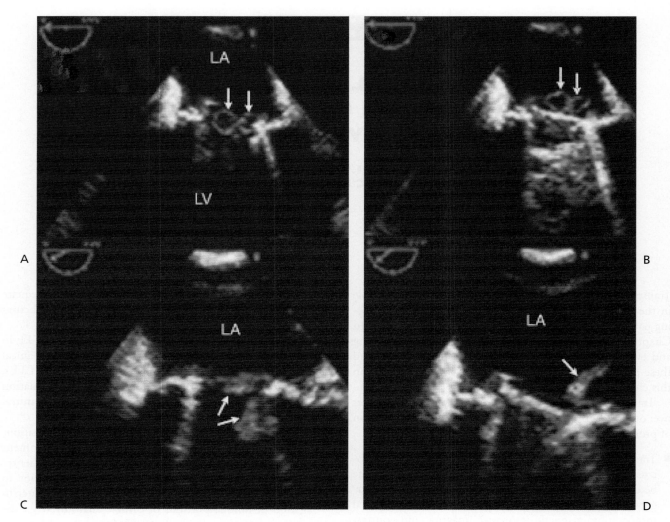

FIGURE 20.1. A 45-year-old woman with a St. Jude Medical mitral prosthesis (case 1). Transesophageal echocardiographic images obtained with a multiplane transducer positioned posterior to the LA, demonstrating a close-up of the transverse plane four-chamber view at 0 degrees **(A and B)** and at 30 degrees **(C and D)**. The left atrium (*LA*) is at the top of each figure, with the more anterior left ventricle (*LV*) at the bottom of each figure. In all figure parts, the bright echodensity separating the LA from the LV is created by the mechanical prosthetic mitral valve. **A:** The two disc occluders of the prosthetic mitral valve extend into the LV during diastole, seen as two bright linear echodensities in the LV aligned parallel to the transducer beam, with two hollow-appearing echodensities protruding into the orifice of the prosthetic valve (*arrows*). These hollow echodensities represent multiple thrombi adherent to the prosthetic valve. **B:** The two disc occluders are now perpendicular to the transducer beam, in the closed position during ventricular systole. The hollow-appearing thrombi (*arrows*) have prolapsed into the LA but still appear adherent to the valve. **C:** With the transducer crystal rotated to 30 degrees, a different irregularly shaped solid-appearing echodensity is seen protruding through the orifice of the prosthetic valve into the LV (*arrows*) during diastole, and prolapsing back into the LA during ventricular systole **(D)**, consistent with a third thrombus.

manifested a hypercoagulable state with pulmonary and systemic emboli, and she was known to abuse alcohol and intravenous drugs. Physical examination revealed stable vital signs, clear lungs, and a regular rhythm without an audible valve click or murmur. Transesophageal echocardiography was performed for presumed prosthetic valve thrombosis. The study revealed a bileaflet tilting disc valve, trivial valvular and perivalvular mitral regurgitation, and normal-

appearing disc excursion. Increased echodensities were detected along the mitral annulus, and several mobile echodensities attached to the LA aspect of the prosthetic mitral valve were noted. The patient underwent mitral valve replacement with a Carpentier-Edwards porcine bioprosthesis, at which time examination of the explanted mechanical prosthesis confirmed multiple thrombi adherent to the LA aspect of its discs and annulus.

As seen in Fig. 20.1A and B, with the transesophageal multiplane probe positioned posterior to the LA, two hollow-appearing echodensities consistent with thrombi protrude into the orifice of the valve during ventricular diastole, and prolapse into the LA with valve closure during ventricular systole. Abnormal echodensities are also noted along the annulus consistent with pannus formation or thrombus. Figure 20.1C and D shows a third irregularly shaped solid-appearing echodensity protruding into the left ventricle during diastole and prolapsing into the LA with ventricular systole consistent with a third thrombus on the valve disc. Figure 20.2A and B shows normal-appearing leaflet motion in diastole and systole, despite the thrombi associated with the valve. There was trivial valvular regurgitation noted on color Doppler imaging.

Role of Echocardiography

Prosthetic valve thrombosis is an infrequent but potentially life-threatening complication, occurring in 0.1% to 4% of patients per year. Clinical presentation can vary from mild heart failure symptoms to acute pulmonary edema, and from transient ischemic attacks to massive systemic or cerebral embolization. Although TTE or cinefluoroscopy can be used to diagnose severe thrombosis of a prosthetic valve, nonobstructive thrombi may be missed by TTE due to extraneous ultrasound reflections off the prosthesis or inadequate ultrasound penetration due to acoustic shadowing of the LA. If valve leaflet motion is not impeded by the thrombus, then cinefluoroscopy and TTE Doppler studies may appear normal. Transesophageal echocardiography provides a more accurate assessment of prosthetic mitral valve dysfunction with improved visualization of the LA aspect of the prosthetic valve, allowing better visualization of small thrombi, pannus formation, leaflet excursion, and valvular or perivalvular regurgitation (1,2). The differentiation between thrombus and pannus formation is critical to the management of valve thrombosis, if thrombolysis is contemplated. Both thrombus and pannus formation result in similar severity of valve obstruction, as measured by Doppler-derived peak transvalvular gradients and valve areas for both aortic and mitral valves. In contrast, pannus formation on prosthetic mitral valves is associated with slightly lower mean gradients than are seen with thrombosis. Size, shape, and mobility are not criteria that can be used to significantly differentiate between pannus and thrombi, but the ultrasound video intensity ratio is lower for thrombi compared with pannus, and thrombi appear to have a softer echodensity closer to the appearance of myocardium (3).

Treatment alternatives for prosthetic valve thrombosis include conservative anticoagulation therapy, thrombolysis, and surgical exploration, whereas obstructive pannus formation requires surgical resection. Assessment of thrombus size by TEE may be helpful in determining appropriate treatment. In general, thrombolytic therapy of patients with involvement of left-sided prosthetic valves is reserved for high-risk surgical candidates, because thrombolysis carries a significant risk for systemic or cerebral embolization (12%–17%), up to a 5% death rate, and only an 82% initial success rate with 11% recurrence of thrombosis (4). Success of thrombolysis (and determination of the duration of therapy) is measured by resolution of abnormal valve gradients by Doppler echocardiography and evidence of clot dissolution by TEE imaging. Thrombolysis is continued for a maximum of 72 hours of infusion, and is discontinued after 24 hours if no clinical or hemodynamic improvement is noted (4,5). If thrombolytic therapy is used, serial TEE examinations can be performed to assess initial success of thrombolysis within the first 48 hours of treatment, and to determine further management with repeat thrombolysis or surgical intervention, if thrombolysis is incomplete (6). Conservative management with anticoagulation can be reserved for patients with small nonobstructive thrombi less than 5 mm in size, with serial TEE examinations to confirm resolution of thrombi within 1 to 2 weeks. Patients whose thrombi do not resolve with conservative treatment, or in whom thrombi are larger than 5 mm in length, have a high risk for experiencing systemic embolism and should be referred for surgical treatment (2).

This patient was treated aggressively by surgical replacement of the mechanical mitral valve with a bioprosthetic valve due to symptoms of embolization, multiple large thrombi 7 to 12 mm in length, and a history of noncompliance with anticoagulation therapy.

PROSTHETIC MITRAL PERIVALVULAR REGURGITATION
Case 2

A 70-year-old man with severe obstructive lung disease and mechanical mitral valve replacement 3 months previously for endocarditis presented with severe orthopnea and dyspnea on exertion. Physical examination was significant for coarse breath sounds, mild expiratory wheezing, and prolonged expiratory phase, but no obvious rales on the lung examination. Cardiovascular examination revealed the presence of a soft valve click without systolic murmur or third heart sound, and no evidence of right or left heart failure. Chest radiography showed a normal cardiac silhouette, flattened diaphragms with evidence of emphysema, and minimal pulmonary vascular redistribution. Transthoracic echocardiography revealed normal left ventricular function with normal prosthetic mitral valve gradient, but mitral regurgitation was not adequately evaluated due to acoustic shadowing of the LA from the prosthetic mitral valve. A TEE was initially deferred due to marked dyspnea with mild hypoxia. The patient's respiratory status deteriorated, requiring intubation, after which TEE was performed to further assess the function of the prosthetic mitral valve. Despite the TTE findings,

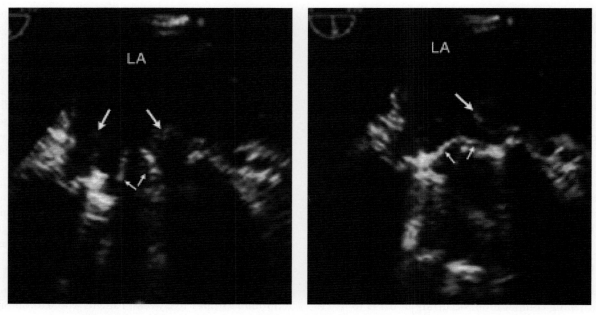

FIGURE 20.2. A 45-year-old woman with a St. Jude Medical mitral prosthesis (case 1). Transesophageal echocardiographic images obtained with a multiplane transducer positioned posterior to the left atrium, demonstrating a close-up of the longitudinal plane two-chamber view at 100 degrees. The left atrium (*LA*) is at the top of each figure, with the more anterior left ventricle (*LV*) at the bottom of each figure. **A:** During ventricular diastole, both occluder discs of the prosthetic mitral valve appear to open normally, seen as two linear densities (*small arrows*) protruding into the LV cavity parallel to the transducer beam. Two large linear densities (*large arrows*) appear adherent to the prosthetic valve annulus and prolapse into the LA, consistent with thrombi. **B:** The occluder discs (*small arrows*) are now in the closed position during ventricular systole, forming a shallow inverted "v." The *large arrow* points to a large mobile thrombus attached to the prosthetic mitral valve annulus, prolapsing into the LA. Despite multiple thrombi associated with the prosthetic valve, the images demonstrate unencumbered prosthetic leaflet motion in both systole and diastole.

prosthetic valve dysfunction with valvular or perivalvular regurgitation was suspected as the cause of the patient's dyspnea, orthopnea, and subsequent respiratory distress leading to intubation.

Role of Echocardiography

Transesophageal echocardiography of the prosthetic mitral valve in the esophageal five-chamber view (Fig. 20.3A and B) revealed excessive tissue density at the mitral-aortic intervalvular fibrosa with a rocking motion of the mitral valve at its anterior suture line as it abuts the aortic annulus, consistent with prosthetic valve dehiscence. Initial color Doppler imaging did not reveal significant mitral regurgitation, despite the apparent valvular dehiscence. Peak early diastolic transmitral inflow velocities of 1.6 to 1.8 m/s by pulsed-wave Doppler (Fig. 20.4A) were consistent with an acceptable degree of relative obstruction with this prosthesis. The rapid deceleration of the mitral inflow and its short pressure half-time (<120 msec), however, suggested that increased forward transvalvular flow due to significant mitral regurgitation (and not relative prosthetic obstruction) explained the

peak early diastolic flow velocities seen in this patient (7). Further interrogation of the prosthesis with anteroflexion (large wheel control) and severe lateral flexion (small wheel control) of the TEE transducer tip was necessary to reveal severe mitral regurgitation through the area of dehiscence (Fig. 20.3C and D). This regurgitant jet was clearly perivalvular, originating outside the valvular sewing ring. The color Doppler map also reveals multiple "aliased" signals (indicating proximal isovelocity surface areas) on the ventricular side of the regurgitant leak. Such findings suggest high flow rates in the flow convergence zone, consistent with significant mitral regurgitation (7). In normal patients, pulmonary venous return detected by TEE pulsed-wave Doppler reveals a triphasic to quadriphasic pattern with one to two forward systolic peaks, forward diastolic flow, and a small atrial reversal of flow. Progressive degrees of severity of mitral regurgitation are associated with increases in the peak velocity of diastolic pulmonary venous inflow and its integral. In reciprocal fashion, the peak velocity of systolic inflow and its integral decrease. A highly sensitive and specific finding in severe mitral regurgitation is the finding of reversal of pulmonary venous systolic flow (8). Figure 20.4B

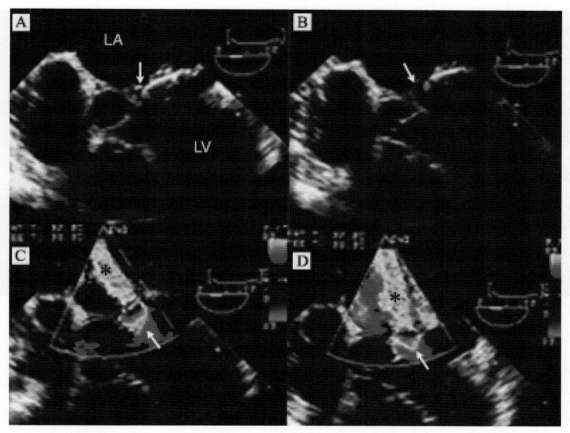

FIGURE 20.3. A 70-year-old man with a mechanical mitral prosthesis (case 2). Transesophageal images obtained in the esophageal five-chamber view at 0 degrees with the transesophageal echocardiography (TEE) probe positioned just posterior to the left atrium (*LA*) and the left ventricle (*LV*) at the bottom of the image. The bright echodensity separating the LA from the LV, and abutting the aortic valve, is the mechanical mitral prosthesis. **A:** Excessive tissue density is noted at the mitral-aortic intervalvular fibrosa (*arrow*), between the prosthetic mitral valve and the aortic valve. **B:** Rocking motion of the mitral prosthesis at the anterior suture line (*arrow*) was noted throughout the cardiac cycle (on review of real-time images), with the prosthesis prolapsing into the LA during ventricular systole, consistent with prosthetic valve dehiscence. **C:** Initial color Doppler imaging at this plane revealed mild perivalvular mitral regurgitation (*asterisk*). **D:** Further rotation of the TEE probe with anteroflexion and severe lateroflexion revealed an area of severe perivalvular mitral regurgitation (*asterisk*) through the area of dehiscence. Proximal isovelocity surface areas (*PISAs*) are noted on the ventricular side of the regurgitant leak (*arrows* in **C** and **D**), consistent with high flow rates of significant regurgitation.

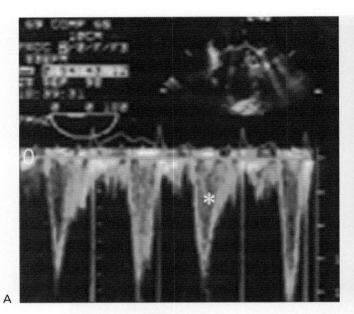
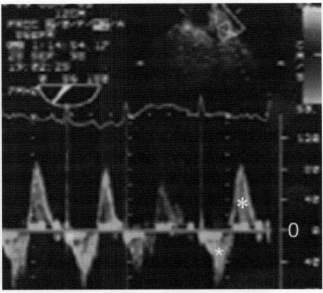

A

B

FIGURE 20.4. A 70-year-old man with a mechanical mitral prosthesis (case 2). **A:** Transesophageal image obtained in the transverse plane four-chamber view at 0 degrees. Pulsed-wave Doppler echocardiography through the mechanical mitral prosthesis (*asterisk*) reveals an acceptable peak early diastolic transmitral inflow velocity of 1.6 to 1.8 m/s, with rapid deceleration of the mitral inflow and a short pressure half-time (<120 msec), suggesting increased forward transvalvular flow from significant mitral regurgitation. **B:** Pulsed-wave Doppler spectrum of the left upper pulmonary vein, obtained at 60 degrees with the transesophageal echocardiography probe anteroflexed into the basal short-axis position. Severe mitral regurgitation is demonstrated with reversal of pulmonary venous systolic inflow velocity (*small asterisk*) and an increase in the peak diastolic inflow velocity and flow velocity integral (*large asterisk*).

demonstrates in our patient the effect of severe mitral regurgitation on pulmonary venous flow with reversal of systolic flow velocity seen in this pulsed-wave Doppler spectrum from the left upper pulmonary vein.

Transesophageal echocardiography provides a superior means of assessing prosthetic mitral valve function and anatomy over TTE due to the close proximity of the probe to the posterior wall of the LA. This view of the LA aspect of the prosthesis improves visualization of the valve discs and sewing ring with clearer definition of the origin and extension of perivalvular regurgitant jets, obviating acoustic shadowing of the LA by the mitral prosthesis (9). In addition, TEE has been shown to be highly accurate in predicting the surgical location of periprosthetic mitral regurgitation mapped about the mitral annulus into four quadrants (anterior, medial, posterior, and lateral) defined by the anterior mitral annulus abutting the aortic root in the basal short-axis view (9). Figure 20.5A and B demonstrates an intervalvular pseudoaneurysm with prosthetic mitral valve dehiscence in the anterior quadrant of the mitral valve annulus, with Fig. 20.5C and D demonstrating a perivalvular regurgitant jet through this pseudoaneurysm. The pseudoaneurysm most likely represents a perivalvular abscess that now communicates with the left ventricle. The patient's condition rapidly worsened over the next 24 hours, blood cultures grew *Staphylococcus epidermidis,* and he subsequently died.

PROSTHETIC MITRAL VALVULAR REGURGITATION

Case 3

A 51-year-old man with rheumatic heart disease who underwent porcine mitral valve replacement 10 years earlier presented with new-onset congestive heart failure. He had moderate systolic dysfunction of the left ventricle despite normal bioprosthetic valve function by TTE performed 1 year earlier. Physical examination revealed a loud holosystolic murmur heard best at the apex with a soft S3, and basilar rales in the lungs. Transthoracic echocardiography revealed severe mitral regurgitation, which was new in comparison with the study performed a year earlier. The images raised the possibility of a flail bioprosthetic leaflet or vegetation. A TEE was performed to better assess the anatomy of the bioprosthetic valve and the cause of the mitral regurgitation.

Role of Echocardiography

As discussed in the two prior cases, TTE with a mitral valve prosthesis in place is often associated with significant reverberation artifact from the valve, limiting assessment of valve anatomy (particularly visualization of the valve leaflets) and

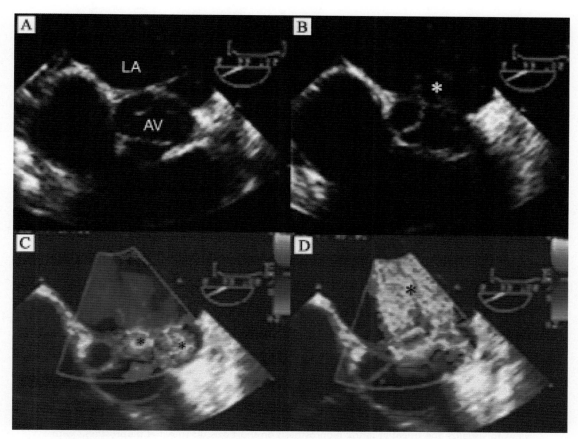

FIGURE 20.5. A 70-year-old man with a mechanical mitral prosthesis (case 2). Images obtained with the TEE probe posterior to the left atrium (*LA*), at the level of the aortic valve (*AV*), with rotation of the transducer to 33 degrees from the basal short-axis view. **A:** An intervalvular pseudoaneurysm is seen at the anterior suture line of the prosthetic mitral valve where it abuts the aortic root. **B:** Disruption of the anterior suture line (*asterisk*) with dehiscence of the prosthetic mitral valve. **C:** Evidence of perivalvular flow (*asterisk*) into the pseudoaneurysm. **D:** Severe perivalvular regurgitant jet through the pseudoaneurysm demonstrating communication between the left ventricle and the left atrium (*asterisk*).

interfering with both qualitative and quantitative assessment of mitral regurgitation (10). With the TEE probe in the esophagus just posterior to the LA, visualization of the mitral bioprosthesis on short axis in the transverse plane revealed a trileaflet valve with one partially flail leaflet (Fig. 20.6A). This view was obtained by marked anteroflexion of the probe in the four-chamber view. Color Doppler interrogation at the mitral valve level revealed severe mitral regurgitation originating predominantly from the flail leaflet (Fig. 20.6B). No perivalvular mitral regurgitation was noted. Figure 20.7A and B shows normal-appearing bioprosthetic stents in the longitudinal two-chamber view, but a flail leaflet prolapsing into the LA (Fig. 20.7C). The resultant mitral regurgitant jet is seen in Fig. 20.7D, with proximal flow acceleration of the jet on the left ventricular side of the valve consistent with volumetrically significant mitral regurgitation (as described in case 2). This patient was also found to have systolic flow reversal of the pulmonary venous inflow consistent with hemodynamically severe mitral regurgitation.

Durability of bioprosthetic valves is known to be a major limitation to their use. Rapid progression of valve degeneration, caused by either tissue degeneration or calcification, may occur within 7 to 10 years of implantation. Increased valve failure rates are seen in children and adults under 35 years of age. Recent modifications in the preservation of the tissue leaflets with use of low-pressure gluteraldehyde fixation methods may prolong the life of bioprosthetic valves, but long-term data are presently not available (11).

PROSTHETIC AORTIC VALVE ENDOCARDITIS WITH PERIVALVULAR ABSCESS

Case 4

A 36-year-old man with rheumatic heart disease and a history of intravenous drug abuse underwent aortic valve replacement 17 months earlier for symptomatic moderate to severe aortic insufficiency. His first prosthesis was explanted and

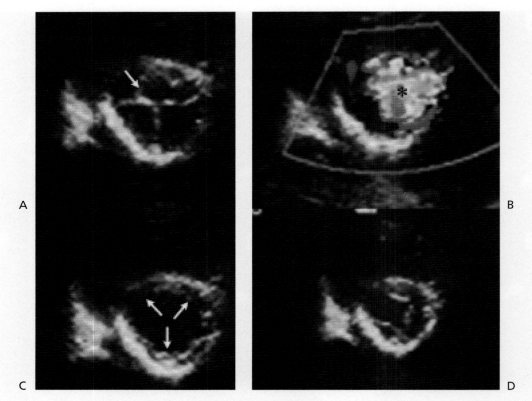

FIGURE 20.6. A 51-year-old man with porcine mitral valve replacement 10 years ago (case 3). Images obtained by severe anteroflexion of the probe from the transverse plane four-chamber view, to visualize the trileaflet mitral bioprosthesis on short axis. **A:** Trileaflet bioprosthesis with two cusps coapting normally. The third leaflet (*arrow*), however, fails to coapt normally during ventricular systole and was subsequently demonstrated to be flail. **B:** Color Doppler demonstration of severe valvular mitral regurgitation originating predominantly through the flail leaflet (*asterisk*). **C:** Trileaflet mitral bioprosthesis during ventricular diastole with all three leaflets appearing structurally normal in the fully opened position (*arrows*). **D:** Evidence of structural deformity of one leaflet of the bioprosthetic valve as the leaflets return to their closed position.

a repeat aortic valve replacement was performed 3 months later with an aortic homograft to treat prosthetic fungal endocarditis, perivalvular abscess, and perivalvular aortic regurgitation. He presented 14 months following his second operation with septic emboli to his left leg requiring embolectomy. A TTE revealed a 2 × 2 cm vegetation on the aortic valve with mild aortic insufficiency, normal left ventricular size, and normal systolic function. After 28 days of antifungal therapy for recurrent fungal prosthetic valve endocarditis, a TEE was performed to further assess homograft anatomy and response to medical therapy. During this time period the patient remained essentially asymptomatic and hemodynamically stable.

The TEE revealed trivial to mild valvular aortic insufficiency with mild thickening of the cusps of the trileaflet aortic homograft. A large perivalvular cavity was noted between the aorta and LA, and posterior to the left main coronary artery, in the region of the mitral-aortic continuity or intervalvular fibrosa (Fig. 20.8A) with amorphous echodense

material on the wall of the cavity. The basal short-axis views of the aortic valve during systole suggest destruction of the aortic annulus with a flail homograft leaflet or vegetation prolapsing into the abscess cavity (Fig. 20.8B and C). Figure 20.8D shows apparent flow through the aortic valve by color Doppler. The longitudinal plane long-axis view, however, demonstrates that these structures actually represent prolapse of the wall of the abscess cavity into the left ventricular outflow tract, with an intact aortic valve (Fig. 20.9A–C). Competency of the valve with trivial to mild aortic insufficiency was noted during diastole, but Fig. 20.9D demonstrates communication between the left ventricular outflow tract and the abscess cavity by color Doppler imaging during systole. The abscess cavity was noted to extend between the aorta and pulmonary artery, compressing the main pulmonary artery during ventricular systole, as noted in the sequential stop-frame images in Fig. 20.10.

At the time of surgery, multiple small vegetations were noted on the leaflet tips of each cusp of the homograft

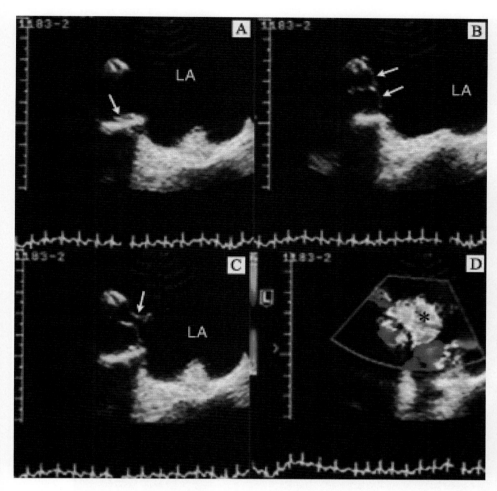

FIGURE 20.7. A 51-year-old man who had undergone porcine mitral valve replacement 10 years ago (case 3). Images obtained from the longitudinal two-chamber view with the transesophageal echocardiography probe just posterior to the left atrium (*LA*). **A:** Normal-appearing bioprosthetic valve during ventricular diastole with normal cusp opening and a bright echodense stent (*arrow*) projecting into the left ventricle. **B:** Normal-appearing bioprosthetic cusp coaptation (*arrows*) during ventricular systole with thin leaflets. **C:** The third leaflet (*arrow*) of the bioprosthetic valve, which was not imaged in **B**, is flail and swings into the LA during systole. **D:** Color Doppler demonstrates mitral regurgitation (*asterisk*) with proximal flow acceleration of the jet on the left ventricular side of the valve. These findings are consistent with volumetrically significant mitral regurgitation.

aortic valve. A large old thrombus or vegetation was discovered beneath the noncoronary cusp of the homograft, and it projected into the left ventricular outflow tract. There was also an abscess cavity from the base of the heart projecting over the LA and behind the pulmonary artery, with complete separation of the anterior mitral valve leaflet from the aortic root. Dissection of the aortic homograft revealed dense adhesions with indistinct tissue planes between the aortic root and the pulmonary artery.

Role of Echocardiography

Prosthetic valve endocarditis remains a serious complication of surgical valve replacement, occurring in 3% to 6% of the patients. Endocarditis early after valve replacement is associated with a mortality rate of up to 30% to 80%, whereas endocarditis more than 60 days following valve replacement has a 20% to 40% mortality rate (12). Endocarditis is a rare complication with homograft valves, with only a 2% occurrence at 15 years in several large studies (13). Preoperative evaluation of prosthetic valve endocarditis with TEE can help direct

the surgical plan by guiding the choice between valve repair and replacement of the valve and surrounding structures. Accurate preoperative assessment of the surgical anatomy also facilitates choice of strategies for myocardial protection during cardiopulmonary bypass, and anesthetic management. These benefits translate into improved immediate survival and long-term outcome after valve surgery (14).

Doppler assessment of prosthetic aortic valvular disease with TEE may be limited by the inability to properly orient the Doppler beam parallel to transvalvular flow for assessment of the gradient due to the limited available imaging planes. In addition, acoustic shadowing created by the prosthetic valve may limit assessment of aortic insufficiency. This is especially common when both aortic and mitral prostheses are in place. In such cases, combining TTE and TEE examinations of prosthetic aortic valves allows comprehensive assessment of aortic prosthetic obstruction and regurgitation, and elucidation of the cause of prosthetic valve dysfunction (15).

Evaluation of pseudoaneurysms of the aortic valve or root is best accomplished with TEE. Although computed

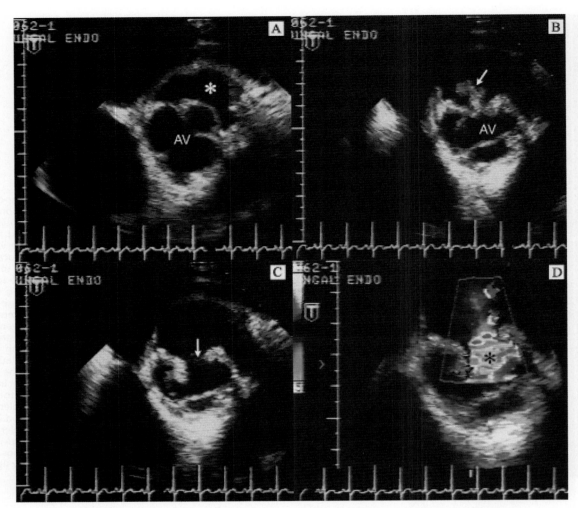

FIGURE 20.8. A 36-year-old man with an aortic homograft for recurrent prosthetic valve endo-carditis (case 4). All images were obtained in the basal short-axis view of the aortic valve in the transverse plane. **A:** Trileaflet aortic valve (AV) in ventricular diastole with a large perivalvular cavity posterior to the left main coronary artery, at the mitral-aortic continuity or intervalvular fibrosa (*asterisk*), with amorphous echodense material on the wall of the cavity. **B:** During ventric-ular systole, the images raise the possibility that either the homograft leaflet is flail or there is a vegetation (*arrow*) prolapsing into the abscess cavity (see further discussion in **C**). **C:** Apparent de-struction (*arrow*) of the aortic annulus noted during ventricular systole. Later images (see Fig. 20.9) clarify these findings by demonstrating the integrity of the aortic valve, with hypermobility of the wall of the abscess cavity, which prolapses into the left ventricular outflow tract. **D:** Color Doppler of the aortic valve at end systole shows blood flow (*asterisk*) through the region of apparent aortic annular destruction, representing flow from the left ventricle into the abscess cavity.

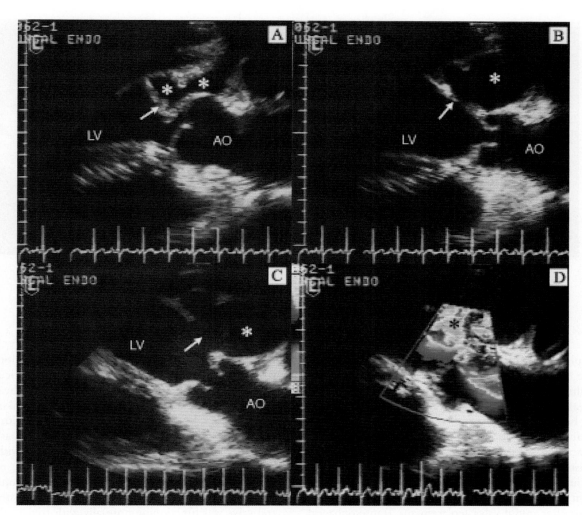

FIGURE 20.9. A 36-year-old man with an aortic homograft for recurrent prosthetic valve endocarditis (case 4). All images obtained in the longitudinal two chamber view of the aortic valve and aortic root (*AO*). **A:** Collapse of the abscess cavity (*asterisk*) during ventricular diastole, with prolapse of the wall of the abscess cavity (*arrow*) into the left ventricular (*LV*) outflow tract. **B:** During ventricular systole, the wall of the abscess cavity (*arrow*) moves upward, as the LV outflow tract expands, and the abscess cavity enlarges (*asterisk*). **C:** At end ventricular systole, there is evidence of destruction of the cavity wall (*arrow*) with communication between the subaortic left ventricular outflow tract and the abscess cavity (*asterisk*). **D:** Color flow Doppler imaging shows systolic blood flow (*asterisk*) between the LV and the abscess cavity through the discontinuity. Only trivial aortic insufficiency was noted during ventricular diastole (images not provided), implying functional integrity of the aortic valve (consistent with the anatomic integrity of the valve noted in **A–C**).

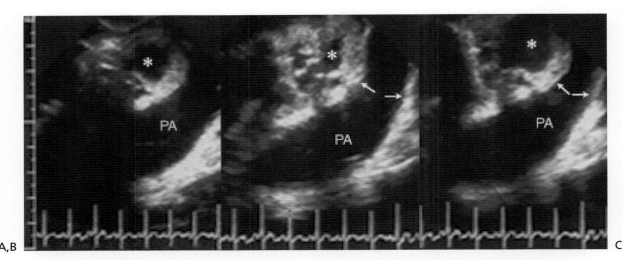

FIGURE 20.10. A 36-year-old man with aortic homograft for recurrent prosthetic valve endocarditis (case 4). All images were obtained in the longitudinal plane at the level of the right ventricular outflow tract and pulmonary artery (*PA*). The abscess cavity (asterisk) extends between the aorta and pulmonary artery, compressing the main pulmonary artery (*arrows*) during sequential systolic stop-frame images.

tomography with contrast and aortography can help identify these lesions, it is difficult to assess dynamic flow patterns within the outflow tract with these techniques. Transesophageal echocardiography can accurately demonstrate the dynamic behavior of these pseudoaneurysms with characteristic expansion and contraction during systole and diastole (7). Intracardiac fistulae also may occur after valve replacement. Fistulae may develop between the aorta and left or right atrium (RA) or right ventricle after aortic valve replacement, and between the left ventricle and RA or coronary sinus after mitral valve replacement. Transesophageal echocardiographic imaging and Doppler techniques provide superior techniques for anatomic correlation and assessment of shunt flow between the various cavities (7).

The extensive distortion of this patient's cardiac anatomy identified preoperatively on TEE helped guide the surgical approach for this patient. The surgery involved removal of the old homograft, and replacement with a new homograft, as well as anterior mitral valve reconstruction and reanastomosis of the coronary arteries. His initial clinical course was uncomplicated as he was rapidly weaned from cardiopulmonary bypass, but later he developed severe delayed bleeding from the right coronary anastomosis and distal aortic root anastomosis. Despite returning to the operating room for reexploration of the valve and aortic root, bleeding could not be controlled and the patient died.

INTRAOPERATIVE COMPLICATIONS OF PROSTHETIC VALVE SURGERY

Case 5

A 66-year-old man with a history of porcine mitral valve replacement 10 years previously presented for repeat mi-

tral valve replacement and tricuspid valve annuloplasty to treat severe prosthetic mitral regurgitation and tricuspid regurgitation. A new no. 29 porcine Carpentier-Edwards bioprosthetic valve was implanted to replace the leaking prosthetic mitral valve, and a tricuspid annuloplasty with a no. 33 St. Jude ring was performed. Postoperatively the patient had difficulty coming off cardiopulmonary bypass with persistent hypotension and left ventricular dilatation, requiring high-dose norepinephrine and epinephrine infusions. Emergent intraoperative TEE revealed that the bioprosthetic mitral valve was functioning normally with trivial valvular or perivalvular leak, but its septal strut appeared to abut the proximal left ventricular septum. Doppler studies revealed turbulence in the left ventricular outflow tract during ventricular systole and peak systolic velocities of 2 to 2.5 m/s. There was persistent severe tricuspid regurgitation despite the tricuspid annuloplasty. At least moderate aortic insufficiency was noted, but shadowing from the bioprosthetic mitral valve limited accurate visualization of the aortic regurgitant jet. Direct visualization of the aortic valve revealed a trileaflet valve with immobility of the noncoronary cusp during both systole and diastole (Fig. 20.11A and B) with at least moderate aortic insufficiency through the noncoronary cusp (Fig. 20.11C).

Role of Echocardiography

Intraoperative TEE has become increasingly popular over the past decade, now being used in the vast majority of all cardiac surgical cases (16). Intraoperative TEE prior to cardiopulmonary bypass can accurately define valvular anatomy, leading to changes in the operative plan in up to 19% of valvular surgical procedures (17,18). Findings unanticipated by other

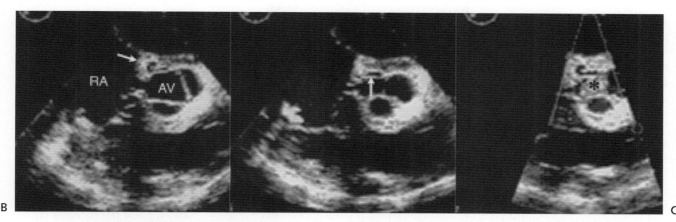

A,B   C

FIGURE 20.11. A 66-year-old man undergoing repeat bioprosthetic mitral valve surgery with tricuspid valve annuloplasty (case 5). All images were obtained with the transducer rotated 40 degrees from the basal short-axis view of the aortic valve. **A:** A bright echodensity noted adjacent to the aortic valve (*AV*) annulus represents the tricuspid valvuloplasty ring (*arrow*) protruding into the right atrium (*RA*). Two of the three aortic valve leaflets appear to open normally during ventricular systole, but the noncoronary cusp appears adherent to the aortic annulus, snared by a suture from the tricuspid valvuloplasty ring. **B:** During ventricular diastole, the right and left coronary cusps coapt normally, but the noncoronary cusp (*arrow*) appears severely restricted in motion. **C:** Color Doppler of the aortic valve reveals at least moderate aortic insufficiency (*asterisk*) through the noncoronary cusp during ventricular diastole.

diagnostic procedures, changes in the severity of regurgitant (and occasionally stenotic) lesions due to evolving clinical conditions or alterations in cardiac loading, and concomitant valvular problems (e.g., secondary tricuspid regurgitation) are often first appreciated by prebypass TEE. A recent study of intraoperative TEE in patients undergoing aortic valve replacement revealed the magnitude of concomitant mitral regurgitation to be significantly different than previously anticipated, leading to a change in the planned concomitant mitral valve surgery (repair or replacement) in 13% of the cases (17). Intraoperative TEE has proved most useful in the assessment of patients undergoing mitral valve surgery, with the use of both two-dimensional imaging of the valvular structure to design the repair and Doppler color flow imaging of the extent and direction of the regurgitant jet (as well as Doppler measurement of pulmonary venous flow) to determine the severity of the regurgitation. These evaluations influenced the final surgical plan in up to 41% of patients at the time of surgery (18). Intraoperative TEE can then be used to assess the immediate success of mitral valve repair, the proper function of prosthetic valve function, the occurrence of abnormal amounts of intracardiac air, global and segmental ventricular function, and other immediate surgical complications (19). Assessment of residual tricuspid regurgitation following mitral valve surgery may deem tricuspid repair unnecessary in as many as 10% of patients in whom tricuspid repair was anticipated preoperatively. Alternatively the finding of significant residual tricuspid regurgitation after mitral valve repair can prompt a return to a second bypass run and immediate surgical intervention (19).

Specific operative complications following mitral valve surgery that should be evaluated include new wall motion abnormalities due to inadequate myocardial protection and segmental myocardial ischemia [from coronary artery air embolism (most commonly the right coronary artery in up to 5% of mitral valve cases) or accidental left circumflex coronary artery ligation during mitral annuloplasty, leading to lateral wall motion abnormalities]. Less frequent complications include new-onset aortic insufficiency due to deformity of the aortic valve from deeply placed sutures at the fibrous trigone (16). Other immediate complications following mitral valve surgery include new-onset left ventricular outflow tract obstruction in 4% to 14% of patients following mitral valve repair. Obstruction is often multifactorial but may result from excessive billowing of posterior or anterior mitral leaflet tissue, small ventricular cavity (relative to the mitral prosthesis), or a narrow mitral-aortic angle resulting in systolic anterior motion of the anterior leaflet of the mitral valve (20). Turbulent blood flow in the left ventricular outflow tract with proximal flow convergence just prior to the point of obstruction, along with mitral regurgitation, should lead one to suspect this problem. Left ventricular outflow tract obstruction also can be seen when a bioprosthetic mitral valve (or other bulky prosthesis such as the Starr-Edwards caged ball prosthesis) is positioned such that a strut abuts the ventricular septum running perpendicular rather than parallel to the outflow tract. Continuous-wave Doppler can be used to assess the maximum instantaneous and mean gradients, whereas pulsed-wave Doppler can be used to localize the point of flow acceleration at the obstruction. Assessment of left ventricular outflow tract obstruction can be very difficult to achieve with TEE due to the inability to correctly orient the Doppler beam parallel to the outflow tract. The best TEE views for Doppler beam alignment with the outflow tract are the deep transgastric transverse or longitudinal imaging planes. The turbulence and proximal flow acceleration seen on color Doppler imaging can aid in positioning the cursor for pulsed-wave or continuous-wave Doppler interrogation. Pharmacologic intraoperative manipulation of left ventricular loading conditions can be used to assess the dynamic nature of left ventricular outflow tract obstruction (16,19).

Other immediate complications following valve repair or replacement that should be routinely assessed include valvular and perivalvular regurgitation, prosthetic valve disc or leaflet mobility, and transvalvular gradients. Clinically meaningful information can only be obtained if strict attention is directed to approximating physiologic loading conditions and stable cardiac rate and rhythm during the TEE study. Rare complications following mitral valve replacement include rupture of the left ventricular wall (0.5%–2% incidence). This may occur immediately coming off cardiopulmonary bypass (55% of cases) with excessive bleeding or hemodynamic collapse, or after a delay of hours to days with a similar presentation (34% of cases with only an 11% survival rate) (21,22). "Contained" left ventricular rupture following mitral valve replacement also may present days to years later, often as a pseudoaneurysm of the left ventricle detected on TTE or TEE (21). The clinical presentation of patients with such pseudoaneurysms is similar to the clinical picture seen with severe mitral regurgitation, congestive heart failure, and postoperative debilitation. Transesophageal echocardiography can be extremely helpful in distinguishing perivalvular defects, prosthetic valve dysfunction, or true left ventricular aneurysm as the cause for such clinical syndromes. The posterior location of pseudoaneurysms renders TEE to be superior to all other forms of cardiac imaging for accurate diagnosis (23).

Recurrent replacement of aortic or mitral valve prostheses is known to be associated with higher intra- and postoperative morbidity and mortality due to pericardial adhesions, friable tissue, distortion of anatomy, fistulae formation, LA dissection, and aneurysms or pseudoaneurysms of the aorta, ventricles, or atrium with potential rupture at time of surgery. Preoperative or intraoperative identification of these abnormalities by TEE significantly alters the surgical plan, often improving the surgical outcome (24–27).

In this patient, an extremely unusual complication of tricuspid valve repair was demonstrated. A deeply imbedded suture from the tricuspid valve annuloplasty apparently snared the noncoronary cusp of the aortic valve, leading to leaflet immobility and significant aortic insufficiency (Fig. 20.11). The close proximity of the aortic, mitral, and tricuspid annuli at the cardiac crux predisposes to a variety of iatrogenic complications. Other TEE investigators have reported another rare complication of mitral valve replacement and tricuspid annuloplasty: an iatrogenic left ventricle to RA fistula (28). In our patient, hemodynamic instability was probably related to acute aortic insufficiency (Fig. 20.12), residual tricuspid regurgitation, and possible

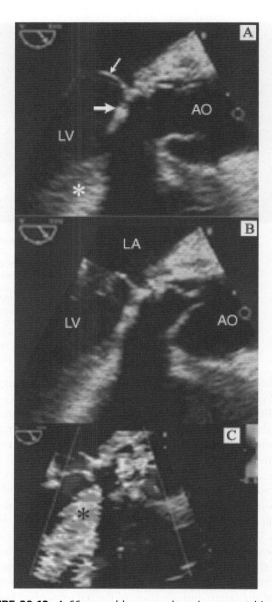

FIGURE 20.12. A 66-year-old man undergoing repeat bioprosthetic mitral valve surgery with tricuspid valve annuloplasty (case 5). All images were obtained with the transducer rotated to 120 degrees at the left ventricular outflow tract and aortic root (*AO*), with the left atrium (*LA*) at the top of each image, and the bioprosthetic mitral valve separating the LA from the left ventricle (*LV*). **A:** Transesophageal echocardiographic imaging of a normal-appearing bioprosthetic mitral valve with a thin leaflet (*small arrow*) coapting normally in ventricular systole, the linear bright echodensity of the mitral valve strut (*large arrow*), and the heavy shadowing artifact (*asterisk*) produced by the bioprosthesis in the LV cavity. Two leaflets of the aortic valve appear to open normally. **B:** Same orientation as in **A**, during ventricular diastole, with incomplete coaptation of the aortic valve cusps. **C:** Same image orientation as in **A and B**, with color Doppler imaging of moderate to severe aortic insufficiency (*asterisk*).

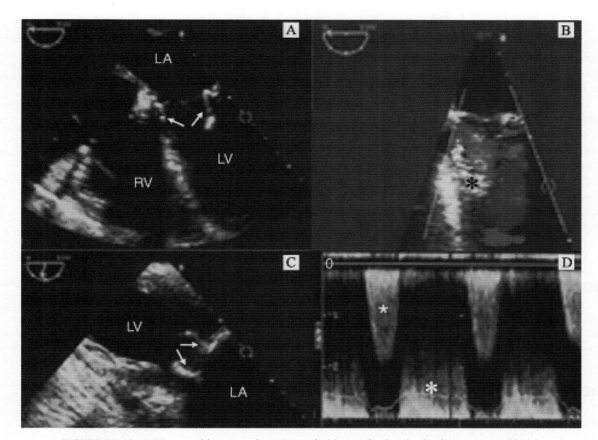

FIGURE 20.13. A 66-year-old man undergoing redo bioprosthetic mitral valve surgery with tricuspid valve annuloplasty (case 5). Images **A and B** were obtained in the transverse four-chamber view, with the left atrium (*LA*) at the top, the left ventricle (*LV*) at the right, and the right ventricle (*RV*) at the left part of the image. **A:** Two echodense struts (*arrows*) of the bioprosthetic mitral valve are seen directed toward the LV septum with one strut appearing to abut the proximal LV septum. **B:** Color Doppler map superimposed on the image seen in **A** during ventricular diastole shows aortic insufficiency (*asterisk*). **C:** Transgastric two-chamber view obtained with the transducer rotated to 77 degrees, with the transducer near the left ventricular apex and the LA at the bottom of the image. Two of the struts (*arrows*) from the bioprosthetic mitral valve project into the LV cavity. The LV outflow tract appears partially obliterated by one of the struts, which encroaches on the LV septum. A continuous-wave Doppler beam oriented along this image of the LV outflow tract produced the spectrum in **D. D:** Continuous-wave Doppler spectrum demonstrating aortic insufficiency (*large asterisk*) noted as diastolic Doppler signal directed toward the transducer (bottom of the image). A 2 m/s peak forward systolic velocity signal across the LV outflow tract and aortic valve (*small asterisk*) is noted as a systolic Doppler signal below the zero baseline (directed away from the transducer). The true magnitude of LV outflow tract obstruction was probably underestimated by these Doppler studies because the Doppler cursor could not be aligned parallel with blood flow in the LV outflow tract (see image orientation in **C**).

left ventricular outflow tract obstruction secondary to encroachment of the bioprosthetic mitral valve on the outflow tract (Fig. 20.13). Although a significant outflow tract gradient could not be demonstrated in this patient intraoperatively, ideal cursor alignment of the Doppler beam could not be achieved on the TEE examination due to limited probe positioning. Hemodynamic changes associated with varied left ventricular loading conditions (achieved by inotropic infusions, blood volume replacement, and vasopressors) suggested at least a moderate degree of inducible outflow tract obstruction when the left ventricle was underfilled and receiving beta-adrenergic stimulation. The

patient was finally weaned from cardiopulmonary bypass with careful titration of alpha- and beta-agonist–stimulating drugs, but had persistent hemodynamic instability with hypotension, low cardiac output, and pulmonary edema. By 48 hours postsurgery the patient developed multiorgan system failure and died.

CONCLUSIONS

Transesophageal echocardiography offers three unique advantages as a cardiac diagnostic technique: (a) adaptability to severely ill patients in a variety of critical care settings, including the operating room, (b) dynamic correlation of anatomic and physiologic information, and (c) high-resolution imaging of cardiac structures not well captured by other techniques. In this chapter we have explored some unique applications of this technology to the diagnosis and management of prosthetic valvular disease. Prosthetic valvular regurgitation, obstruction, thrombosis, infection, and iatrogenic complications are but a few of the many conditions that can be diagnosed by TEE. Intelligent integration of clinical reasoning with high-resolution TEE images of the pathologic anatomy and unique Doppler measurement of intracardiac flow events opens the door to understanding a wide array of clinical problems associated with prosthetic valves.

ACKNOWLEDGMENT

We gratefully acknowledge the excellent technical support provided by Eric R. Reynertson on the echocardiographic images provided in this chapter.

REFERENCES

1. Dzavik V, Cohen G, Chan K. Role of transesophageal echocardiography in the diagnosis and management of prosthetic valve thrombosis. *J Am Coll Cardiol* 1991;18:1829.
2. Gueret P, Vignon P, Fournier P, et al. Transesophageal echocardiography for the diagnosis and management of nonobstructive thrombosis of mechanical mitral valve prosthesis. *Circulation* 1995;91:103.
3. Barbetseas J, Nagueh S, Pitsavos C, et al. Differentiating thrombus from pannus formation in obstructed mechanical prosthetic valves: an evaluation of clinical, transthoracic and transesophageal echocardiographic parameters. *J Am Coll Cardiol* 1998;32:1410.
4. Lengyel M, Fuster V, Keltai M, et al. Guidelines for management of left-sided prosthetic valve thrombosis: a role for thrombolytic therapy. *J Am Coll Cardiol* 1997;30:1521.
5. Silber H, Khan S, Matloff J, et al. The St. Jude valve: thrombolysis as the first line of therapy for cardiac valve thrombosis. *Circulation* 1993;87:30.
6. Om A, Sperry R, Paulsen W. Transesophageal echocardiography for evaluation of thrombosed mitral valve prosthesis during thrombolytic therapy. *Am Heart J* 1992;124:781.
7. Barbetseas J, Zoghbi W. Evaluation of prosthetic valve function and associated complications. *Cardiol Clin* 1998;16:505.
8. Castello R, Pearson A, Lenzen P, et al. Effect of mitral regurgitation on pulmonary venous velocities derived from transesophageal echocardiography color-guided pulsed Doppler imaging. *J Am Coll Cardiol* 1991;17:1499.
9. Meloni L, Aru G, Abbruzzese P, et al. Localization of mitral periprosthetic leaks by transesophageal echocardiography. *Am J Cardiol* 1992;69:276.
10. Alam M, Serwin J, Rosman H, et al. Transesophageal echocardiographic features of normal and dysfunctioning bioprosthetic valves. *Am Heart J* 1991;121:1149.
11. Wernly J, Crawford M. Choosing a prosthetic heart valve. *Cardiol Clin* 1998;16:491.
12. Vongpatanasin W, Hillis D, Lange R. Prosthetic heart valves. *N Engl J Med* 1996;335:407.
13. Otto C. Prosthetic valves. In: Otto CM, ed. *Valvular heart disease,* 1st ed. Philadelphia: WB Saunders, 1999:17.
14. Lytle B. Surgical treatment of prosthetic valve endocarditis. *Semin Thorac Cardiovasc Surg* 1995;7:13.
15. Karalis D, Ross J, Brown B, et al. Transesophageal echocardiography in valvular heart disease. In: Frankl WS, Brest AN, ed. *Valvular heart disease: comprehensive evaluation and treatment.* Philadelphia: FA Davis, 1993:6.
16. Grimm R, Stewart W. The role of intraoperative echocardiography in valve surgery. *Cardiol Clin* 1998;16:477.
17. Nowrangi S, Connolly H, Freeman W, et al. Impact of intraoperative echocardiography among patients undergoing aortic valve replacement for aortic stenosis. *J Am Soc Echocardiogr* 2001;14:863.
18. Sheikh K, DeBruijn N, Rankin J, et al. The utility of transesophageal echocardiography and Doppler color flow imaging in patients undergoing cardiac valve surgery. *J Am Coll Cardiol* 1990;15:363.
19. Bryan A, Barzilai B, Kouchoukos N. Transesophageal echocardiography and adult cardiac operations. *Ann Thorac Surg* 1995;59:773.
20. Jebara V, Mihaileanu S, Acar C, et al. Left ventricular outflow tract obstruction after mitral valve repair. *Circulation* 1993;88(Part 2):30.
21. Karlson K, Ashraf M, Berger R. Rupture of left ventricle following mitral valve replacement. *Ann Thorac Surg* 1988;46:590.
22. Azariades M, Lennox S. Rupture of the posterior wall of the left ventricle after mitral valve replacement: etiologic and technical considerations. *Ann Thorac Surg* 1988;46:491.
23. Alam M, Glick C, Garcia R, et al. Transesophageal echocardiographic features of left ventricular pseudoaneurysm resulting after mitral valve replacement surgery. *Am Heart J* 1992;123:226.
24. Carrel T, Pasic M, Jenni R, et al. Reoperations after operation on the thoracic aorta: etiology, surgical techniques, and prevention. *Ann Thorac Surg* 1993;56:259.
25. Ballal R, Nanda N, Sanyal R. Intraoperative transesophageal echocardiographic diagnosis of left atrial pseudoaneurysm. *Am Heart J* 1992;123:217.
26. Hamilton D, Firmin R, Millar-Craig M. Pseudoaneurysm of the thoracic aorta presenting with angina: a late complication of aortic valve replacement. *Heart* 1998;79:310.
27. Gallego P, Oliver J, Gonzalez A, et al. Left atrial dissection: pathogenesis, clinical course, and transesophageal echocardiographic recognition. *J Am Soc Echocardiogr* 2001;14:813.
28. Benisty J, Roller M, Sahar G, et al. Iatrogenic left ventricular-right atrial fistula following mitral valve replacement and tricuspid annuloplasty: diagnosis by transthoracic and transesophageal echocardiography. *J Heart Valv Dis* 2000;9:732.

NATIVE AORTIC VALVE ENDOCARDITIS

ADAM B. ROSENBLUTH
LORI BRAY CROFT
EDWARD A. FISHER
MARTIN E. GOLDMAN

Infectious endocarditis (IE) is a potentially lethal disease in which the endothelial surface of the heart (most commonly a heart valve) is infected, and whose complications include congestive heart failure (1), systemic emboli (2,3), sepsis, and death (4,5). Infectious endocarditis usually is a clinical diagnosis based on the presence of fever, a new or changing heart murmur, bacteremia, and classic peripheral signs. Infectious endocarditis can then be classified, on the basis of duration and severity prior to treatment, as acute or chronic (subacute) (6).

The diagnosis of IE is suspected clinically and confirmed pathologically or echocardiographically by the presence of a vegetation, an aggregate of microorganisms, inflammatory cells, fibrin, and platelets. Vegetations can be large, especially when associated with *Staphylococcus aureus,* fungi, and gram-negative organisms. They can cause hemodynamic consequences, most commonly regurgitation, on the basis of their size and location. Leaflet coaptation can be disrupted, prolapse of a leaflet secondary to the weight of a vegetation can occur, and there can be destruction of the valve leaflets, chordae, or papillary muscles. In the most severe cases, paravalvular or myocardial abscesses may develop and can rupture. All of these complications are potential causes of regurgitation. Larger vegetations can obstruct flow and also are more likely to produce emboli (7).

In his Gulstonian lectures in 1885, Osler noted that 75% of patients with IE had preexisting abnormal cardiac valves (8). However, recent studies have demonstrated that acute IE can be associated with previously normal cardiac valves

---

A. B. Rosenbluth: Department of Cardiology, Mount Sinai Hospital, New York, New York.

L. Bray Croft: Department of Cardiology, The Mount Sinai Medical Center, New York, New York.

E. A. Fisher: Department of Medicine, Mount Sinai Hospital, New York, New York.

M. E. Goldman: Department of Medicine/Cardiology, Mount Sinai Medical School; and Department of Cardiology, Mount Sinai Hospital, New York, New York.

(Fig. 21.1) and that it is characterized by a septic, fulminant course classically caused by virulent *Staphylococcus aureus, Streptococcus pneumoniae,* or *Neisseria gonorrhoeae.* The bacteremia usually originates from a focus remote from the heart. Subacute or chronic IE generally is associated with underlying valvular disease and is characterized by an insidious onset and slowly progressive course, with low-grade fever, sweats, weight loss, and vague constitutional symptoms. Chronic IE usually develops within a few weeks of the bacteremia caused by viridans streptococci or by enterococci.

SCIENTIFIC PRINCIPLES

Pathophysiology

Several factors probably are involved in the development of IE on a native valve. Regurgitant or stenotic native valves may generate a high-velocity turbulent jet flowing from a high- to a low-pressure chamber that disrupts the endothelial surface and results in the deposition of platelets and fibrin, causing nonbacterial thrombotic endocarditis. Transient bacteremia then causes adherence of microorganisms to these sterile areas of platelet and fibrin deposition. Immunologic factors, including preformed circulating antibodies to the microorganisms, and interaction between the organism and an endothelial receptor also play a role (9).

Underlying valve pathology is a critical factor in the pathophysiology of IE. In the industrialized world, with increasing longevity, the incidence of valvular heart disease remains high; however, rheumatic heart disease has been replaced by degenerative valve disease, particularly aortic valvular stenosis in the elderly and mitral annular calcification as the dominant causes (10). The mitral valve is more likely to become infected if there is underlying pathology (i.e., rheumatic mitral stenosis). At present, mitral valve prolapse is the most common cardiac diagnosis predisposing patients to valvular endocarditis, but if there is no premorbid abnormality, the aortic valve is more commonly involved. Native aortic valve endocarditis is more often related to infection

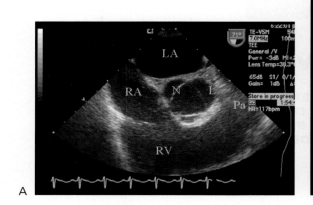
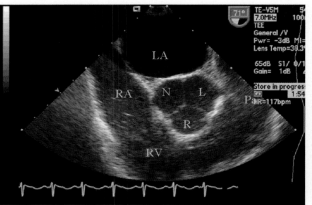

FIGURE 21.1. Transverse plane view at the base of the heart of the three leaflets of the aortic valve. **A:** The left (*L*), right (*R*), and noncoronary (*N*) cusps are visualized open in systole. **B:** The leaflets are seen closed in diastole. *LA,* left atrium; *Pa,* pulmonary artery; *RA,* right atrium; *RV,* right ventricle.

on a pathologically abnormal valve (including rheumatic heart disease, aortosclerosis, or stenosis), a bicuspid valve (Fig. 21.2), or a regurgitant valve.

Finally, nosocomial infections are now reaching rates of 7% to 29% in various studies (6). Over half of these cases of nosocomial IE are thought to arise in the setting of implanted intravascular devices such as central lines and Swan-Ganz catheters (11). With constant increase in the number and virulence of resistant organisms, this class of IE microorganisms is the most feared.

Anatomy

The vegetation can form on one or all of the valve leaflets. The side of the leaflet involved usually is on the low-pressure side of the jet lesion onto which the turbulent jet is directed (i.e., the ventricular side of the valve in aortic regurgitation, and the aortic side in aortic stenosis). Endocarditis complicating a ventricular septal defect develops on the low-pressure side

of the shunt flow (i.e., in the right ventricle in a left-to-right shunt, but in the left ventricle in a patient with Eisenmenger physiology and a right-to-left shunt). The destruction of the valve tissue results from the infecting organism's invasion into the valve and surrounding tissue, and from the subsequent immunologic response.

Because of its central location, the aortic valve and its sinuses are in contact with all four cardiac chambers. When an abscess develops in the aortic annulus, the clinical presentation depends on which cusp is involved. A ventricular septal myocardial abscess can form, producing a large abscess cavity, or it can rupture into either ventricle, producing a fistula. An annular abscess can expand into the pericardial cavity, producing purulent pericarditis or hemopericardium, or it can form a fistula between the aorta and a nearby structure, such as the right atrium, the left atrium, or the pulmonary artery. An abscess of the mitral valve can involve the conduction system, causing PR segment prolongation on the electrocardiogram, or even heart block.

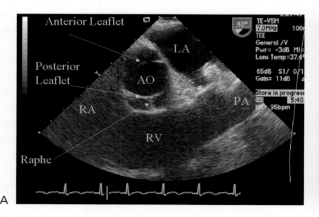
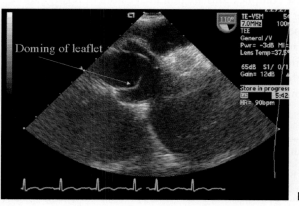

FIGURE 21.2. A: Bicuspid aortic valve with anterior and posterior cusps open in systole (short-axis view). *AO,* aorta; *LA,* left atrium; *Pa,* pulmonary artery; *RA,* right atrium; *RV,* right ventricle. **B:** Doming of leaflet in long-axis view.

Complications

Before the introduction of penicillin in the 1930s, the mortality rate of patients with IE was almost 100%, with sepsis being the leading cause of death. Today, congestive heart failure is the leading cause of death (up to 85%) in patients with IE (12–14). However, despite the availability of effective antibiotics, as well as earlier and improved surgical intervention (15–17), morbidity and mortality rates are still significant. Because its resolution is superior to that of transthoracic echocardiography (TTE), transesophageal echocardiography (TEE) is better able to differentiate a sclerotic or calcified valve from one that is infected. Thus, by detecting smaller vegetations earlier in the course of diseases, TEE can be used to expedite treatment before extensive damage is done.

Complications of IE include both cardiac (heart failure caused by valvular regurgitation, myocardial abscess and rupture, conduction defects, myocardial infarction, and pericarditis) and extracardiac (emboli; mycotic aneurysm; metastatic infection; and central nervous system, cutaneous, renal, and musculoskeletal abnormalities) problems (18). Emboli are detected clinically in 15% to 35% of patients, most commonly involving the spleen, brain, kidneys, and coronary vessels (12,19–21). Silent microemboli occur in a larger percentage of patients.

Patients with aortic valve vegetations are more likely to have a major complication, develop congestive heart failure, or require surgery compared to patients with vegetations on other valves (22–24).

Abscesses

Infectious endocarditis, most often caused by staphylococci and gram-negative bacilli, can produce valve ring abscesses (Fig. 21.3) with the formation of fistulae into the myocardium or pericardium. Aneurysms of the valve leaflet or

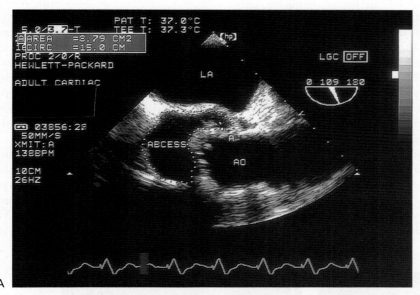

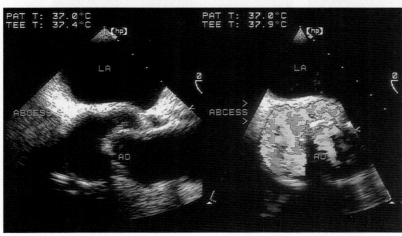

FIGURE 21.3. A: Aortic abscess. Longitudinal view demonstrating abscess space. **B:** Abscess space with color flow in the right plane. *LA*, left atrium; *AO*, aorta.

sinus of Valsalva also can occur. Myocarditis or myocardial infarction from coronary artery emboli can be found at autopsy. Myocardial abscesses have been reported in up to 30% of surgical and autopsy cases (25–29). These abscesses can be associated with conduction disturbances and rhythm abnormalities, and with rapid onset of congestive heart failure. Purulent pericarditis, from rupture of an abscess or contiguous extension, occurs more commonly with acute than chronic IE.

Ellis and colleagues (30) studied 46 patients with native and prosthetic valve IE documented by surgery, 22 with associated abscesses and 24 without, and recommended four diagnostic criteria for the diagnosis of abscesses: prosthetic valve rocking, aneurysm of the sinus of Valsalva, thickness of the anterior or posterior wall of the aortic root greater than 10 mm, and perivalvular density in the septum greater than 14 mm. The presence or absence of one or more of these criteria had positive and negative predictive value for an abscess of 86% and 87%, respectively. However, these abnormalities can be seen in diseases other than abscess associated with IE.

Because of its higher resolution due to its proximity to the heart and its higher frequency (7 or 5 MHz vs. 2.5 to 3.5 MHz in TTE), TEE is superior to TTE for abscess detection. Transthoracic echocardiography detected 13 of 46 areas of abscess, whereas TEE detected 40 of 46 areas (31). The sensitivity and specificity were 28.3% and 98.6% with TTE, respectively, compared with 87% and 94.6% with TEE. Therefore, TEE led to significant improvement in the detection of abscesses associated with endocarditis, and facilitated earlier treatment. Because antibiotics may not penetrate into an abscess effectively, early identification and surgery can improve outcome (32). Daniel and colleagues found a hospital mortality rate of 22.7% in patients with abscesses compared with 13.5% in patients without abscesses (30).

Myocardial abscess occurs most commonly in patients with prosthetic valve endocarditis, but when they involve a native valve, they usually are associated echocardiographically demonstrable vegetations. Preoperative TTE detected 41% of myocardial abscesses in patients with native valve IE but only 15% of those in patients with prosthetic valve IE, probably because the metal components of the prosthesis cause extensive shadowing, which can obscure visualization of an abscess (33).

CLINICAL ASPECTS

About 8,000 cases of IE occur annually in the United States, with an incidence of 1.7 to 6.2 cases per 100,000 person-years. The median age of patients with endocarditis has gradually increased from 30 to 40 years in the preantibiotic era to 47 to 69 years at present (34). The likely cause of the increase in age of patients with IE is the decreased incidence of rheumatic fever and the increased incidence of degenerative heart disease in the elderly. Calcified mitral or aortic valves (Fig. 21.4) predispose to IE by providing a nidus for circulating bacteria. Up to 30% to 40% of patients without any demonstrable underlying valvular heart disease who develop IE have degenerative cardiac valvular disease (35). The most common predisposing factors in patients over 65 years of age who have native valve endocarditis are these degenerative valve lesions, including mitral annular calcification and aortosclerosis, with or without a bicuspid valve. In this population, the mitral valve is involved more frequently than is the aortic valve, but the aortic valve is involved in two thirds of male cases versus one third of female cases.

In pediatric patients, after the neonatal period, there usually is an identifiable lesion predisposing to IE (36,37). During the 1980s, only 1.5% to 10% of IE occurred on valves affected by rheumatic fever (5,38,39). There also is an association between congenital heart disease and IE. Of 181 children with congenital heart disease who were examined at

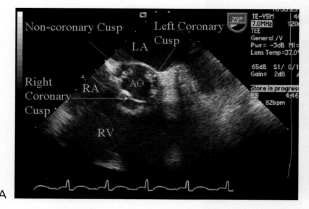
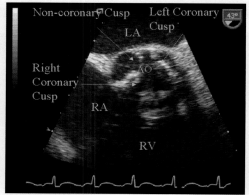

FIGURE 21.4. Longitudinal plane view of calcific aortic stenosis. **A:** Open. **B:** Closed. Valve area measures 1.26 cm². Calcium and fibrosis of the valve can be difficult to differentiate from a vegetation. However, the lack of mobility and the diffuse nature of the infiltration of the valve are more suggestive of calcific stenosis, especially given the limited excursion of the valve. *LA,* left atrium; *RA,* right atrium; *RV,* right ventricle; *AO,* aorta.

autopsy in the preantibiotic era, 16.5% had IE (40). The frequency of known underlying congenital heart disease varies from 6% to 24% of patients with IE (41). Those with cyanotic heart disease who have shunts and stenotic valves are at highest risk. Patients with ventricular septal defects, patent ductus arteriosus, and tetralogy of Fallot are infected much more commonly than are patients with coarctation of the aorta and bicuspid aortic valves. Aortic valve disease accounts for 9% of children with IE. Importantly, unrestricted atrial septal defects without turbulent jet flow are not associated with an increased risk for IE.

Underlying lesions in the adult population include, in decreasing order, mitral valve prolapse, no underlying heart disease, degenerative disease of the aortic and mitral valves, congenital heart disease, and rheumatic heart disease (42).

Rheumatic heart disease accounted for most cases of IE until the 1970s, but now is responsible for only about 30% of lesions in patients with IE (43). With rheumatic heart disease, the mitral valve is involved in over 85% of cases (41). If there is isolated rheumatic mitral valve disease, the female to male ratio is 2:1, but if there is isolated aortic valve disease, there is a 4:1 male predominance. The mitral valve is involved in most patients (85%), followed by the aortic valve (50%) (41). Congenital heart disease occurs in about 15% of adult patients with IE (42). A bicuspid aortic valve is an important risk factor, especially in men over 60 years of age. Patients with hypertrophic cardiomyopathy can develop IE on the aortic valve because of turbulence of the jet crossing the aortic valve distal to the subvalvular obstruction, or on the mitral valve if there is associated mitral regurgitation. Patients with Marfan syndrome and aortic regurgitation also can develop IE, although the vegetations are found primarily on the mitral valve from the jet of aortic regurgitation (44). Luetic aortic valves are now uncommon. There is a significantly increased incidence of IE in the elderly, probably due to longer survival of patients with underlying heart disease and the increased incidence of degenerative valve disease (45).

The clinical course of a patient with IE depends on several factors. If there was prior ventricular adaptation to volume overload (prior aortic regurgitation with aortic valve IE), the further hemodynamic burden of the additional valvular regurgitation may be well tolerated. However, if the underlying valve was normal and there was no previous regurgitation, a new large regurgitant volume can precipitate symptoms. Patients can deteriorate quickly because acute severe mitral regurgitation causes pulmonary edema, which can be treated pharmacologically, whereas acute aortic regurgitation can cause a marked decrease in cardiac output and pulmonary congestion.

CONTRIBUTION OF ECHOCARDIOGRAPHY

The clinical course of IE can be predicted by echocardiographic determination of the size (46–48), extent, and mo-

bility of the vegetations (Fig. 21.5) (23,24,49), as well as by the severity of the regurgitation (50). Transthoracic echocardiography offers a rapid and noninvasive technique with specificity as high as 98%; however, secondary to technical difficulties in obtaining images such as obesity or hyperinflated lungs in patients with chronic obstructive pulmonary disease, the sensitivity may be less than 60% to 70% (51). Vegetations can be adherent but are distinct from the underlying valve leaflet, chord, or endocardium. Echocardiography sometimes can distinguish the tissue density of the vegetation from the underlying valve, and the mobility of the vegetation usually is independent or lags from the underlying tissue. Echocardiographic demonstration of disruption of the aortic valve tissue, premature closure of the mitral valve, or diastolic mitral regurgitation indicates significant hemodynamic decompensation secondary to severe aortic regurgitation with marked elevation of left ventricular and diastolic pressures that often requires valve replacement.

Extra echoes on a valve can be caused by calcium, fibrosis, myxomatous degeneration, excrescences, tumor (i.e., papillary fibromas and fibroelastomas, Fig. 21.6), thrombus, or healed or active vegetations. A mobile, echogenic, pedunculated mass visualized on a leaflet is most often a vegetation. Abnormal echoes seen on the left ventricular outflow tract can represent a vegetation (Fig. 21.7) or part of a flail aortic valve.

Both M-mode and two-dimensional echocardiography can be used to detect valvular vegetations (9,20,52–57). Transesophageal echocardiography is able to image closer to cardiac structures using a high-frequency transducer (up to 7 MHz), providing better resolution of small structures and spatial relationships than do standard 2- to 3.5-MHz TTE transducers. Because of its much higher sampling rate, color M-mode facilitates the resolution of subtle abnormalities (i.e., fluttering of the anterior leaflet of the mitral valve in aortic endocarditis) that are not easily perceived with routine two-dimensional echocardiography.

Transesophageal echocardiography technology has improved two-dimensional image quality and color flow mapping, which facilitates the recognition of even smaller vegetations (Fig. 21.8) than was possible with earlier equipment and is invaluable in differentiating sclerotic from calcific aortic valves (Fig. 21.4) and excrescences from infected valves. Transesophageal echocardiography increases sensitivity for detection of valve lesions to 75% to 95%, while maintaining a specificity of 85% to 98% (58). By detecting smaller vegetations earlier in the course of IE, TEE can facilitate prompt therapy before extensive damage is done to the valve. Studies have reported improved sensitivity of TEE versus TTE (100% vs. 3%) in the detection of native and prosthetic IE (57). All vegetations larger than 10 mm were detected by both techniques, but because of poorer image resolution, TTE could visualize only 69% of moderately sized vegetations (6–10 mm) and 25% of small vegetations (<5 mm), all of which were detected with TEE. In general, a vegetation

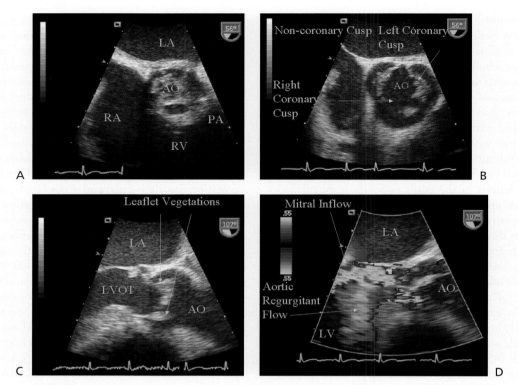

FIGURE 21.5. Aortic vegetation. Note the irregularly shaped and echogenic densities on the aortic valve leaflets that appear heterogeneous in density with some mobility. **A:** Short axis closed. **B:** Short axis open. **C:** Long axis open. **D:** Long axis with color flow Doppler demonstrating mitral inflow in blue and aortic regurgitation in red resulting from vegetation preventing appropriate coaptation of valve leaflets. *LA,* left atrium; *RA,* right atrium; *RV,* right ventricle; *AO,* aorta; *PA,* pulmonary artery; *LVOT,* left ventricular outflow tract.

must be at least 2 to 3 mm to be visualized accurately through the thorax.

Aortic Valve Imaging

There are various approaches to TEE imaging. We perform a complete study on all patients. However, if a patient is

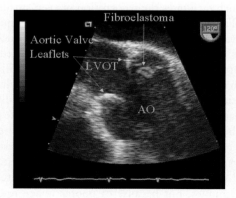

FIGURE 21.6. Long-axis view of the aortic valve in systole demonstrating a fibroelastoma on the valve, which can be difficult to differentiate from a vegetation. *AO,* aorta; *LVOT,* left ventricular outflow tract.

clinically unstable, we initiate the study to image the region of interest first and then complete the study as time allows. For example, in a patient with suspected aortic dissection, we image the ascending and descending aorta and the aortic arch initially, then assess left ventricular function and the severity of the aortic insufficiency and evaluate the coronary arteries. If the patient remains stable, we then complete the study.

We routinely initiate imaging of the aortic valve in the transgastric five-chamber view, which is similar to the transthoracic apical five-chamber view in which the apex is at the top of the screen, the left ventricular area is on the right, and the aortic leaflets are well seen. From this plane, any subvalvular gradient or gradient across a stenotic aortic valve or prosthesis can be measured. Because imaging originates from the apex of the ventricle, the left ventricular outflow tract is not shadowed by a prosthetic valve or by calcium on the aortic valve. This view allows visualization of the ventricular surface of the leaflets. Slightly higher in the transgastric view, imaging at about 75 degrees, a modified long-axis view is seen with the aorta toward the lower portion of the screen. We then raise the probe above the diaphragm and evaluate the aortic valve and its three leaflets at a 45 to 60 degree plane. The mobility of the leaflets, the number of

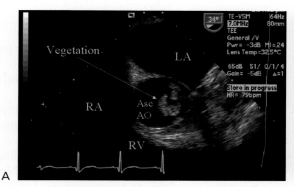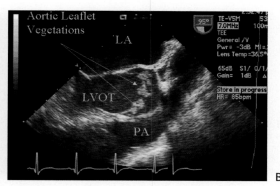

FIGURE 21.7. A longitudinal plane view of an aortic vegetation extending into the ascending aorta (*Asc AO*) on the aortic side of the aortic valve. In short-axis **(A)** and long-axis **(B)** views. *LA*, left atrium; *RA*, right atrium; *RV*, right ventricle; *LVOT*, left ventricular outflow tract; *PA*, pulmonary artery.

leaflets, and the presence and severity of aortic insufficiency can be assessed by continuing to rotate and image toward a 90 degree plane as the left ventricular outflow tract, the ascending aorta, and the aortic valve are seen. The presence of an aortic abscess can be diagnosed as the probe is maneuvered from 90 degrees back toward 0 degrees and the aortic valve is fully imaged.

A vegetation usually is visualized by TEE as an irregularly shaped, mobile, or sessile density that protrudes from the normal valve contour. Its location on the leaflet depends on the underlying pathology. As previously described, the inciting infection develops in the area of the jet flow and turbulence. Therefore, with aortic insufficiency, the turbulence is directed toward the ventricular side of the aortic valve, whereas in aortic stenosis, vegetations form on the aortic side of the valve.

The differential diagnosis of a mass on the valve includes an infectious, degenerative, thrombotic, or neoplastic etiology. Most commonly, a patient's history provides insight into whether infection is more likely. Patients who develop

endocarditis usually have underlying valvular disease, which can include rheumatic disease, congenital disease (bicuspid, Fig. 21.2), degenerative aortic sclerosis, or redundant prolapsing leaflets.

Lambl excrescences are fine endothelial strands seen on the ventricular side of the valve related to shear forces eroding the fine endothelial layer of the valve tissue itself. These fine mobile strands have embolic potential. Papillomas may form on the valve and can be a source of embolization. They usually are bulbous structures on a fine stalk and are denser than a vegetation.

The likelihood of identifying a vegetation on echocardiography depends partially on its duration. Earlier in its course, when it consists more of inflammatory cells and bacteria, the vegetation can be less dense than the underlying valve tissue and may be smaller than the resolution of TEE imaging. However, as the lesion evolves, it can become denser, with more fibrous tissue, as well as less mobile. Embolic potential increases with increasing vegetation size and mobility.

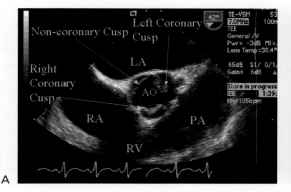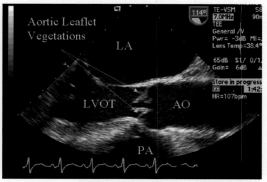

FIGURE 21.8. A vegetation that prolapses into the left ventricular (*LV*) outflow tract on short-axis **(A)** and long-axis **(B)** views. Smaller vegetations need to be differentiated from excrescences. *LA*, left atrium; *RA*, right atrium; *RV*, right ventricle; *PA*, pulmonary artery; *AO*, aorta; *LVOT*, left ventricular outflow tract.

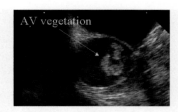

FIGURE 21.9. Case 1. A 73-year-old man who was seen for evaluation of a fever and new murmur. *AV,* aortic valve.

Case 1

A 73-year-old man was seen for evaluation of a fever and new murmur. Blood cultures were positive for *Staphylococcus epidermidis* and the patient was referred for TEE, which revealed aortic valve vegetation and regurgitation (Fig. 21.9).

Case 2

A 46 year-old woman presented with fever, chills, and a new murmur on examination. On admission, white blood cell count was 25, erythrocyte sedimentation rate was 97, and blood cultures grew out *Enterococcus faecalis.* Transesophageal echocardiography revealed moderate to severe aortic regurgitation with poor coaptation of the leaflets, and multiple echodensities consistent with vegetations on all three cusps of the aortic valve (Fig. 21.10).

CONCLUSION

Transesophageal echocardiography is the imaging technique of choice to confirm the presence of vegetations or abscesses involving native or prosthetic valves. Multiple imaging planes can be used to differentiate vegetations from other valvular abnormalities, including excrescences, redundant leaflets, and degenerative calcification. By facilitating early diagnosis and prompt treatment, TEE can prevent the development of more serious complications of endocarditis.

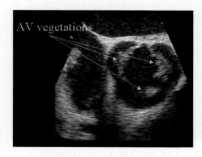

FIGURE 21.10. Case 2. A 46-year-old woman who presented with fever, chills, and a new murmur on examination. *AV,* aortic valve.

KEY POINTS

- Underlying pathology or prostheses predispose patients to endocarditis.
- Infectious endocarditis is a clinical diagnosis, and echocardiographic findings are often not diagnostic.
- Echocardiography is useful in defining the complications of endocarditis, including perforation, regurgitation, and abscess formation.
- The differential diagnosis of valvular findings other than endocarditis include excrescences, redundant leaflets, thrombus, neoplasm, and degenerative calcification.

REFERENCES

1. Varma MP, et al. Heart failure associated with infective endocarditis. A review of 40 cases. *Br Heart J* 1986;55:191–197.
2. Salgado AV, et al. Neurologic complications of endocarditis: a 12-year experience. *Neurology* 1989;39(2 Part 1):173–178.
3. Ting W, et al. Splenic septic emboli in endocarditis. *Circulation* 1990;82(5 suppl IV):105–109.
4. Weinstein L, Rubin RH. Infective endocarditis—1973. *Prog Cardiovasc Dis* 1973;16:239–274.
5. Von Reyn CF, et al. Infective endocarditis: an analysis based on strict case definitions. *Ann Intern Med* 1981;94(4 Part 1):505–518.
6. Mylonakis E, Calderwood SB. Infective endocarditis in adults. *N Engl J Med* 2001;345:1318–1330.
7. Vilacosta I, et al. Risk of embolization after institution of antibiotic therapy for infective endocarditis. *J Am Coll Cardiol* 2002;39(9):1489–1495.
8. Osler W. The Gulstonian lectures on malignant endocarditis. *BMJ* 1885;1:467.
9. Steckelberg JM, et al. Emboli in infective endocarditis: the prognostic value of echocardiography. *Ann Intern Med* 1991; 114(8):635–640.
10. Soler-Soler J, Galve E. Worldwide perspective of valve disease. *Heart* 2000;83(6):721–725.
11. Fernandez-Guerrero ML, et al. Hospital-acquired infectious endocarditis not associated with cardiac surgery: an emerging problem. *Clin Infect Dis* 1995;20(1):16–23.
12. Mills J, Utley J, Abbott J. Heart failure in infective endocarditis: predisposing factors, course, and treatment. *Chest* 1974; 66(2):151–157.
13. Richardson JV, et al. Treatment of infective endocarditis: a 10-year comparative analysis. *Circulation* 1978;58(4):589–597.
14. Steckelberg JM, Giuliani ER, Wilson WR. Infective endocarditis. In: Giuliani ER, Gersh BJ, McGoon MD, eds. *Cardiology: fundamentals and practice.* Vol. 2. Boston: Mosby-Year Book, 1991:1740.
15. Brandenburg RO, et al. Infective endocarditis—a 25 year overview of diagnosis and therapy. *J Am Coll Cardiol* 1983;1(1):280–291.
16. Alsip SG, et al. Indications for cardiac surgery in patients with active infective endocarditis. *Am J Med* 1985;78(6B):138–148.
17. Wilson WR, et al. Cardiac valve replacement in congestive heart failure due to infective endocarditis. *Mayo Clin Proc* 1979;54(4):223–226.
18. Wilson WR, et al. Management of complications of infective endocarditis. *Mayo Clin Proc* 1982;57(3):162–170.

19. Wann LS, et al. Echocardiography in bacterial endocarditis. *N Engl J Med* 1976;295(3):135–139.

20. Wann LS, et al. Comparison of M-mode and cross-sectional echocardiography in infective endocarditis. *Circulation* 1979;60(4):728–733.

21. Lerner PI, Weinstein L. Infective endocarditis in the antibiotic era. *N Engl J Med* 1966;274(4):199–206.

22. **Sanfilippo AJ, et al. Echocardiographic assessment of patients with infectious endocarditis: prediction of risk for complications. *J Am Coll Cardiol* 1991;18(5):1191–1199.**

23. **Rohmann S, et al. Clinical relevance of vegetation localization by transoesophageal echocardiography in infective endocarditis. *Eur Heart J* 1992;13(4):446–452.**

24. Krause JR, Levison SP. Pathology of infective endocarditis. In: Kaye D, ed. *Infective endocarditis.* Baltimore: University Park Press, 1976:55.

25. Roberts W. Characteristics and consequences of infective endocarditis (active or healed or both) learned from morphologic studies. In: Rahimoola SH, ed. Infective endocarditis. New York: Grune & Stratton, 1978:55.

26. Buchbinder NA, Roberts WC. Left-sided valvular active infective endocarditis. A study of forty-five necropsy patients. *Am J Med* 1972;53(1):20–35.

27. Arnett EN, Roberts WC. Valve ring abscess in active infective endocarditis. Frequency, location, and clues to clinical diagnosis from the study of 95 necropsy patients. *Circulation* 1976;54(1):140–145.

28. Arnett EN, Roberts WC. Prosthetic valve endocarditis: clinico-pathologic analysis of 22 necropsy patients with comparison observations in 74 necropsy patients with active infective endocarditis involving natural left-sided cardiac valves. *Am J Cardiol* 1976;38(3):281–292.

29. Ellis SG, Goldstein J, Popp RL. Detection of endocarditis-associated perivalvular abscesses by two-dimensional echocardiography. *J Am Coll Cardiol* 1985;5(3):647–653.

30. **Daniel WG, et al. Improvement in the diagnosis of abscesses associated with endocarditis by transesophageal echocardiography. *N Engl J Med* 1991;324(12):795–800.**

31. Croft CH, et al. Analysis of surgical versus medical therapy in active complicated native valve infective endocarditis. *Am J Cardiol* 1983;51(10):1650–1655.

32. Enzler MJ, Wilson WR, Giuliani ER. Noninvasive detection of cardiac abscesses complicating infective endocarditis. *Am J Non-invasive Cardiol* 1987;1:109.

33. Scheld WM, Sande MA. Endocarditis and intravascular infections. In: Douglas RG, Mandell GL, Bennett JE, eds. *Principles and practice of infectious disease.* New York: John Wiley & Sons, 1985:504.

34. Hogevik H, et al. Epidemiologic aspects of infective endocarditis in an urban population. A 5-year prospective study. *Medicine (Baltimore)* 1995;74(6):324–339.

35. Saiman L, Prince A. Infections of the heart. *Adv Pediatr Infect Dis* 1989;4:139–161.

36. Johnson CM, Rhodes KH. Pediatric endocarditis. *Mayo Clin Proc* 1982;57(2):86–94.

37. Sholler GF, Hawker RE, Celermajer JM. Infective endocarditis in childhood. *Pediatr Cardiol* 1986;6(4):183–186.

38. Schollin J, Bjarke B, Wesstrom G. Infective endocarditis in Swedish children. I. Incidence, etiology, underlying factors and port of entry of infection. *Acta Paediatr Scand* 1986;75(6):993–998.

39. Cutler JG, Ongley PA, Shwachman H, et al. Bacterial endocarditis in children with heart disease. *Pediatrics* 1958;22:706.

40. Kaye D. Definitions and demographic characteristics. In: Kaye D, ed. *Infective endocarditis.* Baltimore: University Park Press, 1976:1.

41. McKinsey DS, Ratts TE, Bisno AL. Underlying cardiac lesions in adults with infective endocarditis. The changing spectrum. *Am J Med* 1987;82(4):681–688.

42. Griffin MR, et al. Infective endocarditis. Olmsted County, Minnesota, 1950 through 1981. *JAMA* 1985;254(9):1199–1202.

43. Soman VR, et al. Bacterial endocarditis of mitral valve in Marfan syndrome. *Br Heart J* 1974;36(12):1247–1250.

44. Kaye D. Changing pattern of infective endocarditis. *Am J Med* 1985;78(6B):157–162.

45. Bardy G, Talano J, Reisberg B, et al. Sensitivity and specificity of echocardiography in a high-risk population of patients for infective endocarditis: significance of vegetation size. *J Cardiovasc Ultrasonogr* 1983;2:83.

46. Buda AJ, et al. Prognostic significance of vegetations detected by two-dimensional echocardiography in infective endocarditis. *Am Heart J* 1986;112(6):1291–1296.

47. Wong D, et al. Clinical implications of large vegetations in infectious endocarditis. *Arch Intern Med* 1983;143(10):1874–1877.

48. **Mugge A, et al. Echocardiography in infective endocarditis: reassessment of prognostic implications of vegetation size determined by the transthoracic and the transesophageal approach. *J Am Coll Cardiol* 1989;14(3):631–638.**

49. Jaffe WM, et al. Infective endocarditis, 1983–1988: echocardiographic findings and factors influencing morbidity and mortality. *J Am Coll Cardiol* 1990;15(6):1227–1233.

50. Roy P, et al. Spectrum of echocardiographic findings in bacterial endocarditis. *Circulation* 1976;53(3):474–482.

51. Shively BK, et al. Diagnostic value of transesophageal compared with transthoracic echocardiography in infective endocarditis. *J Am Coll Cardiol* 1991;18(2):391–397.

52. Martin RP, et al. Clinical utility of two dimensional echocardiography in infective endocarditis. *Am J Cardiol* 1980;46(3):379–385.

53. Rubenson DS, et al. The use of echocardiography in diagnosing culture-negative endocarditis. *Circulation* 1981;64(3):641–646.

54. Mintz GS, et al. Comparison of two-dimensional and M-mode echocardiography in the evaluation of patients with infective endocarditis. *Am J Cardiol* 1979;43(4):738–744.

55. **Klodas E, Edwards WD, Khandheria BK. Use of transesophageal echocardiography for improving detection of valvular vegetations in subacute bacterial endocarditis. *J Am Soc Echocardiogr* 1989;2(6):386–389.**

56. Dillon JC, et al. Echocardiographic manifestations of valvular vegetations. *Am Heart J* 1973;86(5):698–704.

57. Erbel R, et al. Improved diagnostic value of echocardiography in patients with infective endocarditis by transoesophageal approach. A prospective study. *Eur Heart J* 1988;9(1):43–53.

58. **Werner GS, et al. Infective endocarditis in the elderly in the era of transesophageal echocardiography: clinical features and prognosis compared with younger patients. *Am J Med* 1996;100(1):90–97.**

ECHOCARDIOGRAPHIC ASSESSMENT OF AORTIC DISSECTION

DAVID L. REICH

CLINICAL ISSUES

Aortic dissection is one of the areas in cardiothoracic surgery where the anesthesiologist-echocardiographer will have important contributions to make to the diagnosis and intraoperative management of the patient. The causes of aortic dissection include hypertension, trauma, atherosclerosis, iatrogenic causes such as aortic manipulation, and Marfan syndrome. The complications and sequelae of the aortic pathology include aortic rupture, hemothorax, pericardial effusion/tamponade, aortic valve insufficiency, and ischemia of various tissues (coronary, cerebral, renal, mesenteric, limb, etc.). As a consequence of these problems, the patients are often hemodynamically unstable and in respiratory failure. In order to prevent rupture of the aorta, the patients are usually placed on pharmacologic therapy to reduce aortic wall stress and shear forces (beta-adrenergic blockers and vasodilators). Excellent topical or general anesthesia is required to perform a diagnostic transesophageal echocardiography (TEE) examination to blunt the hemodynamic responses to instrumentation of the upper airway. A case of rupture of the false lumen during TEE has been reported that was presumably related to the hemodynamic response to echo probe insertion or manipulation (1). Other diagnostic examinations, such as magnetic resonance imaging and computed tomography (CT) scanning, may not be possible in these patients, who are frequently unstable.

The diagnosis of an acute dissection involving the ascending aorta (type A) with or without aortic insufficiency necessitates urgent surgery, whereas a dissection limited to the descending aorta (type B) usually is managed conservatively (2). Intraoperatively, the assessment of cardiopulmonary bypass (CPB) perfusion in the true lumen of the aorta at the initiation of CPB is extremely important to ensure the adequacy of end-organ perfusion (especially cerebral perfusion). Additionally, TEE will aid in the assessment of intravascular volume repletion, myocardial perfusion, and the quality of the surgical repair.

SCIENTIFIC PRINCIPLES

Anatomy

The aorta is composed of intimal, medial, and adventitial layers. The proximal third of the ascending aorta arises from the left ventricle posterior to the right ventricular infundibulum and pulmonary valve. The middle third of the aorta lies to the right of the main pulmonary artery, anterior to the right pulmonary artery, and anteromedial to the superior vena cava. The distal third of the ascending aorta and the proximal portion of the transverse aortic arch lie anterior to the trachea and right main-stem bronchus. The remainder of the transverse and descending thoracic aorta lies in close proximity to the esophagus in the left thoracic cavity.

Pathology and Pathophysiology

Aortic dissection has an incidence of approximately 5.2 per million per year in the general population. Predisposing factors are thought to include age, hypertension, connective tissue disorders, congenital aortic stenosis and other malformations of the valve and aorta, iatrogenic causes, trauma, and pregnancy (3). The clinical presentation of acute aortic dissection usually includes pain described as tearing or ripping. The pain remains constant rather than fluctuating, but may change in location. Syncope, usually transient in nature, is thought to be related to temporary ischemia of the central nervous system. Dyspnea and hemoptysis are more common in chronic dissections, but can be seen with acute dissections that impinge on the tracheobronchial tree. On physical examination, acute onset differential or absent pulses in the extremities is reliable indicator of acute dissection; this may accompany limb ischemia.

An aortic dissection consists of a tear (often referred to as a rent) in the intimal layer that allows blood to flow between

D. L. Reich: Department of Anesthesiology, The Mount Sinai Medical Center, New York, New York.

the intimal and the medial/adventitial layers. One or more secondary (reentry) tears also may be present more distally. As the blood separates (dissects) the intimal from the medial/adventitial layers, the intima that gives rise to blood flow to coronary, cerebral, and other vascular beds is compressed. Thus, one of the major complications of aortic dissection is ischemia or infarction in one or more of the myocardial, cerebral, mesenteric, renal, or limb tissues. The terminal event in untreated aortic dissection patients is usually rupture of the adventitia that leads to hemorrhage into the pericardium or pleural spaces. Aortic root dilatation with severe aortic insufficiency also may be associated with aortic dissection. Severe aortic insufficiency may lead to pulmonary edema and a low cardiac output state.

Aortic dissections are classified according to two systems (4,5). The DeBakey classification system is described in Fig. 22.1. The dissection is classified as type A if the intimal tear is in the ascending aorta. Type A dissections are subdivided into type IA if the dissection extends from the ascending through the descending aorta and type IIA if the dissection is limited

to the ascending aorta. Type B dissections involve an intimal tear distal to the origin of the left subclavian artery and are also known as type III dissections. The Daily classification system is described in Fig. 22.2. A type A dissection is any dissection involving the ascending aorta, regardless of the site of the tear. A type B dissection involves the descending aorta alone. The acute mortality rate associated with a Daily type A dissection is 90% to 95% without surgical intervention. The acute mortality rate associated with a Daily type B dissection is approximately 40% (Table 22.1) (6).

CLINICAL INFORMATION

History

A 60-year-old man with a history of hypertension that was poorly controlled on enalapril and atenolol complained of excruciating back pain and shortness of breath. He presented to another hospital hypotensive and diaphoretic. His condition improved with volume resuscitation using crystalloid

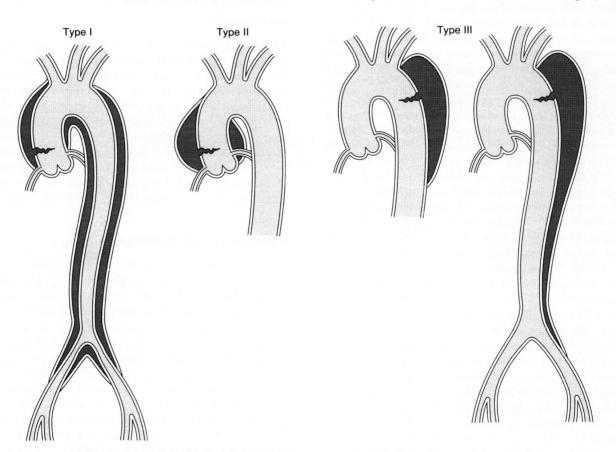

FIGURE 22.1. The DeBakey classification of aortic dissections. Type I: intimal tear in the ascending aorta with extension of the dissection to the descending aorta. Type II: ascending intimal tear with dissection limited to the ascending aorta. Type IIIA: intimal tear in the descending aorta with proximal extension of the dissection to involve the ascending aorta. Type IIIB: intimal tear in the descending aorta with dissection limited to the descending aorta. (Reprinted from Larson EW, Edwards WD. Risk factors for aortic dissection: a necropsy study of 161 cases. *Am J Cardiol* 1984;3:849, with permission.)

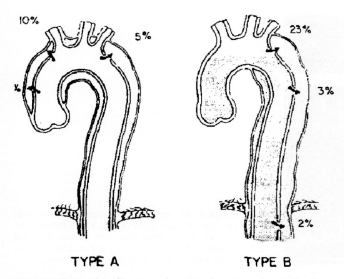

FIGURE 22.2. Classification of aortic dissections by Daily. Type A is any involvement of the ascending aorta, regardless of the location of the intimal tear. Type B is dissection limited to the descending aorta. (Reproduced from Ergin MA, Galla JD, Lansman S, et al. Acute dissections of the aorta: current surgical treatment. *Surg Clin North Am* 1985;63:721, with permission.)

replacement solution. Following a chest radiograph showing mediastinal widening, he was transferred for evaluation and treatment of a possible aortic dissection. The patient was placed on intravenous esmolol and sodium nitroprusside to diminish the shear stresses on the aortic wall in order to reduce the progression of the dissection.

Physical Examination

On arrival, the patient was cyanotic and in acute respiratory distress with severe pulmonary edema. He remained diaphoretic, but the hypoxia resolved with tracheal intubation and mechanical ventilation with positive end-expiratory pressure. The blood pressure was 90/60 mm Hg in the right arm and 130/80 mm Hg in the left arm. Left-sided

TABLE 22.1. CHARACTERISTICS OF DAILY TYPE A AND TYPE B AORTIC DISSECTIONS

	Type A	Type B
Frequency (%)	65–70	30–35
Male: Female ratio	2:1	3:1
Average age	50–55	60–70
Associated hypertension (%)	50	80
Hypertension on admission	±	++
Associated atherosclerosis	±	++
Aortic insufficiency (%)	50	10
Intimal tear	Always present	Absent in 5%–10%
Acute mortality (%)	90–95	40

From Ergin MA, Galla JD, Lansman S, et al. Acute dissections of the aorta: current surgical treatment. *Surg Clin North Am* 1985;63:721, with permission.

hemiplegia was present and breath sounds were diminished over the left lung field. A urinary catheter was placed, and oliguria was present.

Preoperative Laboratory and Diagnostic Studies

Chest radiography: Chest radiography was repeated and showed mediastinal widening, alveolar infiltrates, and a left pleural effusion.

Electrocardiography (ECG): Sinus tachycardia at 130 beats/min; left ventricular hypertrophy with "strain" pattern.

Transesophageal echocardiography: The patient was considered too unstable to be transported to the cardiac catheterization laboratory or the CT scan suite. A magnetic resonance imaging study also is not practical in an unstable intubated patient. A TEE was ordered to confirm the presumptive diagnosis of acute aortic dissection. Transesophageal echocardiography was performed by the anesthesiologist, with the use of propofol and opioid sedation, beta-adrenergic blockade, and sodium nitroprusside, in order to control hemodynamic responses to the upper airway instrumentation. The TEE examination demonstrated a Daily type A aortic dissection with an intimal tear above the sinuses of Valsalva, intussusception of the intimal flap, and severe aortic insufficiency (Fig. 22.3).

Intraoperative Course

The patient was brought to the operating room, where a large-bore femoral venous catheter was placed for fluid administration. Intraoperative monitoring lines placed included a pulmonary artery catheter via a right internal jugular introducer, a left radial intraarterial line, and a right jugular bulb catheter. A TEE probe was inserted after the induction of anesthesia using fentanyl, midazolam, vecuronium, and 100% oxygen.

The patient underwent a Bentall procedure, which is replacement of the aortic valve and ascending aorta (with reimplantation of the coronary arteries) with a composite graft consisting of a mechanical valve and a tube of synthetic material. Extracorporeal circulation was achieved using right atrial–to–right axillary arterial bypass. At the initiation of CPB, TEE was used to confirm that the true lumen was being perfused by the right axillary arterial cannula. The replacement of the aortic valve with the composite graft was completed on hypothermic CPB following placement of an aortic cross-clamp at the distal ascending aorta and cardioplegia. During the latter portion of this period, the blood was cooled to 8°C. Repetitive sampling of jugular bulb oxyhemoglobin saturation demonstrated an increase from 58% (at normothermic baseline) to 97%, accompanied by a reduction in the urinary bladder temperature to 14°C. The anastomosis of the distal end of the composite

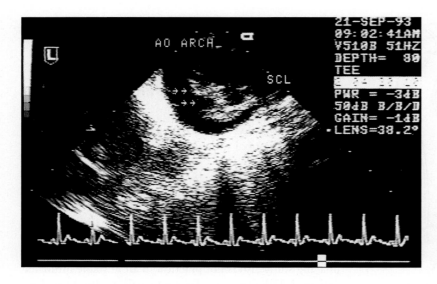

FIGURE 22.3. An upper esophageal aortic arch short-axis view showing aortic dissection with intussusception of the intimal flap. The *arrows* indicate the redundant flap; note its close proximity to the origin of the subclavian artery (*SCL*). *AO,* aorta.

graft to the dissected layers of the distal ascending aorta was performed during a 20-minute period of hypothermic circulatory arrest. The reimplantation of the coronary arteries to the graft and the evacuation of air from the heart and graft was performed during slow rewarming of the patient on CPB.

After weaning from CPB, sodium nitroprusside was used to control the arterial pressure to limit bleeding from anastomotic sites. Transesophageal echocardiography showed good ventricular function. The false lumen in the descending aorta had no blood flow on color-flow Doppler mapping and demonstrated spontaneous echo contrast ("echo smoke") on two-dimensional imaging (consistent with stasis).

Contribution of Transesophageal Echocardiography

In this section we describe the rationale for and use of TEE in the perioperative period for this patient. The standard examination of the aorta in multiple planes is described in the normal patient and in aortic dissection. The clinical problems addressed in this section include the origin of the intimal tear and extent of the dissection (and the implications for surgical vs. medical management), the adequacy of perfusion of the true lumen during CPB, and the monitoring of left ventricular loading conditions, left ventricular function, and air evacuation.

Relative Value of Diagnostic Modalities for Aortic Dissection

Investigation of a suspected aortic dissection should start with a high degree of suspicion. The chest radiograph may reveal widening of the mediastinum, changes in the aortic knob, or a left pleural effusion (hemothorax). A CT scan, especially with intravenous contrast, can aid in determining the extent of the lesion, and can show the tear and the true and false lumens. One major draw back to the contrast CT, however, is the volume of dye required, especially in the face of compromised renal function. Another major problem with CT is that it lacks the temporal resolution to detect a mobile flap. Magnetic resonance imaging has the advantage of not requiring dye, but may not be readily available, and is difficult to perform in patients with hemodynamic and respiratory compromise. Aortography is infrequently used, but is an extremely helpful tool in elucidating anatomy. It can demonstrate involvement of the ascending aorta, the intimal tear location, the extent and patency of false lumen, and the condition of major arteries. However, it is a time-consuming and invasive technique. Transesophageal echocardiography is a minimally invasive technique that can be performed quickly (7).

There have been several comparisons of these modalities for the diagnosis of acute aortic dissection. Erbel et al. compared TEE with CT scanning and aortography (6). In 164 patients, there was only one false-negative study and only two false-positive studies with TEE; thus, the sensitivity was 99% and the specificity was 98%. Similar detection rates were found by Nienaber et al., but they noted a higher false-positive rate (specificity 68.2%) for TEE (8). This was particularly true for lesions located in the ascending aorta. In a subsequent study, Nienaber et al. reported a sensitivity of 97.7% for TEE and a specificity of 76.9% in 110 patients (Table 22.2) (9). The low specificity was mainly caused by false-positive findings in the ascending aorta. Nevertheless, the researchers recommended TEE as the sole diagnostic study in unstable patients with suspected aortic dissection.

A limitation of these last two studies is that the researchers used a monoplane (transverse) probe that only offers extremely limited views of the ascending aorta. Either a biplane or multiplane probe would have offered additional tomographic images of the ascending aorta, which may have

TABLE 22.2. SENSITIVITY AND SPECIFICITY OF DIAGNOSTIC STUDIES FOR AORTIC DISSECTION

	Sensitivity (%)	Specificity (%)
TEE[a]	97.7	76.9[b]
Transthoracic echocardiography	59.3[c]	83.0[b]
Radiographic CT scanning	93.8	87.1
Magnetic resonance imaging	98.3	97.8

[a]Note that multiplane TEE was not available during the era when these data were collected.
[b]$P < 0.05$ compared with radiographic CT scanning and magnetic resonance imaging.
[c]$P < 0.005$ compared with TEE, radiographic CT scanning, and magnetic resonance imaging.
TEE, transesophageal echocardiography; CT, computed tomography. Modified from Nienaber CA, von Kodolitsch Y, Nicolas V, et al. The diagnosis of thoracic aortic dissection by noninvasive imaging procedures. *N Engl J Med* 1993;328:1–9, with permission.

improved the specificity. Despite these additional views, there are some limitations in visualization from the distal ascending aorta to the mid-transverse aortic arch because of the interposition of the trachea and right main-stem bronchus between the esophagus and the ascending aorta (10). The extent of the "blind spot" varies from patient to patient.

In addition to merely detecting the presence and extent of an aortic dissection (i.e., the intimal membrane), a number of important features of the dissection need to be defined: (a) differentiation of the true and false lumens and determination of the flow pattern, (b) the location of the intimal tears, (c) coronary artery integrity, (d) aortic valve function, and (e) the presence of pleural or pericardial effusions. Among the

various diagnostic modalities available, with its combination of two-dimensional imaging and Doppler color flow mapping, TEE is uniquely suited to answer all of these relevant questions (11–13).

Transesophageal and Epicardial Echocardiographic Examination of the Aorta

Whenever possible, we have used the standardized nomenclature for multiplane TEE established by the American Society of Echocardiography and the Society of Cardiovascular Anesthesiologists (14).

Transverse Imaging Views (0 Degrees)

Only a very short segment of the ascending aorta is visualized using transverse TEE in the mid-esophageal aortic short-axis view. However, by advancing and withdrawing the probe near where this view is optimal, the aortic annulus, the sinuses of Valsalva, the left coronary ostium, and the proximal half of the ascending aorta are reliably imaged (Figs. 22.4 and 22.5). Despite the limited views obtainable, many aortic dissections originate just above the level of the sinuses of Valsalva and are well visualized. It is also relatively easy to determine which is the true lumen in the ascending aorta because of the true lumen's continuity with the aortic valve leaflets.

Although it would seem logical to image the transverse arch of the aorta next, it is easier to do this following examination of the descending aorta. The descending thoracic

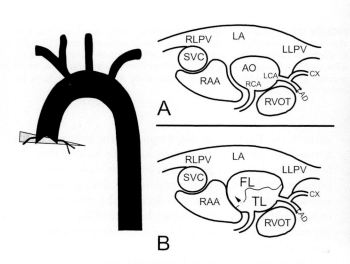

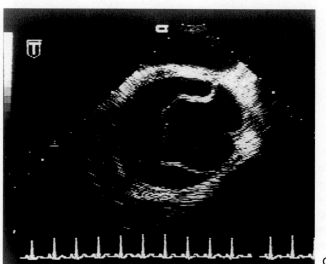

FIGURE 22.4. Diagram of the short-axis view of the aorta (at 0 degrees) at the level of the sinuses of Valsalva in the normal patient **(A)** and the patient with an aortic dissection **(B)**. The *arrow* indicates the direction of blood flow through the intimal tear. **C:** The corresponding echocardiogram. *RLPV,* right lower pulmonary vein; *LLPV,* left lower pulmonary vein; *LA,* left atrium; *SVC,* superior vena cava; *RAA,* right atrial appendage; *AO,* aorta; *RCA,* right coronary artery; *LCA,* left coronary artery; *CX,* circumflex coronary artery; *LAD,* left anterior descending coronary artery; *RVOT,* right ventricular outflow tract; *FL,* false lumen; *TL,* true lumen.

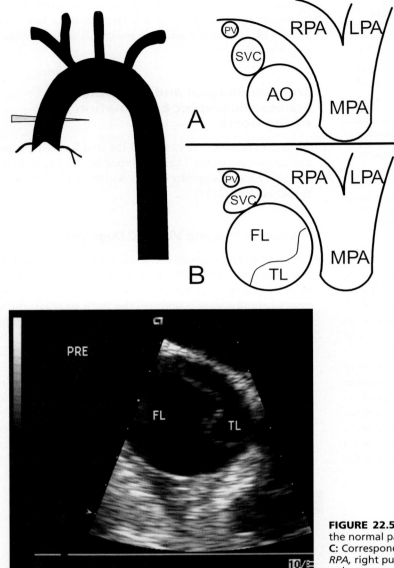

FIGURE 22.5. Mid-esophageal ascending aortic short-axis view in the normal patient **(A)** and the patient with an aortic dissection **(B)**. **C:** Corresponding echocardiogram. *PV,* right upper pulmonary vein; *RPA,* right pulmonary artery; *LPA,* left pulmonary artery; *MPA,* main pulmonary artery; *SVC,* superior vena cava; *AO,* aorta; *FL,* false lumen; *TL,* true lumen.

aorta is in close proximity to the left atrium. At the level of the four-chamber view of the heart, rotation of the probe in the counterclockwise direction brings the descending thoracic aorta into view. This is known as the descending aortic short-axis view (Fig. 22.6). Advancement of the probe toward the stomach will continue to show the descending aorta superior and inferior to the diaphragm as well as left pleural fluid collections. Withdrawal of the probe will usually image the entire descending aorta up to the level of the subclavian artery takeoff. The probe will have to be rotated gradually to maintain the descending aortic view because the esophagus is posterior to the aorta in the superior thorax, to the right of the aorta in the mid-thorax, and anterior to the

aorta at the level of the diaphragm. In the presence of an aortic dissection, the true lumen is usually smaller than the false lumen, has more prominent color with color flow mapping, and bulges toward the false lumen during ventricular systole. It may be necessary to decrease the color-flow scale to observe flow in the true lumen because of the suboptimal alignment of aortic flow for Doppler interrogation from the transesophageal approach.

The transverse aortic arch is imaged from a point near the innominate artery origin to a point distal to the left carotid origin using transverse imaging. This is known as the upper esophageal aortic arch long-axis view. It is more difficult to determine which is the true lumen in this view, although

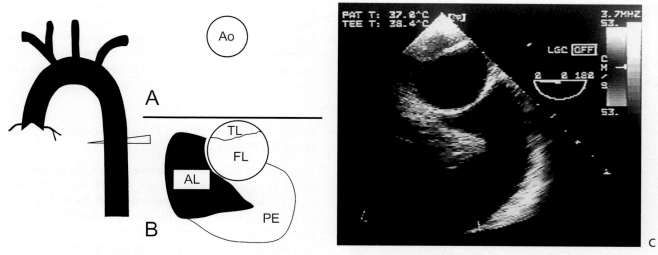

FIGURE 22.6. Descending aortic short-axis view in the normal patient **(A)** and the patient with an aortic dissection **(B). C:** Corresponding echocardiogram. *Ao,* aorta; *FL,* false lumen; *TL,* true lumen; *AL,* atelectatic lung; *PE,* pleural effusion.

the same principles apply. Intimal tears may be seen in this plane.

Longitudinal (Orthogonal) Imaging Views (90 Degrees)

The descending aorta is well imaged in the longitudinal plane by rotating the axis of the probe leftward (counterclockwise) toward the left hemithorax. This is known as the descend-

ing aortic long-axis view (Fig. 22.7). Color flow mapping of the flow in the true lumen usually demonstrates a laminar flow pattern. This is characterized by a single color on color flow mapping without a "mosaic" pattern caused by velocities that exceed the Nyquist limit ("aliasing"). Pulsed-wave Doppler shows flow moving toward the probe in the proximal descending aorta, and away from the probe in the distal descending aorta. Reversal of this flow pattern on the initiation of femoral extracorporeal perfusion is a convincing way

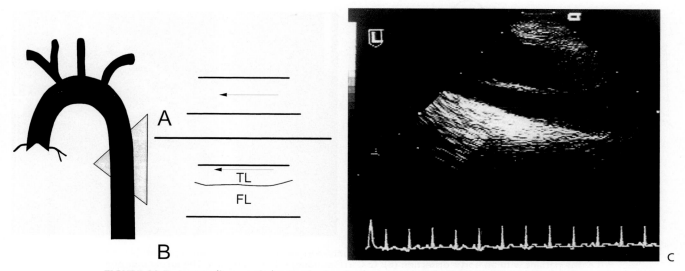

FIGURE 22.7. Descending aortic long-axis view in the normal patient **(A)** and the patient with an aortic dissection **(B). C:** Corresponding echocardiogram. The *arrow* indicates the direction of blood flow in the true lumen. *FL,* false lumen; *TL,* true lumen; *LA,* left atrium; *RA,* right atrium; *ASC AO,* ascending aorta; *RPA,* right pulmonary artery.

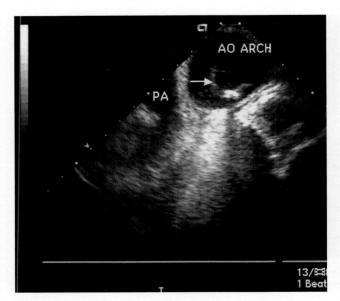

FIGURE 22.8. Upper esophageal aortic arch short-axis view in a patient with an aortic dissection. *AO,* aorta; *PA,* pulmonary artery, The *arrow* points to the dissection flap.

of demonstrating that the true lumen is being adequately perfused in a retrograde fashion.

The use of the longitudinal imaging plane to visualize the transverse aortic arch is a valuable tool in aortic dissection. Withdrawing the probe while imaging the descending aorta long-axis view, the aortic image ends superiorly at the level of the subclavian artery origin. From this point, the probe is rotated clockwise (to the right), yielding cross-sectional im-

ages of the aortic arch from the region near the left carotid origin until the region just distal to the innominate artery origin. This is known as the upper esophageal aortic arch short-axis view (Fig. 22.8). The true lumen gives rise to the brachiocephalic vessels and may be identified by this criterion.

Other Transesophageal Echocardiography Imaging Planes

Longitudinal scanning of the ascending aorta between 100 and 130 degrees usually images 5 to 10 cm of the vessel from the level of the aortic valve through the middle to distal ascending aorta (10). This is a slight modification of the mid-esophageal aortic valve long-axis view that is obtained at a slightly shallower depth of insertion than the standard view (Fig. 22.9). Posterior and anterior intimal tears are better visualized than lateral ones. Color flow mapping may help to visualize communications between the lumens when two-dimensional imaging is suboptimal. The distal ascending aorta and the region near the innominate artery origin remains obscured in nearly all patients by the airway structures (10). The same view yields excellent images of the left-ventricular outflow tract, where the degree and cause of aortic insufficiency (if present) can be assessed.

Optimal short-axis images of the semi-lunar leaflets of the aortic valve are best visualized in the mid-esophageal aortic valve short-axis view (Fig. 22.10). This view is usually obtained at an angle of 30 to 45 degrees. Advancing and withdrawing the probe from this view yields views of the coronary artery origins and the sinuses of Valsalva. It is

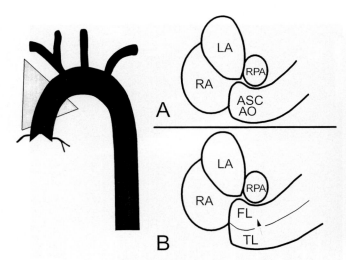

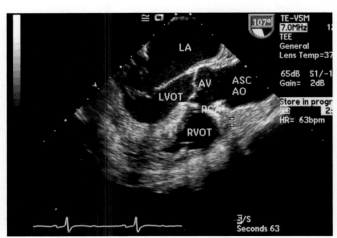

FIGURE 22.9. Modified mid-esophageal aortic valve long-axis view in the normal patient **(A)** and the patient with an aortic dissection **(B)**. **C:** Corresponding echocardiogram. The *arrow* indicates the direction of blood flow through the intimal tear. *LA,* left atrium; *RA,* right atrium; *ASC AO,* ascending aorta; *RPA,* right pulmonary artery; *FL,* false lumen; *TL,* true lumen; *LVOT,* left ventricular outflow tract; *RVOT,* right ventricular outflow tract; *AV,* aortic valve; *RCA,* right coronary artery.

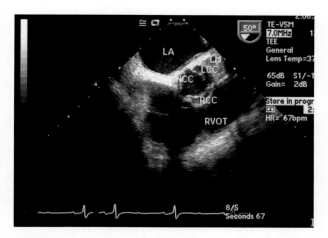

FIGURE 22.10. Mid-esophageal aortic valve short-axis view in the normal patient. *LA,* left atrium; *NCC,* non-coronary cusp; *RCC,* right coronary cusp; *LCC,* left coronary cusp; *LM,* left main coronary artery; *RVOT,* right ventricular outflow tract.

important to determine whether aortic dissection involves this region.

Epiaortic Scanning

Surgeon-assisted scanning of the ascending aorta is of particular use in intimal tears of the distal ascending aorta. This is the most common site for iatrogenic aortic dissections related to aortic cannulation and clamping that occurs during cardiac surgery. A 7- to 9-MHz probe is placed in a lubricated sterile sheath passed into the sterile field. The aorta is imaged in transverse, longitudinal, and intermediate planes to see whether aortic dissection is present proximal to the aortic arch. An example of a short-axis epiaortic image in a patient with a dilated aorta and aortic dissection is present in Fig. 22.11. A sterile setback is needed to image the near field (objects within 5 mm of the probe). Flooding the surgical field with saline, a saline-filled sterile surgical glove or gel setback is useful for this purpose.

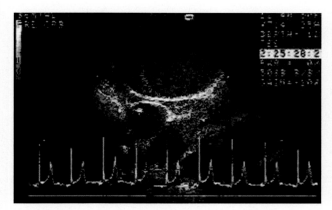

FIGURE 22.11. Epiaortic short-axis view of the patient with a dilated aorta with dissection present.

Implications for Surgical versus Medical Management

For the past several years, the prevalent surgical opinion is that type A dissections require urgent surgical management with resection of the intimal tear. Type B dissections, however, may be managed conservatively with vasodilators and beta-adrenergic blockers, and followed with serial CT scans. The advantages of using preoperative TEE to differentially diagnose type A and type B aortic dissections is that it is a minimally invasive, portable, sensitive, and specific tool that may be used in hemodynamically unstable patients. The data of Erbel et al. suggest that rapid initiation of therapy based on TEE examinations may improve outcome and that thrombosis of the false lumen is a good prognostic sign (15).

Assessment of Ventricular Function and Loading Conditions

Patients with aortic dissection may have myocardial ischemia due to underlying coronary artery disease or dissection at the origin of one or both coronary arteries. During aortic root replacement surgery (Bentall procedure), the coronary arteries are reimplanted, leading to the potential for myocardial ischemia following the surgical repair if technical difficulties are encountered. In addition to ECG monitoring, TEE provides a highly sensitive method of detecting acute changes in coronary perfusion. In the future, contrast echocardiography also may be used to detect regional myocardial ischemia.

The pre-CPB period may be complicated by massive hemorrhage in patients with aortic dissection due to partial or complete rupture of the false lumen. The extensive number of anastomoses, extensive surgical dissection, prolonged CPB times, profound hypothermia, and use of cardiotomy suction all contributes to post-CPB hemorrhage. The potential for hypovolemia is thus present during both the pre- and post-CPB periods. Filling pressures may not be informative regarding ventricular preload in patients with aortic dissection, because the patients frequently have associated left ventricular hypertrophy and ventricular noncompliance. TEE of the left ventricle provides another means of assessing the left ventricular preload. In the transgastric mid short-axis view of the left ventricle, a normal end-diastolic area is in the range of 12 to 17 cm^2. Additionally, if the ventricle is seen to have no end-systolic volume (the ventricle seems to collapse upon itself in systole), this is another reliable sign of clinical hypovolemia that is independent of filling pressures.

CONCLUSION

Transesophageal echocardiography is one of the most useful tools for the diagnosis and perioperative management of patients with aortic dissection. Its portability, minimally invasive nature, and excellent diagnostic sensitivity and specificity have been well documented. This particular indication for TEE is so well established that TEE is nearly indispensable in the management of these patients in the preoperative and intraoperative periods.

KEY POINTS

- In the majority of cases, type A dissections require urgent repair while type B dissections are managed medically.
- Transesophageal echocardiography has high sensitivity and specificity for detecting aortic dissection.
- Transesophageal echocardiography should be performed with excellent analgesia or general anesthesia and vasoactive medications in the patient with suspected aortic dissection to prevent acute hypertension during the diagnostic examination.
- A thorough examination of short-axis and long-axis views of the aortic valve, ascending aorta, transverse arch, and descending thoracic aorta is required to determine whether aortic dissection is present.
- Epiaortic scanning is valuable for detecting ascending aortic dissections in the region where transesophageal echocardiographic imaging is limited by airway interposition.

REFERENCES

1. Silvey SV, Stoughton TL, Pearl W, et al. Rupture of the outer partition of aortic dissection during transesophageal echocardiography. *Am J Cardiol* 1991;68:286–287.
2. Estrera AL, Huynh TT, Porat EE, et al. Is acute type A aortic dissection a true surgical emergency? *Semin Vasc Surg* 2002;15:75–82.
3. Troianos CA, Savino JS, Weiss R. Transesophageal echocardiographic diagnosis of aortic dissection during cardiac surgery. *Anesthesiology* 1991;75:149–153.
4. Larson EW, Edwards WDP. Risk factors for aortic dissection: a necropsy study of 161 cases. *Am J Cardiol* 1984;53:849.
5. Ergin MA, Galla JD, Lansman S, et al. Acute dissections of the aorta, current surgical treatment. *Surg Clin North Am* 1985;63:721.
6. Erbel R, Daniel W, Visser C, et al. Echocardiography in diagnosis of aortic dissection. *Lancet* 1989;1:457–461.
7. Hudak AM, Konstadt SN. Aortic intussusception: a rare complication of aortic dissection. *Anesthesiology* 1995;82:1292–1294.
8. **Nienaber CA, Spielmann RP, von Kodolitsch Y, et al. Diagnosis of thoracic aortic dissection. Magnetic resonance imaging versus transesophageal echocardiography. *Circulation* 1992;85:434–447.**
9. **Nienaber CA, von Kodolitsch Y, Nicolas V, et al. The diagnosis of thoracic aortic dissection by noninvasive imaging procedures. *N Engl J Med* 1993;328:1–9.**
10. Konstadt SN, Reich DL, Quintana C, et al. The ascending aorta: how much does transesophageal echocardiography see? *Anesth Analg* 1994;78:240–244.
11. **Simon P, Owen AN, Havel M, et al. Transesophageal echocardiography in the emergency surgical management of patients with aortic dissection. *J Thorac Cardiovasc Surg* 1992;103:1113–1117.**
12. Ballal RS, Nanda NC, Gatewood R, et al. Usefulness of transesophageal echocardiography in assessment of aortic dissection. *Circulation* 1991;84:1903–1914.
13. Pepi M, Campodonico J, Galli C, et al. Rapid diagnosis and management of thoracic aortic dissection and intramural haematoma: a prospective study of advantages of multiplane vs. biplane transoesophageal echocardiography. *Eur J Echocardiogr* 2000;1:72–79.
14. **Shanewise JS, Cheung AT, Aronson S, et al. ASE/SCA guidelines for performing a comprehensive intraoperative multiplane transesophageal echocardiography examination: recommendations of the American Society of Echocardiography Council for Intraoperative Echocardiography and the Society of Cardiovascular Anesthesiologists Task Force for Certification in Perioperative Transesophageal Echocardiography. *Anesth Analg* 1999;89:870–884.**
15. **Erbel R, Oelert H, Meyer J, et al. Effect of medical and surgical therapy on aortic dissection evaluated by transesophageal echocardiography. Implications for prognosis and therapy. *Circulation* 1993;87:1604–1615.**

23

AORTIC ATHEROSCLEROSIS

ELLISE DELPHIN
MARC KANCHUGER

AORTIC ATHEROSCLEROSIS

Atherosclerosis, a disorder that results in thickening and hardening of the walls of larger arteries, is responsible for most coronary artery disease, cerebrovascular disease, peripheral vascular disease, and diseases of the aorta. Atherosclerosis is the leading cause of death in the United States both above and below the age of 65 years and in both genders (1). The National Health Examination survey estimates that 5 million Americans have ischemic heart disease, the most reliable indicator for atherosclerotic disease (2).

Aortic atherosclerosis may be regarded as a continuum of development from early lesions (fatty streaks) to intermediate lesions (fibrous plaque) through complicated lesions. Fatty streaks are visible in the aorta of young children and increase in size and number at puberty. Fibrous plaques, elevated areas of intimal thickening, are characteristic of advancing atherosclerosis. These lesions appear in the abdominal aorta and in coronary and carotid arteries in the third decade of life and increase with age. Complicated lesions are calcified fibrous plaques that contain degrees of ulceration and thrombus. Penetrating aortic ulcer or intramural hematoma may weaken the intimal wall, resulting in aneurysm or dissection. Complicated lesions are also a source of arterial emboli and have been implicated in stroke as well as peripheral embolization (3).

Recognition of atherosclerosis is difficult, and detection usually awaits clinical manifestation of the disease. Evidence suggests that all patients with ischemic heart disease have atheromatous disease of the aorta. Perioperative identification and monitoring of thoracic aortic lesions is useful for the identification of patients at risk for stroke or peripheral embolization. Transesophageal echocardiography (TEE) and epiaortic echocardiography (EAE) are sensitive and specific methods for the detection and grading of aortic plaque intraoperatively. Diagnosis of the surgical population at high risk may allow for modification of the surgical approach in order to prevent emboli and improve outcome.

SCIENTIFIC PRINCIPLES

Screening for aortic atherosclerotic disease by angiography or computed tomography (CT) is not feasible in all patients undergoing cardiac surgery. Prior to the routine use of TEE and EAE intraoperatively, digital palpation of the aorta by the surgeon was the only method of assessing plaques. Identification of atheroma by this method is not reliable, with 83% of plaques identified by TEE missed by palpation (4). A combination of TEE and EAE is the most sensitive way to evaluate the thoracic aorta. Transesophageal echocardiography provides a thorough examination of the descending aorta and arch but has been found to have a poor predictive value in detecting disease of the ascending aorta. Epiaortic echocardiography of the ascending aorta is superior to TEE (5).

The three-stage grading system devised by Tunick et al. is the simplest and most commonly used system to categorize aortic atheroma (6–9). Intraluminal projections are composed of cholesterol plaque and may contain calcification or hemorrhage. Plaque may appear smooth or irregular. Calcification appears as high amplitude linear echoes. Grade I (insignificant) plaque is intimal thickening of less than 2 mm; grade II (moderate disease) is intimal plaque or thickening of 2 to 5 mm; and grade III (severe disease) is plaque or intimal thickening of greater than 5 mm or mobile protruding atheroma. Computed tomography scanning used to evaluate patients who also had TEE was found to have a sensitivity of 87% and a specificity of 82%. Gated magnetic resonance imaging studies found fewer grade III plaques when compared with TEE (10).

The incidence of perioperative stroke correlates with the TEE grade of atherosclerotic plaque. In a small prospective study, Hartman et al. found a stroke rate of 45.5% (5 of 11) in patients with severe atheromatous disease of the thoracic

E. Delphin: Department of Anesthesiology, UMDNJ–New Jersey Medical School; and Department of Anesthesiology, UMDNJ–University Hospital, Newark, New Jersey.

M. Kanchuger: Department of Anesthesiology, New York University School of Medicine, New York, New York.

aorta (11). Ribacove et al. studied 97 patients, and 3 of 10 with mobile atheroma had intraoperative stroke (30%). The incidence of stroke in the remaining patients was 1.1% (8). Surgical technique was not modified in either of these studies. Katz et al. studied 130 patients with TEE: 35 had grade III disease, 12 with mobile atheroma. Surgical technique was modified in 5 with no perioperative complications. Of the 7 without surgical modification, 3 had perioperative stroke (43%) (4).

The identification and location of atheromas with TEE and EAE has implications for patients undergoing open heart surgery. If cardiopulmonary bypass is necessary, the location of lesions may modify the placement of the aortic cross clamp, aortic cannula, and proximal vein grafts. If surgery can be performed with a minimally invasive technique or off pump, the degree of aortic atherosclerotic disease may guide the decision-making process.

LOGISTICS

Most segments of the thoracic aorta can be clearly imaged with multiplane TEE as the aorta descends along the esophagus. Two blind spots, the distal ascending aorta and the proximal arch, occur due to the intervening trachea and left main-stem bronchus. Epiaortic echocardiography may be useful during surgery in order to observe these two areas.

Examination of the ascending aorta begins with the mid-esophageal aortic valve long-axis view at approximately 120 degrees (Fig. 23.1). Rotation of the multiplane angle in this position to between 100 and 150 degrees provides a view where the anterior and posterior walls of the vessel appear as parallel lines. Slight withdrawal of the probe and rotation of the angle back to 0 degrees allows further visualization of

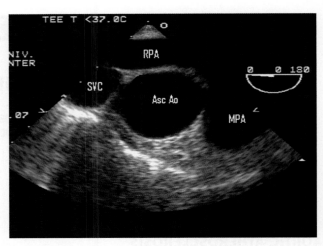

FIGURE 23.2. Transverse (0 degree) view of the ascending aorta (*Asc Ao*) at the base of the heart, just superior to the sinotubular ridge. Note the relationship of the right pulmonary artery (*RPA*), superior vena cava (*SVC*), and main pulmonary artery (*MPA*).

the ascending aorta (Fig. 23.2). This view displays the main and right pulmonary arteries as longitudinal structures and the aorta as a circular section. The diameter of the aorta may be measured in either the long or short-axis view. Further rotation of the angle to 30 to 40 degrees with deeper insertion reveals the aortic root (Fig. 23.3).

Examination of the descending thoracic aorta begins by turning the probe to the left from the mid-esophageal four-chamber view until a circular structure appears in the upper center of the echo image. This view is called the descending aorta short-axis view and is best viewed with an enlarged picture with a depth of 6 to 8 cm (Fig. 23.4). The rotation of the multiplane probe to 90 degrees produces a horizontal long-axis view of the descending aorta (Fig. 23.5). The entire descending aorta and upper abdominal aorta can be

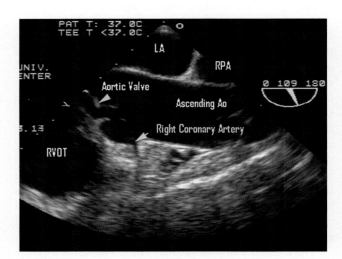

FIGURE 23.1. Longitudinal (109 degree) view of the ascending aorta (*Ascending Ao*) demonstrating an open aortic valve and the right coronary artery off the right coronary sinus. Note the relationships to the right pulmonary artery (*RPA*), left atrium (*LA*), and the right ventricular outflow tract (*RVOT*).

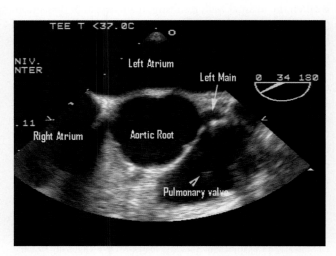

FIGURE 23.3. Slightly oblique transverse (34 degree) view of the base of the heart through the aortic root demonstrating the left main coronary artery arising from the left coronary sinus. The tip of the pulmonic valve is above the *arrow*.

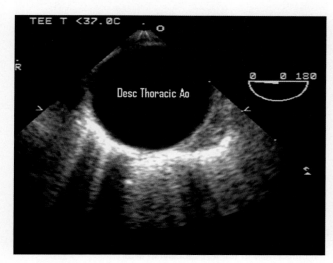

FIGURE 23.4. Transverse (0 degree) view of the descending thoracic aorta (*Desc Thoracic Ao*).

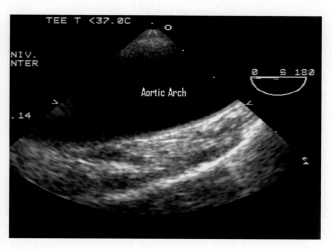

FIGURE 23.6. Transverse (0 degree) view of the distal aortic arch (*Ao Arch*).

imaged in either the long or short axis by slowly advancing and withdrawing the probe. It is difficult to pinpoint the exact location of a descending aortic lesion due to the changing positional relationship of the esophagus and the aorta. Localization of aortic wall lesions is often marked in terms of their distance from the left subclavian artery.

As the probe is withdrawn at an angle of 0 degrees, the circular descending aorta becomes an elliptical structure, the aortic arch (Fig. 23.6). This view is called the upper esophageal aortic arch long-axis view. The distal arch is to the right of the image and the proximal arch to the left, with the posterior wall at the top and the anterior wall below. Turning the probe to the right and left allows full visualization of the length of the arch. A short-axis aortic arch view may be obtained by rotating the multiplane angle to 90 degrees (Fig. 23.7). Visualization of the proximal portions of the arch major vessels is often difficult to obtain. The left

subclavian and carotid arteries may be seen in the 90 degree view. Color flow and pulsed Doppler help distinguish the two (Fig. 23.8–23.12).

Atheroma may be visualized and graded during execution of the entire preliminary examination and may be relocated during the procedure to guide surgical decisions about cannula, cross clamp, and graft placement (Figs. 23.1–23.12) (12–15).

CLINICAL INFORMATION

Case 1

A 78-year-old man with severe triple vessel coronary artery disease is about to undergo coronary artery bypass grafting via median sternotomy with cardiopulmonary bypass. He has a history of hypertension and smoking but no previous history of cerebrovascular disease. After induction of anesthesia, TEE examination of the thoracic aorta reveals severe

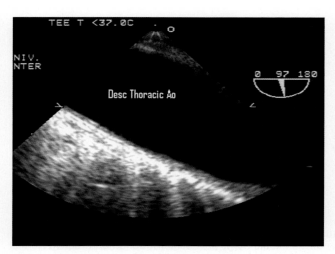

FIGURE 23.5. Longitudinal (97 degree) view of the descending thoracic aorta (*Desc Thoracic Ao*).

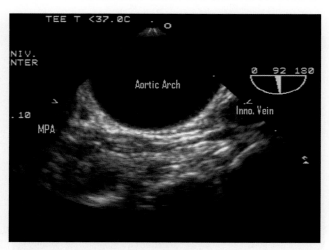

FIGURE 23.7. Longitudinal (92 degree) view of the middle aortic arch demonstrating its relationship to the main pulmonary artery (*MPA*) and the innominate (*Inno*) vein.

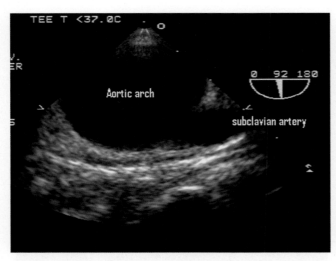

FIGURE 23.8. Longitudinal (92 degree) view of the middle aortic arch demonstrating the takeoff of the left subclavian artery. Notice it is smaller in diameter than the left carotid artery shown in Fig. 23.12.

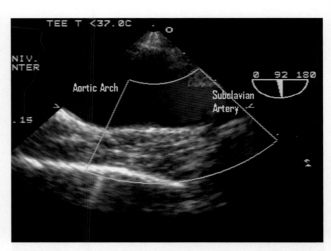

FIGURE 23.9. Color flow Doppler in the longitudinal (92 degree) view of the middle aortic arch demonstrating nonturbulent normal blood flow in the left subclavian artery.

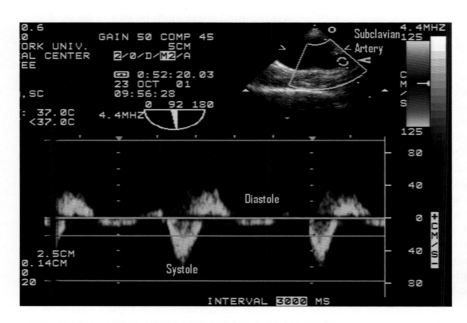

FIGURE 23.10. Pulsed Doppler interrogation of the left subclavian artery demonstrating absence of diastolic flow characteristic of blood flow in a systemic artery.

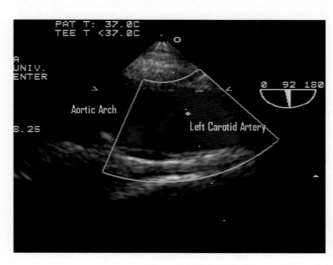

FIGURE 23.11. Color flow Doppler in the longitudinal (92 degree) view of the middle aortic arch demonstrating nonturbulent normal blood flow in the left carotid artery takeoff.

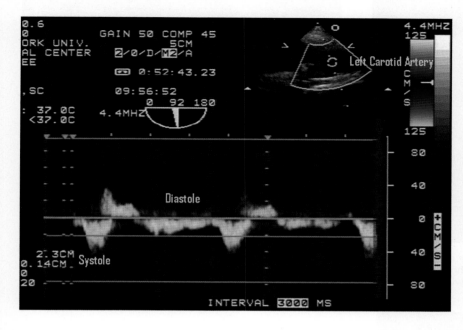

FIGURE 23.12. Pulsed Doppler interrogation of the left carotid artery demonstrating diastolic flow, characteristic of blood flow in the cerebral circulation.

(grade III) atheroma in the descending aorta and arch. The arch atheroma has mobile components. These findings led to modification of the initial surgical plan. The surgery was performed off pump, and bilateral internal mammary artery grafts and one saphenous vein graft were placed. Epiaortic echocardiography guided the placement of the proximal vein graft in the ascending aorta. The patient did well with no complications postoperatively (Figs. 23.13–23.15).

Clinical Decision Making

The incidence of stroke increases with age, rising from 0.42% in the 40- to 50-year-old population to greater than 7% in individuals over 75 years of age. Severe, grade III aortic atherosclerotic disease seen on TEE examination of the thoracic aorta correlates with a high (30%–43%) incidence of stroke in patients undergoing open heart surgery with cardiopulmonary bypass if the surgical technique is not modified (8). The TEE findings in this case resulted in modification of the surgical technique to reduce the risk of a poor outcome. The use of cardiopulmonary bypass incurs the risks of aortic cannulation and aortic cross clamping in a patient with severe disease of the ascending aorta and arch. Both types of aortic manipulation carry the risk for plaque rupture and embolic phenomena. The decision to use bilateral mammary artery grafts and one saphenous vein graft also spared extra manipulation and disturbance in the aortic root. The use of EAE intraoperatively guided the placement of the one proximal graft to an area that was free of disease (15,16).

Case 2

A 60-year-old woman with severe mitral regurgitation and mild congestive heart disease is admitted for minimally inva-

sive repair of her mitral valve. She is a nonsmoker and has no history of cerebrovascular or peripheral vascular disease. The planned repair involves cardiopulmonary bypass with retrograde cannulation of the aorta via the femoral artery and retrograde perfusion. Transesophageal echocardiography of the thoracic aorta after induction of anesthesia reveals moderate disease (grade II) of the descending aorta and arch with a normal ascending aorta. The surgical plan was changed to central aortic cannulation (Figs. 23.16 and 23.17).

Clinical Decision Making

Mitral valve repair requires the use of cardiopulmonary bypass. Minimally invasive surgery with retrograde cannulation of the femoral artery and vein permits a smaller surgical incision in the chest with less pain and less recovery time. The TEE findings of moderate disease (2–5 mm plaque) in the descending thoracic aorta and arch posed a problem for retrograde perfusion of the aorta. The turbulence of retrograde flow in a diseased vessel makes the possibility of plaque rupture and embolic phenomena, either peripheral or central, high. Epiaortic echocardiography of the ascending aorta was not performed in this case because the patient was felt to be at low risk for ascending aortic disease and finding of multiplane TEE of the ascending aorta were negative. Known risk factors for ascending aortic disease are severe (grade III) disease of the arch, age greater than 70 years, a history of heavy smoking, and known peripheral or cerebrovascular disease. Central cannulation in the ascending aorta, which was free of disease, was the safest method to employ.

Case 3

An 80-year-old hypertensive, diabetic man is scheduled for coronary artery bypass grafts. He has a past medical history

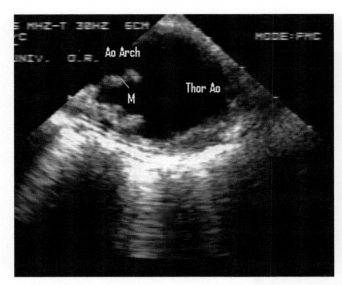

FIGURE 23.13. Case 1. Transverse view of the distal aortic arch (*Ao Arch*) as it meets the proximal descending thoracic aorta (*Thor Ao*), demonstrating a large complex atheroma with a mobile component (*M*).

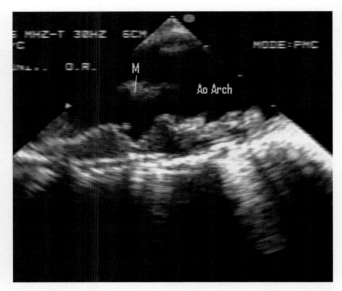

FIGURE 23.14. Case 1. Transverse view of the middle aortic arch with the same large complex atheroma with a mobile component (M) as shown in Fig. 23.13. *Ao Arch,* aortic arch.

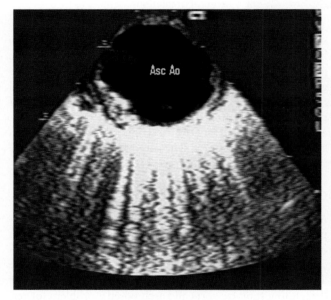

FIGURE 23.15. Case 1. Transverse epiaortic scan of the ascending aorta (*ASC Ao*) demonstrating a large protruding atheroma.

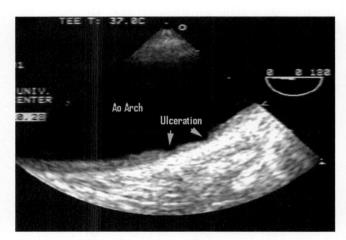

FIGURE 23.16. Case 2. Transverse (0 degree) view of the aortic arch (*Ao Arch*), demonstrating diffuse thickening of the intima with small ulcerations (*arrows*).

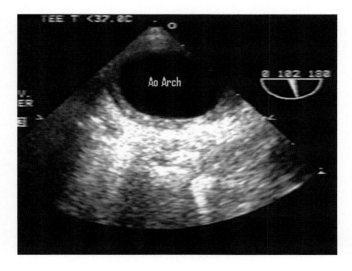

FIGURE 23.17. Case 2. Longitudinal (102 degree) view of the aortic arch (*Ao Arch*) demonstrating diffuse thickening of the intima.

of a stroke 2 years prior to this admission. Coronary artery bypass grafts are planned via median sternotomy with cardiopulmonary bypass. A multiplane TEE examination of the thoracic aorta reveals moderate to severe disease of both the descending aorta and distal arch, and the ascending aorta has mild disease in the proximal portion. An EAE of the ascending aorta and arch reveals minimal to no disease. A long aortic cannula is placed in the distal arch under EAE guidance with its tip positioned distal to the left subclavian artery. A single soft aortic cross clamp is placed with EAE guidance. The decision is made to do only two grafts, right and left mammary arteries (Figs. 23.18–23.20).

Clinical Decision Making

Using the criteria of age, diabetes, and past history of cerebrovascular disease that was possibly embolic, the patient is at high risk for perioperative stroke during his cardiac surgery (17,18). The procedure is modified after his TEE reveals moderate to severe arch disease and mild ascending aortic disease. Mechanisms of dislodgement of aortic debris and subsequent embolization include aortic manipulation, aortic cannulation, the use of side-biting aortic clamps to place proximal vein grafts, cross clamping the aorta, and a "sand-blasting effect" from flow from the aortic cannula. Transesophageal echocardiography and EAE were used in this case to alter management in order to avoid disruption of plaque (17). The long arch aortic cannula was positioned distal to the left subclavian artery to avoid sand blasting of debris into the cerebral vessels (19,20). The aortic cross clamp was positioned with echo guidance, avoiding diseased areas of the ascending aorta. Bilateral mammary artery grafts were used to avoid placement of proximal grafts on the aortic root. If vein grafts had been required, anastomosis of these proximally to the mammary grafts or the

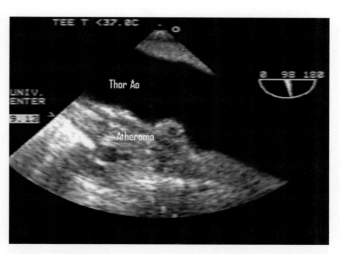

FIGURE 23.19. Case 3. Longitudinal (98 degree) view of the middle thoracic aorta (*Thor Ao*) demonstrating the same large protruding atheroma as shown in Fig. 23.18.

innominate artery would avoid further manipulation of the aorta.

CONTRIBUTIONS OF ECHOCARDIOGRAPHY

Neurologic complications continue to be a major cause of morbidity and mortality after cardiac surgery. With the increasing population of elderly patients undergoing surgery, atherosclerotic disease of the aorta with the risk of embolic cerebrovascular disease is increasing in incidence. Moderate to severe atheromatous disease of the aorta correlates with an increased incidence of perioperative stroke. In a nonsurgical setting Tunick et al. first described the independent association of aortic atheroma with stroke (6). Quickly thereafter the correlation of aortic atheroma with neurologic events in the perioperative period of cardiac surgery became established by Davila-Roman et al. and others. The recognition of this association makes the accurate diagnosis of thoracic aortic atheroma very important. A traditional approach of palpation of the aorta is highly inaccurate when compared with TEE. Transesophageal echocardiography and EAE have emerged as the most useful methods of identifying aortic pathology. Transesophageal echocardiography and EAE are complementary methods that may be used in the evaluation of thoracic aortic disease, and have a use in the modification and guidance of surgical technique.

Multiplane TEE has been shown to be a sensitive and specific method of evaluating the thoracic aorta. Its limitation lies in the inadequate visualization of the distal aortic arch, the most common site for cross clamping and aortic cannula placement. Epiaortic echocardiography may be used with great success to visualize this portion of the aorta. The most successful approach to high-risk patients is an initial diagnostic examination, modification of the surgical technique, if required, and echocardiography-guided

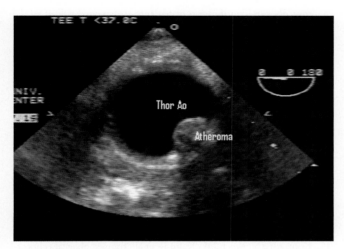

FIGURE 23.18. Case 3. Transverse (0 degree) view of the middle thoracic aorta (*Thor Ao*) demonstrating a large protruding atheroma.

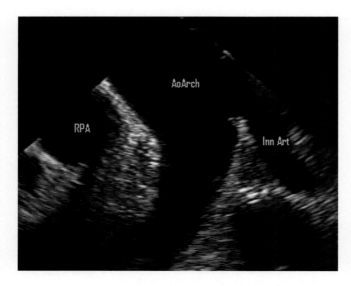

FIGURE 23.20. Case 3. Epiaortic echo of the proximal aortic arch (*Ao Arch*) demonstrating a normal proximal arch and innominate artery (*Inn Art*). The right pulmonary artery (*RPA*) is posterior to the ascending aorta and proximal aortic arch.

placement of cannulas or cross clamps by TEE and EAE (17,21). This will help to decrease the risk of neurologic events due to embolization of plaque during open heart surgery.

KEY POINTS

- Perioperative identification of thoracic aortic lesions is useful for the identification of patients at high risk for stroke or peripheral embolization.
- Transesophageal echocardiography and epiaortic echocardiography are sensitive and specific methods for the detection and grading of aortic plaque intraoperatively.
- Transesophageal echocardiography and epiaortic echocardiography are complementary methods that together allow the most comprehensive view of the aorta in order to visualize plaque.
- The approach to the high-risk patient is an initial diagnostic examination, modification of the surgical technique, if necessary, and echocardiography-guided placement of cannulas and cross clamps.
- Modification of technique in high-risk patients may modify the risk of neurologic sequelae in cardiac surgery
- Modification of surgical technique and echocardiography-guided placement of aortic cannulas and cross clamps in high-risk patients will modify the risk of neurologic sequelae in cardiac surgery.

REFERENCES

1. National Center of Health Statistics, Vital Statistics Report, Final Mortality Statistics, 1989.
2. National Center for Health Statistics, Monthly Vital Statistics Report. Advance Report of Final Mortality Statistics, 1990.
3. Bierman EL. Atherosclerosis and other forms of arteriosclerosis. In: Braunwald E, Fauci A, Hausers, et al. *Principles of internal medicine,* 13th ed. New York: McGraw Hill, 2001.
4. Katz E, Tunick P, Rusinek H, et al. Protruding aortic atheromas predict stroke in elderly patients undergoing cardiopulmonary bypass: experience with intraoperative transesophageal echocardiography. *J Am Coll Cardiol* 1992;20:70–77.
5. Davila-Roman VG, Phillips KJ, Daily BB, et al. Intraoperative transesophageal echocardiography and epiaortic ultrasound for assessment of atherosclerosis of the thoracic aorta. *J Am Coll Cardiol* 1996;28:942–947.
6. Tunick P, Perez JL, Kronzon I. Protruding atheromas in the thoracic aorta and systemic embolization. *Ann Intern Med* 1991;115:423–427.
7. Amerenco P, Cohen A, Tzourio C, et al. Atherosclerotic disease of the aortic arch and the risk of ischemic stroke. *N Engl J Med* 1994;331:1474–1479.
8. Ribacove GH, Katz ES, Galloway AC, et al. Surgical implications of transesophageal echocardiography to the grade atheromatous aortic arch. *Ann Thor Surg* 1992;53:758–764.
9. Marschall K, Kanchuger M, Kessler K, et al. Superiority of transesophageal echocardiography in detecting aortic arch atheromatous disease: identification of patients at increased risk of stroke during cardiac surgery. *J Cardiothorac Vasc Anesth* 1994;8:5–13.
10. Willens HJ, Kessler KM. Transesophageal echocardiography in the diagnosis of diseases of the aorta. *Chest* 1999;116:1772–1779.
11. Hartman GS, Fun-Sun F, Bruefach M, et al. Severity of aortic atheromatous disease diagnosed by transesophageal echocardiography predicts stroke and other outcomes associated with coronary artery surgery: a prospective study. *Anesth Analg* 1996;83:701–708.
12. Marshall WG, Barzilai B, Kouchoukos NT, et al. Intraoperative ultrasonic imaging of the ascending aorta. *Ann Thorac Surg* 1989;48:339–344.
13. Karalis DG, Chandrasekaran K, Victor MF, et al. Recognition and embolic potential of intra-aortic atherosclerotic debris. *J Am Coll Cardiol* 1991;17:73–76.
14. Konstadt SN, Reich DL, Quintana C, et al. The ascending aorta: how much does transesophageal echocardiography see? *Anesth Analg* 1994;78:240–244.
15. Konstadt SN, Reich DL, Kahn R, et al. Transesophageal echocardiography can be used to screen for ascending aortic atherosclerosis. *Anesth Analg* 1995;81:225–228.

16. Trehan N, Mishra M, Kasliwal RR. Reduced neurological injury during CABG in patients with mobile aortic atheromas: a five year follow-up study. *Ann Thor Surg* 2000;70:1558–1564.

17. Grigore AM, Grocott HP. Pro: epiaortic scanning is routinely necessary for cardiac surgery. *J Cardiothorac Vasc Surg* 2000;14:87–90.

18. Peterson E, Cowper P, Jollis J, et al. Outcomes of coronary artery bypass surgery in 24,461 patients aged 80 years or older. *Circulation* 1995;92(suppl II):85–91.

19. Culliford AT, Colvin SB, Rohrer K, et al. The atherosclerotic ascending aorta and transverse arch: a new technique to prevent cerebral injury during bypass: experience with 13 patients. *Ann Thorac Surg* 1986;41:27–31.

20. Grossi EA, Kanchuger MS, Schwartz DS, et al. Effect of cannula length on aortic arch flow: protection of the atheromatous aortic arch. *Ann Thorac Surg* 1995;59:710–712.

21. Ostrowski JW, Kanchuger MS. Con: epiaortic scanning is not routinely necessary for cardiac surgery. *J Cardiothorac Vasc Surg* 2000;14:91–94.

DIAGNOSIS OF MYOCARDIAL ISCHEMIA

KRISTINE J. HIRSCH

Transesophageal echocardiography (TEE) is now recognized as a sensitive tool for the detection of myocardial ischemia, allowing for the rapid diagnosis and treatment of perioperative ischemic left ventricular (LV) dysfunction. This role for TEE holds out the promise of real-time, quality assessment of coronary artery bypass surgery (CABG) analogous to its well-established role in valvular heart surgery. Its use has been expanding from the operating suite to the intensive care unit (ICU), and from cardiac surgical application to noncardiac surgical patients.

Perioperative myocardial ischemia is strongly associated with short and long-term adverse outcomes, with a ninefold increase in the occurrence of unstable angina, nonfatal myocardial infarction (MI), or cardiac death (1,2). In patients undergoing CABG surgery, ischemia detected in the post-bypass period is strongly associated with adverse outcomes (3). Rapid and accurate perioperative diagnosis of cardiac ischemia allows optimization of hemodynamic management and offers the opportunity to correct inadequate surgical revascularization with subsequent improvement in patient outcomes.

Transesophageal echocardiography has been demonstrated to be superior in sensitivity and specificity to either electrocardiographic (ECG) or pulmonary artery catheter (PAC) monitoring techniques in the detection of myocardial ischemia (4,5). Changes in LV regional wall motion have been shown experimentally to occur earlier and more consistently in response to coronary occlusion than changes in the ECG (6), and are more specific to ischemia than PAC data (7). In addition, myocardial ischemia can result in TEE-detectable changes in global LV function, ventricular volumes, mitral regurgitation (MR), and mitral inflow patterns related to changes in diastolic function. The unobtrusive nature of TEE allows intraoperative, real-time assessment to discern myocardial ischemia from other causes of hemodynamic instability and allow for rapid corrective measures to restore adequate perfusion.

Recently, assessment of myocardial viability with dobutamine stress echocardiography (DSE) has been established as an accurate predictor of recruitable, hibernating myocardium and can differentiate ischemic from nonischemic dysfunction. New advances in TEE will soon permit intraoperative assessment of coronary perfusion using myocardial contrast echocardiography (MCE). Transesophageal echocardiography combined with MCE can demonstrate successful graft placement, adequacy of cardioplegia delivery, and integrity of myocardial microvasculature. Refinements in echocardiographic technology such as automatic border detection (ABD) and Color Kinesis (CK) permit automatic identification and tracking of endocardial border motion and will enhance the ability of TEE to automatically quantify and map ventricular segmental dysfunction.

Perioperative TEE allows for the detection and localization of myocardial ischemia with superior sensitivity and specificity to standard techniques. In addition, there is an expanding role for TEE in discerning recoverable from nonviable myocardium. Finally, new techniques may allow direct assessment of myocardial perfusion. This chapter reviews the scientific principles relevant to these TEE capabilities, describes the techniques required to obtain this information during a TEE examination, and illustrates by way of case scenarios the clinical utility of these techniques.

SCIENTIFIC PRINCIPLES

It is well established that a close relationship between myocardial blood flow and mechanical function exists, so that a rapid loss of regional contraction occurs with acute ischemia. Regional wall motion abnormalities (RWMAs) are the hallmark of myocardial ischemia, with systolic impairment of myocardial thickening and inward wall motion immediately discernible by TEE (8). Experimentally, coronary artery ligation leads to a rapid progression of wall motion abnormalities from mild hypokinesis to severe hypokinesis, and finally to outward bulging (dyskinesis) of the ventricular wall in the area subtended by the occluded coronary

K. J. Hirsch: Department of Anesthesia, Halifax Infirmary, Queen Elizabeth II Health Sciences Center, Halifax, Nova Scotia, Canada.

artery (9). These mechanical changes are associated with tissue hypoxia, depletion of cardiomyocyte energy substrate, and ultimately impaired delivery of calcium to the contractile units (10). Consequently, contraction abnormalities can be detected within seconds of an ischemic event. Hauser and colleagues have documented the exquisite sensitivity of TEE to discern RWMA resulting from coronary ischemia. In patients undergoing percutaneous transluminal coronary angioplasty, balloon inflation in noncollateralized arteries resulted in rapid TEE-detectable RWMA in 19 of 22 patients. By contrast, ECG abnormalities were only detectable in 8 of 22 patients (11).

The severity of RWMA has been shown to correlate with the degree of coronary stenosis and extent of the perfusion deficit. Subtotal coronary occlusion producing subendocardial ischemia will result in segmental hypokinesis, whereas total coronary occlusion producing transmural ischemia will result in akinesis or dyskinesis of a myocardial segment (6).

Regional wall motion abnormalities associated with myocardial ischemia are found not only in the area of coronary insufficiency, but also in adjacent areas of normal myocardium. Adjacent normal myocardium will exhibit compensatory hyperactivity and transitional wall motion abnormalities known as "tethering" in areas adjacent to ischemic areas (12). Compensatory hyperactivity in normal myocardial segments is likely the reason for preserved LV ejection fraction (EF) and the lack of changes in filling pressures, making PAC measurements relatively insensitive to ischemia.

Not all RWMAs are indicative of myocardial ischemia. Areas of infarction, "stunning," or hibernation all may appear as impairment in segmental myocardial thickening, and a decrease in endocardial excursion by TEE. Whereas acute ischemia is due to a dynamic supply/demand insufficiency in viable myocardium, chronically infarcted myocardium generally denotes nonviable tissue. Two other categories of viable myocardium have been described: stunned myocardium denotes a temporary postischemic dysfunction in which flow is preserved, and hibernating myocardium describes contractile dysfunction regarded as an adaptive mechanism to chronic hypoperfusion (13–15). Differentiating these conditions in the setting of impaired ventricular function detected by RWMAs has important prognostic and therapeutic implications.

In acutely infarcted myocardium, coronary occlusion results in myocardial ischemia and ultimately cellular necrosis. This is a time-dependent phenomenon whereby increasing the duration of ischemia results in a greater extent of transmural necrosis. Pockets of viable myocardial cells may exist in regions of acute infarction. Reperfusion up to 3 hours (and possibly 6 hours) after coronary occlusion has been shown to rescue critically ischemic cells, limit MI size, and preserve ventricular function (16). This dysfunctional or stunned myocardium salvaged by coronary reperfusion may

exhibit prolonged postischemic dysfunction. After an ischemic insult—either caused by acute MI or perioperative ischemia due to inadequate myocardial protection—full recovery of normal segmental contraction may occur hours to days after restoration of blood flow. Acute ischemia induces an inflammatory response with resultant cardiomyocyte swelling and cellular dysfunction. Ventricular dysfunction due to myocardial stunning often requires inotropic support following cardiopulmonary bypass (CPB) and improves over a period of hours to days concomitant with recovery of myocyte function. Viability of myocardial cells (stunning) within infarct zones has been noted in many studies reviewed by Lualdi and Douglas (17). Dobutamine stress echocardiography can detect contractile reserve (improvement in wall motion of hypocontractile segments in response to low-dose dobutamine) in settings of myocardial stunning and predict salvage of jeopardized myocardium with early revascularization (18,19). Although no studies have addressed the question of whether identification and revascularization of stunned myocardium improves patient outcome, Barilla and colleagues have reported that patients with viable myocardium treated medically had less recovery of systolic function than those who were revascularized (20). This finding suggests that revascularization of stunned myocardium identified by DSE can have a positive impact on LV function and hence, patient outcome.

Wall motion abnormalities due to hibernating myocardium occur in the setting of chronic coronary artery disease with LV dysfunction. Hibernating myocardium is a result of chronic underperfusion of viable myocardial cells, rendering them noncontractile, resulting in regional myocardial dysfunction. Hibernating myocardial segments are recruitable with improvement in regional perfusion and demonstrate contractile reserve. This state may be detected as a reversible RWMA by the use of low-dose dobutamine or nitroglycerin (by improving the myocardial oxygen supply/demand ratio). Demonstration of contractile reserve predicts recovery of segmental function in hibernating myocardium with revascularization. Histopathologic analysis of segments demonstrating a lack of contractile reserve generally reveals significant myocardial fibrosis, whereas segments with contractile reserve (reversible RWMA) may indicate the presence of a nontransmural MI with minimal muscle loss or even normal myocardium histologically. Contractile reserve has been demonstrated even with akinetic or (rarely) dyskinetic segments. Ultimate recovery of function after revascularization defines hibernating myocardium, although improvement in segmental wall motion may take place over a period of months. Dobutamine stress echocardiography can be used to identify hibernating myocardium and predict improvement in regional LV function after coronary revascularization (20). Chronic, transmurally infarcted myocardium with scarring appears as segmental thinning with akinesis or dyskinesis. These findings most commonly involve the inferobasal and anteroapical areas (21). The infarcted areas generally do not contribute to ventricular ejection and may decrease ventricular performance through loss of normal cardiac architecture (remodeling). Early remodeling or infarct expansion is an acute dilatation and thinning of the involved segment likely due to side-by-side slippage of cardiomyocytes rather than by additional cell necrosis. Infarct expansion predisposes to asymmetrical ventricular geometry, increased cavity size, abnormal wall stress, and, eventually, ventricular dysfunction and clinical heart failure. Extreme infarct expansion can result in profound wall thinning with aneurysmal dilatation and ventricular rupture.

Although the diagnosis of myocardial ischemia by intraoperative TEE evaluation is heavily dependent on the detection of RWMA, this modality requires continuous operator attention to avoid missing ischemic episodes. The fact that ischemic episodes also have been shown to affect chamber size has allowed a continuous, automated system of monitoring potential episodic ischemic events. In anesthetized patients undergoing CABG, myocardial ischemia induced by atrial pacing results in increases in LV dimensions compared with nonischemic patients. Changes demonstrated included an increase in LV end-systolic area (ESA) and end-diastolic area (EDA) and a resultant decrease in fractional area change (FAC; FAC, [EDA − ESA]/EDA) (22). Recent advances in acoustic data analysis have allowed the development of ABD systems that provide continuous, automatic online monitoring of ventricular dimensions. The use of this technique to diagnose ischemia intraoperatively must be used with caution, because changes in volume and loading conditions commonly occur and can significantly confound ventricular dimension data. Although the diagnostic value of intraoperative TEE-measured changes in LV dimensions as a marker of ischemia has yet to be definitively demonstrated, intraoperative use of ABD-capable TEE is a promising modality (22,23).

Transesophageal echocardiography evaluation of mitral inflow and pulmonary venous flow patterns by pulsed-wave Doppler (PWD) techniques also permits real-time monitoring of diastolic function. Diastolic dysfunction as evidenced by impairment of LV relaxation and a decrease in LV compliance is known to precede systolic dysfunction in the cascade of ischemic events (24,25). For example, Koolen and colleagues demonstrated that during balloon inflation for percutaneous transluminal coronary angioplasty, there was a marked reversal of the early (E) to late (A) transmitral peak Doppler flow velocity ratio (E/A), a change that preceded the development of RWMAs by several seconds (26). Because mitral inflow patterns are influenced by changes in preload, afterload, heart rate, rhythm, and left atrial (LA) pressure gradient, the dynamic environment of the operating room makes the evaluation of diastolic function by this technique challenging and often unreliable. Therefore, the detection

of diastolic dysfunction indicating myocardial ischemia remains primarily a research tool and valuable particularly in more stable settings.

TECHNIQUES

Scanning

Intraoperative TEE evaluation of myocardial ischemia is typically initiated following induction of general anesthesia, a time of increased stress and thus risk for myocardial ischemia. It is imperative that the baseline evaluation takes into consideration the effects of general anesthetic induction, positive pressure ventilation, and the pharmacologic milieu on loading conditions. For example, new RWMAs that are unrelated to ischemia have been shown to occur with the acute reductions in preload associated with initiating CPB in patients with preexisting abnormalities of LV contraction (27). In addition, new RWMAs have been observed with acute increases in afterload following supraceliac aortic clamping (28).

In order to assess and monitor myocardial ischemia, a comprehensive TEE evaluation of the entire heart must first be performed. By obtaining a baseline evaluation with reproducible views, the onset of myocardial ischemia may be detected as a new RWMA. Any baseline RWMA should be noted and recorded. Most echocardiography consoles allow the saving of loop segments to be displayed for comparison with subsequent images. The side-by-side analysis for RWMAs is invaluable because it allows the echocardiographer to evaluate the adequacy of the comparison views as well as any changes in wall motion/segmental thickening. Baseline RWMAs may indicate areas of infarcted, hibernating, or stunned myocardium. Differentiation of these conditions is an area of intense interest and investigation that is rapidly producing techniques of clinical importance. New RWMAs will most commonly signify myocardial ischemia. Once high-quality scans are obtained of both ventricles, continuous monitoring using reproducible landmarks will permit assessment of new-onset myocardial ischemia.

Views

The guidelines established by the American Society of Echocardiography (ASE) and the Society of Cardiovascular Anesthesiologist (SCA) recommend the use of a 16-segment model to describe the location of the RWMA (Fig. 24.1) (29). This model is anatomically referenced based on the coronary artery supply to various regions. Figure 24.2 depicts the LV divided into three levels from base to apex. The base and mid-ventricular levels are divided into six segments: anterior, anteroseptal, septal, inferior, posterior, and lateral. The apex is divided into four segments: anterior, septal, inferior, and lateral. A popular modification is the 12-segment model, simplified by having only four divisions in the short

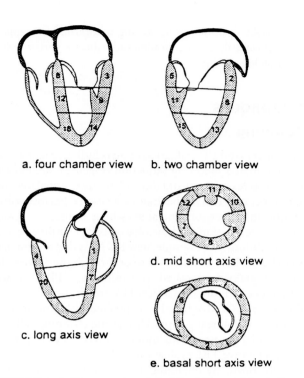

a. four chamber view   b. two chamber view

c. long axis view

d. mid short axis view

e. basal short axis view

FIGURE 24.1. A 16-segment model of the left ventricle. **A:** Four-chamber views show the three septal and three lateral segments. **B:** Two-chamber views show the three anterior and three inferior segments. **C:** Long-axis views show the two anteroseptal and two posterior segments. **D:** Middle short-axis views show all six segments at the middle level. **E:** Basal short-axis views show all six segments at the basal level. The basal segments are as follows: *1,* basal anteroseptal; *2,* basal anterior; *3,* basal lateral; *4,* basal posterior; *5,* basal inferior; *6,* basal septal. The middle segments are as follows: *7,* mid-anteroseptal; *8,* mid-anterior; *9,* mid-lateral; *10,* mid-posterior; *11,* mid-inferior; *12,* mid-septal. The apical segments are as follows: *13,* apical anterior; *14,* apical lateral; *15,* apical inferior; *16,* apical septal. (Reproduced from Shanewise JS, Cheung AT, Aronson S, et al. ASE/SCA guidelines for performing a comprehensive intraoperative multiplane transesophageal echocardiography examination: recommendations of the American Society of Echocardiography Council for Intraoperative Echocardiography and the Society of Cardiovascular Anesthesiologists Task Force for Certification in Perioperative Transesophageal Echocardiography. *Anesth Analg* 1999;89:875, with permission.)

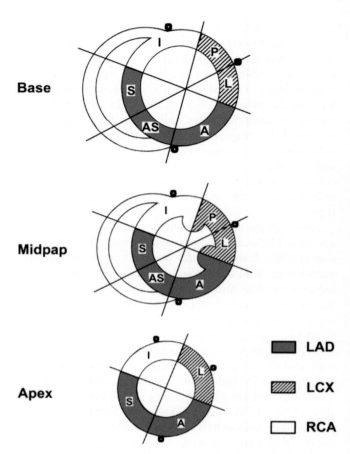

FIGURE 24.2. Cross-sectional views of the left ventricle from base (*top*) and midpap (*middle*) to apex (*bottom*). The coronary distribution of a typical right-dominant circulation is indicated by shading: *LAD,* left anterior descending coronary artery; *LCX,* left circumflex coronary artery; *RCA,* right coronary artery. The various segments are labeled as follows: *I,* inferior; *P,* posterior; *L,* lateral; *A,* anterior; *AS,* anteroseptal; *S,* septal. *Midpap,* mid-papillary.

axis representing the anterior, septal, inferior, and lateral walls at the base and mid-papillary levels. Rouine-Rapp and colleagues evaluated the utility of TEE for detecting segmental dysfunction and found the most useful views to be a combination of both transverse and longitudinal views at the mid-esophageal (ME) and transgastric (TG) levels, demonstrating 86% of all RWMAs. Apical and deep gastric views were more difficult to obtain and had a low yield in depicting wall motion abnormalities (30).

In practice, the intraoperative detection of RWMAs depends on a rapid and systematic method of scanning that allows correlation of myocardial regions with coronary supply. As suggested in Fig. 24.3, the TEE probe can be positioned at the ME depth to obtain the four-chamber view (at 0 degrees)

depicting the right ventricle (RV) and LV. The ME four-chamber view allows visualization of the septum [left anterior descending coronary artery (LAD) distribution] and lateral wall [left circumflex coronary artery [LCx] distribution]. At 90 degrees from the ME four-chamber view, the ME two-chamber view reveals the inferior wall perfused by the right coronary artery (RCA), the anterior wall perfused by the LAD, and the apex supplied by the distal LAD. Further multiplane rotation to 120 degrees permits visualization of the anterior septal wall perfused by the LAD and the posterior wall typically supplied by the LCx. These initial views permit the acquisition of an overall assessment of global LV and RV function with concomitant visualization of the basal, middle, and apical segments. The probe is then advanced to a TG position with a variable degree of anteflexion to obtain the mid-papillary short-axis view (TG mid-SAX). This view is often called the "mid-papillary view" with the well-defined posterior (PPM) and anterior (APM) papillary muscle heads serving as useful landmarks. The middle portions of the

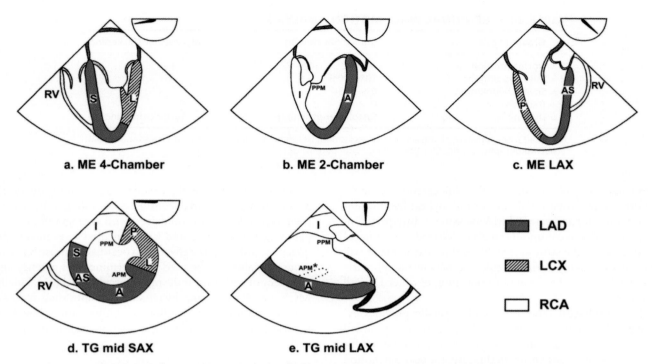

FIGURE 24.3. Views for intraoperative scanning for regional wall motion abnormalities. **A:** Mid-esophageal four-chamber (*ME 4-Chamber*). **B:** Mid-esophageal two-chamber (*ME 2-Chamber*). **C:** Mid-esophageal long axis (*ME LAX*). **D:** Transgastric mid-papillary short axis (*TG mid SAX*). **E:** Transgastric mid-papillary long axis (*TG mid LAX*). The coronary distribution of a typical right-dominant circulation is indicated by shading: *LAD,* left anterior descending coronary artery; *LCX,* left circumflex coronary artery; *RCA,* right coronary artery. The various segments are labeled as follows: *I,* inferior; *P,* posterior; *L,* lateral; *A,* anterior; *AS,* anteroseptal; *S,* septal; *PPM,* posterior papillary muscle; *APM,* anterior papillary muscle; *RV,* right ventricle. (Modified from Shanewise JS, Cheung AT, Aronson S, et al. ASE/SCA guidelines for performing a comprehensive intraoperative multiplane transesophageal echocardiography examination: recommendations of the American Society of Echocardiography Council for Intraoperative Echocardiography and the Society of Cardiovascular Anesthesiologists Task Force for Certification in Perioperative Transesophageal Echocardiography. *Anesth Analg* 1999;89:875, with permission.)

inferior wall (RCA distribution), lateral wall (LCx distribution), and anterior wall and septum (LAD distribution) are seen in this view. The TG mid-SAX view with its prominent landmarks is the most commonly used view for continuous ischemia monitoring because it is relatively easy to acquire, reveals more RWMAs than other views, and is easiest to interpret as evidenced by multiple studies (31). From this view, the TG two-chamber view may be obtained by multiplane rotation to 90 degrees. The PPM and its basal attachment to the inferior wall (RCA territory) are often well visualized in this view, although the APM is more variably seen. This is an important view to identify ischemic papillary muscle rupture and resultant mitral valve dysfunction. The regions seen here are the basal and middle portions of the inferior wall perfused by the RCA, and the anterior wall perfused by the LAD. The LV apex in this view is typically not seen.

These five views allow detection of the majority of RWMAs and have the advantages of minimal probe manipulation and visualization of good landmarks for ease of reproducibility. Other cross-sections may be obtained at the basal and apical SAX views (Fig. 24.2), but diagnostic yield is lower and reproducibility is less reliable.

Assessment of Regional Function

Analysis of LV segmental function is based on a qualitative visual assessment of myocardial regional motion and thickening during systole. Radial shortening is defined as the percentage shortening of an imaginary radius from the endocardial border to the center of the LV. The ASE/SCA standards recommend a grading scale of 1 to 5 for describing RWMAs, as shown in Table 24.1 (29).

The diagnosis of myocardial ischemia requires worsening of segmental function by two grades from normal or mild hypokinesis to at least severe hypokinesis or akinesis.

There are several potential pitfalls in the diagnosis of myocardial ischemia by TEE. Marked global movements of the heart and uncoordinated contractions due to bundle branch block or ventricular pacing frequently confound RWMA assessment. The use of a floating frame of reference will help

TABLE 24.1. REGIONAL WALL MOTION ANALYSIS

Grading Scale	Radial Shortening	Myocardial Thickening
1 = Normal motion	>30%	+++
2 = Mild hypokinesis	10%–30%	++
3 = Severe hypokinesis	0%–10%	+
4 = Akinesis	0	0
5 = Dyskinesis	Systolic lengthening	Systolic thinning

Modified from Sutton et al. Intraoperative assessment of left ventricular function with transesophageal echocardiography. *Cardiol Clin* 1993;11:395, with permission.

compensate for global cardiac motion, but careful assessment of both inward endocardial motion and myocardial thickening is critical for accurate RWMA assessment. Interpretation of septal motion is commonly confounded by discoordinated contraction. If the septum is viable and nonischemic, it will thicken appreciably during systole, but may be notably early or late relative to the timing of thickening of other LV wall segments.

Transesophageal echocardiography usually provides excellent views of the LV, although frequently the epicardial portion of the lateral wall cannot be viewed, making it difficult to assess wall thickening. In this case, endocardial motion alone may be used to assess the lateral segment for RWMAs.

Pulsed-Wave Doppler

Mitral inflow variables used in determining diastolic function are best obtained in the ME four-chamber view using PWD echocardiography. The PWD sample volume should be placed between the tips of the mitral valve leaflets in diastole. A normal diastolic flow pattern reveals a prominent E wave in early diastole and a smaller A wave in late diastole due to atrial contraction. Commonly evaluated variables include E/A, deceleration time (DT), and deceleration rate (DR) of the E wave, and the isovolumic relaxation time (IVRT) measured at the end of the aortic outflow signal to the beginning of the E wave. Characteristic findings in myocardial ischemia are a decrease in DR, increase in DT and IVRT, and a reduction in the E/A ratio (32).

Myocardial Contrast Echocardiography

Myocardial contrast echocardiography (MCE) is a technique in which ultrasound echoes are enhanced by injecting microbubbles into the blood vessels. The microbubbles consist of a shell with a gas-filled core that create an acoustic interface and change the local scattering of ultrasound energy. These microbubbles are smaller than red cells (<10 μm) and can pass freely through the coronary circulation. Clinical applications include the enhancement of intracardiac shunts and intracavitary masses, such as LA and LV thrombi. By opacification of the LV cavity, endocardial borders are better delineated to assist the detection of RWMAs and better evaluate regional as well as global ventricular function. Exciting new applications of MCE lie in the area of myocardial per-

fusion analysis and are of particular interest in the operating room setting. Myocardial contrast echocardiography may be used to correlate perfusion defects with angiographic data in planning bypass grafts and has been used to evaluate adequacy of cardioplegia delivery. Myocardial contrast echocardiography also may be used to determine graft patency and adequacy of perfusion at the microvascular level (31). Finally, MCE may permit clinically relevant decisions such as differentiating stunned (normal flow) and hibernating (low flow) myocardium from infarcted (no flow) myocardium (33).

Dobutamine Stress Echocardiography

Dobutamine stress echocardiography has been used preoperatively to diagnose myocardial ischemia and more recently to identify viable myocardium. Barilla and colleagues have shown that the response of abnormal myocardial segments to low-dose dobutamine in patients following acute MI (representing stunned myocardium) can predict the magnitude of improvement in regional function in response to coronary revascularization. Previously, RWMAs were regarded as irreversible, representing infarcted, scarred tissue. However, viable myocardium may be present within areas of myocardial dysfunction and may be functionally salvageable. This distinction is important for clinical decisions regarding revascularization procedures because rescue of viable tissue could have a significant impact on patient outcome (34). This is of particular importance in patients with poor ventricular function (EF <35%) who are candidates for CABG. Although these patients have higher surgical morbidity and mortality rates, their long-term survival is improved with surgical revascularization compared with medical therapy. The use of DSE to differentiate patients with reduced EF as a result of reversible ischemia from those with irreversible myocardial injury will allow more appropriate patient selection for high-risk CABG with improvement in overall outcomes in this population.

Dobutamine stress echocardiography involves comparison of regional LV wall motion during basal conditions and with incremental doses of intravenous dobutamine. A common protocol for performing DSE is to start with 5 μg/kg/min and to subsequently increase the dose to 10, 20, 30, and ultimately 40 μg/kg/min as tolerated in 3-minute stages. Normally perfused myocardium will exhibit normal resting wall motion and develop hyperdynamic function with increasing doses of dobutamine due to beta-adrenergic stimulation. Myocardial ischemia is identified by the development of new RWMAs or decline of baseline systolic function with increasing doses of dobutamine. Contractile reserve (in the setting of postischemic insult or stunned myocardium) is characterized by baseline RWMAs that improve with low-dose dobutamine. Several studies have shown that identification of contractile reserve by DSE in the setting of acute MI is specific, and is sensitive in the stable hemodynamic setting (18,35). A biphasic response in which an RWMA improves with low-dose dobutamine and subsequently worsens with high-dose dobutamine suggests hibernating myocardium in the setting of chronic ischemia, and may predict recovery of segmental LV function after coronary revascularization (20,36,37). LV segments that remain akinetic or dyskinetic despite dobutamine infusion are nonviable and likely reflect scarring.

Although intraoperative DSE is not routinely performed, it has the potential to help direct management in revascularization procedures. Dobutamine stress echocardiography can identify or confirm areas of normally functioning myocardium that are underperfused, or areas of akinetic myocardium that are viable and would benefit from revascularization. This information may be useful in interpreting the significance of borderline angiographic lesions that may benefit from revascularization as well as for determining the potential benefit of grafting apparently nonfunctioning myocardium.

PROBLEM-ORIENTED CASE DISCUSSIONS

Case 1: Coronary Artery Bypass Graft Complicated by Cardiovascular Collapse

An 81-year-old man presented with unstable angina requiring intravenous nitroglycerin. Angiography revealed diffuse three-vessel coronary artery disease (CAD) with preserved LV function. He was taken to the operating room where pre-CPB TEE revealed normal anterior, septal, and inferior wall function with severe hypokinesis of the lateral wall. Quadruple CABG was performed, with the left internal mammary artery (LIMA) to the LAD diagonal and LAD sequentially (anterior wall) and the radial artery from the side of the LIMA (T-graft) to the posterior left ventricular (PLV) and the posterior descending (PDA) branches (lateral and inferior walls). Although the LIMA was small, the initial sluggish flow improved following administration of intraarterial papaverine. The patient was weaned from CPB on low-dose dopamine with normal wall motion in all regions as visualized by TEE. However, during chest closure systemic hypotension developed and TEE revealed a newly akinetic anterior wall (Fig. 24.4A and B). Hemodynamics deterioration continued

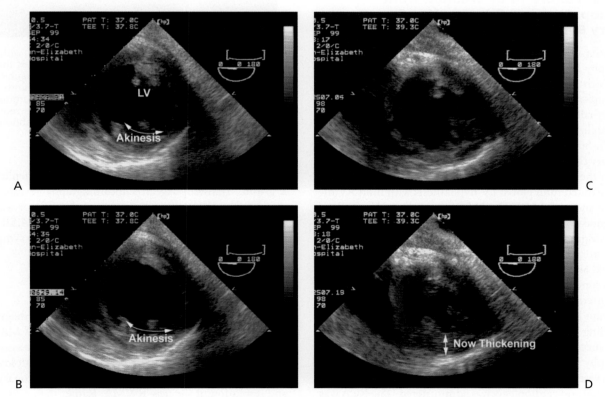

FIGURE 24.4. Transgastric mid-papillary short-axis view of the left ventricle (*LV*). A newly akinetic anterior wall was detected during chest closure, as indicated in **A** (diastole) and **B** (systole). With regrafting of the anterior wall circulation, normal anterior wall motion returned, as indicated in **C** (diastole) and **D** (systole).

despite inotropic support. The heart was recannulated and CPB reestablished. The distal LIMA was in spasm, reducing flow to the anterior wall via the LAD and diagonal grafts, whereas the T-graft to the PLV and PDA appeared intact and of good caliber. Cardioplegia was administered, and the anterior wall was regrafted via an aortocoronary saphenous vein graft. The T-graft supplying the lateral and inferior walls was left intact. The patient was weaned from CPB on moderate doses of inotropes. Transesophageal echocardiographic images verified the return of anterior LV wall function (Fig. 24.4C and D). Although the patient recovered hemodynamically, he suffered a perioperative stroke. He was subsequently discharged from the hospital and was reportedly intact neurologically at the time of his postoperative follow-up visit.

Discussion

This case demonstrated the utility of TEE in accurately identifying the cause of post-CPB cardiovascular collapse. The identification of a new RWMA in the anterior wall territory allowed the rapid diagnosis of a failed graft due to spasm of the small distal LIMA. Regrafting with vein remedied the problem and allowed a successful outcome. In the absence of these data, the decision to regraft may have been delayed, thus contributing to further perioperative morbidity.

Case 2: Failure to Be Weaned from Cardiopulmonary Bypass after Coronary Artery Bypass Grafting

A 60-year-old woman presented with unstable angina. Angiography revealed critical three-vessel CAD and an EF of 49% with mild global hypokinesis, moderate anterior and anteroapical hypokinesis, and severe MR. She developed pulmonary edema in the cardiac catheterization laboratory but was stabilized with insertion of an intraaortic balloon pump (IABP). Subsequent transthoracic echocardiography in the coronary care unit revealed only trivial MR. The patient was sent to the operating room for CABG. The pre-CPB TEE demonstrated mild global LV hypokinesis with mild RV dilatation and trivial MR. The IABP was confirmed by TEE to be in good position with the tip just below the left subclavian artery origin. Quadruple CABG was performed with three aortocoronary grafts using saphenous vein to the LAD, circumflex, and PLV branches. Because a LIMA was not available as conduit (prior radiotherapy for breast cancer), a small right internal mammary (RIMA) was used to graft a large, dominant RCA supplying the inferior wall. Elevated ventricular filling pressures and systemic hypotension prevented an initial successful wean from CPB. Transesophageal echocardiography revealed inferior wall and inferior septal akinesis with severe MR (Fig. 24.5A). Cardiopulmonary bypass was reinitiated and cardioplegia was administered. The RCA was regrafted with a saphenous vein conduit. The subsequent attempt to wean the patient from CPB was successful with

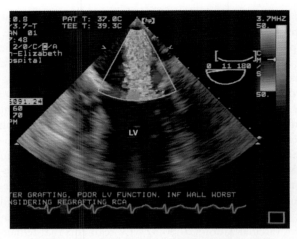

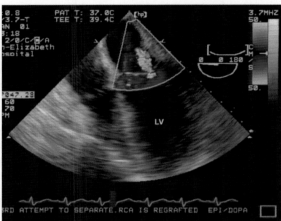

FIGURE 24.5. Mid-esophageal four-chamber view with color flow Doppler across the mitral valve. After grafting of the right coronary artery (*RCA*), transesophageal echocardiographic imaging revealed inferior wall akinesis. **A:** Concomitant with a new regional wall motion abnormality, severe mitral regurgitation is shown. **B:** Resolution of the mitral regurgitation after regrafting of the RCA and reversal of the inferior wall motion abnormality. *LV,* left ventricle.

dopamine administered at 5 g/kg/min and epinephrine at 2 g/min. Transesophageal echocardiography revealed dramatic improvement in wall motion of the inferior wall and inferior septum with resolution of the MR (Fig. 24.5B). The patient was discharged with an EF of 48% and no symptoms of congestive heart failure.

Discussion

This case demonstrates the utility of TEE in diagnosing failure to be weaned from CPB. Here a new RWMA indicated graft insufficiency in the RCA territory. The associated episodic severe MR indicated an acute ischemic etiology and was predicted to resolve with restoration of coronary flow and resolution of the new RWMA. Rather than persevering with increasing inotropes in the face of hemodynamic compromise or attempting valve surgery, the surgical team was rapidly and accurately informed by the TEE data that the critical issue was inadequate flow in a large dominant RCA. Subsequent regrafting with a saphenous vein conduit was effective.

Case 3: Regional Dysfunction in the Setting of Ischemia Improves after Grafting (Rescue of Stunned Myocardium)

A 77-year-old woman sustained an inferior MI and was treated with thrombolysis. Her course was complicated by pulmonary edema requiring intubation. Transthoracic echocardiography revealed an EF of 41%, inferoposterior akinesis, and moderate MR. She recovered, and was mobilized and discharged only to have recurrent pulmonary edema and unstable angina. She was admitted to the ICU, was intubated, and required inotropic support to treat congestive heart failure with hemodynamic instability. Cardiac catheterization revealed three-vessel CAD, inferior wall akinesis and anterior wall hypokinesis with an EF of 30%, moderate MR, and a left ventricular end-diastolic pressure of 27 mm Hg. She was taken to the operating room, where TEE revealed inferior and posterior wall akinesis consistent

with her prior inferior MI and akinesis of the anterior and lateral LV walls (Fig. 24.6A and B). She also had moderate MR with normal mitral valve anatomy. Triple CABG was performed with LIMA to the LAD, and saphenous vein grafts to the PDA and circumflex marginal branch. She was weaned from CPB on 5 g/kg/min of dopamine and 3 g/min of epinephrine. Postgrafting TEE revealed reversal of the RWMA in the anterior and lateral walls, with no change in the inferior akinesis (Fig. 24.6C and D). Hemodynamics improved steadily, and the patient was weaned from epinephrine over the following few hours. Follow-up echocardiographic examination 3 months postsurgery revealed preserved anterior wall function with an EF estimated at 40% and persistent moderate MR.

Discussion

This case demonstrates reversibility of anterior and lateral wall motion abnormalities with revascularization. Confounding this interpretation is the inotropic support in the post-CPB period, although the patient was rapidly weaned from this support with no alteration in the anterolateral wall recovery. Furthermore, the patient was receiving

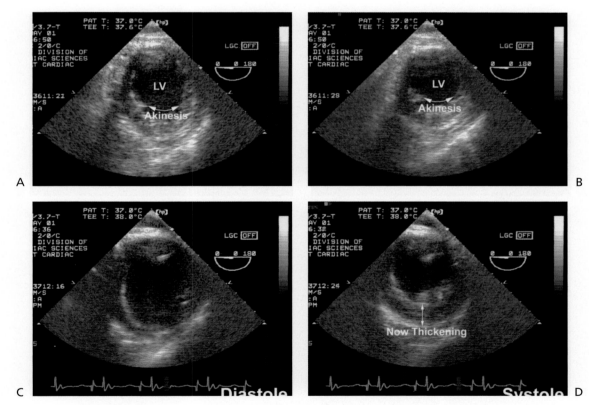

FIGURE 24.6. Transgastric mid-papillary short-axis view of the left ventricle (*LV*). This unstable patient was taken to the operating room with new anterior wall akinesis as depicted in **A** (diastole) and **B** (systole). After grafting of her left anterior descending coronary artery, reversal of her anterior regional wall motion abnormality was observed, as depicted in **C** (diastole) and **D** (systole), indicating salvage of ischemic myocardium.

inotropic support preoperatively. The anterolateral walls remained functionally normal 3 months postsurgery, suggesting rescue of stunned myocardium through revascularization rather than altered inotropic support.

Case 4: Post-induction Hemodynamic Instability

A 65-year-old man presented with an acute anterolateral MI complicated by cardiogenic shock requiring intubation, inotropic support, and insertion of an IABP. Cardiac catheterization revealed inferior and anteroapical akinesis with an EF of 31%. Transthoracic echocardiography revealed severe LV dysfunction but visualization was limited because of poor acoustic windows. RV function was normal. The patient was taken urgently to the operating room. Following induction of general anesthesia, the patient's systemic blood pressure markedly deteriorated without a concomitant rise in pulmonary artery pressure. Increasing the dopamine dose resulted in a further deterioration of his hemodynamic status. A TEE probe was inserted and revealed severe LV dilatation and global severe hypokinesis (Fig. 24.7A and B). Nitroglycerin was begun, and dopamine was reduced with marked improvement in LV function by TEE. Triple CABG was

performed with LIMA to the LAD, and vein grafts to the PDA and obtuse marginal (OM) branches. The patient was weaned from bypass on 2 g/min of epinephrine and low-dose dopamine. Transesophageal echocardiography revealed normal RV and anterior wall function, with persistent inferior wall motion abnormalities but improved global LV function (Fig. 24.7C and D). The patient sustained a postoperative stroke and TEE was performed on postoperative day 6 to rule out a thrombus. This study verified normal RV and LV anterior wall function off inotropic support. A late postoperative RWMA study revealed an EF of 54% with normal anterior wall function.

Discussion

This case demonstrates the utility of TEE in the management of postanesthetic induction hemodynamic instability. Hemodynamic data alone suggested possible cardiac depression, decrease in preload, or loss of vasomotor tone due to anesthetic induction. Transesophageal echocardiography gave clear evidence of depressed LV function with escalating inotropic stimulation in the setting of acute ischemia. Initial treatment with escalating inotropic support likely increased myocardial oxygen demand and only with the institution of

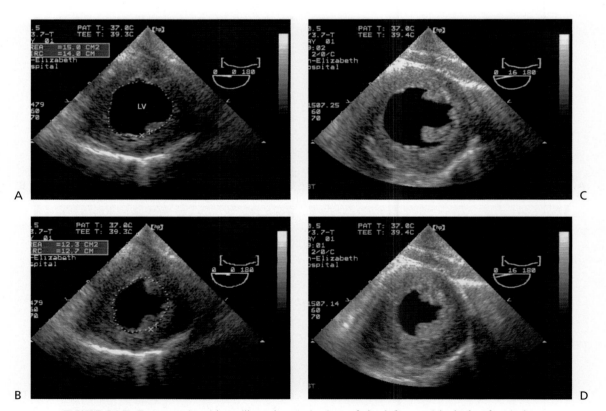

FIGURE 24.7. Transgastric mid-papillary short-axis view of the left ventricle (*LV*). After induction of anesthesia and significant hemodynamic deterioration, severe LV failure was diagnosed by transesophageal echocardiography (TEE), as depicted in **A** (diastole) and **B** (systole). With antiischemic therapy, TEE showed marked improvement in LV function, which was maintained after grafting, as depicted in **C** (diastole) and **D** (systole).

nitroglycerin and reduction in the inotropes dose did the patient's hemodynamic status improve. Rapid stabilization of this patient's hemodynamic status averted "crashing" onto CPB and allowed the surgeon time to dissect the left internal mammary artery for optimal conduit and perform a careful, complete revascularization.

Case 5: Regional Wall Motion Abnormality Detected on Separation from Bypass

A 65-year-old woman presented with typical exertional angina and a positive stress test and was found to have critical stenosis of the origin of a very large RCA without other significant CAD. She was taken to the operating room for single-vessel grafting of her RCA. Pre-CPB TEE revealed normal RV and LV function without RWMAs. She had undergone previous vein stripping, so a small RIMA was used as conduit. On separation from CPB, she had persistent ECG changes in the inferior leads and TEE revealed severe inferobasal hypokinesis with no other RWMAs (Fig. 24.8). Although there was no hemodynamic instability, the decision was made to redo the RCA graft with a radial artery as conduit. The patient was subsequently weaned from CPB without inotropic support, and TEE revealed normal RV and LV function with normal inferobasal wall motion. She was taken to the ICU in stable condition and made an uneventful recovery.

Discussion

This case demonstrates the utility of TEE in intraoperative clinical decision making. Reinstitution of CPB to redo a CABG is often reserved for the hemodynamically unstable patient. In this stable patient, with ECG changes indicating ischemia in the inferior wall, TEE confirmed a new and persistent RWMA in the RCA territory. These data clearly indicated the insufficiency of using a small RIMA to a large RCA. Since this was her only significant CAD, it seemed imperative to redo this graft. Intraoperative detection of RWMA postgrafting in this setting gave the surgeon clear direction and allowed for successful revascularization in this patient. The patient made a full recovery and remained symptom free at postoperative follow-up.

Case 6: New Ischemia Detected as a Regional Wall Motion Abnormality During Repair of a Complex Congenital Heart Lesion

A 32-year-old woman had undergone a complete repair for tetralogy of Fallot (TOF) at age 6 after initial palliation with a Blalock-Taussig shunt. Although asymptomatic, serial echocardiography revealed increasing RV diameter with new hypokinesia in association with significant pulmonary insufficiency. She was referred for pulmonary valve replacement

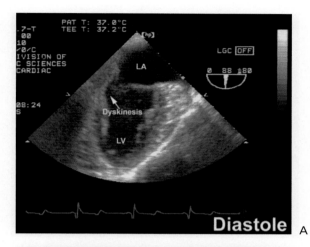

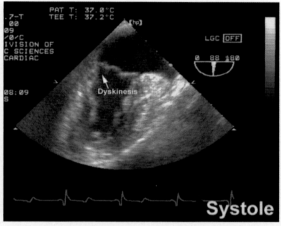

FIGURE 24.8. Mid-esophageal two-chamber view of the left ventricle (*LV*). After grafting the right coronary artery (*RCA*), transesophageal echocardiography revealed a persistent inferior basal area of dyskinesis, as depicted in **A** (diastole) and **B** (systole). The RCA graft was redone, and the regional wall motion abnormality resolved entirely. *LA*, left atrium.

to correct chronic RV volume overload. Preoperative cardiac catheterization revealed normal LV function (EF 67%) and no residual stenosis of the RV outflow tract or pulmonary artery. Coronary angiography was omitted. Intraoperative, prebypass TEE revealed severe pulmonary insufficiency, moderate RV dilatation with mildly depressed function, and normal LV function. Surgically, a transannular right ventriculotomy was made, which divided a moderate sized conal branch of the RCA. A pulmonary valve replacement with a bioprosthetic valve was performed and a transannular patch of bovine pericardium was used to close the RV defect. Post-CPB TEE revealed new anteroapical and anteroseptal akinesis (Fig. 24.9). These akineses were accompanied by episodes of ventricular tachycardia and anterior ECG ST-segment changes. Although the ST changes persisted, the irritability resolved and she remained hemodynamically stable. Therefore, no additional intervention was attempted and she made an uneventful recovery.

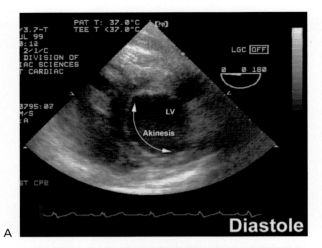

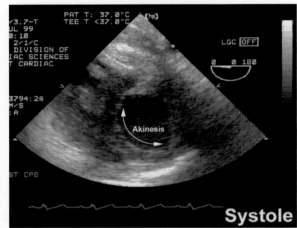

FIGURE 24.9. Transgastric apical short-axis view of the left ventricle (*LV*). During pulmonary valve replacement in a patient with repaired tetralogy of Fallot, division of a conal branch of the right coronary artery compromised distal left anterior descending coronary artery perfusion. The resultant wall motion abnormality in the apical septal and anterior wall regions is shown in **A** (diastole) and **B** (systole).

Long-term follow-up echocardiographic examination revealed persistent distal anteroseptal akinesis with marked hypokinesis of the distal anterior wall and apex. She remained symptom free with an EF of 50%.

Discussion

This case demonstrates the exquisite sensitivity of TEE for diagnosing acute ischemia. Anomalous origin of the LAD from the RCA is known to occur in 5% of TOF patients, and in this case division of the conal RCA branch compromised distal LAD perfusion. Preoperative coronary angiography would have alerted the surgeons to the contribution of this RCA conal branch to the distal LAD supply. The new RWMA detected by TEE accurately localized the ischemic area and offered the surgeon the opportunity to perform distal LAD coronary artery bypass grafting.

Case 7: New Regional Wall Motion Abnormality after Coronary Artery Bypass Grafting Indicating Graft Failure

A 78-year-old man with a history of prior CABG surgery presented with recurrent angina. Cardiac catheterization revealed native triple-vessel CAD and compromise of all previous grafts, including a LIMA with a mid-portion critical lesion but an otherwise normal distal vessel. Reoperative CABG surgery was undertaken with a sequential vein graft from aorta to distal LIMA, first obtuse marginal branch of the circumflex (OM-1), and RCA continuation. On separation from CPB, a newly akinetic lateral wall was noted by TEE concomitantly with lateral ECG changes (Fig. 24.10). The surgeon confirmed that atherosclerotic debris had been present in one of the OM grafts and hypothesized that

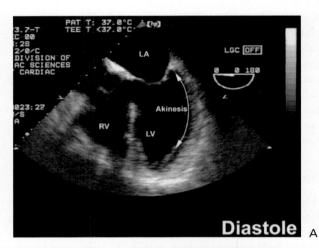

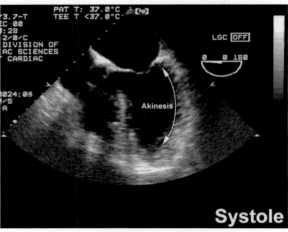

FIGURE 24.10. Transesophageal mid-esophageal four-chamber view. A newly akinetic left ventricular (*LV*) lateral wall was noted after reoperative coronary artery bypass grafting, as depicted in **A** (diastole) and **B** (systole). The obtuse marginal branch of the left circumflex coronary artery had contained significant atherosclerotic debris noted intraoperatively, and postoperative cardiac catheterization revealed poor run-off in this branch, consistent with embolization. *LA*, left atrium; *RV*, right ventricle.

embolization may have occurred. The patient was separated from CPB on inotropic support and was taken to the cardiac ICU postoperatively. He could not be weaned from inotropic support and was reevaluated with TEE, which showed overall depressed LV function and an akinetic lateral wall. He therefore underwent repeat cardiac catheterization, which revealed that all three anastomoses were patent but that runoff in the OM-1 was poor, consistent with distal embolization of the native OM-l. The decision not to reintervene was made based on the quality of native vessels in this region. He was subsequently weaned from inotropic support with an estimated EF of 35% and was discharged from the hospital.

Discussion

The use of TEE during reoperative CABG surgery allowed for rapid diagnosis of graft failure in this instance. This information provided an accurate diagnosis substantiated by the surgeon's analysis and confirmed by cardiac catheterization. Although regrafting of the lateral territory in this patient was not possible, TEE provided information that narrowed the differential diagnosis and allowed for more informative surgical decision making, thus preventing other interventions with potentially deleterious results.

KEY POINTS

- Transesophageal echocardiography has been demonstrated to be superior in sensitivity and specificity to either ECG or PAC monitoring techniques in the detection of myocardial ischemia.
- Not all RWMAs are indicative of myocardial ischemia. Areas of infarction, stunning, or hibernation all may appear as impairment in segmental myocardial thickening and a decrease in endocardial excursion by TEE. Ventricular pacing, and changes in loading conditions also can affect regional wall motion.
- The guidelines established by the ASE/SCA recommend the use of a 16-segment model to describe the location of the RWMA.
- The diagnosis of myocardial ischemia requires worsening of segmental function by at least two grades: from normal or mild hypokinesis to at least severe hypokinesis or akinesis.
- Most echocardiography consoles allow the saving of loop segments to be displayed for comparison with subsequent images. The side-by-side analysis for RWMA is invaluable because it allows the echocardiographer to evaluate the adequacy of the comparison views as well as any changes in wall motion/segmental thickening.
- Diastolic dysfunction as evidenced by impairment of LV relaxation and a decrease in LV compliance is known to precede systolic dysfunction in the cascade of ischemic

events. Characteristic findings in acute myocardial ischemia include a reduction in the E/A ratio, and an increase in DT and IVRT. The dynamic environment of the operating room makes the evaluation of diastolic function by this technique challenging.
- Assessment of myocardial viability with DSE has been established as an accurate predictor of recruitable, hibernating myocardium and can differentiate ischemic from nonischemic dysfunction.
- Transesophageal echocardiography combined with MCE can demonstrate successful graft placement, adequacy of cardioplegia delivery, and integrity of myocardial microvasculature.

REFERENCES

1. Mangano DT, Browner WS, Hollenberg M, et al., SPI Research Group. Association of perioperative myocardial ischemia with cardiac morbidity and mortality in men undergoing noncardiac surgery. *N Engl J Med* 1990;323:1781–1788.
2. Mangano DT, Browner WS, Hollenberg M, et al. Long-term cardiac prognosis following noncardiac surgery. The Study of Perioperative Ischemia Research Group. *JAMA* 1992;268:233–239.
3. Leung JM, O'Kelly B, Browner WS, et al., SPI Research Group. Prognostic importance of postbypass regional wall-motion abnormalities in patients undergoing coronary artery bypass graft surgery. *Anesthesiology* 1989;71:16–25.
4. Fleisher LA, Weiskopf RB. Real-time intraoperative monitoring of myocardial ischemia in noncardiac surgery. *Anesthesiology* 2000;92:1183–1188.
5. Wohlgelernter D, Jaffe CC, Cabin HS, et al. Silent ischemia during coronary occlusion produced by balloon inflation: relation to regional myocardial dysfunction. *J Am Coll Cardiol* 1987;10:491–498.
6. Battler A, Froelicher VF, Gallagher KP, et al. Dissociation between regional myocardial dysfunction and ECG changes during ischemia in the conscious dog. *Circulation* 1980;62:735–744.
7. **van Daele ME, Sutherland BR, Mitchell MM, et al. Do changes in pulmonary capillary wedge pressure adequately reflect myocardial ischemia during anesthesia? A correlative preoperative hemodynamic, electrocardiographic and transesophageal echocardiographic study. *Circulation* 1990;81:865–871.**
8. Perrino AC Jr, McCloskey G. Detection of intraoperative myocardial ischemia. *Int Anesthesiol Clin* 1996;34:37–56.
9. Tennant R, Wiggers CJ. The effect of coronary occlusion on myocardial contraction. *Am J Physiol* 1935;112:351–361.
10. Massie BM, Botvinick EH, Brundage BH, et al. Relationship of regional myocardial perfusion to segmental wall motion: a physiological basis for understanding the presence of reversibility of asynergy. *Circulation* 1978;58:1154–1163.
11. **Hauser AM, Gangaharan V, Ramos RG, et al. Sequence of mechanical, electrocardiographic and clinic effects of repeated coronary artery occlusion in human beings: echocardiographic observations during coronary angioplasty. *J Am Coll Cardiol* 1985;5:193–197.**
12. Noma S, Askenase AD, Weintraub WS, et al. Augmentation of contraction in remote nonischemic zone during acute ischemia. *Am J Physiol* 1988;255:H301–H310.
13. Braunwald E, Kloner RA. The stunned myocardium: prolonged,

post-ischemic ventricular dysfunction. *Circulation* 1982;66:1146–1149.

14. Rahimtoola SH. The hibernating myocardium. *Am Heart J* 1989;117:211–221.

15. Braunwald E, Ruterford JD. Reversible ischemic left ventricular dysfunction: evidence for the "hibernating myocardium." *J Am Coll Cardiol* 1986;8:1467–1470.

16. Yousef ZR, Marber MS. The open artery hypothesis: potential mechanisms of action. *Prog Cardiovasc Dis* 2000;42:41.

17. **Lualdi JC, Douglas PS. Echocardiography for the assessment of myocardial viability. *J Am Soc Echocardiogr* 1997;10:772–781.**

18. **Barilla F, Gheorghiade M, Alam M, et al. Low-dose dobutamine in patients with acute myocardial infarction identifies viable but not contractile myocardium and predicts the magnitude of improvement in wall motion abnormalities in response to coronary revascularization. *Am Heart J* 1991;122:1522–1531.**

19. Smart SC, Sawada S, Ryan T, et al. Low-dose dobutamine echocardiography detects reversible dysfunction after thrombolytic therapy of acute myocardial infarction. *Circulation* 1993;88:405–415.

20. **Cigarroa CB, deFilippi CR, Brickner E, et al. Dobutamine stress echocardiography identifies hibernating myocardium and predicts recovery of left ventricular function after coronary revascularization. *Circulation* 1993;88:430–436.**

21. Pfeffer MA, Braunwald E. Ventricular remodeling after myocardial infarction: experimental observations and clinical implications. *Circulation* 1990;81:1161.

22. **Hogue CW, Davila-Roman VG. Detection of myocardial ischemia by transesophageal echocardiographically determined changes in left ventricular area in patients undergoing coronary artery bypass surgery. *J Clin Anesth* 1997;9:388–393.**

23. **Cahalan MK, Ionescu P, Melton HE et al. Automated real-time analysis of intraoperative transesophageal echocardiograms. *Anesthesiology* 1993;78:477–485.**

24. Nishimura R, Abel M, Hatle L, et al. Assessment of diastolic function of the heart: background and current applications of Doppler echocardiography. Part II: clinical studies. *Mayo Clin Proc* 1989;64:131–204.

25. Nishimura R, Housmans P, Hatle L et al. Assessment of diastolic function of the heart: background and current application of Doppler echocardiography. Part I: Physiological and pathophysiological features. *Mayo Clin Proc* 1989;64:71–81.

26. Koolen JJ, Visser CA, David GK. Transesophageal echocardiographic assessment of systolic and diastolic dysfunction during percutaneous transluminal coronary angioplasty. *J Am Soc Echocardiogr* 1990;3:374–383.

27. Seeberger MD, Cahalan MK, Rouine-Rapp K, et al. Acute hypovolemia may cause segmental wall motion abnormalities in

the absence of myocardial ischemia. *Anesth Analg* 1997;85:1252–1257.

28. Roizen MF, Beaupre PN, Alpert RA, et al. Monitoring with 2D transesophageal echocardiography: comparison of myocardial function in patients undergoing supraceliac, suprarenal-infraceliac, or infrarenal aortic occlusion. *J Vasc Surg* 1984;1:300–305.

29. **Shanewise JS, Cheung AT, Aronson S, et al. ASE/SCA guidelines for performing a comprehensive intraoperative multiplane transesophageal echocardiography examination: recommendations of the American Society of Echocardiography Council for Intraoperative Echocardiography and the Society of Cardiovascular Anesthesiologists Task Force for Certification in Perioperative Transesophageal Echocardiography. *Anesth Analg* 1999;89:870–884.**

30. **Rouine-Rapp K, Ionescu P, Balea M, et al. Detection of intraoperative segmental wall motion abnormalities by transesophageal echocardiography: the incremental value of additional cross sections in the transverse and longitudinal planes. *Anesth Analg* 1996;83:1141–1148.**

31. Villanueva FS, Spotnitz WD, Jayaweera AR, et al. On-line intraoperative quantification of regional myocardial perfusion during coronary artery bypass graft operations with myocardial contrast two-dimensional echocardiography. *J Thorac Cardiovasc Surg* 1992;104:1524–1531.

32. Kolev N, Berkemeir G, Mayer IN, et al. A new scoring system using Doppler transmitral diastolic measurement identifies transient myocardial ischemia. *Eur J Anaesth* 1995;13:49–55.

33. **Aronson S, Savage R, Toledano A, et al. Identifying the cause of left ventricular systolic dysfunction after coronary artery bypass surgery: the role of myocardial contrast echocardiography. *J Cardiothorac Vasc Anesth* 1998;12:512–518.**

34. Baer FM, Voth E, LaRosee K, et al. Comparison of dobutamine transesophageal echocardiography and dobutamine magnetic resonance imaging for detection of residual myocardial viability. *Am J Cardiol* 1996;78:415–419.

35. Pierard LA, de Landsheere CM, Berthe C, et al. Identification of viable myocardium by echocardiography during dobutamine infusion in patients with myocardial infarction after thrombolytic therapy: comparison with positron emission tomography. *J Am Coll Cardiol* 1990;15:1021–1031.

36. Senior R, Lahiri A. Enhanced detection of myocardial ischemia by stress dobutamine echocardiography utilizing the "biphasic" response of wall thickening during low and high dose dobutamine infusion. *J Am Coll Cardiol* 1995;26:26–32.

37. Afridi I, Kleiman NS, Raizner AE, et al. Dobutamine echocardiography in myocardial hibernation: optimal dose and accuracy in predicting recovery of ventricular function after coronary angioplasty. *Circulation* 1995;91:663–670.

HYPERTROPHIC OBSTRUCTIVE CARDIOMYOPATHY

ROBERT M. SAVAGE
RANDALL CORREIA

NATURE OF HYPERTROPHIC CARDIOMYOPATHY

Hypertrophic obstructive cardiomyopathy (HOCM) is a rare progressive cardiac abnormality associated with dynamic systolic left ventricular outflow tract (LVOT) obstruction and diastolic dysfunction. The pathology may be distinguished from the more general, hypertrophic cardiomyopathy, which is a heterogeneous group of diseases that includes those without obstructive features. Clinically, the entity of obstructive hypertrophic cardiomyopathy is defined by the extent of hypertrophy and its functional consequences. Hypertrophic obstructive cardiomyopathy was initially described more than 100 years ago, but its classic features were not clarified until the 1960s (1–3). The pathophysiologic features of LVOT obstruction in HOCM (Table 25.1) include a decreased diameter of the LVOT and an increased velocity of blood flow to a critical level. This results in systolic anterior motion of the coapted mitral valve leaflets into the LVOT and contact with the interventricular septum, producing a subvalvular stenosis and systolic LVOT gradient. Symptoms of HOCM include syncope or sudden death, ischemic chest pain, and pulmonary congestion (Table 25.2).

Because of its asymptomatic nature, the prevalence of HOCM is difficult to estimate. It is thought to occur in 0.2% (by electrocardiographic screening) to 5% (echocardiographic screening) of the population (4–6). The average annual mortality rate of patients with HOCM under medical management alone has been estimated to be 3% to 4% (3). This chapter reviews the underlying nature of HOCM, gives an overview of the clinical presentation and management of HOCM, and emphasizes the role of intraoperative echocardiography in the surgical management of HOCM

and of postoperative evaluation in the search for potential surgical complications.

Definition and Classification

Classically, HOCM has been defined as an unexplained hypertrophy of the left ventricle (LV) associated with LVOT obstruction and abnormal diastolic function (7–9). However, it has been recognized that HOCM also may include those patients with secondary ventricular hypertrophy and dynamic LVOT obstruction. Hypertrophic obstructive cardiomyopathy has two anatomic presentations classified as either asymmetric hypertrophy or symmetric hypertrophy (Table 25.3).

Hypertrophic obstructive cardiomyopathy is thought to be familial, being genetically transmitted as an autosomal-dominant trait with variable or incomplete penetrance in more than 50% of patients with this abnormality (10). Studies have reported a dominant inheritance pattern with incomplete penetrance. Deoxyribonucleic acid (DNA) probe studies have demonstrated that familial hypertrophic cardiomyopathy is a genetically heterogenous disease (11). The incidence of familial hypertrophic cardiomyopathy is somewhat confounded in that, in many patients, the disease does not become apparent until after adolescence (3). Histologically, familial asymmetric hypertrophic cardiomyopathy is characterized microscopically by large numbers of bizarrely shaped muscle cells in a disorganized architectural arrangement involving the interventricular septum and associated with extensive fibrosis. This segment of hypertrophied interventricular septum imposes on the LV cavity and decreases the distance between the ventricular septum and the anterior edge of the mitral valve during systole.

There are other forms of asymmetric septal hypertrophy besides the familial type. Those types of asymmetric septal hypertrophy not necessarily associated with obstruction include right ventricular hypertrophy, chronic hypertension with LV hypertrophy and posterior wall myocardial

---
R. M. Savage and R. Correia: Department of Anesthesiology, Cleveland Clinic Foundation, Cleveland, Ohio.

TABLE 25.1. LEFT VENTRICULAR OUTFLOW TRACT (LVOT) OBSTRUCTION: PATHOPHYSIOLOGIC FEATURES

Decreased diameter of LVOT
  Small ventricular cavity
  Decreased LV volume
  Hypovolemia
  Tachycardia

Left ventricular hypertrophy
  Diastolic dysfunction
  Septal hypertrophy → LVOT narrowing

Abnormal mitral valve apparatus or motion
  Anteriorly displaced papillary muscle
  Redundancy of mitral valve leaflets
  Systolic anterior motion of mitral valve leaflets

Increased velocity of blood flow in LVOT
  Hypercontractility
    Increased sympathetic tone
    Inotrope administration
  Decreased afterload
    Exercise
    Pharmacological agents
      Vasodilators
      β_2 agonists
      Inodilators
    Systemic shunts
      Hepatic disease
      Atrioventricular malformations
      Pregnancy
  Medical comorbidities
    Anemia
    Thyroid disease
    Pheochromocytoma
    Paget disease
    Hypovolemia

---

infarction, interventricular septal sarcomas, amyloidosis, glycogen and mucopolysaccharides storage diseases, Friedreich ataxia, and myxedema. The fetal heart typically demonstrates asymmetric septal thickening, which usually disappears within the first 2 years of life. Newborns of mothers with insulin-dependent diabetes mellitus also may demonstrate a temporary condition of asymmetric septal hypertrophy with LVOT obstruction and heart failure in some

TABLE 25.2. HYPERTROPHIC OBSTRUCTIVE CARDIOMYOPATHY PATHOPHYSIOLOGY AND PRESENTING SYMPTOMS

Left ventricular outflow tract obstruction
  Syncope
  Sudden death
Myocardial ischemia
  Chest pain
  Ectopy
Diastolic dysfunction with increased left atrial pressures
  Pulmonary congestion
  Dyspnea

TABLE 25.3. HYPERTROPHIC OBSTRUCTIVE CARDIOMYOPATHY MORPHOLOGIC CLASSIFICATION

Asymmetrical hypertrophy
  Familial
  Sigmoid-shaped septum associated with elderly
  Apical variant, spadelike appearance
  Mid: ventricular rings
  Miscellaneous
    Eisenmenger Syndrome with septal hypertrophy
    Septal sarcoma
    Left ventricular hypertrophy with lateral wall infarction
    Neonates of diabetic mothers
    Pulmonary hypertension and right ventricular hypertrophy
    Transient stage during fetal development
Symmetrical hypertrophy
  Concentric left ventricular hypertrophy
    Associated with chronic hypertension
    Associated with aortic stenosis
  Miscellaneous comorbidities
    Cardiac amyloidosis
    Friedereich ataxia
    Myxedema
    Glycogen storage diseases
    After mitral valve repair
    After lung transplantation
    Hepatic disease

---

instances (12). Patients with long-standing pulmonary hypertension, D-transposition of the great vessels, and valvular pulmonic stenosis may demonstrate asymmetric septal hypertrophy (13).

Symmetric hypertrophy of the LV is another anatomic class of hypertrophic cardiomyopathy. Patients who have had chronic untreated hypertension may develop concentric LV hypertrophy and LVOT obstruction. When symmetric ventricular hypertrophy is associated with obstruction, it is always associated with systolic anterior motion (SAM) of the mitral valve with a dynamic functional subvalvular stenosis. Patients who have undergone aortic valve replacement for severe aortic stenosis also may manifest LVOT obstruction in the presence of concentric LV hypertrophy, secondary to a chronic aortic valve gradient. Such obstruction is associated with a diminished LVOT diameter and SAM of the mitral valve.

The features of HOCM that are common to the various forms of this entity are dynamic LVOT obstruction and diastolic dysfunction characterized by an abnormal relaxation and a noncompliant restricted LV with impaired ventricular filling. Consequently, the most common clinical presentation of patients with this abnormality include symptoms of LVOT obstruction such as chest pain, syncope, and sudden death in addition to those symptoms associated with poor LV compliance resulting in LV end-diastolic pressure and manifested as symptoms associated with pulmonary edema (14).

Etiology

The exact cause of hypertrophy in patients with familial HOCM is unknown. Defects have been identified in several of the genes that encode sarcomeric proteins, including myosin, heavy-chain actin, and tropomyosin, and these may provide the molecular basis for hypertrophic disease. Varieties of mutations have been identified with varying genotypic degrees of hypertrophy and risks for mortality, but the correlation between risk for hypertrophy and risk for mortality is poor. Specific tropomyosin defects, for example, are associated with only mild hypertrophy, little LVOT obstruction, but high risk for sudden cardiac death.

Several potential mechanisms have been suggested (Table 25.4). Increased concentrations of intracellular calcium can stimulate hypertrophy of the myocardium and the characteristic cellular disarray that is associated with hypertrophic cardiomyopathy (15). Other potential causes of HOCM are thought to include myocardial ischemia with resulting abnormalities in calcium flux leading to diminished LV compliance, abnormal intramural coronary arteries contributing to myocardial ischemia, and abnormal adrenergic stimulation of the heart (16). Although atherosclerotic coronary disease has been associated with HOCM, the penetrating coronary arteries within the myocardium demonstrate a small lumen size and thickening of the vascular wall (17).

Pathophysiology

The anatomic and functional features of LVOT obstruction include (a) a diminished LVOT diameter, (b) an increased velocity of blood flow proceeding out the ventricle to a critical level, producing a Venturi effect in the LVOT, and (c) anterior and central displacement of the papillary muscles with typically elongated chordae (18,19). With the onset of systole, the anterior displacement of the papillary muscle positions the mitral valve leaflets in the stream of flow proceeding from the ventricular cavity into the LVOT. This draws the coapted leaflets into the LVOT, resulting in SAM of the coapted mitral valve leaflets and development of a Venturi mechanism with a pressure differential between the ventricular and LVOT sides of the coapted mitral leaflets. This further promotes the anterior motion of the mitral leaflets and eventual contact with the interventricular septum and produces a subvalvular stenosis at the point of leaflet SAM–septal contact and a dynamic LVOT gradient. Reduction of

TABLE 25.4. PATHOGENESIS OF FAMILIAL HYPERTROPHIC OBSTRUCTIVE CARDIOMYOPATHY

Abnormal calcium metabolism
  Increased calcium flux in the sarcoplasmic reticulum associated with abnormal and asymmetric growth
Abnormal penetrating coronary arteries producing focal ischemia
Abnormal adrenergic stimulation of the heart

the anatomic diameter of the LVOT and anterior displacement of the papillary muscles are the first key elements in the development of LVOT obstruction. An LVOT diameter of less than 20 mm is associated with LVOT obstruction in up to 66% of patients (20).

Functional factors such as increased contractility or decreased afterload may further contribute to a diminished LVOT diameter. Hyperdynamic LV function may result from anemia, hyperthyroidism, increased sympathetic tone, inotropes, and exercise. With anterior displacement of the papillary muscles or mitral valve leaflet elongation or chordal laxity, the potential diameter of the LVOT is further diminished during systole as the leaflet tips of the mitral valve are moved closer to the LVOT. Higher blood outflow velocities result, thereby increasing the potential for the Venturi effect.

An increased velocity of blood flow proceeding out the LVOT is the second key substrate of LVOT obstruction. For every LVOT diameter there is a critical velocity threshold above which a Venturi effect is established. The flow in the LVOT proceeds across the coapted mitral valve leaflet tips, producing a pressure differential similar to that applied to an airplane wing, with the subsequent production of aerodynamic lift. With lower pressure on the LVOT surface and higher pressure on the posterior surface, the leaflet flies into the LVOT. As the SAM of the mitral valve leaflets continues, the pressure gradient persists and the leaflet tip may eventually contact the interventricular septum. The severity of the LVOT obstruction has been associated with both the diameter of the LVOT and the duration of leaflet SAM, as well as the presence of leaflet SAM–septal contact and the length of the leaflet SAM–septal contact (20). The initial anterior motion of the mitral valve with the onset of systole is thought to be related to a more anterior placement of the anterior and posterior papillary muscles in the ventricular chamber. The tendency for the SAM of the mitral valve and obstruction is further enhanced by the presence of elongated mitral leaflets and laxity of the chordal structures. Systolic anterior motion of the mitral valve and mitral valve prolapse are thought to represent two manifestations of chordal laxity. In the presence of anterior displacement of the papillary muscles, the chordal laxity may result in the LVOT Venturi effect, whereas in the absence of anterior displacement of the papillary muscles, the chordal laxity may cause the mitral valve leaflets to prolapse into the left atrial (LA) cavity (19).

The pathophysiology of ischemia in hypertrophic cardiomyopathy is attributed to several mechanisms (Table 25.5): (a) an increased ratio of muscle mass to blood vessel area; (b) compression of intramural coronary arteries; (c) abnormal regulation of vascular resistance; and (d) increased myocardial oxygen demand due to increased wall stress associated with the outflow tract obstruction. The development of syncope is attributed to periods of increased LVOT obstruction brought about by hypovolemia, tachycardia with diminished LV filling, decreased afterload,

TABLE 25.5. HYPERTROPHIC OBSTRUCTIVE CARDIOMYOPATHY MECHANISMS OF ISCHEMIA

Increased muscle mass to blood vessel ratio
Intramural coronary artery compression
Abnormal vascular resistance regulation
Increased wall stress due to obstruction

paradoxic vasodilatation associated with the Bezold-Jarisch reflex, and hypercontractility due to increased sympathetic tone and hyperresponsiveness of the myocardium to sympathetic stimulation.

CLINICAL PRESENTATION

History and Physical Examination

Most patients with HOCM are asymptomatic until syncope or sudden death occurs as the initial manifestation of this disease. The incidence of sudden death is higher in younger patients. Patients are usually in their third or fourth decade of life and are asymptomatic. When symptoms are present, they are associated with shortness of breath, chest pain, and the more ominous symptoms of syncope and dizziness. Pulmonary congestion and edema have been attributed to the increase in LA pressure, which is associated with diastolic dysfunction.

There are a number of proposed mechanisms to account for the ischemia in these patients (Table 25.5), including: (a) an increased muscle mass to blood vessel area ratio; (b) compression of the intramural coronary arteries; (c) abnormal vascular resistance regulation; and (d) increased myocardial oxygen demand caused by increased wall stress associated with the outflow tract obstruction. Syncope has been attributed to periods of increased severity of LVOT obstruction associated with hypovolemia, tachycardia with diminished LV filling, decreased afterload, inappropriate vasodilatation associated with the Bezold-Jarisch reflex, and hypercontractility associated with increased sympathetic tone and responsiveness of the myocardium to sympathetic stimulation.

The physical examination in individuals with LVOT obstruction frequently does not reflect the severity of the obstructive gradient and may demonstrate only an accentuated fourth heart sound (S4) due to the diminished ventricular compliance and reliance on the atrial contraction for LV filling. In addition to a prominent S4, however, the patient may demonstrate a harsh mid-systolic murmur (which increases with the Valsalva maneuver, when standing, or with inhalation of amyl nitrate) and rales consistent with pulmonary edema. The typical harsh mid-systolic murmur is accentuated with changes that diminish LV filling, reduce LV afterload, or increase contractility. A sustained apical impulse is associated with the mid-systolic outflow tract obstruction. As opposed to the physical findings of aortic valvular obstruc-

tion, those associated with LVOT obstruction are a brisk "bifid" carotid upstroke and an increase in murmur harshness associated with those same maneuvers that diminish LV filling.

Laboratory Evaluation

Routine Laboratory Data

In patients with HOCM, a chest radiograph may demonstrate a normal to markedly enlarged cardiac silhouette, LA enlargement associated with diminished LV compliance, and mitral regurgitation. Electrocardiography typically demonstrates prominent septal Q waves in the inferolateral leads, QRS voltage consistent with LV hypertrophy, and ST-segment and T-wave abnormalities. Large negative T waves in the V3 through V5 leads may be noted in the apical variant forms of HOCM. Ventricular dysrhythmias are frequently found on ambulatory electrocardiographic monitoring, with ventricular tachycardia being reported in up to 25% of patients with HOCM (21). Ventricular preexcitation also has been reported in a small portion of patients with hypertrophic cardiomyopathy manifested as a short PR interval and aberrant conduction that is shown as a widened QRS complex.

Cardiac Catheterization

Cardiac catheterization typically demonstrates a spike and dome arterial pressure tracing consistent with mid-systolic LVOT obstruction. The typical LA pressure tracing demonstrates a prominent A wave, and the LV diastolic pressure tracing may demonstrate the "square root sign" consistent with reduced ventricular compliance. A pressure gradient across the LVOT is commonly seen in patients with HOCM. In patients with the apical form of hypertrophic cardiomyopathy, a mid-ventricular gradient may be present. Pulmonary hypertension has been reported in as many as 25% of patients with hypertrophic cardiomyopathy and may or may not be associated with mitral regurgitation, pulmonary hypertension, and right ventricular dysfunction.

Due to the dynamic nature of the LVOT obstruction, many factors may influence its severity. Among these are the filling of the LV cavity, the LV afterload, and the contractile state of the LV. In patients in whom the SAM of the mitral valve is a prominent feature of the LVOT obstruction, there may be severe mitral regurgitation. In addition, the inhalation of amyl nitrate, which reduces LV preload and afterload, accentuates the dynamic LVOT obstruction. Postextrasystolic potentiation, which enhances LV contractility, also increases the degree of dynamic LVOT obstruction. Beta-adrenergic agents, such as isoproterenol, enhance contractility while reducing afterload, thereby accentuating LVOT obstruction.

Nuclear Studies

Typical findings with radionuclide thallium scanning include those associated with focal myocardial fibrosis or subendocardial fibrosis. Gated pool scanning may demonstrate an abnormal septal configuration and hypercontractile ventricular function, and blood pool scanning may show impaired diastolic relaxation, which is confirmed with magnetic resonance imaging.

ECHOCARDIOGRAPHIC EVALUATION OF HYPERTROPHIC OBSTRUCTIVE CARDIOMYOPATHY

Echocardiography has unique attributes that make it the procedure of choice for the diagnosis and assessment of severity of HOCM during the perioperative period (Table 25.6). Among these features are the ability to define the anatomic abnormalities associated with HOCM (including ventricu-

TABLE 25.6. INTRAOPERATIVE ECHOCARDIOGRAPHIC EVALUATION OF HYPERTROPHIC OBSTRUCTIVE CARDIOMYOPATHY

Characterization of anatomy
  Septal appearance and thickness
  Relationship between septum and mitral valve apparatus
  Left atrial enlargement

Quantification of structural and hemodynamic features
  LVOT gradient measurement with a continuous-wave Doppler
  Anatomic measurements
    Septal thickness
    Distance between aortic valve and point of mitral leaflet
      and septal contact
    Length of mitral leaflet and septal contact

Evaluation of the mitral valve
  Morphology and redundancy of leaflets
  Systolic anterior motion of mitral leaflets
  Mitral regurgitation
  Intrinsic mitral valve disease
  Anterior papillary muscle displacement

Characterization of diastolic dysfunction with pulsed-wave
    Doppler transmitral flow
  Abnormal relaxation
  Pseudonormal pattern
  Restriction

Avoidance of interference with surgical procedure unless
  epicardial echocardiography is required

Immediate evaluation of surgical intervention
  Identification of complications
    Persistence of significant LVOT gradient
    Detection of iatrogenic ventricular septal defect
    Detection of coronary artery–ventricular communication
  Provocative testing
    Response to isoproterenol
    Evaluation under various loading conditions

LVOT, left ventricular outflow tract.

lar wall thickness), and the functional relationship between the mitral valve and interventricular septum, which produces the dynamic obstruction associated with this abnormality. In addition, Doppler echocardiography can measure the severity of the pressure gradient in the LVOT, characterize the hemodynamic pattern of diastolic dysfunction, and determine the severity of the leaflet SAM-induced mitral regurgitation without interfering with the surgical procedure.

Anatomy

The anatomic abnormalities associated with HOCM include ventricular hypertrophy (Fig. 25.1) (symmetric or asymmetric); an enhanced acoustic reflective pattern involving the hypertrophied septum; SAM of the coapted mitral valve leaflets (Fig. 25.2); an echogenic patch at the point of leaflet SAM–septal contact (Fig. 25.3); LA enlargement; and a diminished LV cavity size and LVOT diameter. Echocardiography also can show an abnormal mitral valve apparatus, including anterior displacement of the papillary muscles, myxomatous degeneration, and redundancy of the coapted mitral leaflets or chordal structures. During systole, the functional hallmarks of HOCM with LVOT obstruction include SAM of the coapted mitral valve, LVOT obstruction, diminished systolic LV cavity size, leaflet SAM–septal contact, and turbulent blood flow in the LVOT (Fig. 25.4) with a late peaking gradient in the LVOT, mitral regurgitation associated with the mitral valve SAM (Fig. 25.5), and early closure of one or more of the aortic cusps.

Left Ventricular Hypertrophy

The hypertrophy associated with HOCM is pleomorphic, in that there are a variety of patterns associated with the production of dynamic outflow tract obstruction. Most commonly, the hypertrophy is asymmetric, involving the interventricular septum or anterior septum in the basal and middle portions of the ventricle. Other patterns of asymmetric septal hypertrophy, however, may involve the anterolateral wall of the LV and a variant apical hypertrophic pattern that gives a characteristic spadelike appearance on left ventriculography. A classic sigmoid-shaped septum has been reported to occur in elderly patients. Hypertrophy of the entire interventricular septum may result in a crescent-shaped appearance of the left ventricular cavity on angiography. Rarely, mid-ventricular hypertrophy produces circumferential rings. Medial and lateral hypertrophy of the ventricle also may result in a dumb-bell ventricular configuration.

Asymmetric septal hypertrophy commonly involves the basal and medial portions of the interventricular septum with a septal to free-wall thickness ratio of greater than or equal to 1.3:1. Upper septal hypertrophy associated with a concentric pattern of hypertrophy of the LV may produce significant gradients, whereas localized septal hypertrophy may produce only a latent obstruction in the setting of hypovolemia,

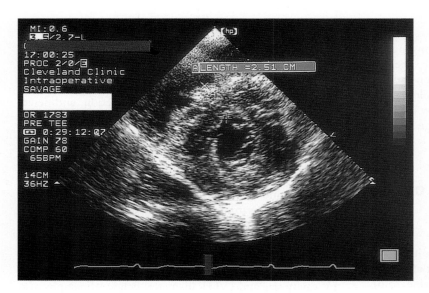

FIGURE 25.1. Left ventricular hypertrophy.

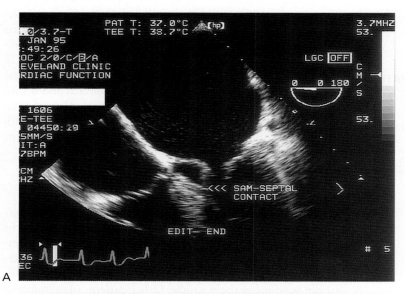

A

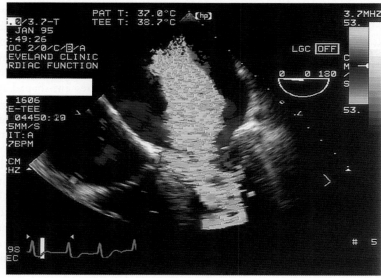

B

FIGURE 25.2. Systolic anterior motion of the coapted mitral valve leaflets. **A:** Real-time image. **B:** Color Doppler.

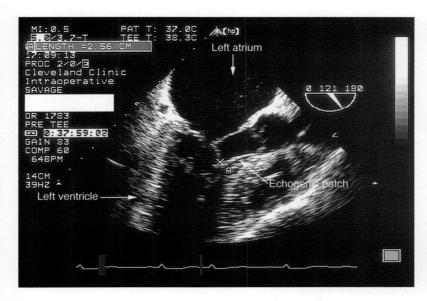

FIGURE 25.3. An echogenic patch at the point of leaflet systolic anterior motion (SAM)–septal-contact. This image also illustrates the distance between right coronary cusp and SAM septal contact.

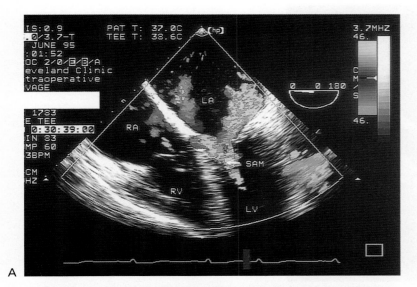

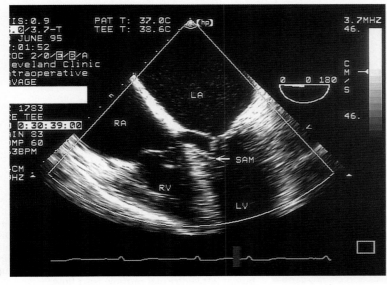

FIGURE 25.4. Systolic anterior motion (*SAM*)–septal contact with the production of LVOT obstruction and turbulent flow in the left ventricular outflow tract. **A:** Color Doppler image. **B:** Real-time image. *LA,* left atrium; *RA,* right atrium; *LV,* left ventricle; *RV,* right ventricle.

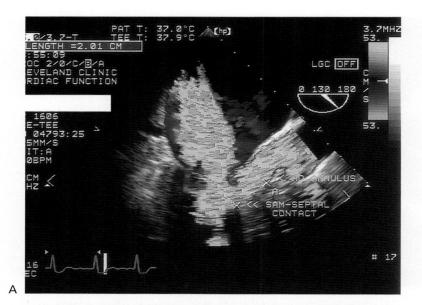

A

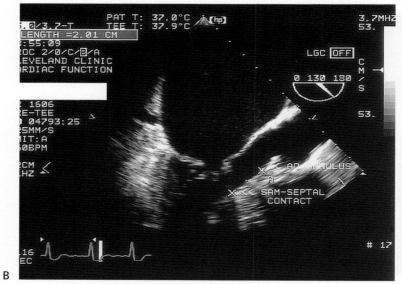

B

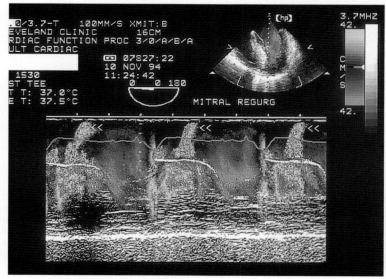

C

FIGURE 25.5. A: Mitral regurgitation associated with systolic anterior motion of the mitral valve. **B:** Distance from right coronary cusp to point of systolic anterior motion–septal contact. **C:** Color M-mode indicating mitral regurgitation flow (*arrows*) and turbulent left ventricular outflow tract flow.

increased sympathetic tone, or provocation with isoproterenol or amyl nitrate. The thickness of the interventricular septum typically is measured in the four-chamber transesophageal view, the transgastric transverse imaging plane, the short axis, or the parasternal long-axis equivalent epicardial imaging plane. A septal thickness of greater than 15 mm is considered abnormal.

In many instances, the hypertrophied septum has an enhanced echogenic pattern described as a speckled ground glass appearance similar to that seen more homogeneously with amyloidosis. It has been hypothesized that this acoustic reflective pattern is associated with the abnormal architectural swirling of the muscle cells and fibrosis within the interventricular septum. The presence of ventricular hypertrophy, whether asymmetric or symmetric, results in a diminished overall size of the LV cavity as well as a diminished size of the dynamic diameter of the LVOT. The diameter of the LVOT is measured between the medial surface of the interventricular septum and the anteriormost displacement of the mitral valve apparatus, including the leaflets in the four-chamber transesophageal transverse and longitudinal imaging planes.

Systolic Anterior Motion of the Coapted Mitral Valve and Left Ventricular Outflow Tract Obstruction

The presence of SAM of the mitral valve, as typically demonstrated in the imaging planes of the LVOT, is often associated with dynamic LVOT obstruction. Systolic anterior motion of the coapted mitral valve leaflets may involve the anterior mitral valve leaflet, the posterior mitral valve leaflet, the chordal structures, or any combination of the mitral valve apparatus. The most frequent form of SAM of the mitral valve apparatus involves the lax chordal structures. The form of SAM of the mitral valve most commonly associated with obstruction, however, involves anterior motion of the mitral valve leaflets distal to the point of coaptation and more commonly involves the anterior mitral valve leaflet. Grigg and colleagues noted that, in comparison with normal control subjects, patients with dynamic LVOT obstruction had longer mitral leaflets (31 ± 4 vs. 22 ± 3 mm), the annulus–coaptation point was more distal (20 ± 2 vs. 15 ± 3 mm), and the coaptation point was in the body of the leaflets (mean 9 ± 2 mm from the anterior leaflet tip vs. within 3 mm of the leaflet tip) (22). During early systole, the more distal portion of the anterior mitral leaflet moved anteriorly and superiorly, resulting in leaflet–septal contact with an incomplete mitral leaflet coaptation in mid-systole. Not only does this anterior and superior angulation of the mitral valve leaflets diminish the overall diameter of the LVOT, but the lack of complete coaptation of the anterior and posterior mitral valve leaflets in mid-systole resulted in a posteriorly directed jet of mitral regurgitation. The typical sequence of mitral regurgitation is ejection, followed by LVOT obstruction, and subsequent regurgitant leak. After coaptation of

the anterior and posterior mitral valve leaflets during systole, the plane of the mitral leaflets is fixed in position by the pressure gradient between the LA and LV. The presence of myxomatous changes in the mitral valve, including leaflet and chordal elongation, may predispose the patient to the occurrence of SAM of the coapted mitral valve apparatus. In many circumstances, the SAM of the coapted mitral valve is associated with a leaflet–septal contact and the production of a significant gradient as well as a sudden decrease of flow from the LVOT into the aortic root.

Left Atrial Enlargement

Left atrial enlargement (LA diameter >4 cm or area >20 cm^2) is frequently seen in the four-chamber transesophageal imaging plane in patients with HOCM and is secondary to both the diastolic dysfunction (abnormal relaxation and diminished compliance) and the presence of varying degrees of mitral regurgitation.

Doppler Interrogation of Hypertrophic Obstructive Cardiomyopathy

Obstruction Severity

Color-flow Doppler examination of LVOT obstruction demonstrates the presence of high-velocity turbulent flow distal to the point of LVOT obstruction (septal–mitral valve leaflet contact), the presence of proximal flow convergence just prior to the point of LVOT obstruction, and the associated occurrence of mitral regurgitation. Whereas pulsed-wave Doppler examination permits the localization of the point of obstruction in the LVOT, continuous-wave Doppler examination permits the determination of the maximum instantaneous and mean gradients associated with LVOT obstruction.

The development of systolic LVOT obstruction during mid- to late systole results in an abrupt decrease of blood flow from the LVOT across the aortic valve into the aorta (23,24). By positioning the pulsed-wave cursor parallel to the axis of the LVOT, specific points progressing from the LV cavity to the upper LVOT may be interrogated to assess the exact point of obstruction. At the point of maximal obstruction, the peak velocity of flow is shown to be greatly increased. This examination may be directed using color Doppler interrogation to search for the point of maximal flow conversion and high-velocity turbulent flow in the LVOT. Given the lower "aliasing" velocities of pulsed-wave Doppler and the high-flow velocity associated with LVOT obstruction, it is often necessary to use continuous-wave Doppler studies to accurately measure the obstructive gradient across the LVOT. Again, using color flow Doppler studies, the cursor is positioned parallel to the LVOT axis.

The best alignment for transesophageal interrogation of the LVOT is usually obtained from the deep transgastric imaging planes. If the cursor is parallel to the LVOT and parallels the leaflet SAM–septal contact, color flow Doppler techniques may be used to define the leaflet SAM–septal contact, with proximal flow acceleration and turbulent post-stenotic flow. Continuous-wave Doppler studies may then be used to further define the severity of obstruction. The Doppler spectral characteristic for LVOT is that of a dagger-shaped spectral envelope with mid- to late systolic peaking (Fig. 25.6). Provocative maneuvers, such as a prolonged positive pressure breath (analogous to the Valsalva maneuver) or administration of isoproterenol, may accentuate the severity of the gradient and are typically used in borderline degrees of LVOT obstruction or after surgical repair to ensure that there is no significant gradient under awake exercising clinical circumstances. The peak instantaneous gradient may be estimated based on the modified Bernoulli equation, which characterizes the peak instantaneous gradient between two chambers as equal to four times the square of the maximal velocity, or $PG = 4V^2$. The mean gradient across the LVOT may be calculated by integrating or planimetering the area under the continuous-wave spectral envelope. Patients with obstructive leaflet SAM demonstrate gradients across the LVOT and simultaneously have mitral regurgitation. If the continuous-wave cursor is incorrectly angled across the mitral valve, a spectral envelope of mitral regurgitation may be demonstrated and incorrectly confused with the envelope of the LVOT gradient. The spectral envelope of mitral regurgitation must not be confused with that of the LVOT (Table 25.7). Such confusion could result in erroneous surgical decision making. The spectral envelope of mitral

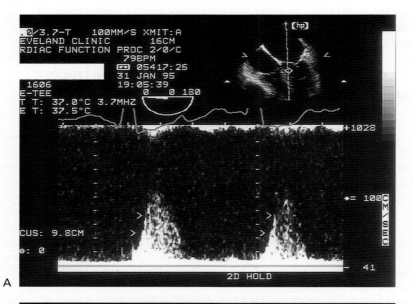

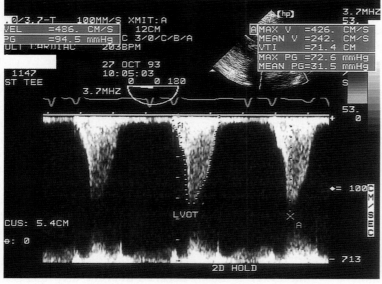

FIGURE 25.6. A: Late peaking continuous Doppler velocity with "dagger-shaped" spectral wave. **B:** Late peaking continuous-wave Doppler recording from deep transgastric interrogation of LVOT.

TABLE 25.7. DISTINGUISHING MITRAL REGURGITATION FROM LEFT VENTRICULAR OUTFLOW TRACT (LVOT) OBSTRUCTION BY CONTINUOUS-WAVE DOPPLER ENVELOPE

	LVOT Spectral Envelope	Mitral Regurgitation Spectral Envelope
Onset	Aortic valve opening	Initiation of systole
Duration	Left ventricular ejection	Holosystolic
Peak velocity	<4.5 m/sec	>4.5 m/sec
Contour	Dagger-shaped	Symmetrical
Timing of peak velocity	Delayed	Early systole

regurgitation occurs earlier than that of LVOT obstruction due to the onset of mitral regurgitation commensurate with ventricular systole and the later onset of LVOT obstruction. The peak velocity obtained with the mitral regurgitant jet is much earlier and greater than that associated with LVOT obstruction. In addition, another potential error in the estimation of the LVOT gradient is nonparallel orientation of the Doppler beam and the flow.

Typically, the gradient obtained from the continuous-wave Doppler examination is 15 to 25 mm Hg greater than that obtained by cardiac catheterization. It is thought that the disparity between these two techniques resides in the phenomenon of pressure recovery distal to the stenosis (25). The continuous-wave Doppler technique, when correctly performed, can detect the highest flow velocity at the point of LVOT obstruction (vena contracta). The pressure gradient obtained at cardiac catheterization, however, is based on the comparison of intercavitary LV pressure and the downstream post-stenotic aortic pressure once the vena contracta has expanded and there is pressure recovery. Consequently, the pressure is higher downstream than it is just distal to the LVOT obstruction (26). A peak instantaneous gradient of greater than 36 mm Hg is indicative of significant LVOT obstruction.

In addition to localizing the turbulence in the LVOT, color-flow Doppler studies are also useful in assessing associated mitral regurgitation. The mitral regurgitation may be related to either the presence of SAM of the coapted mitral valve leaflets or the presence of intrinsic mitral valve disease, such as myxomatous degeneration of the mitral valve leaflets.

It is believed that SAM of the mitral valve distorts the configuration of the leaflet coaptation with resulting mitral

regurgitation. The mitral regurgitant jet is directed posteriorly and occurs concomitantly with the onset of LVOT obstruction in mid- to late systole. The classic cycle of systolic ejection, LVOT obstruction, and mitral regurgitation has been characterized in other studies (27). These studies have demonstrated that virtually 100% of patients with obstructive leaflet SAM demonstrate mitral regurgitation. With provocative testing in LVOT obstruction, the gradient is usually increased. Increased severity of mitral regurgitation also has been demonstrated with such provocative testing, further demonstrating the association between obstructive leaflet SAM and mitral regurgitation (28). With disruption of the normal coaptation configuration of the anterior and posterior mitral valve leaflets caused by the SAM of the mitral valve, the mitral leaflets are exposed to the increased LV pressure caused by the LVOT obstruction. With the increased LV–LA pressure gradient, the severity of mitral regurgitation may be accentuated, even in the presence of a small regurgitant orifice area. Classically, the mitral regurgitation begins early in systole and is greatest in mid- to late systole, similar to the timing of LVOT obstruction.

Hemodynamic Patterns of Diastolic Dysfunction and Hypertrophic Obstructive Cardiomyopathy

Doppler interrogation of the LV inflow pattern permits characterization of the pattern of diastolic dysfunction commonly seen in patients with HOCM (Table 25.8). Determination of the isovolumetric relaxation time, E-wave deceleration time, peak E wave, and peak atrial filling wave is necessary for characterization of the three hemodynamic

TABLE 25.8. PATTERNS OF DIASTOLIC DYSFUNCTION AND DIAGNOSIS

Pattern	Deceleration Time	IVRT	Atrial Wave	Systolic Wave	Diastolic Wave
Normal					
Abnormal relaxation	Prolonged	Prolonged	Normal	Normal	Normal
Pseudonormal	Normal	Normal	Increased	Depressed	Depressed
Restrictive	Shortened	Shortened	Increased	Depressed	Depressed

IVRT, isovolumic relaxation time.

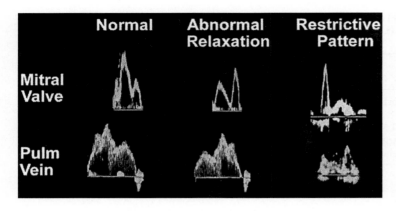

FIGURE 25.7. Doppler pulsed-wave flow patterns.

patterns of diastolic dysfunction associated with hypertrophic cardiomyopathy (Fig. 25.7).

Abnormal relaxation features a delayed relaxation of the ventricle during the period of isovolumetric relaxation (aortic valve closure to mitral valve opening). Because of the continued delayed relaxation of the ventricle after opening of the mitral valve, the flow gradient between the LA and the LV is diminished, resulting in a decreased early filling velocity and prolongation of the deceleration time of the early filling wave.

The second pattern, or pseudonormalization, is characterized by more normal filling velocities of the E and A waves and a normalization of the isovolumetric relaxation time and deceleration times due to the increase in LA pressures, resulting in a decreased isovolumetric relaxation time and deceleration time (increased LA-LV gradient). The pseudonormalization pattern may be distinguished from the normal pattern by evaluating the pulmonary vein flow with pulsed-wave Doppler techniques. Normally, the systolic pulmonary vein flow velocities are greater than the diastolic flow velocities with a small amount of atrial reversal. In the pseudonormalization pattern, however, due to elevation of the LA pressures caused by the combined abnormal relaxation and diminished LV compliance, the systolic wave is markedly accentuated and there is accentuation of the atrial reversal.

The restrictive diastolic filling pattern demonstrates an accentuated E wave due to the elevation of LA pressures and rapid increase of pressure in the LV and subsequent rapid decrease of gradient between the LA and the LV. Consequently, the elevated LA pressure leads to a decreased isovolumetric relaxation time. The rapid decrease in LA-LV pressure gradient following mitral valve opening causes a decreased deceleration time of the E wave. With the rapid increase in LV pressure, the gradient during LA contraction is markedly diminished with a diminished A wave.

Even though the pulsed-wave Doppler spectral patterns may not be pathognomonic for individual pathologic conditions, they are diagnostic of specific hemodynamic patterns of diastolic dysfunction. The abnormal relaxation pattern is indicative of a delayed relaxation of the ventricle with prolonged isovolumetric relaxation time and deceleration time, whereas the more restrictive pattern of diastolic dysfunction is indicative of elevated LA pressures (decreased isovolumetric relaxation time and decreased deceleration time) and a rapid increase in LV pressure following opening of the mitral valve with a diminished deceleration time. The presence of LA enlargement implies that there is a pattern of diastolic dysfunction that has progressed from a relaxation abnormality to a more restrictive pattern of diastolic dysfunction.

Case Report

A 14-year-old white girl, who was otherwise healthy, had increasing shortness of breath and chest tightness. She had a known history of hypertrophic cardiomyopathy that was first diagnosed by transthoracic echocardiography after the incidental discovery of a heart murmur during a viral illness at 6 years of age. Her family history is significant for a brother who died during summer football practice of an unknown cardiac condition and a father who has had a known asymptomatic hypertrophic cardiomyopathy for the past 10 years.

On physical examination, she had a heart rate of 60 beats/min and blood pressure of 90/50 mm Hg with no orthostatic changes. A grade 2/6 holosystolic murmur was auscultated with an audible S4 at the left lower sternal border. Results of her laboratory tests, including a complete blood count and blood urea nitrogen, creatinine, and liver enzymes, were all normal. Her chest radiograph showed mild cardiomegaly with LV predominance and clear lung fields. Electrocardiography showed a sinus bradycardia with incomplete left bundle branch block.

Transthoracic echocardiography demonstrated asymmetric septal hypertrophy with enhanced reflectance of the septum and SAM of the coapted anterior and posterior mitral valve leaflets. Continuous-wave Doppler interrogation of the LVOT from the apical two-chamber view demonstrated a peak LVOT velocity of 3 m/s, which increased to 4.5 m/s after the inhalation of amyl nitrate. The color-flow Doppler study demonstrated moderate mitral regurgitation with a posteriorly directed regurgitant jet. Because the transthoracic echocardiogram was technically difficult, a transesophageal echocardiogram was performed to clarify the severity of outflow tract obstruction and to exclude intrinsic mitral valve disease.

Transesophageal echocardiography revealed severe septal hypertrophy, with the interventricular septum measuring 3.5 cm (normal range for the patient's weight, 0.7–0.9 cm). She also demonstrated systolic obliteration of the LV cavity, with an LVOT velocity of 3.5 m/s and a gradient of 49 mm Hg. With inhalation of amyl nitrate, she had an increase in the LVOT velocity to 5 m/s, and the gradient increased to 100 mm Hg. She also developed SAM of the mitral leaflets with 3+ mitral regurgitation. Pulsed-wave Doppler interrogation at the level of the mitral valve leaflet tips was used to characterize the diastolic inflow hemodynamic pattern of the LV. There was a pseudonormal pattern of combined abnormal relaxation and restriction (normal isovolumetric relaxation time, normal early wave deceleration time) and a pulmonary vein flow pattern demonstrating a depressed systolic wave, increased diastolic wave, and increased atrial reversal.

After approximately 6 months of medical therapy with increasing doses of verapamil (up to 60 mg four times per day) and the addition of Inderal (Wyeth-Ayerst, Philadelphia, PA, U.S.A.; 40 mg four times per day), the patient continued to have increasing symptoms, and operative repair was considered.

In the operating room, a precardiopulmonary bypass transesophageal echocardiogram confirmed the diagnosis of severe septal hypertrophic cardiomyopathy, with systolic chamber obliteration, an LVOT velocity of 5.5 m/s, and a gradient of 121 mm Hg across the LVOT. Systolic anterior motion of the coapted mitral valve leaflets was also seen with a posteriorly directed 3+ mitral regurgitant jet. The distances from the aortic annulus to the proximal and distal points of leaflet SAM–septal contact were 23 and 27 mm, respectively, with a septal thickness of 32 mm and a contact length of 4 mm. M-mode echocardiography of the aortic valve demonstrated premature closure of the right coronary cusp of the aortic valve. Epicardial echocardiography confirmed the transesophageal echocardiographic findings, except it showed a maximal septal thickness of 27 mm. The smaller septal thickness shown by epicardial echocardiography suggested that the transesophageal echocardiographic measurement was tangential to the septum.

The patient underwent septal myomectomy, with a 15-mm thick by 3.0-cm long triangular wedge of septal myocardium being removed from the septum directly under the right coronary cusp. After the patient was separated from cardiopulmonary bypass, an echocardiographic study showed widening of the LVOT with a surgical trough, a peak velocity of 1.8 m/s, and a peak instantaneous gradient of only 16 mm Hg. The residual septum measured 12 mm. There was no SAM of the mitral leaflets and a marked improvement in the degree of mitral regurgitation. There was no demonstrable ventricular septal defect or coronary ventric-

ular fistula by color flow Doppler examination. The patient had a stable postoperative course and was discharged after 7 days with no complications. Subsequent periodic follow-up examinations and transthoracic echocardiograms have not demonstrated a recurrence of the LVOT obstruction.

Clinical Course

As discussed, HOCM typically presents in patients in their third or fourth decade of life; however, HOCM also occurs in children. The presence of LVOT obstruction and LV diastolic dysfunction over a chronic course may be manifested as myocardial fibrosis. Once patients become symptomatic, the annual mortality rate is 6% per year in children and 2.5% per year in adults (29). Sudden death is a not infrequent manifestation of asymptomatic patients with HOCM. Risk factors associated with sudden death include age younger than 30 years and a family history of HOCM culminating in sudden death (29). In children, a history of syncope is associated with increased risk of sudden death; not so in adults. In adults, the presence of nonsustained ventricular tachycardia is associated with an increased risk. In young athletes who die suddenly, HOCM is the most common autopsy finding.

Clinical Management

Medical

The goals in treatment of patients with HOCM are to reduce the risk of death and to reduce the symptoms associated with pulmonary congestion and outflow tract obstruction (30). Most importantly, medications that enhance myocardial contractility (e.g., digoxin), medications that reduce preload and afterload (nitrates), and diuretics that reduce preload should be avoided. The cornerstone of therapy includes beta-receptor blockade, which reduces both the inotropic and chronotropic response of the heart. In addition, calcium channel antagonists such as verapamil have been used to depress myocardial contractility, improve diastolic function, and provide potential beneficial effects on myocardial perfusion. Disopyramide also may be used because of its depressant effect on systolic ventricular function. More recently, dual-chamber (atrioventricular sequential) pacing has been used in the management of patients who are refractory to initial medical treatment. Patients should avoid strenuous physical activity, and any supraventricular dysrhythmias should be aggressively treated. Bacterial endocarditis has been seen in a small percentage of HOCM patients. Consequently, prophylaxis is indicated.

Surgical

In patients who remain symptomatic despite medical therapy, transaortic septal myomectomy or mitral valve replacement has been used in their surgical treatment. Transaortic septal myomectomy entails the surgical removal of portions of the abnormal septum beneath the right coronary cusp. Two parallel incisions of the septum are made that are approximately 1 cm in depth and 2 cm in width, extending 3 to 5 cm toward the LV apex to the base of the papillary muscles. The extent of resection is directed by the intraoperative presurgical transesophageal echocardiogram (Table 25.9 and Fig. 25.8). The success of the myomectomy and the evaluation for potential complications of the procedure are assessed by postsurgical intraoperative echocardiography (Table 25.10).

Between 1975 and 1993, 178 patients underwent surgical management of HOCM at the Cleveland Clinic. Operations included transaortic septal myomectomy alone or combined with coronary artery bypass grafting (76%) or a concomitant aortic or mitral valve procedure (22%). After myomectomy, the mean LVOT gradient decreased from 93 to 21 mm Hg. Twenty percent of patients required a second pump run for a more extensive septal resection (31). Complications following septal myomectomy included complete heart block

TABLE 25.9. INTRAOPERATIVE ECHOCARDIOGRAPHIC EVALUATION OF HYPERTROPHIC OBSTRUCTIVE CARDIOMYOPATHY: PRESURGICAL ASSESSMENT

Two-dimensional examination of chambers
  Regional wall motion abnormalities
  Left ventricular wall thickness
    Septum
    Lateral wall
  Left atrial size
  Right ventricular function

Two-dimensional assessment of left ventricular outflow tract
    (LVOT) obstruction
  LVOT diameter
  Systolic anterior motion (SAM) of mitral valve
  SAM–septal contact
    Distance from aortic valve to point of SAM–septal contact
    Length of SAM–septal contact
    Intrinsic mitral valve disease

Color Doppler assessment
  Systolic LVOT turbulence
  Mitral regurgitation
  Direction of jet: anterior, central, or posterior

Pulsed- and continuous-wave Doppler assessment
  Peak gradient localization
  Peak instantaneous and mean gradient measurements
  Left ventricular inflow pattern and assessment of diastolic
    function
  Normal, abnormal relaxation, pseudonormal pattern, or
    restriction
  Pulmonary vein flow assessment
  Mitral regurgitation quantification

Routine comprehensive examination of all valves, chambers and
  the aorta

(10%), iatrogenic ventricular septal defects (0.6%), LV rupture (1%), right ventricular rupture (0.5%), reoperation (1% myomectomy, 1% mitral valve replacement), and ventricular (7.3%) or atrial (26%) dysrhythmias. Mitral regurgitation was present in a large portion of these patients and was related to SAM of the mitral valve. With septal myomectomy alone in patients with moderate or severe mitral regurgitation, regurgitation was improved to acceptable levels in 75% of patients. The remainder of patients had underlying mitral valve pathology that required mitral valve replacement.

Surgical alternatives to transaortic septal myomectomy include mitral valve replacement, even in the absence of intrinsic mitral valve disease. However, because of the risks of bleeding, thromboembolism, and infections associated with valve replacement, this mode of surgical therapy should be considered primarily in those patients with an intrinsic mitral valve disease.

Intraoperative Echocardiography in Surgical Management

The role of intraoperative echocardiography in the surgical treatment of patients with HOCM may be divided into the presurgical and postsurgical assessment (Tables 25.9 and 25.10). Due to the individual anatomic orientation and inability to optimize the interrogation angle, the determination of the maximal LVOT gradient may not be possible in all patients undergoing surgical myomectomy with transesophageal echocardiography alone. Consequently, it may be necessary to perform both transesophageal and epicardial Doppler examinations in patients undergoing surgical resection (Table 25.11). Some experts insist that epicardial imaging and Doppler interrogation of the LVOT be performed both before and after surgery in all patients undergoing surgical repair.

Preoperative Assessment

Preoperatively, transesophageal echocardiography is used in the anatomic characterization of LV hypertrophy, the assessment of mitral valve abnormalities, and the detailed characterization of obstructive SAM of the coapted mitral valve leaflets. It is important to provide the surgeon with an accurate measurement of the septal thickness. Due to potential angulation through the interventricular septum (tangential orientation), it is possible to obtain septal thickness measurements that are greater than the true value. Consequently, the probe must be oriented perpendicular to the septum to obtain the most accurate septal thickness measurement. Because perpendicular transducer orientation to the septum can be achieved in epicardial echocardiography, it is frequently used to provide the most accurate measurement of septal thickness. If an inaccurate measurement is obtained, the

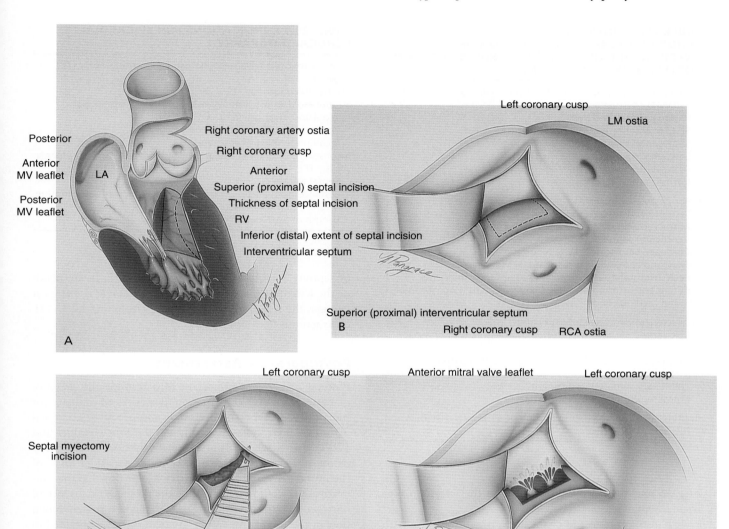

FIGURE 25.8. Septal incision from the surgical perspectives. **A:** Cross section of heart demonstrating superior and inferior borders of septal incision. **B:** Superior (proximal) interventricular septum directly beneath the right coronary cusp. **C:** Septal myomectomy incision. **D:** Septal myomectomy relationship to anterior mitral valve leaflet. *LA,* left atrium; *RV,* right ventricle; *RCA,* right coronary artery; *MV,* mitral valve; *LM,* left main coronary artery.

TABLE 25.10. INTRAOPERATIVE ECHOCARDIOGRAPHIC EVALUATION OF HYPERTROPHIC OBSTRUCTIVE CARDIOMYOPATHY: POSTSURGICAL ASSESSMENT

Two-dimensional assessment of left ventricular outflow tract (LVOT) obstruction
  Residual septal thickness
  Systolic anterior motion (SAM) of mitral valve
  SAM–septal contact
  Left ventricular function
  Right ventricular function
  Intrinsic mitral valve disease

Color Doppler assessment
  Systolic LVOT turbulence
  Mitral regurgitation associated with SAM
  Ventricular septal defect
  Coronary–ventricular cavity blood flow
Pulsed- and continuous-wave Doppler assessment
  Peak instantaneous and mean gradient measurements
  Before and after provocative maneuvers with isoproterenol and loading conditions

Characterization of diastolic function
  Left ventricular inflow pattern and assessment of diastolic function
  Normal, abnormal relaxation, pseudonormal pattern, or restriction
  Pulmonary vein flow assessment
  Mitral regurgitation quantification

Routine comprehensive examination of all valves, chambers and the aorta

TABLE 25.11. INDICATIONS FOR EPICARDIAL ECHOCARDIOGRAPHY

Inability to insert a transesophageal echocardiographic (TEE) probe
Contraindications for TEE
Suboptimal Doppler interrogation of the left ventricular outflow tract gradient
  Poor cursor alignment with flow
  Incomplete spectral envelope
Inconsistent two-dimensional echocardiographic measurements by TEE
  Septal thickness
  Distance from aortic valve to point of systolic anterior motion (SAM)–septal contact
  Length of SAM–septal contact

surgeon may perform a septal resection that creates a ventricular septal defect.

It is also important to characterize the mitral valve with regard to any intrinsic disease (such as myxomatous degeneration) as well as to identify the functional presence of mitral regurgitation. Mitral regurgitation associated with leaflet SAM–septal contact classically is associated with a posteriorly directed jet. The presence of an anterior or central jet often implies an intrinsic disease valve. In addition, the presence of a flail scallop of the posterior leaflet or ruptured chordae also implies an intrinsic mitral valve involvement, which may need to be corrected surgically.

The surgeon should know not only the size of the thickness of the interventricular septum but also the exact point of leaflet SAM–septal contact. This point is marked with an endocardial fibrotic patch (Fig. 25.9A). The absence of the fibrotic patch at the time of surgical exposure may suggest the absence of significant LVOT obstruction. It is important for the surgeon to know the distance between the aortic annulus and the point of septal contact, the length of leaflet SAM–septal contact, and the distal point of septal contact (aortic annulus to distal leaflet SAM–septal contact) to determine the length of septal myomectomy to be performed (Fig. 25.9). Classically, a triangular wedge

of septum is removed to enlarge the LVOT. If the depth or the length of the three-dimensional triangle is not great enough, the resection may be insufficient to prevent LVOT obstruction.

Postoperative Assessment

Postoperatively, it is important to determine the presence of persistent LVOT obstruction as well as to evaluate for the presence of potential complications related to septal myomectomy (Table 25.12). Using the four-chamber and 120 degree views, two-dimensional echocardiography may demonstrate the presence or absence of persistent SAM of the mitral valve and septal contact. Color flow Doppler interrogation would further define the presence or absence of obstruction by demonstrating the absence of turbulent blood flow in the LVOT. An LVOT gradient must be obtained to determine the degree of success of the surgical myomectomy. Furthermore, because patients do not live at resting baseline conditions, it is advisable to measure the LVOT gradient during provocative maneuvers such as by administering isoproterenol (increasing the heart rate by 20%) and by dropping the patient's afterload. In some circumstances, only the epicardial or epiaortic Doppler interrogation can accurately assess the LVOT gradient due to angulation of flow and the Doppler beam in the TEE views.

Intraoperative echocardiography has a great value in the evaluation of potential complications associated with septal myomectomy when performed for HOCM (29). Complications associated with this procedure include not only persistence of the obstruction but the presence of a ventricular septal defect, persistent mitral regurgitation, the creation of a coronary artery (septal perforator) ventricular arteriovenous connection, and the presence of significant postsurgical diastolic dysfunction.

The area of surgical myomectomy may easily be visualized in the esophageal and transgastric views of the LVOT (Fig. 25.10). The presence of a thin interventricular

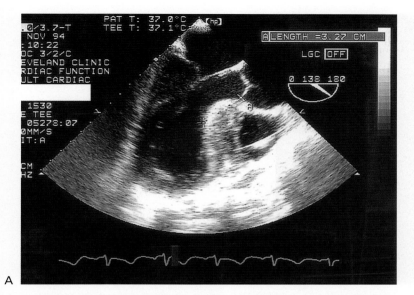

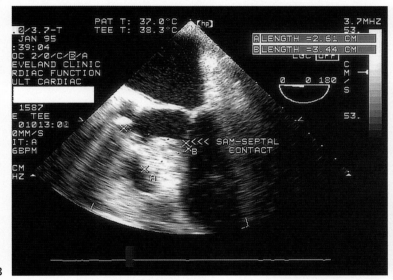

FIGURE 25.9. A: Longitudinal plane view of left ventricular outflow tract illustrating the distance from the right coronary cusp (*A*) to the point of systolic anterior motion (SAM)–septal contact (*B*). **B:** Five-chamber transesophageal view demonstrating (in a different patient) septal thickness measurement and right coronary cusp to SAM–septal contact distance.

septum (<3 mm) following surgical myomectomy leads to a high index of suspicion for a potential ventricular septal defect (Fig. 25.11). The presence of a ventricular septal defect intraoperatively can be ascertained by color flow Doppler images showing a high-velocity blood flow between the left

and right ventricles. Pulsed-wave Doppler interrogation of the interventricular septum may reveal a high-velocity flow from the left to the right ventricle. Coronary artery blood flow should not be confused with that of an interventricular septal defect. Color M mode may be used in characterizing the timing pattern of any flow in the interventricular septum. Classically, coronary flow occurs during diastole, whereas a surgical ventricular septal defect occurs in both diastole and systole.

Coronary artery–left ventricular connections are uncommon, but potential findings are associated with a septal myomectomy (Fig. 25.12); such "fistulae" are characterized by color-flow Doppler images demonstrating localized diastolic flow from a point in the interventricular septum into the LV cavity. The differential diagnosis of this abnormality includes a small ventricular septal defect. As mentioned above,

TABLE 25.12. HYPERTROPHIC OBSTRUCTIVE CARDIOMYOPATHY COMPLICATIONS OR FINDINGS ASSOCIATED WITH SURGICAL MYOMECTOMY

Persistence of a significant pressure gradient across left ventricular outflow tract
Persistence of systolic anterior motion of mitral valve leaflets
Persistence of significant mitral valve regurgitation
Evidence of coronary artery–ventricular fistula
Evidence of ventricular septal defect

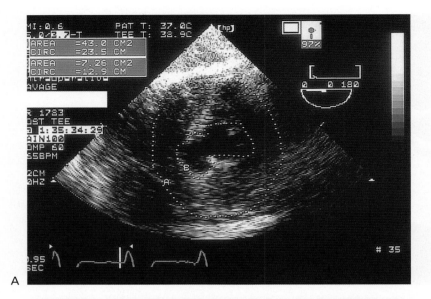

A

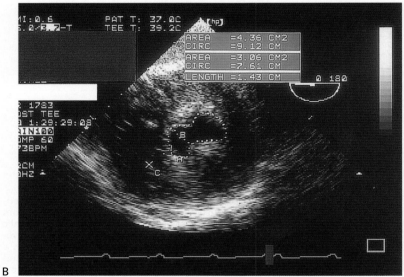

B

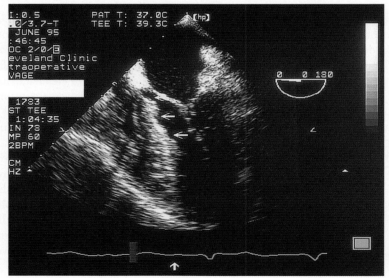

C

FIGURE 25.10. A: Transgastric cross section of left ventricle indicating area of septal resection. **B:** Transgastric cross section with residual septal thickness of 14 mm. **C:** Area of septal resection from four-chamber transesophageal view.

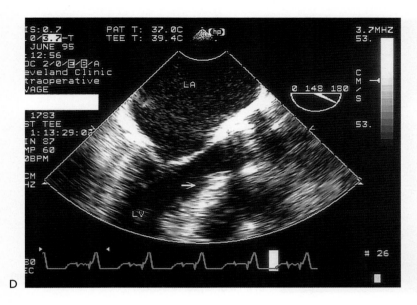

FIGURE 25.10. (*continued*) **D:** Area of septal resection from longitudinal esophageal view. *LA,* left atrium; *LV,* left ventricle.

color M-mode may be of great benefit in determining the flow characteristics of the abnormality. A coronary artery LV connection would demonstrate dominant diastolic flow, whereas the ventricular septal defect would demonstrate systolic greater than diastolic flow.

The persistence of mitral regurgitation in the absence of leaflet SAM–septal contact implies the presence of an underlying mitral valve disease. The echocardiographic Doppler examination of such a mitral valve should include an examination of the anterior and posterior mitral valve leaflets in all of the possible views and characterization of the severity and direction of the mitral regurgitant jet. Transgastric cross-sectional evaluation of the mitral valve is also helpful. The transgastric cross-sectional view of the mitral valve permits evaluation of the scallops of the posterior leaflet (P1, P2, and P3) as well as the anterior mitral valve leaflet. Not only

should the severity of regurgitation be determined, but also its underlying mechanism should be ascertained to optimally assist the surgical decision-making process. Examination for papillary muscle or chordal disruption should be included in the comprehensive examination.

Postoperatively, transesophageal echocardiography is of great value in determining potential complications in the intensive care unit. Because LVOT obstruction is dynamic, changing conditions such as hypovolemia, cardiac tamponade, and reduced afterload may result in significant LVOT obstruction despite an adequate surgical myomectomy. Consequently, in patients who have undergone surgical myomectomy for LVOT obstruction or in patients who have undergone aortic valve replacement with the potential for latent LVOT obstruction, postoperative transesophageal echocardiography is of great value in the immediate

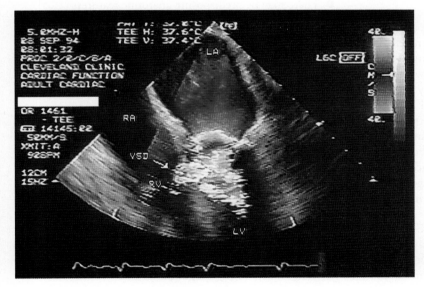

FIGURE 25.11. Postmyomectomy ventricular septal defect (*VSD*). *LA,* left atrium; *LV,* left ventricle; *RA,* right ventricle; *RV,* right ventricle.

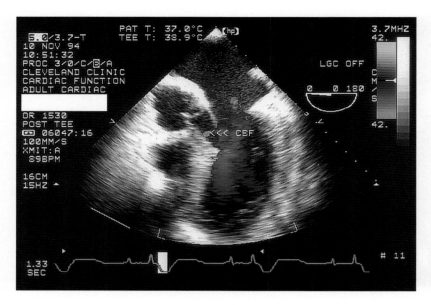

FIGURE 25.12. Diastolic coronary blood flow (*CBF*) in area of septal resection.

assessment of hemodynamic instability in the intensive care unit.

CONCLUSION

Intraoperative echocardiography, consisting of transesophageal and epicardial echocardiography, is an integral part of the surgical treatment of outflow tract obstruction caused by HOCM. Echocardiography is an accurate means of establishing the diagnosis in patients with unrecognized LVOT obstruction as well as confirming the diagnosis of LVOT obstruction in patients presenting for surgical management of HOCM.

Intraoperative echocardiography provides the surgical team guidance in their operative management by accurately documenting the septal thickness, the location and depth of mitral valve–septal contact, and the intrinsic function and anatomy of the mitral valve. It also provides a method of intraoperative assessment of the surgical approach. Patients with HOCM may have a septal thickness ranging from 15 mm to more than 30 mm. This represents a wide range of variability in possible depths of myomectomy incisions without creating an iatrogenic ventricular septal defect. If the patient has a normal mitral valve anatomy, the regurgitation associated with leaflet SAM improves once an effective myomectomy eliminates the substrates for systolic anterior motion of the mitral valve. On the other hand, intrinsic mitral valve abnormalities, such as myxomatous degeneration of the mitral valve with chordal rupture, may necessitate mitral repair or replacement.

The intraoperative echocardiogram after myomectomy demonstrates the effectiveness of the myomectomy in eliminating leaflet SAM and LVOT obstruction before or after provocative testing. It may identify the location and mecha-

nism of residual leaflet SAM if the operative result is imperfect. Intraoperative echo has provided a means for the optimal management of patients undergoing surgical myomectomy for LVOT obstruction. In addition, it has permitted an understanding of the mechanisms and underlying pathophysiologic process in LVOT obstruction, enabling the development and advancement of surgical techniques that will permit more successful management of these patients (32).

KEY POINTS

- Important clinical features:

    Unusual physiology
    Potential for sudden death
    Specific therapies

- There may be predisposing anatomic features:

    Mitral valve: elongation of the mitral valve leaflets, anterior displacement
    Left ventricular outflow tract: narrowing of the outflow tract due to hypertrophy or edema

- Common precipitating events:

    Hyperdynamic
    Hypovolemia, anemia
    Tachycardia

- Echo characteristics:

    Color flow will show turbulence in the LVOT
    Elevated gradient across the LVOT: A peak instantaneous gradient of greater than 36 mm Hg is considered indicative of significant LVOT obstruction
    Restricted closure of the anterior leaflet leads to posteriorly directed mitral regurgitation.

REFERENCES

1. Brock R. Functional obstruction of the LV cavity. *Guys Hosp Rep* 1957;106:221.
2. Braunwald E, Brockenbrough EC, Morrow AG. Hypertrophic subaortic stenosis—a broadened concept. *Circulation* 1962;26: 161.
3. **Maron BJ, Bonow RO, Cannon RO, et al. Hypertrophic cardiomyopathy: interrelations of clinical manifestations, pathophysiology, and therapy. *N Engl J Med* 1987;316:780.**
4. Agnarsson U, Hardaron T, Sigfusson N. Hypertrophic cardiomyopathy identified by echo screening: prevalence and clinical significance. *Circulation* 1988;78:584.
5. Hada Y, Sakamoto T, Amano K, et al. Prevalence of hypertrophic cardiomyopathy in a population of adult Japanese workers as detected by electrocardiographic screening. *Am J Cardiol* 1987;59:183.
6. **Agnarson U, Hardaron T, Sigfusson N. Hypertrophic cardiomyopathy identified by echo screening: prevalence and significance. *Circulation* 1988;78(suppl II):584.**
7. Braunwald E, et al. Idiopathic hypertrophic subaortic stenosis: clinical hemodynamic and angiographic manifestations. *Am J Med* 1960;29:924.
8. Braunwald E. Hypertrophic cardiomyopathy—continued progress. *N Engl J Med* 1989;320:800.
9. Maron J, Epstein SE. Hypertrophic cardiomyopathy: a discussion of nomenclature. *Am J Cardiol* 1979;43:1242.
10. Maron BJ, Mulvihill JJ. The genetics of hypertrophic cardiomyopathy. *Ann Intern Med* 1986;105:610.
11. Solomon SD, Jarcho JA, McKenna W, et al. Familial hypertrophic cardiomyopathy is a genetically heterogeneous disease. *J Clin Invest* 1990;86:993.
12. Gutsgesell HP, Speer ME, Rosenberg HS. Characterization of the cardiomyopathy in infants of diabetic mothers. *Circulation* 1980;61:441.
13. Maron BJ, Cannon RO, Leon MB, et al. Hypertrophic cardiomyopathy: interrelations of clinical manifestations, pathophysiology, and therapy. *N Engl J Med* 1987;16:780.
14. Wynne J, Braunwald E. The cardiomyopathies and myocardites: toxic, chemical, and physical damage to the heart. In: Braunwald E, ed. *Heart disease*. Philadelphia: WB Saunders, 1992.
15. Pearce PC, Hawkey C, Symons C, et al. Role of calcium in the induction of cardiac hypertrophy and myofibrillar disarray. Experimental studies of a possible cause of hypertrophic cardiomyopathy. *Br Heart J* 1985;54:420.
16. Lawson JWR. Hypertrophic cardiomyopathy: current views on etiology, pathophysiology, and management. *Am J Med Sci* 1987; 294:191.
17. Tanaka M, Fujiware H, Onodera T, et al. Quantitative analysis of narrowing of intramyocardial small arteries in normal hearts, hypertensive hearts, and hearts with hypertrophic cardiomyopathy. *Circulation* 1987;75:1130.
18. Wigle ED, Adelman AG, Silver MD. Pathophysiologic considerations in muscular subaortic stenosis. In: Wolstenholme GEW, O'Conner M, eds. *Hypertrophic obstructive cardiomyopathy.* CIBA Foundation Study. London: J & A Churchill, 1971:63.
19. Levine RA. Echocardiographic assessment of the cardiomyopathies. In: Weyman AE, ed. *Principles and practice of echocardiography*, 2nd ed. Philadelphia: Lea & Febiger, 1994.
20. Pollick C, Rakowski H, Wigle ED. Muscular subaortic stenosis; the quantitative relationship between systolic anterior motion and the pressure gradient. *Circulation* 1984;69:43.
21. Fananapazir L, Tracy C, Leon M, et al. Electrophysiologic abnormalities in patients with hypertrophic cardiomyopathy: a consecutive analysis in 155 patients. *Circulation* 1989;80:1259.
22. **Grigg L, Wigle ED, Williams W, et al. Transesophageal Doppler echocardiography in obstructive hypertrophic cardiomyopathy: clarification of pathophysiology and importance in intraoperative decision making. *J Am Coll Cardiol* 1992;20:42.**
23. Maron BJ, Gottdiener JS, Arce J, et al. Dynamic subaortic obstruction in hypertrophic cardiomyopathy: analysis by pulsed Doppler echocardiography. *J Am Coll Cardiol* 1985;6:1.
24. Gardin JM, Dabestani A, Glasgow GA, et al. Echocardiographic and Doppler flow observations in obstructed and nonobstructed hypertrophic cardiomyopathy. *Am J Cardiol* 1985;56: 614.
25. **Stewart WJ, Schiavone WA, Salcedo EE, et al. Intraoperative Doppler echocardiography in hypertrophic cardiomyopathy: correlations with the obstructed gradient. *J Am Coll Cardiol* 1987;10:327.**
26. Levine RA, Jimoh A, Cape EG, et al. Pressure recovery distal to a stenosis: potential cause of gradient "overestimation" by Doppler echocardiography. *J Am Coll Cardiol* 1989;13(3):706.
27. Pollick C, Rakowski H, Wigle ED. Muscular subaortic stenosis: the temporal relationship between systolic anterior motion and the pressure gradient. *Circulation* 1982;66:1087.
28. Jiang L, Levine RA, King ME, et al. An integrated mechanism to explain the systolic anterior motion in hypertrophic cardiomyopathy based on echocardiographic observations. *Am Heart J* 1987;113:633.
29. **Marwick TH, Stewart WJ, Lever HM, et al. Benefits of intraoperative echocardiography in the surgical management of hypertrophic cardiomyopathy. *J Am Coll Cardiol* 1992;20(5):1066.**
30. Wigle ED, Adelman AD, Felderhof CH. Medical and surgical treatment of cardiomyopathy. *Circ Res* 1974;35(suppl II): 196.
31. Heric B, Lytle BW, Rosencranz ER, et al. Surgical management of hypertrophic obstructive cardiomyopathy. Early and late results. *J Thorac Cardiovasc Surg* 1995;110(1):195–206; discussion 206–208.
32. **Cecchi F, Olivotto I. New concepts in hypertrophic cardiomyopathies. *Circulation* 2002;105(23):188.**

THE USE OF TRANSESOPHAGEAL ECHOCARDIOGRAPHY DURING ENDOVASCULAR STENT-GRAFT EXCLUSION OF THORACIC ANEURYSMS AND DISSECTIONS

ALANN SOLINA
RONALD A. KAHN

CASE PRESENTATION

The patient is a 78-year-old woman with past medical history significant for coronary artery disease, severe chronic obstructive pulmonary disease, diabetes mellitus and hypertension, who presented with an extensive thoracic artery aneurysm. After placement of appropriate monitors and a radial arterial line, a 16-gauge Silastic catheter was inserted into the lumbar subarachnoid space for both administration of an anesthetic as well as cerebral spinal fluid drainage. The patient underwent placement of a thoracic aortic endograft without detectable endoleaks by intraoperative fluoroscopy. The patient was sedated and a transesophageal echocardiography (TEE) probe was inserted. A distal type 1 endoleak was detected, which was treated with angioplasty balloon inflations.

INTRODUCTION

Historically, thoracic aortic aneurysms (TAAs) and dissections (TADs) were treated surgically by complex aortic reconstruction through either a thoracotomy or a thoracoabdominal incision. Because of the need for extensive intrathoracic and intraabdominal dissection, fluid shifts, hemodynamic changes (as a result of fluid shifts, extensive blood loss, and aortic cross clamping), and the need for mechanical support during distal perfusion, the morbidity and mortality of these patients are high. In an effort to avoid these risks, and to make

---

A. Solina: Division of Cardiac Anesthesiology, UMDNJ-Robert Wood Johnson Medical School, New Brunswick, New Jersey.
R. A. Kahn: Department of Anesthesiology, The Mount Sinai Medical Center, New York, New York.

procedural intervention possible for those patients that were previously deemed inoperable because of prohibitive surgical risk, the technique of transcatheter stent graft placement was developed.

Preoperative and intraoperative imaging of the anatomy of the TAA/TAD and the stent graft is critically important to the success of the procedure. Preoperative imaging defines the anatomy of the aortic pathology, which is necessary for determination of the feasibility of endovascular repair as well as the customization of the endograft to be implanted. Intraoperative imaging is critical for proper deployment of the graft and evaluation of the adequacy of repair. Initially, intraoperative deployment of the stent graft was facilitated by angiography. More recently, perioperative TEE has been described as an important adjuvant to fluoroscopy. This chapter focuses on the use of TEE during endovascular repair of TAAs and TADs.

SCIENTIFIC PRINCIPLES

Demographics, Conventional Surgical Indications, and Outcome

Thoracic aortic aneurysms and TADs are important causes of morbidity and mortality in the United States. The death rate for TAAs and TADs in the United States is approximately 6 per 100,000 (adjusted to the year 2000 population census) (1). With 15,807 deaths attributable to TAAs and TADs in 1999, the Center for Disease Control and Prevention listed TAA/TAD as the 15th most frequent cause of all deaths in the United States (1).

The most common cause of TAA is atherosclerosis. The descending thoracic aorta is involved in approximately 40% of cases of thoracic aortic aneurysms (2). Patients with TAAs and TADs are frequently elderly and have significant comorbidities, including chronic obstructive pulmonary disease (secondary to tobacco abuse) and atherosclerotic coronary artery disease.

Medical treatment of TAA is unsatisfactory; the mean survival time is less than 3 years after diagnosis, and the 5-year survival rate is only 20% (2). Surgery is indicated if the aneurysm is greater than 6 cm in diameter, or if the aneurysm is greater than twice the diameter of the normal adjacent aorta (2). Surgical treatment has historically involved graft interposition through a thoracotomy. Cooley and DeBakey pioneered this operation in 1956 (3). Despite advances in cardiac anesthesia, graft engineering, tissue protection, and surgical technique, the mortality rate approaches 12% in elective cases of relatively low risk (4). These patients have a 5-year survival rate of about 75% (5). However, operative mortality is estimated to be 50% in patients requiring emergent surgery, or in those patients with significant comorbidity (6). Morbidity and mortality typically involve perioperative stroke, renal failure, myocardial infarction, and vascular insufficiency of the spinal cord and distal organs.

Thoracic aortic dissections affect approximately 9,000 patients per year in the United States (5). Aortic dissections proximal to the takeoff of the left subclavian artery (type A) are treated surgically because of the fear of extension of the dissection into the coronary arteries, aortic valve, or pericardium. Indications for surgical repair of aortic dissections distal to the left subclavian artery (type B) include recurrent chest pain, branch vessel involvement, or an expanding false lumen (7). Work by Kato et al. indicates that patients with acute type B TADs who have an aortic diameter greater than 4.0 cm and a patent entry site should be treated surgically, provided that the surgical risk is not too great (7). The current mortality rate for medically manageable type B dissections is 20% (8). The surgical mortality rate is 35%, and may be as high as 50% when there is evidence of end-organ ischemia (8).

Unfortunately, many patients with TAA are not considered to be candidates for conventional surgical repair because of advanced age, other comorbidity (especially cardiac or pulmonary), or previous thoracic surgery. Historically, these patients have been relegated to medical management and its associated dismal prognosis. This particular subset of patients has a 2-year survival rate of only 24% (9).

In 1991, Parodi and his group pioneered the treatment of abdominal aneurysms with endovascular stent graft placement (10). Subsequently, Mitchell, Miller, and Dake from the Stanford group applied this technique to the treatment of TAAs and TADs (2,4–6,8,11,12). This approach involves the transcatheter deployment of a reinforced stent graft that excludes the flow of blood into the aneurysm or false lumen of a dissection. The theoretic advantage to endovascular technique relative to conventional open technique is the avoidance of (a) aortic cross clamping, (b) cardiopulmonary bypass/deep hypothermic circulatory arrest, and (c) thoracotomy. In a relatively large (N = 103) prospective study,

the Stanford group reported an early mortality rate of 9% in TAA patients who had undergone aneurysm repair by the endovascular stent graft technique (12). This mortality rate is impressive when viewed in the context that 60% of these patients were judged to have prohibitive risk for open surgical graft interposition.

The Stent Graft

From a technical perspective, the stent graft is composed of an expandable metallic endoskeleton, which is typically covered with Dacron or a woven polyester fabric graft (Fig. 26.1). These composite grafts are individually crafted for each patient application. The length and diameter are idiosyncratic to the anatomic concerns of the patient. Grafts are retracted into a delivery system, which is usually introduced transfemorally over a guidewire (Fig. 26.2). A retroperitoneal approach is sometimes required for catheter advancement in patients with severe femoral artery disease. When the graft has been advanced to its proper anatomic position, it is deployed (Fig. 26.3). Presently most grafts are self-expanding; however, the first-generation devices required large angioplasty balloons for deployment. Because of the high flows seen in the thoracic aorta, device deployment may be complicated by distal graft migration, with resultant inadequate endovascular repair. Various methods of mitigating this effect have been used, including the use of beta-blockers, adenosine, nitroprusside, and induction of temporary ventricular fibrillation (13).

Preoperative Evaluation

General Anatomic Concerns

Precise anatomic definition of the patient's aortic pathology is essential. A combination of digital subtraction angiography, spiral computed tomography scanning, and magnetic resonance imaging is used. First, it is essential to consider which part of the aorta is involved. Pathology involving tortuous

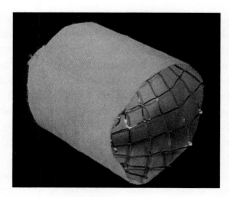

FIGURE 26.1. An endovascular stent graft. From: Kahn R, Marin M, Hollier L, et al. Induction of ventricular fibrillation endovascular stent graft repair of thoracic aortic aneurysms. *Anesthesiology* 1998;88:534, with permission.

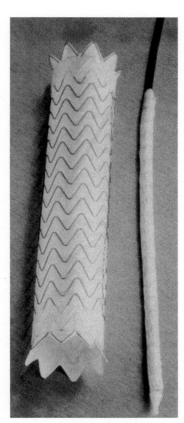

FIGURE 26.2. Fully expanded and retracted stent graft. From: Grabenwoger M, Hutschala D, Ehrich M, et al. Thoracic aortic aneurysms: treatment with endovascular self-expandable stent grafts. *The Annals of Thoracic Surgery* 2000;69:441, with permission.

aortic segments may be complicated by the inability of the stent graft to conform to the geometry of the native segment. Failure to obtain good stent graft–tissue apposition results in the possibility of leak or eventual graft migration (Fig. 26.4). Apposition of the stent graft and native aortic tissue is absolutely necessary to prevent leak, since biologic incorporation of the stent graft is not absolute (14). Perforation of the native vessel is also more likely at the point of curvature. Additionally, the delivery catheter or the stent graft itself may bend or kink when negotiation of the curvature is attempted. In the future, graft engineering improvements may address these concerns.

When sizing the graft for diameter, it is customary to overestimate the diameter by 10% to 15% to ensure adequate radial force transmitted to the native aorta, which prevents perigraft leakage and graft migration. Liberal oversizing of the graft may cause the material of the graft to wrinkle, which could result in poor tissue–graft apposition and leak (15). Additionally, deliberate oversizing could theoretically lead to aortic wall damage. It is sometimes difficult to achieve a leak-proof seal with chronic dissections, because the noncircular geometry precludes the degree of symmetric radial force that is obligatory for a circumferentially tight seal (5). Additionally, important perfusion of distal end organs may

be dependent on false lumen flow, which would be interrupted by complete exclusion of the dissection at this level (5). The size of the largest available graft may limit the application of endovascular technique to patients with aortic landing zones with a diameter of greater than 42 mm.

Branch Vessel Anatomy

Compromise of flow through patent branch vessels is another important concern during stent graft placement. Preoperative angiography is critically important to determine the specific vascular anatomy. If the takeoff of the aortic branch arteries must be incorporated into the stent, alternative surgical methods of aortic branch perfusion must be constructed prior to endovascular repair.

The arterial supply of the anterior part of the spinal cord is another important consideration. The artery of Adamkowicz may arise from intercostal vessels in the segment of aorta that is to be stented. If preoperative angiography indicates that these intercostal vessels are patent, blood flow to the spinal cord could be compromised because it is not possible to reattach these potentially important intercostal vessels when using endovascular technique. Although stent grafts usually involve a shorter segment of aorta then a graft interposition would, it is still possible to impair blood supply to the spinal cord, which could result in paresis or paralysis. In order to minimize the likelihood of spinal cord ischemia, it is necessary to make the stent graft as short as is technically feasible while maintaining adequate landing zones (16). It is possible to use a partially uncovered stent that allows for flow in the area of an important branch vessel takeoff, but the anatomic placement of such a composite graft is technically demanding.

Landing Zones

Another consideration is that of adequate landing zone length for stent graft placement. Generally, at least a 15-mm segment of "normal" aorta is required at each end of the stent graft to serve as a landing zone. Because deployment of the graft is affected by the forward propulsive force of aortic blood flow, and the placement of the graft cannot be manipulated significantly after deployment, it is critically important to have relatively generous landing zones that do not involve important branch vessels, are disease free, and are of appropriate geometric dimension.

Intraoperative Concerns
Placement of the Stent Graft

As described above, the proper anatomic placement of the stent graft is technically demanding, but is absolutely critical in order to achieve proper vascular exclusion and to ensure that the graft is seated within the defined landing zones. Intraoperative fluoroscopy with image intensification and

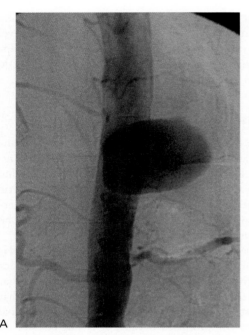

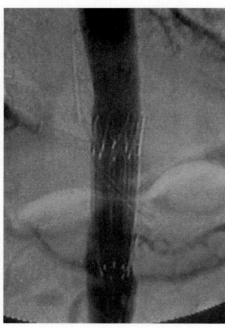

FIGURE 26.3. A: Angiogram of distal descending thoracic aneurysm. **B:** Stent-graft exclusion of the same aneurysm. From: Ishimaru S, Kawaguchi S, Koizumi N, et al. Preliminary report on prediction of spinal cord ischemia in endovascular stent graft repair of thoracic aortic aneurysm by retrievable stent graft. *J Thorac Cardiovasc Surg* 1998;115:811, with pemission.

digital subtraction capabilities is used to guide the placement of the stent graft. The portable C-arm units that are used in the operating room for angiographic fluoroscopy are inferior to the stationary units that are used in the radiology suite (17). These portable units have a diminished capacity to compensate for the various tissue densities in the thorax. Additionally, it may be difficult to achieve the angulation requisite for proper plane of interrogation with the portable C-arm (17). Furthermore, angiography does not reveal the anatomic nature of the vessel lumen, especially in the presence of intramural plaque. However, intraopera-

tive angiography does provide vital information concerning branch vessel anatomy.

Paralysis

Despite advances in adjunctive preservation techniques, postoperative paralysis remains an important cause of morbidity in patients with TADs and TAAs. Paralysis occurs in as many as 4.5% to 21% of patients treated by conventional open graft interposition (18,19), and in as few as 0% to 3% of patients treated with endovascular technique (18,20,21).

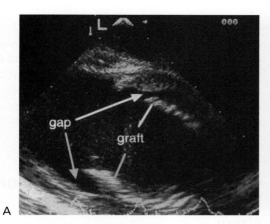 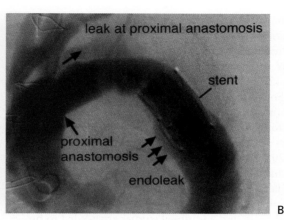

A   B

FIGURE 26.4. A: Transesophageal echocardiographic image demonstrating failure to achieve a seal between the stent-graft and the aortic tissue. Angiogram of the same area. From: Orihashi K, Matsuura Y, Sueda T, et al. Echocardiography-assisted surgery in transaortic endovascular stent grafting: role of transesophageal echocardiography. *The Journal of Thoracic and Cardiovascular Surgery* 2000;120:672, with permission.

Angiography is used to define the patency of intercostals vessels, particularly in the T8 to L2 region. If the stent graft will cover patent intercostal vessels in this area, endovascular stent grafting is precluded. In some cases it may be possible to use a stent graft that has an opening at the takeoff of an important intercostal vessel. Ishimaru et al. (19) reported the use of a retrievable stent in combination with the recording of spinal cord evoked potentials to test for the precipitation of spinal cord ischemia by stent graft placement in 16 patients with TAAs (Fig. 26.5). After the retrievable temporary stent demonstrated that stent graft placement would not precipitate spinal cord ischemia, the temporary stent was removed, and a permanent stent placed in the same position. Despite the reported success of this technique, the obligatory manipulation of the aorta that is involved with expansion and removal of the retrievable stent may cause atheroembolic events. The development of a retrievable permanent stent graft may obviate this concern.

Detection of Leaks

Failure to completely exclude the aneurysm or false lumen of a TAD is called an endoleak, and may occur in as many

as 3% to 44% of patients undergoing endovascular exclusion of TADs and TAAs (21–23). The Stanford group reported a leak incidence of 24% in the first 103 patients that they studied (12). The principal concern about leaks is that they subject that partially excluded segment of aorta to arterial pressure, which increases the risk for expansion or rupture (22). Historically, leaks were detected by angiography. However, angiography has proved to have a relatively low sensitivity for detection of intraoperative and postoperative leaks (22,24,25). Work by Armerding and colleagues indicates that while postoperative conventional angiography has a sensitivity for detecting post—stent graft leakage of 63%, computed tomographic angiography has a sensitivity of 92% (24).

Type 1 endoleaks can occur from an inadequate seal between the endograft and the aortic wall at the proximal or distal graft attachment sites (26). This results in continued leakage of blood from the central aortic flow into the diseased aortic segment. They may occur as a result of intimal plaque distortion during placement of the endovascular stent, short and anatomically difficult aneurysm necks (i.e., severe neck angulation and/or calcification), stent migration, or inappropriate endograft size. Endovascular repair does not address the underlying aortic pathology, and progression of the aortic disease process usually continues after the endovascular procedure. It has been shown that the proximal aneurysm neck diameter continues to grow approximately 1 mm per year after endovascular repair and may result in further endoleaks (27). If a type 1 endoleak is diagnosed at the time of the procedure, further endovascular intervention (e.g., molding the stent graft with balloon distention, or placing an additional graft) can be undertaken immediately to ameliorate the problem. If diagnosed at a later time, it is also possible to correct the problem using endovascular technology.

Type 2 endoleaks occur from filling of the excluded diseased aorta from collateral vessels (backbleeding). Retrograde

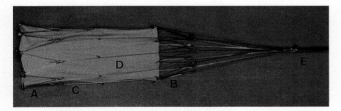

FIGURE 26.5. Retrievable stent-graft. From: Ishimaru S, Kawaguchi S, Koizumi N, et al. Preliminary report on prediction of spinal cord ischemia in endovascular stent graft repair of thoracic aortic aneurysm by retrievable stent graft. *J Thoracic Cardiovasc Surg* 1998;115:811, with permission.

filling of the excluded aortic segments may occur by the lumbar arteries or the inferior mesenteric arteries. Resnikoff et al. reported an incidence of approximately 2% for type 2 endoleaks in 831 patients treated for abdominal aortic aneurysms (28). Treatment of a type 2 endoleak is controversial. Some suggest that persistent type 2 endoleaks caused no further change in aneurysm diameter over an 18-month follow-up, while others have noted that if type 2 endoleaks are treated, there is a decrease on aneurysm diameter (29,30). Current measures to prevent type 2 endoleaks include filling of the aneurysm sac with thrombogenic material at the time of endovascular repair or embolization of the side branches (30,31). These studies have met with some success, and additional studies are needed to further define a proper treatment algorithm for these types of complications.

A type 3 endoleak is a leak from the central component of an endograft. With time, the woven polyester sleeves of endografts display evidence of yarn shifting and distortion, damage, and filament breakage, forming holes that result in endoleaks. Structural graft failure also may be related to compaction and dislocation of the metallic frame (32). It is possible that successful aneurysmal exclusion may result in a decrease in aortic diameter. This shrinkage may cause a physical stress on the endograft, resulting in changes in element alignment or traction with a resultant change in the relationship between graft components (33). These stresses may result in erosion and subsequent loss of endograft integrity by dislocation of individual components of a modular endograft over time.

Hemodynamic Monitoring

As previously described, most TAD and TAA patients are elderly individuals with significant cardiac and pulmonary comorbidity. Even though patients treated with endovascular technique are not subjected to cardiopulmonary bypass or aortic cross clamping, there is still a need to aggressively monitor the hemodynamic state of the patient throughout the procedure.

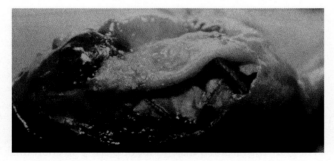

FIGURE 26.6. Gross anatomical specimen of an aneurysmal sac that was perforated by a migrated stent-graft. From: Garbenwoger M, Hutschala D, Ehrich M, et al. Thoracic aortic aneurysms: treatment with endovascular self-expandable stent grafts. *The Annals of Thoracic Surgery* 2000;69:441, with permission.

Postoperative Concerns

The principal postoperative concerns are endovascular leak with resultant failure of vascular exclusion and inadvertent branch vessel compromise with consequent end-organ damage. The Stanford group reported a postoperative stroke rate of 4% to 5% (2,11). Migration of the stent graft is a relatively uncommon occurrence, as is perforation of the aorta (Fig. 26.6) by the stent graft (14).

CONTRIBUTION OF TRANSESOPHAGEAL ECHOCARDIOGRAPHY

Sizing

Measurement of the aorta for proper sizing (diameter and length) of the graft is critically important. When the graft diameter is too small, there is an increased chance of endovascular leak. Transesophageal echocardiography may provide more accurate intraoperative sizing of the internal diameter of the aorta because unlike calibrated angiography, it is able to discriminate intramural plaque and thrombus from true intima (34). Transesophageal echocardiography may allow for intraoperative verification of sizing determined preoperatively by computer tomography. In cases where tomographic images were obtained in an oblique plane relative to the true short axis, TEE may provide for more accurate sizing of the graft (35).

Proper Anatomic Placement of the Stent Graft

The placement of the stent graft is facilitated by intraoperative angiography and TEE. Transesophageal echocardiography may identify branch vessel anatomy and aortic morphology. Once the exact area for graft deployment has been determined, the TEE probe itself can serve as a visual marker during angiographic interrogation (Fig. 26.7). This technique is especially important in cases of dissection, because angiography does not reliably reveal the false lumen entry site. Transesophageal echocardiography can be used to help negotiate the stent graft guidewire into the true lumen in cases of TAD (Fig. 26.8). Transesophageal echocardiography also can be used to detect graft migration and kinking of the stent graft.

Landing Zones

Transesophageal echocardiography is used to determine the morphologic characteristics of the aorta in the anticipated landing zones in an effort to avoid areas with extensive plaque, calcification, or mural thrombus. A study by Fattori and colleagues, which involved 25 patients undergoing endovascular stent placement for TAA, found that TEE was instrumental in determining landing zone in 62% of patients

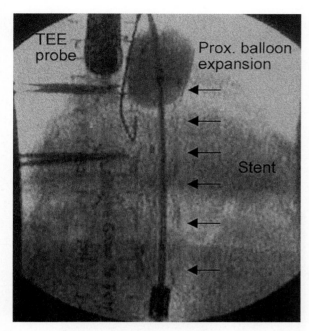

FIGURE 26.7. Fluoroscopic image demonstrating how a transesophageal echocardiographic probe can be used intraoperatively as a landmark to aid in the positioning of the stent-graft. From: Rapezzi C, Rocchi G, Fattori R, et al. Usefulness of transesophageal echocardiographic monitoring to improve the outcome of stent-graft treatment of thoracic aortic aneurysms. *The American Journal of Cardiology* 2001;87:315, with permission.

(35). Rapezzi et al. found that intraoperative TEE findings led surgeons to change the site of stent positioning, which had originally been determined by angiography in 33% of patients undergoing endovascular exclusion of TAAs or TADs (25).

Branch Vessel Avoidance

As previously discussed, it is critical to avoid the takeoff of patent branch vessels that would otherwise be excluded by stent placement. Transesophageal echocardiography can be used to visualize the origin of the subclavian and celiac

arteries. It should be noted that TEE does not reliably enable visualization of intercostal vessels (36).

Detection of Leaks

Vascular leak is the most common complication of endovascular stent graft exclusion. Failure to achieve complete vascular exclusion places the patient at risk for catastrophic rupture. As discussed above, angiography has a relatively low sensitivity for detection of endovascular leaks.

Two-Dimensional Transesophageal Echocardiography

Two-dimensional TEE is used to grossly examine the area of tissue–graft apposition to ensure that the graft is correctly seated in the landing zone (Fig. 26.4). The graft can be molded to better conform to the shape of the aorta with successive balloon inflations. In some cases it may be necessary to use a second stent graft. The appearance of spontaneous contrast or "smoke" in the excluded area after stent graft placement is an indicator of successful exclusion (25,37). In cases of TADs, expansion of the true lumen can be detected by TEE.

Doppler Velocities

Doppler interrogation of the stent graft can provide valuable information concerning anastomotic integrity. Perigraft leaks are characterized by relatively high-velocity Doppler signals, whereas low-velocity signals are seen with flow due to normal graft porosity (Fig. 26.9).

Color-Flow Doppler

Fattori's study demonstrated that color-flow Doppler techniques are a more sensitive indicator of intraoperative perigraft leak than angiography (35). In this study, TEE identified perigraft leak in 8 of 25 patients undergoing thoracic

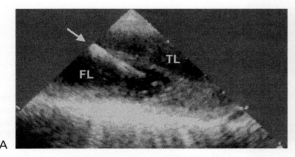
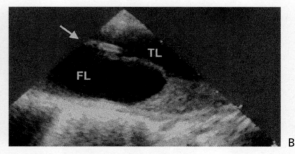

FIGURE 26.8. TEE-assisted guidewire placement for stent-grafting in a patient with a thoracic aortic dissection. **A:** The guidewire is in the false lumen. **B:** The guidewire has been repositioned into the true lumen. From: Rapezzi C, Rocchi G, Fattori R, et al. Usefulness of transesophageal echocardiographic monitoring to improve the outcome of stent-graft treatment of thoracic aortic aneurysms. *The American Journal of Cardiology* 2001;87:315, with permission.

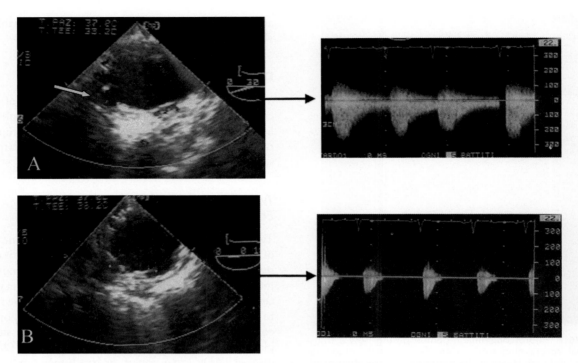

FIGURE 26.9. Doppler TEE as used to detect perigraft leak. **A:** 2-D image and Doppler recording demonstrating perigraftleak. **B:** 2-D image and Doppler recording of the same area after molding of the stent-graft with successive balloon inflations. The low velocity Doppler signals represent graft porosity. From: Fattori R, Caldarera I, Rapezzi C, et al. Primary endoleakage in endovascular treatment of the thoracic aorta: importance of intraoperative transesophageal echocardiography. *The Journal of Thoracic and Cardiovascular Surgery* 2000;120:490, with permission.

endovascular exclusion for TAAs, whereas angiography revealed a perigraft leak in only two of the 8 patients demonstrating leak by TEE (Fig. 26.10).

M-mode Transesophageal Echocardiography

Pulsatile wall movement (PWM) is the excursion of the wall of an aneurysm that corresponds to the pulsatile pressure changes engendered by the cardiac cycle. Malina and colleagues found that there was a 75% reduction in PWM in TAA patients who underwent successful endovascular exclusion of their aneurysms (38). M-mode TEE can be used to detect PWM in aneurysms after placement of the endovascular stent (Fig. 26.11). Unfortunately, it is possible to have a patent endovascular leak and not have detectable PWM.

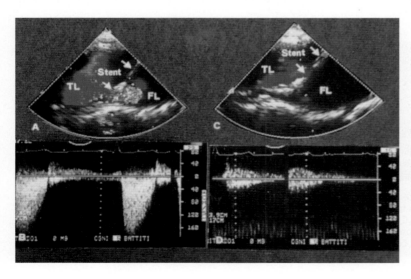

FIGURE 26.10. Color Doppler and pulsed Doppler examination of a patient with a stent-graft repair of a type B aortic dissection. **A and B** demonstrate significant leak proximal to the stent. **C and D** demonstrate resolution of the leak after a second stent was deployed. Note that low velocity signals representing graft porosity remain after the leak has been repaired. From: Rapezzi C, Rocchi G, Fattori R, et al. Usefulness of transesophageal echocardiographic monitoring to improve the outcome of stent-graft treatment of thoracic aortic aneurysms. *The American Journal of Cardiology* 2001;87:315, with permission.

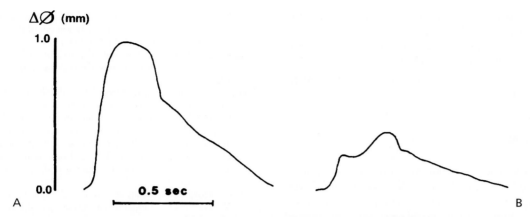

FIGURE 26.11. Change in pulsatile aortic wall motion after stent-graft exclusion of an aortic aneurysm. Aortic diameter change during one cardiac cycle before (**A**) and after (**B**) exclusion. From: Malina M, Lanne T, Ivancer K, et al. Reduced pulsatile wall motion of abdominal aortic aneurysms after endovascular repair. *Journal of Vascular Surgery* 1998;27:624, with permission.

Cardiac Function

As discussed above, most patients undergoing endovascular exclusion of TAAs or TADs are elderly individuals with other significant comorbid conditions. Frequently these patients have coronary artery disease, and may have impaired ventricular function. Despite the fact that aortic cross clamping and cardiopulmonary bypass are avoided with endovascular techniques, patients are still exposed to significant risk of intraoperative and perioperative morbidity and mortality. Transesophageal echocardiography is arguably the most comprehensive monitor of overall cardiac function in the operative setting.

Technical Issues

Transesophageal echocardiography is a useful clinical tool during endovascular vascular exclusion procedures. How-

ever, there are some technical issues that must be considered during its clinical application:

1. The catheter and delivery device may not be readily apparent when the aorta is imaged in long axis, since they may be out of the imaging plane. Short-axis interrogation may be necessary to help locate intraluminal devices.
2. The highly echogenic stent graft may cause significant side-lobe artifacts, confounding efforts to accurately image the graft during placement. It may be necessary to rotate the plane of interrogation 90 degrees to the neck of the aneurysm (Fig. 26.12) to adequately visualize the graft and aneurysm (36).
3. The TEE may cause significant artifacts with fluoroscopy, and thus its use may be limited to times when fluoroscopy is not in use (36).

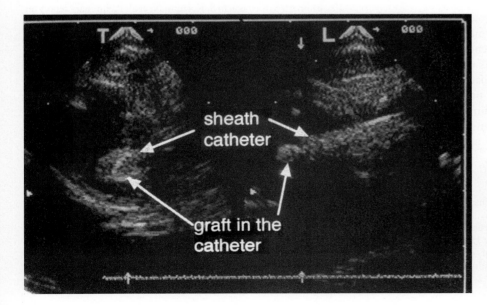

sheath catheter

graft in the catheter

FIGURE 26.12. It may be necessary to rotate the plane of interrogation 90 degrees to the neck of the aneurysm to adequately visualize the stent-graft and aneurysm. From: Orihashi K, Matsuura Y, Sueda T, et al. Echocardiography-assisted surgery in transaortic endovascular stent grafting: role of transesophageal echocardiography. *The Journal of Thoracic and Cardiovascular Surgery* 2000;120:672, with permission.

4. It is difficult to visualize the distal ascending aorta and proximal aortic arch with TEE.
5. Far-field artifacts caused by the stent graft may interfere with TEE detection of leaks (37).
6. Some patients may not be candidates for TEE (e.g., esophageal pathology).

CONCLUSION

Disease of the thoracic aorta is an important cause of mortality in the United States. Unfortunately, patients with TADs and TAAs frequently have significant comorbid conditions, placing them at high or unacceptable risk for conventional open repair. Over the past decade, endovascular exclusion with stent grafting has emerged as a valuable therapeutic modality. During endovascular procedures, proper intraoperative placement of the graft and the ability to identify failure of vascular exclusion are of paramount importance. Additionally, TEE serves as a useful monitor of cardiac function during these procedures. Intraoperative TEE is now considered an invaluable tool during stent graft placement. In the future it is likely that anesthesiologists will be more frequently called upon to provide comprehensive TEE services for these procedures.

KEY POINTS

- Transesophageal echocardiography is used to help determine appropriate sizing of the endovascular graft, which is necessary to reduce the likelihood of endovascular leak.
- Transesophageal echocardiography facilitates the placement of the endovascular stent graft because it defines the anatomic characteristics of the landing zones for graft deployment, including intraluminal pathology, and branch vessel anatomy.
- Transesophageal echocardiography techniques, such as two-dimensional, Doppler, and M-mode interrogation, are extremely sensitive indicators of endovascular leak.
- Transesophageal echocardiography is used as an important intraoperative monitor of cardiac function during endovascular stent graft deployment procedures.
- Technical considerations sometimes limit the clinical utility of TEE during endovascular exclusion procedures.

REFERENCES

1. Hoyert D, Arias E, Smith B, et al. Deaths: final data for 1999. *Natl Vital Stat Rep* 2001;49:8.
2. Mitchell R. Endovascular stent graft repair of thoracic aortic aneurysms. *Semin Thorac Cardiovasc Surg* 1997;9:257.
3. Cooley D, De Bakey M. Resection of the entire ascending aorta in fusiform aneurysm using cardiopulmonary bypass. *JAMA* 1956;162:1158.
4. Dake M, Miller D, Semba C, et al. Transluminal placement of endovascular stent-grafts for the treatment of descending thoracic aneurysms. *N Engl J Med* 1994;331:1729.
5. Fann J, Miller D. Endovascular treatment of descending thoracic aortic aneurysms and dissections. *Surg Clin North Am* 1999;79:551.
6. Semba C, Mitchell R, Miller D, et al. Thoracic aortic aneurysm repair with endovascular stent-grafts. *Vasc Med* 1997;2:98.
7. Kato M, Bai H, Sato K, et al. Determining surgical indications for acute type B dissection based on enlargement of aortic diameter during the chronic phase. *Circulation* 1995;92(suppl II):107.
8. Dake M, Kato N, Mitchell R, et al. Endovascular stent-graft placement for the treatment of acute aortic dissection. *N Engl J Med* 1999;340:1546.
9. Crawford E, DeNatale R. Thoracoabdominal aortic aneurysms: observations regarding the natural course of the disease. *J Vasc Surg* 1986;3:578.
10. Parodi J, Palmaz J, Barone H. Transfemoral intraluminal graft implantation for abdominal aortic aneurysm. *Ann Vasc Surg* 1991;5:491.
11. Mitchell R, Miller D, Dake M. Stent-graft repair of thoracic aneurysms. *Semin Vasc Surg* 1997;10:257.
12. **Dake M, Miller D, Mitchell R, et al. The "first generation" of endovascular stent-grafts for patients with aneurysms of the descending thoracic aorta. *J Thorac Cardiovasc Surg* 1998;116:689.**
13. Kahn R, Marin M, Hollier L, et al. Induction of ventricular fibrillation to facilitate endovascular stent graft repair of thoracic aortic aneurysms. *Anesthesiology* 1998;88:534.
14. Malina M, Brunkwall J, Ivancev K, et al. Late aortic arch perforation by graft-anchoring stent: complication of thoracic aneurysm exclusion. *J Endovasc Surg* 1998;5:274.
15. Nolthenius R, van en Berg J, Moll F. The value of intraoperative intravascular ultrasound for determining stent graft size with a modular system. *Ann Vasc Surg* 2000;14:311.
16. Nienaber C, Fattori R, Lund G, et al. Nonsurgical reconstruction of thoracic aortic dissection by stent-graft placement. *N Engl J Med* 1999;340:1539.
17. Sakai T, Dake M, Semba C, et al. Descending thoracic aortic aneurysm: thoracic CT findings after endovascular stent-graft placement. *Radiology* 1999;212:169.
18. Kasirajan K, Dolmatch B, Ouriel K, et al. Delayed onset of ascending paralysis after thoracic aortic stent graft deployment. *J Vasc Surg* 2000;31:196.
19. Ishimaru S, Kawaguchi S, Koizumi N, et al. Preliminary report on prediction of spinal cord ischemia in endovascular stent graft repair of thoracic aortic aneurysm by retrievable stent graft. *J Thorac Cardiovasc Surg* 1998;115:811.
20. Reidy J, Taylor P. The use of stent-grafts in thoracic aortic disease. *Cardiovasc Int Radiol* 2000;23:249.
21. Temudom T, D'Ayala M, Marin M, et al. Endovascular grafts in the treatment of thoracic aortic aneurysms and pseudoaneurysms. *Ann Vasc Surg* 2000;14:230.
22. Gorich J, Rilinger N, Sokiranski R, et al. Treatment of leaks after endovascular repair of aortic aneurysms. *Radiology* 2000;215:414.
23. Cartes-Zumelzu F, Lammer J, Kretschmert G, et al. Endovascular repair of thoracic aortic aneurysms. *Semin Intervent Cardiol* 2000;5:53.
24. Amerding M, Rubin G, Beaulieu C, et al. Aortic aneurysmal disease: assessment of stent-graft treatment—CT versus conventional angiography. *Radiology* 2000;215:138.
25. **Rapezzi C, Rocchi G, Fattori R, et al. Usefulness of transesophageal echocardiographic monitoring to improve the outcome of stent-graft treatment of thoracic aortic aneurysms. *Am J Cardiol* 2001;87:315.**

26. Wain RA, Marin ML, Ohki T, et al. Endoleaks after endovascular graft treatment of aortic aneurysms: classification, risk factors, and outcome. *J Vasc Surg* 1998;27:69–80.

27. Prinssen M, Wever JJ, Mali WP, et al. Concerns for the durability of the proximal abdominal aortic aneurysm endograft fixation from a 2-year and 3-year longitudinal computed tomography angiography study. *J Vasc Surg* 2001;33:64–69.

28. Resnikoff M, Darling RC 3rd, Chang BB, et al. Fate of the excluded abdominal aortic aneurysm sac: long-term follow-up of 831 patients. *J Vasc Surg* 1996;24:851–855.

29. Resch T, Ivancev K, Lindh M, et al. Persistent collateral perfusion of abdominal aortic aneurysm after endovascular repair does not lead to progressive change in aneurysm diameter. *J Vasc Surg* 1998;28:242–249.

30. Khilnani NM, Sos TA, Trost DW, et al. Embolization of back-bleeding lumbar arteries filling an aortic aneurysm sac after endovascular stent-graft placement. *J Vasc Interv Radiol* 1996;7:813–817.

31. Walker SR, Macierewicz J, Hopkinson BR. Endovascular AAA repair: prevention of side branch endoleaks with thrombogenic sponge. *J Endovasc Surg* 1999;6:350–353.

32. Guidoin R, Marois Y, Douville Y, et al. First-generation aortic endografts: analysis of explanted Stentor devices from the EUROSTAR Registry. *J Endovasc Ther* 2000;7:105–122.

33. May J, White GH, Harris JP. Devices for aortic aneurysm repair. *Surg Clin North Am* 1999;79:507–527.

34. **Orihashi K, Matsuura Y, Sueda T, et al. Echocardiography-assisted surgery in transaortic endovascular stent grafting: role of transesophageal echocardiography.** *J Thorac Cardiovasc Surg* **2000;120:672.**

35. **Fattori R, Caldarera I, Rapezzi C, et al. Primary endoleakage in endovascular treatment of the thoracic aorta: importance of intraoperative transesophageal echocardiography.** *J Thorac Cardiovasc Surg* **2000;120:490.**

36. **Moskowitz D, Kahn R, Konstadt S, et al. Intraoperative transesophageal echocardiography as an adjuvant to fluoroscopy during endovascular thoracic aortic repair.** *Eur J Vasc Endovasc Surg* **1999;17:22.**

37. Abe S, Ono S, Murata K, et al. Usefulness of transesophageal echocardiographic monitoring in transluminal endovascular stent-graft repair for thoracic aortic aneurysm. *Jpn Circ J* 2000;64:960.

38. Malina M, Lanne T, Ivancev K, et al. Reduced pulsatile wall motion of abdominal aortic aneurysms after endovascular repair. *J Vasc Surg* 1998;27:624.

CRITICAL CARE AND TRAUMA

PART I: CRITICAL CARE
Left Ventricular Pseudoaneurysm: A Contained Cardiac Rupture

Scott T. Reeves
A. Jackson Crumbley III

Left ventricular (LV) pseudoaneurysm following myocardial infarction develops after acute rupture of an infarcted area of the LV, usually the inferoposterior wall. Such ruptures are usually fatal unless the pericardium is sufficiently adherent to the epicardium to result in limited egress of blood and a localized hemopericardium. The persistent communication of the hemopericardium with the LV cavity will result in gradual expansion into a large false aneurysm. In addition to myocardial infarction, other causes for pseudoaneurysm include surgery, sharp or blunt trauma, bacterial endocarditis, and syphilis (1–4).

A true aneurysm is defined as a bulging or dyskinetic area of the ventricle in which all layers of the ventricular wall are usually present. This is in contradistinction to a pseudoaneurysm, in which there is an abrupt interruption and thinning of the myocardium at the neck or orifice leading into the aneurysm, and the wall of the aneurysm contains fibrous pericardial tissue with no myocardial elements (1–3).

CASE PRESENTATION

The patient is a 55-year-old white man who sustained an inferior wall myocardial infarction 6 weeks prior to presentation. His infarction was medically managed with aspirin and metoprolol. Upon presentation to his local physician for his 6-week postinfarct stress test, he was found to be in moderate congestive heart failure with progressive fatigue, dyspnea on exertion, bilateral leg edema, and a 35-pound weight loss over the preceding 3 weeks. On physical examination, he had bibasilar rales and a grade III/VI systolic

murmur radiating from the base to the axilla and epigastrium. The patient had an acute syncope episode, which was evaluated with an electrocardiogram (Fig. 27.1). A subsequent transthoracic echocardiogram was reported to show a massively dilated ventricle and severe mitral regurgitation. Emergency cardiac catheterization demonstrated tight proximal stenosis of the left anterior descending coronary artery, subtotal occlusion of the right coronary artery, and subtotal occlusion of the second obtuse marginal coronary artery. Left ventriculography also appeared to show a massively dilated LV and severe mitral regurgitation (Fig. 27.2). He was transferred to the University Hospital for further therapy.

Review of his left ventriculogram suggested instead a small vigorously contracting ventricle with a large pseudoaneurysm. Repeat catheterization with right anterior oblique left ventriculography confirmed this finding (Fig. 27.3).

At operation, transesophageal echocardiography (TEE) clearly demonstrated a 3 × 4 cm inferior pseudoaneurysm involving the mitral valve chordal structures and posteromedial papillary muscle (Figs. 27.4 and 27.5). Spontaneous echo contrast was visible within the pseudoaneurysm, but no thrombus was identified. A high-velocity, mosaic, eccentric jet of mitral regurgitation further complicated the situation (Fig. 27.6). Pulmonary systolic venous flow reversal indicated that the mitral regurgitation was severe.

Operative findings included extensive pericardial adhesions containing a large pseudoaneurysm beneath the diaphragmatic surface of the LV. Upon initiation of cardiopulmonary bypass, the pseudoaneurysm was entered, and the heart was completely mobilized (Fig. 27.7). The mitral valve was carefully inspected from the LV side with no anatomic abnormalities noted. The left anterior descending and obtuse marginal coronary arteries were bypassed. Pledgetted, 2-0 Prolene, horizontal mattress sutures were passed through the thickened and fibrotic edge of the pseudoaneurysm, through a carefully trimmed Hemoshield Dacron graft, and finally through additional pledgets. The patch was lowered into position and all the sutures were tied. An additional running

S. T. Reeves: Department of Anesthesia and Perioperative Medicine, Medical University of South Carolina, Charleston, South Carolina.
A. J. Crumbley III: Department of Surgery, Thoracic Organ Transplantation Service, Medical University of South Carolina, Charleston, South Carolina.

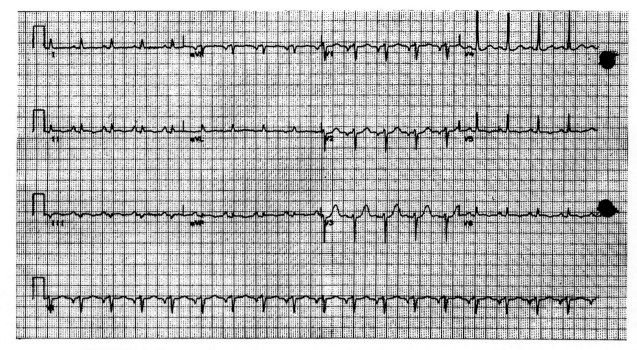

FIGURE 27.1. Electrocardiogram demonstrating possible inferolateral myocardial infarction.

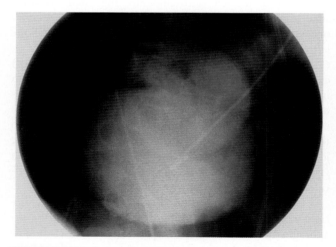

FIGURE 27.2. Left anterior oblique projection of left ventriculography. Note the dilated area at the base of the ventriculogram. This area is actually the pseudoaneurysm with the left ventricle just above it.

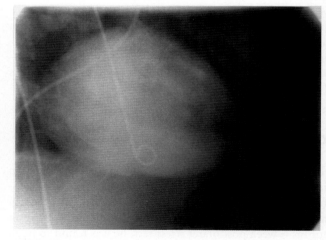

FIGURE 27.3. Right anterior oblique ventriculography demonstrating a small left ventricle with a large pseudoaneurysm.

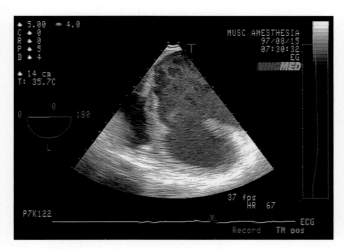

FIGURE 27.4. Two-dimensional transesophageal echocardiography image demonstrating a large inferior wall pseudoaneurysm with spontaneous echo contrast.

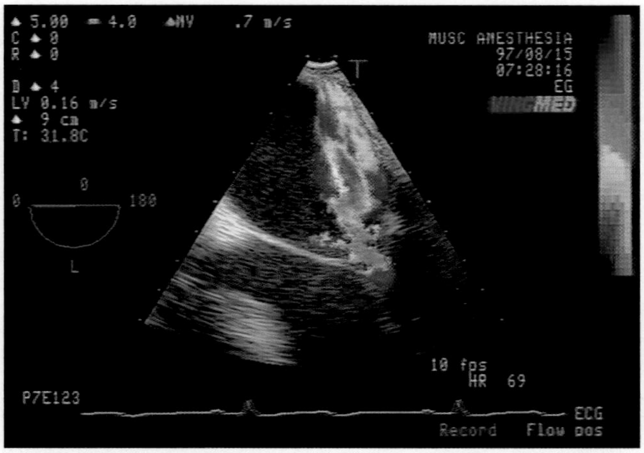

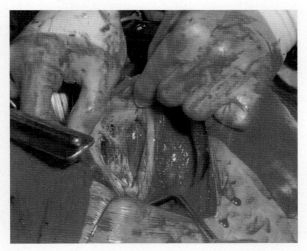

FIGURE 27.6. Color Doppler demonstrating a severe eccentric jet of mitral regurgitation.

Prolene suture around the edge of the patch served as an additional aid in hemostasis (Figs. 27.8 and 27.9).

Because of the echo and ventriculographic findings of mitral regurgitation, the left atrium (LA) was opened through the interatrial groove for inspection of the mitral valve. Careful evaluation, including filling the LV with saline, revealed a fully competent valve. This finding was confirmed by TEE after separating from cardiopulmonary bypass. In addition, the Hemoshield Dacron graft could be clearly visualized in the transgastric short axis view (Fig. 27.10).

The patient was discharged from the hospital on the 6th postoperative day. He returned to work 6 weeks later and remains asymptomatic 4 years postoperatively.

SCIENTIFIC PRINCIPLES

Demographic and Clinical Features

In the largest series to date at a single institution, 48% of patients with pseudoaneurysms were discovered in asymptomatic patients. The majority of asymptomatic pseudoaneurysms were found on follow-up imaging studies performed after staged repairs of complex congenital heart disease. The rest were discovered to have asymptomatic pseudoaneurysms during follow up after valve operations or on evaluation of abnormal electrocardiograms. The presenting symptoms of the remaining 52% were myocardial infarction,

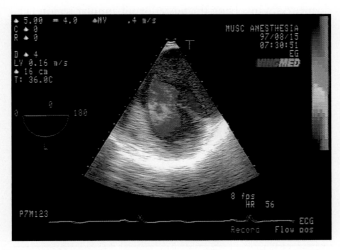

FIGURE 27.5. Color Doppler image of Fig. 27.4 demonstrating classical to-and-fro movement of blood from the left ventricle to the pseudoaneurysm.

FIGURE 27.7. Intraoperative photograph of the left ventricle following debridement of the pseudoaneurysm. Note the mitral valve apparatus and papillary muscles.

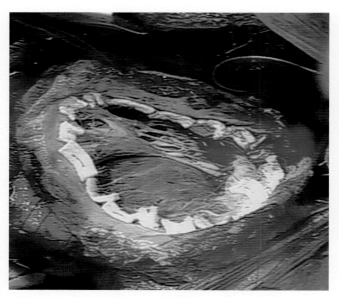

FIGURE 27.8. Intraoperative photograph of the pledgetted mattress sutures in place.

cardiac tamponade, congestive heart failure, chest pain, syncope/arrhythmia, or systemic embolism (Table 27.1).

Location and Etiology

The location of a pseudoaneurysm is directly related to its cause. Pseudoaneurysms resulting from contained rupture of a myocardial infarction are located in the inferior or posterior wall in up to 82% of patients. These are typically diagnosed

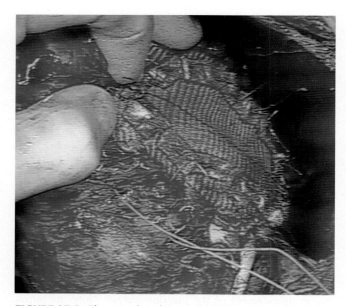

FIGURE 27.9. The completed Hemoshield Dacron patch repair.

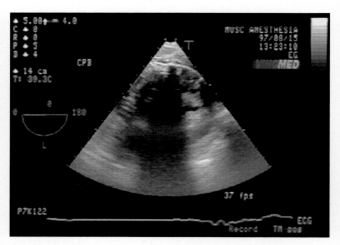

FIGURE 27.10. Transgastric middle short-axis view demonstrating the Hemoshield Dacron patch in the inferior wall.

within the first 6 months following a myocardial infarction; however, intervals of as long as 12 years have been reported (1). The reason for the predominantly inferior or posterior location is currently unknown. In contrast, fatal myocardial ruptures typically occur with infarcts of the anterior and lateral LV walls. Natarajan has postulated that ruptures involving the anterior free wall have significantly more acute hemodynamic effects and result in death, whereas patients experiencing inferior and posterior wall ruptures tend to be contained, resulting in a chronic state once pericardial adhesions develop (5).

Cardiac pseudoaneurysm also may occur following cardiac surgery. This is felt to be most likely secondary to surgical manipulation. It has been hypothesized that removal of excessive leaflet or annular tissue, the placement of a large prosthesis, faulty suturing technique, or previous mitral valve replacement surgery may predispose the patient to a pseudoaneurysm involving the posterior subannular region (1).

If a pseudoaneurysm occurs following aortic valve replacement, it is typically found in the subaortic region. The mechanisms may include an inherent weakness of the aortic root, surgically induced weakness from sutures being tied

TABLE 27.1. PRESENTATION OF CARDIAC PSEUDOANEURYSMS

Asymptomatic	48%
Myocardial infarction	6%
Cardiac tamponade	2%
Congestive heart failure	15%
Chest pain	13%
Syncope/arrhythmia	10%
Systemic embolism	6%

Adapted from Yeo TC, Malouf JF, Oh JK, et al. Clinical profile and outcome in 52 patients with cardiac pseudoaneurysm. *Ann Intern Med* 1998;128:299–305.

TABLE 27.2. CAUSES OF CARDIAC PSEUDOANEURYSMS

Myocardial infraction	42.5%
Congenital heart surgery	29.0%
Mitral valve replacement	7.6%
Aortic valve replacement	5.6%
Mitral and aortic valve replacement	5.6%
Aneurysmectomy	3.8%
Other	5.6%

Adapted from Yeo TC, Malouf JF, Oh JK, et al. Clinical profile and outcome in 52 patients with cardiac pseudoaneurysm. *Ann Intern Med* 1998;128:299–305.

to tightly, extensive decalcification, and the proximity and number of sutures placed (Table 27.2) (1).

Associated Complicating Diagnoses

In patients undergoing inferior/posterior pseudoaneurysm repair, concomitant mitral insufficiency, as in this case report example, is an important operative consideration (2,6,7). Mickleborough in a series of 196 patients undergoing LV true aneurysm repair demonstrated that the resection of the aneurysm actually decreases mitral regurgitation by at least one grade in 81% of patients (6). Possible explanations for this improvement include a decrease in size of the dilated mitral annulus caused by decreased ventricular size, realignment of the papillary muscles due to improved geometry after ventricular repair, and improved function of ischemic papillary muscles related to revascularization (6–8). Transesophageal echocardiography is essential to the evaluation of residual mitral regurgitation after completion of the ventricular repair. This case example demonstrated profound improvement with only trace mitral regurgitation following repair of the ventricular pseudoaneurysm. Had mitral insufficiency persisted, mitral repair or replacement would have been indicated.

Outcome and Natural History

Recently, the need for prophylactic aneurysmectomy in stable, asymptomatic patients has come into question. Van Tassel reported that 50% of pseudoaneurysms rupture within the days to weeks following a myocardial infarction (9). Cardiac rupture has been reported to occur following acute myocardial infarction, resulting in 7% to 10% of all early deaths. Enthusiasm for early surgery is tempered by the 7% to 20% operative mortality (1). Two studies have demonstrated that close observation is possible without substantial mortality. Long-term follow-up of patients who did not undergo operation because of associated medical conditions, small pseu-

doaneurysm, or refusal of surgery revealed that mortality was related to the primary underlying disease or cardiac dysfunction, not rupture (1,5). In the study by Yeo, 10 such patients were identified retrospectively and none died of acute cardiac rupture (1).

ECHOCARDIOGRAPHY

Transesophageal echocardiography demonstrates the unique two-dimensional characteristics of pseudoaneurysms, which include a sharp demarcation of the endocardial image at the site of the pseudoaneurysm communication with the LV cavity and the presence of a relatively narrow orifice when compared with the maximum diameter of the pseudoaneurysm's fundus. This small neck rarely exceeds half the maximum parallel internal diameter of aneurysm sack (3). There is decreasing LV cavity size in systole while the false aneurysm gradually expands. As in our patient, it is not uncommon to see spontaneous echo contrast or thrombus within the pseudoaneurysm cavity (Fig. 27.4). Doppler echocardiography has proven to be useful in difficult-to-diagnosis cases and will demonstrate bidirectional flow of blood between the pseudoaneurysm and the LV (Fig. 27.5). One also may see marked variation in maximal Doppler flow velocity throughout the respiratory cycle, with inspiration causing a significant increase in the maximum flow velocity. Color Doppler echocardiography will usually demonstrate systolic, mosaic jets exiting the LV and entering the pseudoaneurysm cavity, as was seen in our example (10–12). In diastole this mosaic pattern will occur within the LV, confirming turbulent ebb and flow of blood in and out of the pseudoaneurysm. If, after echocardiography, the diagnosis is still within doubt, angiography, computed tomography, and magnetic resonance imaging can be used to establish the diagnosis.

KEY POINTS

- A pseudoaneurysm contains fibrous pericardial tissue with no myocardial elements.
- Almost half of patients with pseudoaneurysms are asymptomatic at presentation.
- Following a myocardial infarction, pseudoaneurysms are predominantly located in the inferior or posterior wall.
- Two-dimensional echocardiographic manifestations of pseudoaneurysms include a narrow orifice, expansion during systole, and the presence of spontaneous echo contrast or thrombus.

PART II: TRAUMA
Pulmonary Embolism with Paradoxic Embolism
Scott T. Reeves

It has been estimated that approximately 10% of victims of major blunt chest trauma sustain cardiac or aortic injuries. Most of these individuals die at the scene. However, an increasing number of patients are arriving at emergency trauma centers secondary to improvement of pre-hospital care, more aggressive resuscitation in the field, and rapid transport to such units (13–16). Trauma physicians are gaining increased awareness that the detection of cardiovascular injuries in patients who have sustained blunt chest trauma is difficult. These injuries often go undetected due to the requirement to stabilize more obvious injuries such as splenic and liver lacerations and long bone or pelvic fractures.

Due to its noninvasiveness, transthoracic echocardiography (TTE) has been used as a screening tool for patients with blunt chest trauma. Unfortunately, TTE provides suboptimal images in up to 60% of patients and usually cannot adequately evaluate areas of concern such as the thoracic aorta. The explanations given for suboptimal image acquisition include the patient being on mechanical ventilation, the presence of subcutaneous emphysema or pneumomediastinum, the presence of multiple chest or abdominal tubes, and obesity (15,16). Transesophageal echocardiography, due to its ability to use a higher frequency transducer that provides better anatomic resolution and the shorter distance from the esophagus to areas of interest, has emerged as a superior method for evaluating patients with significant chest trauma (17).

CASE REPORT

A 35-year-old man sustained severe blunt chest and pelvic trauma following a head-on motor vehicle accident involving a tree. The patient's injuries included multiple facial fractures, a complex pelvic fracture, bilateral femur fractures, and bilateral pulmonary contusions.

Following his initial stabilization, the intubated patient was transferred to the surgical trauma intensive care unit and remained relatively stable for the first 48 hours. The patient then experienced progressively increasing oxygen requirements. Arterial blood gas analysis demonstrated a pH of 7.46, partial pressure of arterial oxygen (PaO_2) of 50, and partial pressure of arterial carbon dioxide ($PaCO_2$) of 34. Increasing the fraction inspired FiO_2 to 100% resulted in a minimum increase in PaO_2. Increasing positive end-expiratory pressure (PEEP) worsened the hypoxemia. The patient's

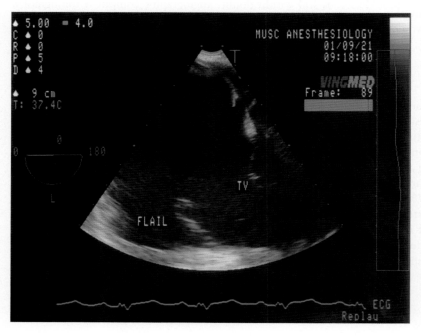

FIGURE 27.11. Image demonstrating rupture and flail of the anterior papillary muscle of the tricuspid valve (*TV*). Note the dilated right ventricle and thinning of the anterior wall indicative of a myocardial contusion.

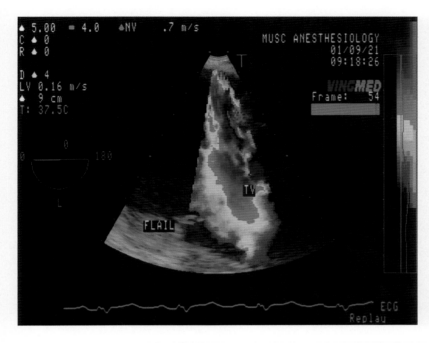

FIGURE 27.12. Color flow Doppler image of Fig. 27.11 demonstrating severe tricuspid regurgitation. *TV,* tricuspid valve.

vital signs and hemodynamic perimeters were as follows: pulse 110 beats/min, arterial blood pressure 85/40 mm Hg, respiratory rate 18 breaths/min, temperature 101.8°F, pulmonary artery pressure (PAP) 30/23 mm Hg, central venous pressure 16 mm Hg, and cordine output (C.O.) 2.3 L/min.

The patient underwent an urgent transthoracic echocardiogram to help delineate his refractory hypoxemia and hypotension. The examination was technically difficult secondary to his bilateral pulmonary contusions and chest tubes, resulting in inadequate acoustic ultrasound windows. Transesophageal echocardiography was immediately performed and demonstrated a profoundly dilated right

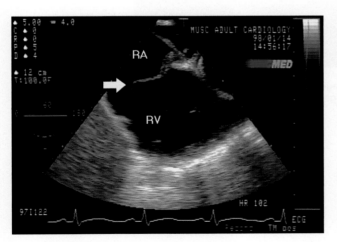

FIGURE 27.13. The arrow points to a paradoxic embolism traversing a patent foramen ovale. Note thrombus in left atrium. *RA,* right atrium; *RV,* right ventricle.

ventricle with hypokinesis of the anterior wall (Fig. 27.11). The tricuspid valve demonstrated a flailing anterior leaflet secondary to papillary muscle rupture with resulting severe tricuspid regurgitation (Fig. 27.12). The patient had right-to-left shunting with a paradoxic embolism involving a patent foramen ovale (PFO) (Fig. 27.13). Right-to-left shunting was further enhanced due to the presence of a sinus venous atrial septal defect (ASD) (Fig. 27.14).

Due to the right-to-left shunting and acute volume overload nature of the right ventricle and right atrium (RA), nitroglycerin was started in an attempt to decrease preload and decrease right-sided filling pressures. Dobutamine was initiated in an attempt to increase cardiac output. The patient's PEEP was decreased from 15 to 0 mm Hg. These maneuvers resulted in a gradual improvement in the patient's cardiac performance and oxygenation, with the cardiac output increasing to 3.5 L per minute and the oxygen saturation SpO_2 increasing to 94%.

This case highlights the multitude of cardiac injuries that are possible within a single patient following blunt chest trauma. Myocardial contusion, ruptured papillary muscles, right-to-left cardiac shunts, and pulmonary embolism are discussed below.

MYOCARDIAL CONTUSION

Scientific Principles

Due to its close proximity to the sternum, the right ventricle is most vulnerable to cardiac contusion. Cardiac contusion is often asymptomatic and frequently undiagnosed. Most echocardiographic studies have indicated an incidence

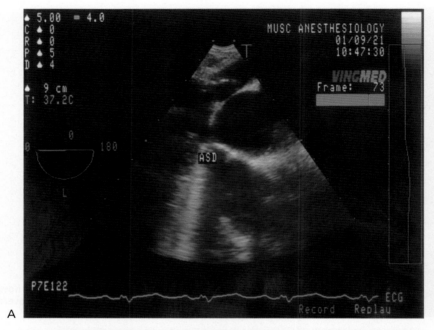

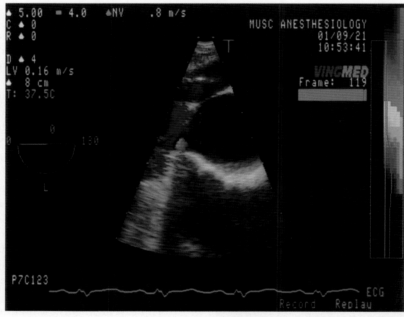

FIGURE 27.14. A: Two-dimensional Doppler image demonstrating a small sinus venosis atrial septal defect. **B:** Color flow Doppler echocardiography through the defect. *ASD,* atrial septal defect.

of right ventricular contusion of 25% to 35% (18–20). In a multicenter prospective trial involving 117 patients, the right ventricle was affected in 32%, the LV in 15%, and both ventricles in 5% of patients (21).

Echocardiography

Pandian et al., in an acute myocardial contusion canine model of blunt chest trauma, demonstrated that echo manifestations of myocardial contusion consist of (a) increased ventricular wall echocardiographic brightness, (b) increased diastolic wall thickness, and (c) impaired regional wall systolic function (22). Clinically, myocardial contusion echo manifestations include the presence of a wall motion abnormality or dilatation of chambers involving either or both ventricles following blunt chest trauma in the absence of a transmural myocardial infarction on ECG (23,24). Figure 27.11 demonstrates a profoundly dilated right ventricle with akinesis of the anterior wall.

TRICUSPID VALVE INJURY/PAPILLARY MUSCLE RUPTURE

Scientific Principles

The most common valve injured owing to blunt chest trauma is the aortic valve, followed by the mitral and then tricuspid valves. The pulmonic valve is infrequently involved. The proposed mechanism for aortic valve involvement deals with the high pressures generated in the aorta and the LV during compressive chest trauma, especially if it occurs during the cardiac cycle, when both the aortic and mitral valves are closed, creating a "blowout" type injury. In addition, the

shearing forces that accompany abrupt deceleration, such as occurs when the chest hits the steering wheel during an automobile accident, also may cause tearing of the aortic valve cusps or cracking of the annulus.

Figures 27.11 and 27.12 demonstrate traumatic disruption of the anterior leaflet of the tricuspid valve resulting in severe tricuspid regurgitation. It is believed that the patient sustained his injury while the tricuspid valve was closed and the right ventricle was maximally distended, resulting in acute papillary muscle rupture.

Echocardiography

The amount of tricuspid regurgitation (TR) can be quantified in the same fashion as performed for mitral insufficiency. Mild TR encompasses less than 33%, moderate 33% to 66%, and severe over 66% of the area of the RA. Severe tricuspid regurgitation also may generate flow reversal during systole in the hepatic veins (Fig. 27.15). It is important to remember that the maximum regurgitant velocity obtained by pulsed- or continuous-wave Doppler reflects the maximum pressure differences across the tricuspid valve and not the severity of tricuspid regurgitation (25).

PULMONARY EMBOLISM WITH A PARADOXIC EMBOLISM

Scientific Principles

Blunt chest trauma can cause severe hypoxemia, usually secondary to a right-to-left shunt within the pulmonary system (i.e., intrapulmonary functional shunt). An intrapulmonary functional shunt can be caused by cardiogenic or

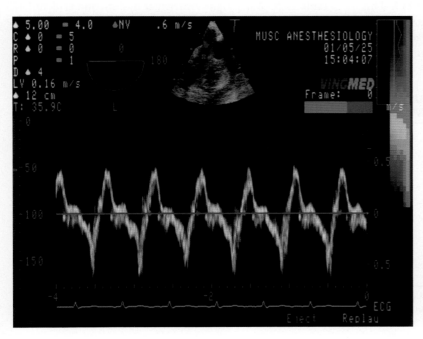

FIGURE 27.15. Continuous-wave Doppler image of hepatic venous flow. Note the profound flow away from the transducer immediately following the QRS complex. This represents profound systolic flow reversal precipitated by the patient's severe tricuspid regurgitation.

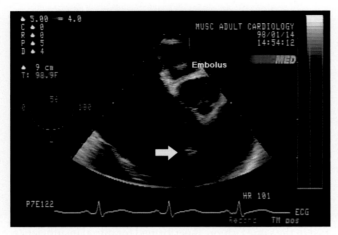

FIGURE 27.16. Two-dimensional Doppler image demonstrating a pulmonary embolism occupying the right ventricular outflow tract (*arrow*). Note the paradoxic embolism within the left atrium (Embolus).

noncardiogenic pulmonary edema, pneumonia, pulmonary embolism, and pulmonary contusion. Fortunately most of these diagnoses can be at least suspected from chest x-ray evaluations. The most common cardiac shunt is secondary to an acute increase in RA pressures, forcing a PFO to open. This is frequently encountered during mechanical ventilation with the use of high PEEP. If one recalls fetal development, oxygenated placental blood flows from the RA across the foramen ovale, into the LA, and onto the systemic circulation. In most individuals this communication fuses shortly after birth. However, a probe PFO has been demonstrated in up to 30% of autopsy patients (25).

In patients with a PFO, the acute elevation in RA pressures that result following a significant pulmonary embolism can precipitate right-to-left shunting across the PFO. This patient's clinical course was not only complicated by a PFO resulting in right-to-left shunting, but also a paradoxic embolus crossing the foramen ovale. Figure 27.16 demonstrates

a pulmonary embolism present in the right ventricular outflow tract. Figure 27.13 is an enhanced view demonstrating thrombus propagating across a PFO.

The incidence of paradoxic embolism following a pulmonary embolism in a patient known to have a PFO is 16%. Aboyans demonstrated in a recent review of 43 published cases of entrapped thrombus through a PFO, that only 47% had clear documentation of a left-sided paradoxic embolism at initial onset of symptoms (Table 27.3) (26).

Konstantinides demonstrated that a right-to-left shunt through a PFO in patients with pulmonary embolism is associated with a mortality rate of 33% compared to 14% without a PFO. Those patients also have significantly higher incidences of ischemic stroke (13%) and peripheral arterial embolism (15%) (27). The magnitude of the right-to-left shunt in this case was increased as a result of an increased RA pressure secondary to severe tricuspid valve regurgitation, and, hence, increased flow through the PFO and the presence of a coexisting sinus venosus ASD.

Treatment strategies consist of anticoagulation, surgery, or thrombolysis. Table 27.4 summarizes the treatment strategies and their outcomes in patients. In our patient, secondary to his long bone and pelvic fractures, thrombolytic therapy was not an option. The patient underwent placement of a Greenfield filter and received systemic heparin.

Echocardiography

Transthoracic echocardiography should be used as an initial rapid diagnostic test in patients suspected of having a pulmonary embolism. Four distinct findings may be found during this initial TTE evaluation and are summarized in Table 27.5. When right ventricular dysfunction is identified in the initial TTE evaluation, Pruszczyk has proposed that patients have three of the following five criteria of right ventricular pressure overload in order to proceed to TEE. They

TABLE 27.3. CLINICAL SEQUELAE OF PATIENTS WITH ENTRAPPED EMBOLUS THROUGH A PATENT FORAMEN OVALE

Clinical Patterns	% of Patients (N = 40)	Embolic Location	No. of Patients
Pulmonary embolism alone	53%	None	
Pulmonary embolism and	40%	Cerebral	8
paradoxical embolism		Limb	5
		Limb and visceral	1
		Coronary	1
		Visceral	1
Paradoxical embolism alone	7%	Cerebral	1
		Limb	1
		Cerebral and limb	1

Modified from Aboyans V, Lacroix P, Ostyn E, et al. Diagnosis and management of entrapped embolus through a patent foramen ovale. *Eur J Cardiothorac Surg* 1998;14:627–628.

TABLE 27.4. TREATMENT STRATEGIES FOR ENTRAPPED EMBOLUS WITH OUTCOME

Treatments	No. of Cases	Outcome (Alive/Dead)
Anticoagulation	11	7/4
Surgery	22	19/3
Thrombocysis	6	5/1

Modified from Aboyans V, Lacroix P, Ostyn E, et al. Diagnosis and management of entrapped embolus through a patent foramen ovale. *Eur J Cardiothorac Surg* 1998;14:624–628.

include: (a) a peak velocity of tricuspid valve insufficiency corresponding to a right ventricular to a RA pressure gradient of more than 30 mm Hg; (b) an enlargement of the diameter of the right ventricle of more than 27 mm measured in the peristernal long axis; (c) a shortened (<80 msec) pulmonary ejection acceleration time measured at the right ventricular outflow track; (d) flattening of the interventricular septum; and (e) distension of the inferior vena cava of greater than 20 mm in diameter. If three of these five criteria are met, then TEE should be performed immediately at the bedside (28).

In contrast to TTE, TEE allows direct visualization of emboli in the right ventricular outflow tract and right main pulmonary artery up to the point of the interlobar trunks and lobar arteries. The left main pulmonary artery may be difficult to image secondary to its location anterior to the left main bronchus but can be imaged in the short-axis aortic arch view. When TEE is performed, the echocardiographer is searching for direct evidence of thrombus. An unequivocal thrombus must have distinct borders that can be imaged in more than one plane. If the thrombus protrudes into the arterial lumen or has distinct movement separate from the vascular wall and blood flow, the echocardiographer can be comfortable with the diagnosis of pulmonary embolism.

The echocardiographic appearance of a paradoxic embolism is similar to those discussed for pulmonary embolism. Figure 27.13 demonstrates a large thrombus passing from the RA through a PFO into the LA (paradoxic embolism). However, the ability to detect a PFO without a thrombus is

TABLE 27.5. TRANSTHORACIC ECHOCARDIOGRAPHIC POSSIBILITIES IN A PATIENT SUSPECTED OF HAVING A PULMONARY EMBOLISM

Normal examination, thereby making the possibility of acute pulmonary embolism extremely unlikely.
Some other diagnosis other than pulmonary embolism.
Right heart thrombus that confirms the diagnosis of pulmonary embolism.
Findings of right ventricular dysfunction, which would support a diagnosis of pulmonary embolism and if it were absent, would make hemodynamically significant pulmonary embolism extremely unlikely.

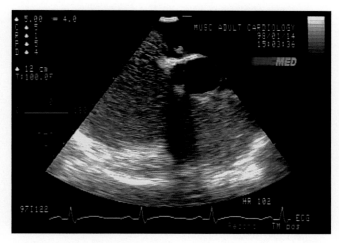

FIGURE 27.17. Mid-esophageal four-chamber view immediately following agitated saline intravenous contrast injection with complete opacification of the right atrium and ventricle. The thrombus completely occludes the foramen, as evidenced by the lack of contrast within the left atrium.

possible with TEE and color flow Doppler in less than 10% of cases. Using an intravenous echo contrast material such as agitated saline can enhance detection of a PFO (28). As demonstrated in Fig. 27.17, complete opacification of the right-sided chambers is necessary to optimize the sensitivity of this diagnostic maneuver. The appearance of bright echo contrast in the LA within one to three beats is diagnostic. By transiently increasing RA pressures during the contrast injection as occurs with a Valsalva maneuver, a PFO can be detected in excess of 25% of patients (29). In this case, the patient had complete opacification of the RA and ventricle without contrast appearing in the LA. The paradoxic embolism was felt to have completely occluded the PFO, resulting in a negative study.

KEY POINTS

Part II

- Transesophageal echocardiography is superior to TTE in the evaluation of patients with significant blunt chest trauma.
- Right ventricular contusion can be present in excess of 30% of patients with blunt chest trauma.
- The aortic valve is the most frequently injured valve following blunt trauma.
- Transthoracic echocardiography is a useful screening test for acute pulmonary embolism in the unstable intensive care unit patient. If findings of right ventricular pressure overload are present, a TEE should be performed immediately.
- Paradoxic embolism occurs frequently in patients with pulmonary embolism and a PFO.

REFERENCES

1. Yeo TC, Malouf JF, Oh JK, et al. Clinical profile and outcome in 52 patients with cardiac pseudoaneurysm. *Ann Intern Med* 1998;128:299–305.
2. Ezzat MA, Abdelmeguid I, Leclerc D, et al. Left ventricular pseudoaneurysm associated with mitral regurgitation. *Ann Thorac Surg* 1992;53:504–506.
3. Saner HE, Asinger RW, Daniel JA, et al. Two-dimensional echocardiographic identification of left ventricular pseudoaneurysm. *Am Heart J* 1986;5:977–985.
4. Fehske W, Kranidis A, Kirchhoff PG, et al. Diagnosis of a posterior left ventricular pseudoaneurysm by multiplane transesophageal echocardiography. *J Clin Ultrasound* 1995;23:59–62.
5. Natarajan MK, Salerno TA, Burke B, et al. Chronic false aneurysms of the left ventricle: management revisited. *Can J Cardiol* 1994;10:927–931.
6. Mickleborough LL, Carson S, Ivanov J. Repair of dyskinetic or akinetic left ventricular aneurysm: results obtained with a modified linear closure. *J Thorac Cardiovasc Surg* 2001;121:675–682.
7. De Paulis R, Zeitani J, Bognolo G, et al. Left ventricular pseudoaneurysm and mitral valve regurgitation. *J Cardiovasc Surg* 1990;40:679–681.
8. Prêtre R, Linka A, Jenni R, et al. Surgical treatment of acquired left ventricular pseudoaneurysms. *Ann Thorac Surg* 2000;70:553–557.
9. Van Tassel RA, Edwards JE. Rupture of heart complicating myocardial infarction. *Chest* 1972;61:104–116.
10. Sutherland GR, Smyllie JH, Roelandt JRTC. Advantages of colour flow imaging in the diagnosis of left ventricular pseudoaneurysm. *Br Heart J* 1989;61:59–64.
11. Roelandt JRTC, Sutherland GR, Yoshida K, et al. Improved diagnosis and characterization of left ventricular pseudoaneurysm by Doppler color flow imaging. *J Am Coll Cardiol* 1988;12:807–811.
12. Olalla JJ, Vazquez de Prada JA, Duran RM, et al. Color Doppler diagnosis of left ventricular pseudoaneurysm. *Chest* 1988;94:443–444.
13. Editorial. Traumatic injury of the heart. *Lancet* 1990;336:1287–1289.
14. LoCicero J, Mattox KL. Epidemiology of chest trauma. *Surg Clin North Am* 1989;69:15–19.
15. Krasna MJ, Flancbaum MJ. Blunt chest trauma: clinical manifestations and management. *Semin Thorac Cardiovasc Surg* 1992;4:192–202.
16. Chirillo F, Oscar T, Cavarzerani A, et al. Usefulness of transthoracic and transesophageal echocardiography in recognition and management of cardiovascular injuries after blunt chest trauma. *Heart* 1996;75:301–306.
17. Johnson SB, Kearney PA, Smith MD. Echocardiography in the evaluation of thoracic trauma. *Surg Clin North Am* 1995;75(2):193–205.
18. Symbas PN. Traumatic heart disease. *Curr Probl Cardiol* 1991;537–582.
19. Spangenthal EJ, Sekovski B, Bhayana JN, et al. Traumatic left ventricular papillary muscle rupture: the role of transesophageal echocardiography in diagnosis and surgical management. *J Am Soc Echocardiogr* 1993;6:536–538.
20. Ellis JE, Bender EM. Intraoperative transesophageal echocardiography in blunt trauma. *J Cardiothorac Vasc Anesth* 1991;5:373–376.
21. Garcia-Fernandez MA, Lopez-Perez JM, Perez-Castellano N, et al. Role of transesophageal echocardiography in the assessment of patients with blunt chest trauma: correlation of echocardiographic findings with the electrocardiogram and creatine kinase monoclonal antibody measurements. *Am Heart J* 1998;135:476–481.
22. Pandian NG, Skorton DJ, Doty DB. Immediate diagnosis of acute myocardial contusion by two-dimensional echocardiography: studies in a canine model of blunt chest trauma. *J Am Coll Cardiol* 1983;2:488–496.
23. Weiss RL, Brier JA, O'Connor W, et al. The usefulness of transesophageal echocardiography in diagnosing cardiac contusions. *Chest* 1996;109:73–77.
24. O'Connor C. Chest trauma: the role of transesophageal echocardiography. *J Clin Anesth* 1996;8:605–613.
25. Otto CM, ed. *Textbook of clinical echocardiography,* 2nd ed, Philadelphia: WB Saunders, 2000:295–296, 367–368.
26. Aboyans V, Lacroix P, Ostyn E, et al. Diagnosis and management of entrapped embolism through a patent foramen ovale. *Eur J Cardiothorac Surg* 1998;14:624–628.
27. Konstantinides S, Geibel A, Kasper W, et al. Patent foramen ovale is an important predictor of adverse outcome in patients with major pulmonary embolism. *Circulation* 1998;97:1946–1951.
28. Konstadt SN, Louie EK, Rao TLK, et al. Intraoperative detection of patent foramen ovale by transesophageal echocardiography. *Anesthesiology* 1991;74(2):212–216.
29. Pruszczyk A, Torbicki A, Kuch-Wocial A, et al. Diagnostic value of transesophageal echocardiography in suspected haemodynamically significant pulmonary embolism. *Heart* 2001;85:628–634.

LUNG TRANSPLANTATION

STEVEN N. KONSTADT

The technique of lung transplantation involves a relatively new set of surgical procedures that have provided another therapeutic option for patients with end-stage lung disease. For anesthesiologists, these patients pose arguably the biggest challenge for providing safe perioperative care. There are several reasons why these patients are difficult to manage. First, their end-stage lung disease can make perioperative oxygenation and ventilation extremely difficult. At the time of anesthesia induction or during the transplantation procedure, it may be necessary to place the patient in a position that severely compromises oxygenation or ventilation. In addition, to eliminate the need for cardiopulmonary bypass and its attendant complications, or just to shorten its duration, it sometimes is necessary to perform one-lung ventilation for an extended period on a patient who had trouble breathing with two lungs. Second, even in the absence of primary cardiac disease, end-stage lung disease frequently precipitates pulmonary hypertension and significant right ventricular (RV) dysfunction. Third, problems in oxygenation can occur during the immediate postoperative period even after a successful transplantation. Some of these problems are self-limited and require only positive-pressure ventilation and positive end-expiratory pressure. In other cases, the presence of anatomic problems necessitates reoperation. For example, reoperation may be required to close a patent foramen ovale with significant right-to-left shunting, to revise a stenotic pulmonary arterial or venous anastomosis, or to remove an obstructing clot. Thus, the three main clinical issues for anesthesiologists are perioperative oxygenation and ventilation, RV contraction and valve function, and differential diagnosis of posttransplantation hypoxia. This chapter focuses on the application of intraoperative echocardiography in the last two areas.

SCIENTIFIC PRINCIPLES

This section addresses the anatomy, physiology, and pathophysiology of the key cardiovascular structures.

Right Ventricle

The RV is a thin-walled, irregular, crescent-shaped structure. Normally it functions as a low-pressure, high-volume pump. Contraction and ejection of the RV begins before that of the left ventricle, and it has its own complex pattern of ejection. There is a small degree of ejection as a result of shortening across the minor axis, but most ejection is a result of shortening along the major axis of the heart. Further ejection is achieved through a wringing action caused by left ventricular shortening in the minor axis of the heart.

Because of its thin-walled architecture, the RV is extremely sensitive to increases in afterload, and severe, acute increases can result in RV failure. The usual adaptive response to a chronic pressure overload is RV thickening, but dilatation also can occur. Ischemia and cardiomyopathy are other common causes of RV dysfunction, and usually are accompanied by ventricular enlargement.

Antegrade ejection of blood into the pulmonary vasculature is dependent on the competence of the tricuspid and pulmonic valves. In comparison with their counterparts on the left side of the heart, these valves are less fibrous and more sensitive to the effects of increased intracavitary pressure (1). Increased intracavitary pressure can result in leaflet prolapse or annular dilatation with poor coaptation of the leaflets. Either of these alterations can lead to valvular incompetence.

Interatrial Septum

The interatrial septum is a blade-shaped structure located in the posteroinferior portion of the medial wall of the right atrium (RA). It extends forward obliquely from right to left and consists of a concave anterior margin, a convex posterior margin, and an inferior margin near the mitral annulus. Within the septum is the fossa ovalis; it comprises about 28% of the septal area (2). The septum primum is a thin

S. N. Konstadt: Department of Anesthesiology, Division of Cardiothoracic Anesthesia, The Mount Sinai Medical Center, New York, New York.

membrane that is closely applied to the left atrial (LA) side of the septum and acts as a flap valve.

Pulmonary Vasculature

The main pulmonary artery courses in a cephalad direction for about 4 cm, then bifurcates at a 90 degree angle into the right and left pulmonary arteries. After coursing through the lungs, the blood returns to the LA through the four pulmonary veins: the right upper, right lower, left upper, and left lower.

CASE REPORT

A 43-year-old woman with end-stage lung disease secondary to sarcoidosis was scheduled for an emergency single-lung transplantation. Sarcoidosis first developed 10 years before and, despite steroid therapy, progressed to end-stage lung disease with dyspnea at rest and the need for supplemental oxygen. The patient had no other known medical problems.

On arrival to the operating room, the patient was sitting upright with a nasal cannula in place providing oxygen at 4 L/min. Her respiratory rate was 26 breaths per minute, and she appeared to be in mild distress. On auscultation, rhonchi were noted over both lung fields.

Preoperative laboratory studies revealed the following results. A chest radiograph showed enlarged right-sided cardiac structures, hilar adenopathy, and increased interstitial markings. An electrocardiogram revealed normal sinus rhythm at 95 beats/min, RV hypertrophy, and right bundle branch block. Transthoracic echocardiography demonstrated RV hypertrophy, RA dilatation, an estimated RV systolic pressure of 55 mm Hg, and mild to moderate tricuspid and pulmonic regurgitation. Cardiac catheterization was performed and showed normal coronary arteries, a pulmonary artery pressure of 50/20 with a mean of 30 mm Hg, a left ventricular pressure of 90/4 mm Hg, and a Fick cardiac output of 4.3 L/min. Gated blood pool scanning revealed RV, RA, and pulmonary arterial enlargement, as well as paradoxic septal motion consistent with RV overload. The left ventricular ejection fraction was 36%.

LOGISTICS AND CONTRIBUTION OF INTRAOPERATIVE ECHOCARDIOGRAPHY

This section describes the actual use of intraoperative echocardiography in this case. The discussion includes the necessary scanning techniques, views, and modalities. The key problems addressed are the evaluation of RV function and the differential diagnosis of perioperative hypoxemia. Guidelines for intraoperative decision making also are presented.

Right Ventricular Function

In contrast to the symmetric left ventricle, the complex geometry and physiology of the RV prevents simple direct assessment of RV function. Because of this complexity, numerous echocardiographic methods have been developed to evaluate RV function. These methods can be divided into geometry-dependent and geometry-independent techniques. The measures of RV function can be divided further into qualitative and quantitative indices. Although most research applications require quantitative indices, most clinical questions can be answered with qualitative measures.

The standard geometry-dependent technique is planimetry of RV end-diastolic and end-systolic dimensions. This evaluation can be performed using a mid-esophageal (ME) four-chamber view of the RV (Fig. 28.1). In normal healthy volunteers, the mean long-axis length of the RV is 2.8 cm/m² at end-diastole and 2.3 cm/m² at end-systole (3). In the same imaging plane, the normal end-diastolic width is 1.6 cm/m² and the normal end-systolic width is 1 cm/m². Transgastric middle short-axis (SAX) images also can be obtained (Fig. 28.2). The intracavitary areas can be traced manually or defined with an automatic border detection system. For more precise determination of RV volume, a combination of long- and short-axis views of the RV can be used to create a crescenteric model of the RV. In a study using this methodology in fixed hearts, a very close correlation ($r = 0.96$) with the actual volume as measured by silicone cast displacement was found (4). Although the results of this study appear promising, in clinical situations this type of modeling and the necessary calculations are impractical. Another approach to determining the RV volume is to measure the total cardiac volume using a combination of long- and short-axis views and then to subtract the left ventricular volume (5). Although a close correlation ($r = 0.935$) with RV volume as determined by radionuclide ventriculography has been demonstrated, this approach also is relatively complicated and may not be suited to use in the operating room.

Regardless of the geometry-dependent measure used to evaluate the RV, the irregularity of the anatomy makes comparison of serial measurements difficult. The transesophageal echocardiography (TEE) probe must be positioned carefully to ensure that the same tomographic plane is obtained on each image. Changes in patient position, ventilatory techniques, and surgical interventions such as pericardiectomy can make it impossible to obtain identical tomographic images, introducing error. Despite these potential problems, reported rates of intraobserver and interobserver variability for these techniques have been less than 8% and 10%, respectively (6).

To avoid these intricate calculations and the problems of complex geometry, Kaul and colleagues (7) proposed the use of tricuspid annular plane systolic excursion to estimate RV function. Based on the concept that most RV ejection is caused by contraction in the long axis, they found a close

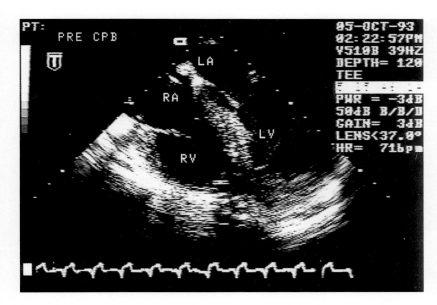

FIGURE 28.1. Mid-esophageal four-chamber, long-axis view of the heart. *RA,* right atrium; *LA,* left atrium; *RV,* right ventricle; *LV,* left ventricle. (With a multiplane probe, this view would be obtained at 0–20 degrees).

correlation between tricuspid annular plane systolic excursion and the radionuclide-determined RV ejection fraction. Proper use of this technique requires careful image orientation to visualize the free-wall septal junction in both end-diastole and end-systole.

Alternatively, there are several qualitative measures of RV function. The RV end-diastolic and end-systolic areas can be assessed visually, and the ejection fraction then can be estimated. The use of paradoxic septal curvature to diagnose acute RV function also has been described (8). Normally, the pressure is lower in the RV than in the left ventricle, so the septum bulges from the left to the right. In patients with RV failure, high right-sided pressure causes the septum to bulge from the right to the left. The timing of the bulge can provide

insight into the mechanism of the RV failure (9). In patients with RV pressure overload, the septal shift occurs at end-systole and early diastole. Conversely, RV volume overload results in late diastolic septal shift.

Doppler echocardiography can be used to provide additional geometry-independent indices of RV function. In situations where right heart catheterization is not possible, continuous-wave Doppler evaluation can be used to estimate the peak pulmonary systolic pressure. Depending on the orientation of the heart, this estimation can be performed in either the ME four-chamber view or the ME RV inflow–outflow view of the heart. The view with the closer alignment of the jet and Doppler beam should be chosen (Fig. 28.3). Color flow imaging is performed to localize the tricuspid

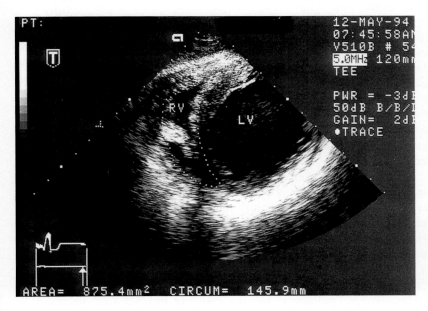

FIGURE 28.2. Transgastric middle short-axis view of the right ventricle (*RV*). The dotted lines define the endocardial border, and the intraventricular area is calculated by the internal analysis software. *LV,* left ventricle. (With a multiplane probe, this view would be obtained at 0 degrees.)

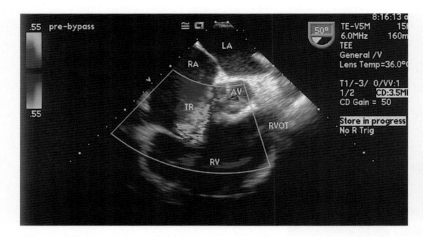

FIGURE 28.3. Mid-esophageal right ventricular (*RV*) inflow–outflow view (*TV*, tricuspid valve). *RA,* right atrium; *LA,* left atrium; *RVOT,* right ventricular outflow tract; *AV,* aortic valve. Note the color flow demonstration of mild aortic insufficiency and severe tricuspid regurgitation.

regurgitation jet (most patients have at least a trivial tricuspid regurgitation jet). The continuous-wave Doppler cursor is positioned on the jet and the peak velocity is noted. The peak pulmonary artery pressure then is calculated using the following formula:

$$\text{Peak pulmonary arterial pressure} = 4$$
$$(\text{peak velocity})^2 + \text{central venous pressure}$$

In some patients, the continuous-wave Doppler signal cannot be visualized adequately. In these cases, the signal can be enhanced by the intravenous injection of a sonicated echocardiographic contrast agent (10).

Another important use of spectral Doppler imaging is in the assessment of pulmonary artery blood flow. In this application, an ME ascending aorta SAX view of the great vessels is obtained (Fig. 28.4). In this view, pulmonary ejection is parallel to the Doppler beam and is easily interrogated. This view is used most often to measure cardiac output (11), but also can be used to detect pulmonic insufficiency or to assess RV ejection. The maximum acceleration of blood in the pulmonary artery can be used as an index of RV ejection (12). The maximum acceleration of pulmonary blood flow is measured easily using the internal calculation software of most clinically used echocardiographic instruments. Changes in the maximum acceleration have been shown to correlate with changes in the thermodilution RV ejection fraction (13). Similar data, obtained with an intravascular probe, have been used in patients undergoing lung transplantation (14). The acceleration data were used in determining the need for cardiopulmonary bypass.

In patients with moderate and severe pulmonary hypertension, lung transplantation results in decreases in mean pulmonary artery pressure, right ventricular end-diastolic area (RVEDA), right ventricular end-systolic (RVESA), and septal flattening (15). However, not every patient improves. Persistent RV failure in the posttransplantation period is caused most commonly by pressure overload of the RV resulting from increased pulmonary vascular resistance. However,

anatomic causes of RV overload must be excluded. In patients with severe hypertrophy of the RV, the dramatic decrease in pulmonary vascular resistance that occurs immediately after lung transplantation can precipitate right ventricular outflow tract (RVOT) obstruction (16). This possibility is evaluated best in the ME RV inflow–outflow view and the transgastric (TG) RVOT view. In addition to using two-dimensional scanning to define the anatomy, color flow mapping can be used to detect turbulence and, in the TG view, continuous-wave Doppler can be used to measure the gradient across the RVOT (Fig. 28.5).

Tricuspid Valve Function

As mentioned earlier, tricuspid jets can be seen in both the transverse and longitudinal planes. It is important to determine the severity of tricuspid regurgitation because this affects the assessment of RV function when ejection phase indices of contraction, such as ejection fraction, are used. If significant regurgitation is present, even a normal RV ejection fraction could accompany severe RV dysfunction. One grading system for tricuspid regurgitation is based on the ratio of the jet area to the RA area: grade I is less than 15%, grade II is less than 30%, grade III is less than 60%, and grade IV is more than 60% (Fig. 28.6).

DIFFERENTIAL DIAGNOSIS OF HYPOXEMIA

Although the most common cause of early postoperative hypoxemia is donor organ malfunction due to ischemia and reperfusion injury, there also are several important potential anatomic causes of hypoxemia. These possibilities fall into two categories: obstruction to normal pulmonary blood flow, and intracardiac shunting at the atrial or ventricular level. Normally, an intracardiac defect results in predominantly left-to-right blood flow, but in the presence of increased pulmonary vascular resistance and high right-sided cardiac

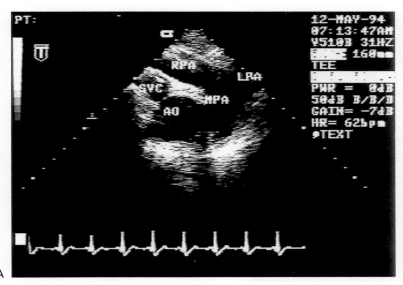

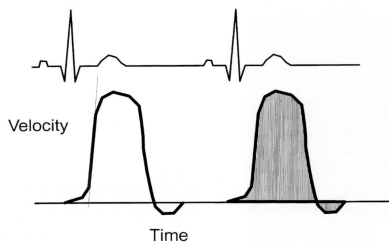

FIGURE 28.4. A: Mid-esophageal ascending aortic short-axis view. *AO,* aorta; *SVC,* superior vena cava; *RPA,* right pulmonary artery; *LPA,* left pulmonary artery; *MPA,* main pulmonary artery. **B:** Diagrammatic representation of the pulmonary artery pulsed-wave Doppler recording of blood flow. In the first velocity profile, the tangent to the upstroke of the velocity recording defines the acceleration of blood flow; in the second velocity profile, the shaded area defines the flow velocity integral. (With a multiplane probe, this view would be obtained at 0 degrees.)

pressures, the defect is more likely to result in right-to-left blood flow and hypoxemia.

Interatrial Septum

The competence of the interatrial septum is an important function that can be evaluated by TEE. Incompetence can be caused by either an atrial septal defect or a patent foramen ovale. Depending on their location, atrial septal defects are classified as primum, secundum, or sinus venosus defects (see Chapter 13). Primum and secundum defects can be visualized in both the ME four-chamber and bicaval views, but sinus venosus defects are visualized best in the bicaval view. All the defects appear as an area of echocardiographic dropout. Although there usually is a minimal pressure gradient across the defect, abnormal shunt flow across the defect often can be detected by either pulsed-wave or color Doppler techniques. Transesophageal echocardiography is an extremely sensitive means of detecting all three types of atrial septal defects,

and can be used to define associated anomalous pulmonary venous drainage (17). Echocardiographic measurement of defect size has been shown to correlate closely (horizontal width, $r = 0.92$; vertical length, $r = 0.85$) with surgical measurement (18). Patent foramen ovale is an anatomic variant that is found in about 25% of the population in autopsy studies and is a potential communication for paradoxic embolism (19). In anesthetized patients with venous air embolism, a patent foramen ovale is a risk factor for paradoxic air embolism, with potentially grave effects (20). In early studies, the frequency with which patent foramen ovale was detected did not approach the prevalence rate found in autopsy studies (21), and two instances of failed detection were reported (22). More recent work has demonstrated that contrast TEE can detect patent foramen ovale with an incidence similar to that found in autopsy studies (23).

The patency of the foramen ovale usually is evaluated by contrast echocardiography, but unenhanced two-dimensional scanning also can provide valuable information.

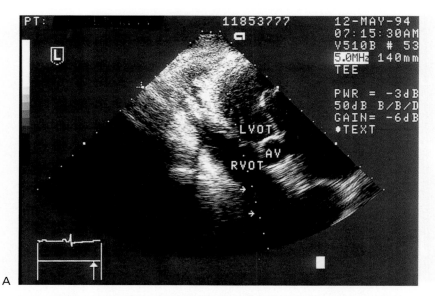

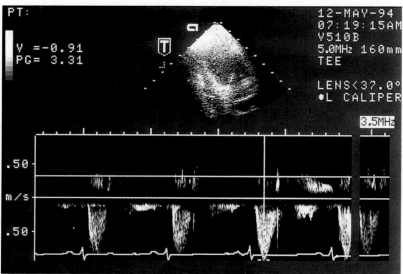

FIGURE 28.5. A: Transgastric right ventricular outflow tract (*RVOT*) view obtained by advancing the probe deep into the stomach and then anteroflexing the tip of the probe and rotating the probe to the right. The arrows point to the interrogating continuous-wave Doppler beam. *AV*, aortic valve; *LVOT*, left ventricular outflow tract. **B:** Continuous-wave Doppler recording from this view. (With a multiplane probe, this view would be obtained at 0 degrees.)

In the transverse plane, the size of the fossa ovalis and the mobility of its flap valve can be assessed. The presence of an actual atrial septal aneurysm or an elongated, highly mobile fossa ovalis indicates a higher likelihood of patency (24). These morphologic measurements, unexplained hypoxemia, or a neurologic event should prompt the performance of contrast echocardiography to confirm the presence of a patent foramen ovale. The use of a longitudinal scanning plane can facilitate direct visualization of the defect, which appears as a separation of the flap valve from the limbus of the fossa ovalis. Color flow mapping of the interatrial septum may be helpful, particularly in patients with markedly elevated LA pressure in whom left-to-right shunting across the defect can be demonstrated (Fig. 28.7). Although the alignment of the Doppler beam relative to the flow is nearly ideal, the low velocity of the flow can make detection difficult. To

optimize the detection of flow, the low-velocity filters must be set at their lowest settings and the velocity scale should be optimized to display low-velocity flow. One confounding variable is that apparent transseptal flow can be confused with flow from nearby venous structures (pulmonary veins and venae cavae).

Contrast echocardiography of the atria can be performed using the bicaval or modified ME four-chamber view. The keys to successful diagnosis are as follows:

1. A contrast agent should be selected that is large enough that it will not pass through the pulmonary capillaries, but small enough that it will not harm the patient if it enters the systemic circulation. Saline agitated by exchange between two syringes interconnected by a stopcock fulfills these criteria. Ultrasonicated solutions are not ideal

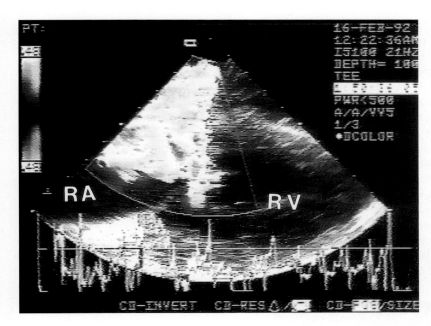

FIGURE 28.6. Severe tricuspid regurgitation seen in a modified mid-esophageal four-chamber view. Note the near-total filling of the right atrium (*RA*) by the regurgitant flow. *RV*, right ventricle. (With a multiplane probe, this view would be obtained at 0 degrees.)

because they can pass through the pulmonary circulation and appear in the left heart.

2. The contrast agent must be injected as a bolus into the venous system (either central or peripheral) such that complete opacification of the RA is achieved.

3. Instrument settings should be adjusted to minimize extraneous background echoes in the blood pool. This will facilitate visualization of the passage of contrast medium and enable partial measurement of the magnitude of right-to-left shunting.

4. Although some patients demonstrate shunting spontaneously during the cardiac cycle, in other patients it is necessary to provoke a reversal of the normal LA–to–

RA pressure differential. In awake patients, this can be achieved by a cough or the release of the Valsalva maneuver after opacification of the RA. In anesthetized patients, the pressure reversal can be obtained after the release of sustained positive airway pressure. After the release of positive airway pressure, systemic venous return increases markedly and RA pressure can exceed LA pressure, driving the contrast medium from the RA to the LA. In the intraoperative setting, the RA and pulmonary capillary wedge pressures can be monitored to ensure that the pressure reversal occurs. Alternatively, the curvature of the interatrial septum can be used to gauge the RA–to–LA pressure gradient. Normally, the septum bulges into the RA. Because

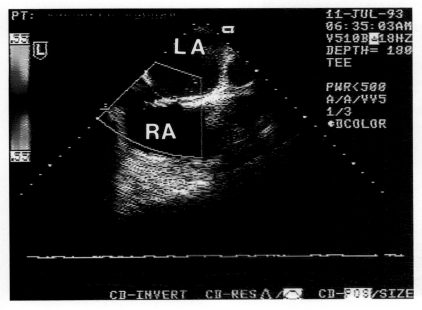

FIGURE 28.7. Mid-esophageal bicaval view with a small jet of left-to-right flow through a patent foramen ovale. *RA*, right atrium; *LA*, left atrium. (With a multiplane probe, this view would be obtained at about 90 degrees.)

the RA pressure transiently exceeds the LA pressure during provocative maneuvers, the septum bulges transiently into the LA.

In the absence of pressure reversal, the diagnosis is uncertain, and in some patients with elevated LA pressure (e.g., those with left ventricular failure or mitral regurgitation), respiratory maneuvers are insufficient to reverse the transatrial septal pressure differential. In these patients, color flow mapping is the preferred technique for detecting left-to-right shunting across a patent foramen ovale (Fig. 28.4). In the evaluation of hypoxemia, it is not merely the presence of a patent foramen ovale that is important, but the amount of contrast medium that passes into the LA. Thus, the density of contrast medium in the RV should be compared with that in the LA. If the interatrial shunt is causing the hypoxemia, the two chambers will be similarly opaque. If there are only a few

microbubbles in the LA, it is unlikely that the interatrial shunt is responsible for the hypoxemia (Fig. 28.8).

Pulmonary Vasculature

After the donor lung has been implanted and blood flow and respiration are resumed, it may be necessary to examine the anastomoses to ensure that there are no obstructions to blood flow. When a single-lung transplantation is performed, the arterial anastomosis is located on the proximal ipsilateral main branch of the pulmonary artery. Transesophageal echocardiography has been reported to show 100% of right pulmonary artery anastomoses and 71% of left pulmonary artery anastomoses (25). Color flow mapping at the suture line can illustrate an area of turbulent flow. In double-lung transplantations, the arterial suture line is on the main

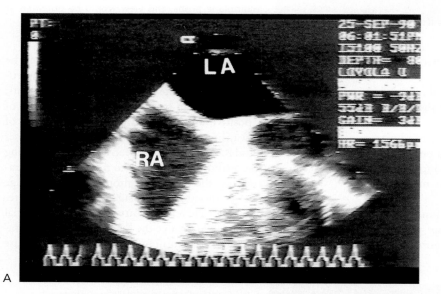

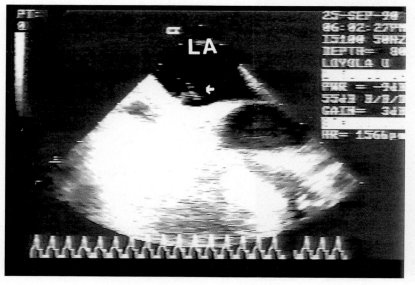

FIGURE 28.8. Two examples of contrast-proven patent foramen ovale. **A and C:** Images obtained before the injection of contrast medium. **B and D:** Images obtained after the injection of contrast medium. Note the significant difference in the amount of right-to-left passage of contrast medium (*arrows*).   *(continued)*

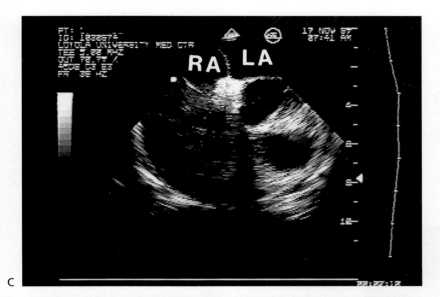

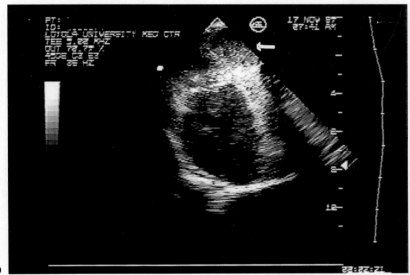

FIGURE 28.8. (*continued*) In the first patient **(B)**, there is only a small amount of contrast medium in the left atrium (*LA*), but in the second patient **(D)**, there is near-total opacification of the left atrium. The second patient had severe hypoxemia because of this right-to-left shunting. *RA*, right atrium.

pulmonary artery. Thus, it often can be seen easily on the ascending aortic SAX view. Furthermore, because of the parallel alignment of the Doppler beam to flow, pulsed-wave Doppler evaluation can be performed above and below the suture line to measure a gradient across the anastomosis.

The venous connections are performed with an atrial cuff in the region of the native pulmonary veins and almost always are visible by TEE. The four main pulmonary veins can be found in the following views. In 0 degree imaging, advancement of the probe an additional 1 to 2 cm deeper than the pulmonary artery view brings the LA and RVOT into view. Anteflexion of the probe usually is necessary. The LA appendage and left upper pulmonary vein are visualized as the probe is rotated slightly counterclockwise (Fig. 28.9). The right upper pulmonary vein is visualized as the probe is rotated slightly clockwise. Advancement of the probe

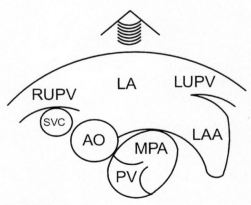

FIGURE 28.9. Diagrammatic representation of the 0 degree plane views of the upper pulmonary veins. *LA*, left atrium; *RUPV*, right upper pulmonary vein; *LUPV*, left upper pulmonary vein; *LAA*, left atrial appendage; *MPA*, main pulmonary artery; *PV*, pulmonic valve; *AO*, aorta; *SVC*, superior vena cava.

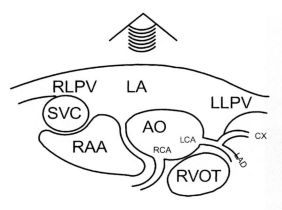

FIGURE 28.10. Diagrammatic representation of the 0 degree imaging views of the lower pulmonary veins. *LA*, left atrium; *RLPV*, right lower pulmonary vein; *LLPV*, left lower pulmonary vein; *RAA*, right atrial appendage; *AO*, aorta; *SVC*, superior vena cava; *RVOT*, right ventricular outflow tract; *RCA*, right coronary artery; *LCA*, left main coronary artery; *LAD*, left anterior descending artery; *CX*, circumflex artery.

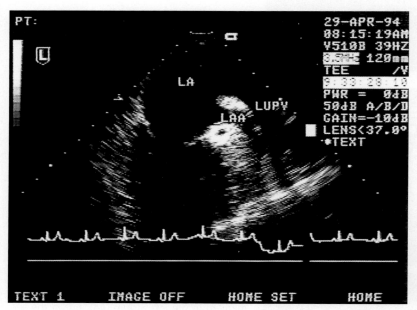

FIGURE 28.11. Mid-esophageal two-chamber view of the left upper pulmonary vein (*LUPV*). *LA*, left atrium; *LAA*, left atrial appendage. (With a multiplane probe, this view would be obtained at about 90 degrees.)

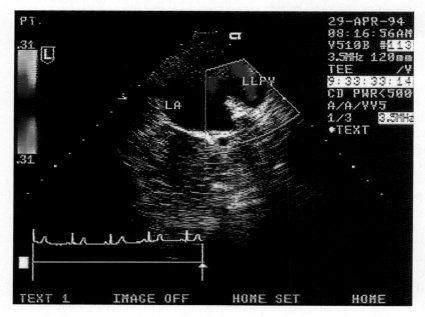

FIGURE 28.12. Mid-esophageal two-chamber view of the left lower pulmonary vein (*LLPV*) obtained by rotating the probe counterclockwise from the view seen in Fig. 28.11. *LA*, left atrium. (With a multiplane probe, this view would be obtained at about 90 degrees.)

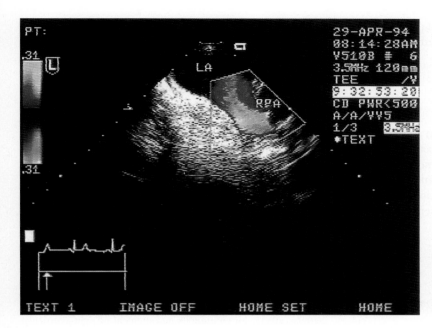

FIGURE 28.13. Modified bicaval view of the right upper pulmonary vein as it enters the left atrium (*LA*) near the right pulmonary artery (*RPA*) obtained by rotating the probe clockwise past the bicaval view. (With a multiplane probe, this view would be obtained at about 90 degrees.)

another 1 to 2 cm brings the coronary arteries and RA appendage into view. The left lower pulmonary vein is seen by rotating the probe counterclockwise, and the right lower pulmonary vein and superior vena cava are seen by rotating it clockwise (Fig. 28.10). Additional views of the pulmonary veins can be obtained in the 90 degree imaging plane (Figs. 28.11–28.14). The left-sided veins can be visualized in variations of the ME long-axis two-chamber view, and the right-sided veins can be visualized by extreme clockwise rotation of the probe from this position.

Once the vein is visualized, three parameters should be examined: diameter, color flow pattern, and pulsed-wave profile. In single-lung transplantations, the diameter and mean pulmonary venous velocity are greater in the allograft (26). In addition, the blood flow measured by echocardiography (the product of the velocity times the diameter) closely correlates ($r = 0.94$) with the values obtained by lung perfusion studies. In addition to anastomotic problems, it is possible for thrombus to obstruct pulmonary venous flow (27). In one study of 87 adult lung transplantation patients, TEE detected early thrombosis in 15% of the patients (28). This can be seen by two-dimensional imaging of the transplanted pulmonary veins and with turbulent color flow. Also, the lack of increased flow in the transplanted lung may be

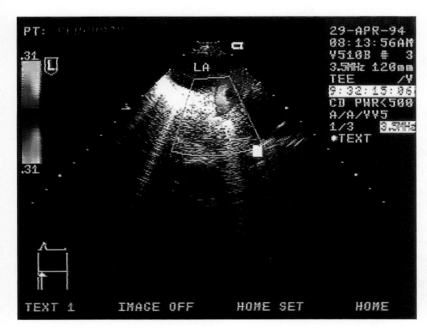

FIGURE 28.14. View of the right lower pulmonary vein obtained by rotating the probe clockwise from the view seen in Fig. 28.13. *LA*, left atrium. (With a multiplane probe, this view would be obtained at about 90 degrees.)

a sign of thrombosis (29). In the event of severe posttransplantation hypoxia, these techniques can be used to assess allograft blood flow.

CONCLUSION

Providing anesthesia for lung transplantation is an extremely difficult challenge. The intraoperative TEE examination should evaluate RV function, tricuspid and pulmonic valve competence, interatrial and interventricular septal continuity, and the anastomotic sites. This valuable physiologic and anatomic information can facilitate the management of these challenging patients.

KEY POINTS

- Lung transplantation is a family of operations on critically ill patients.
- Transesophageal echocardiographic examination of these patients should include the RV, the tricuspid valve, the interatrial septum, and the pulmonary veins.
- Postoperatively, TEE can aid in the diagnosis and management of ventricular failure and the differential diagnosis of hypoxemia.
- Right ventricular function is best evaluated by geometry independent or semiquantitative means.
- Right-to-left shunting through a PFO can be detected by contrast echocardiography.
- Pulmonary vein thrombosis can be readily detected by a comprehensive two-dimensional and color interrogation of the pulmonary veins.

REFERENCES

1. Schant RC, Silverman ME.Anatomy of the heart. In: Hurst JW, ed. *The heart.* New York: McGraw-Hill, 1986:16.
2. Sweeny LJ, Rosenquist GC. The normal anatomy of the atrial septum. *Am Heart J* 1979;98:194.
3. Drexler M, Erbel R, Muller U, et al. Measurement of intracardiac dimensions and structures in normal young adult subjects by transesophageal echocardiography. *Am J Cardiol* 1990;65:1491.
4. Aebisher N, Czegledgy F. Determination of right ventricular volume by two-dimensional echocardiography with a crescenteric model. *J Am Soc Echocardiogr* 1989;2:110.
5. Tomita M, Masuda H, Sumi T, et al. Estimation of right ventricular volume by modified echocardiographic subtraction method. *Am Heart J* 1992;123:1011.
6. Rafferty T, Durkin M, Harris S, et al. Transesophageal two-dimensional echocardiographic analysis of right ventricular systolic performance indices during coronary artery bypass grafting. *J Cardiothorac Vasc Anesth* 1993;7:1160.
7. **Kaul S, Tei C, Hopkins JM, et al. Assessment of right ventricular function using two-dimensional echocardiography. *Am Heart J* 1984;107:526.**

8. Ellis JE, Lichtor JL, Feinstein SB, et al. Right heart dysfunction, pulmonary embolism and paradoxical embolization during liver transplantation. *Anesth Analg* 1989;68:777.
9. **Louis EK, Rich S, Levitsky S, et al. Doppler echocardiographic demonstration of the differential effects of right ventricular pressure and volume overload on left ventricular geometry and filling. *J Am Coll Cardiol* 1992;19:84.**
10. Beppu S, Tanabe K, Shimizu T, et al. Contrast enhancement of Doppler signals by sonicated albumin for estimating right ventricular systolic pressure. *Am J Cardiol* 1991;67:1148.
11. **Savino J, Troianos C, Aukberg S, et al. Measurement of pulmonary blood flow with transesophageal two-dimensional and Doppler echocardiography. *Anesthesiology* 1991;75:445.**
12. Dickstein ML, Jackson DT, Delphia E, et al.Validation of maximum acceleration of pulmonary blood flow as an index of right ventricular function in the dog [Abstract]. In: *Proceedings of the 14th Annual Meeting of the Society of Cardiovascular Anesthesiologists.* 1992:191.
13. Reich DL, Resnick A, Shore-Lesserson L, et al. Doppler assessment of right ventricular function [Abstract]. *Anesthesiology* 1992;77:110.
14. Heerdt PM, Pond CG, Kussman MK, et al. Use of a pulmonary artery catheter for continuous measurement of right ventricular pump function and contractility during single lung transplantation. *J Heart Lung Transplant* 1993;12:686.
15. **Katz WE, Gasior TA, Quinlan JJ, et al. Immediate effects of lung transplantation on right ventricular morphology and function in patients with variable degrees of pulmonary hypertension. *J Am Coll Cardiol* 1996;27(2):384–391.**
16. Gorscan J III, Redd SCB, Armitage JM, et al. Acquired right ventricular outflow tract obstruction after lung transplantation: diagnosis by transesophageal echocardiography. *J Am Soc Echocardiogr* 1993;6:324.
17. Kronzon I, Tunick PA, Freedberg RS, et al. Transesophageal echocardiography is superior to transthoracic echocardiography in the diagnosis of sinus venosus atrial septal defect. *J Am Coll Cardiol* 1991;17:537.
18. Morimoto K, Matsuzaki M, Tohma Y, et al. Diagnosis and quantitative evaluation of secundum-type atrial septal defect by transesophageal Doppler echocardiography. *Am J Cardiol* 1990;66:85.
19. Lechat PH, Mas JL, Lascault G, et al. Prevalence of patent foramen ovale in patients with stroke. *N Engl J Med* 1988;318:1148.
20. Gronert GA, Messick JM, Cucchiara RF, et al. Paradoxical air embolism from a patent foramen ovale. *Anesthesiology* 1979;50:548.
21. Black S, Muzzi DA, Nishimura RA, et al. Preoperative and intraoperative echocardiography to detect right-to-left shunt in patients undergoing neurosurgical procedures in the sitting position. *Anesthesiology* 1990;72:436.
22. Cucchiara RF, Nishimura RA, Black S. Failure of preoperative echo testing to prevent paradoxical air embolism: report of two cases. *Anesthesiology* 1989;71:604.
23. **Konstadt SN, Louie EK, Black S, et al. Intraoperative detection of patent foramen ovale by transesophageal echocardiography. *Anesthesiology* 1991;74:212.**
24. Louie EK, Konstadt SN, Rao TK, et al. Transesophageal echocardiographic diagnosis of right to left shunting across the patent foramen ovale in adults without prior stroke. *J Am Coll Cardiol* 1993;21:1231.
25. Hausmann D, Daniel WE, Mugge A, et al. Imaging of pulmonary artery and vein anastomoses by transesophageal echocardiography after lung transplantation. *Circulation* 1992;86:11251.

26. Ross D, Vassolo M, Kass R, et al. Transesophageal echocardiographic assessment of pulmonary venous flow after single lung transplantation. *J Heart Lung Transplant* 1993;12:689.

27. Sarsam MA, Yonan NA, Deton D, et al. Early pulmonary vein thrombosis after single lung transplantation. *J Heart Lung Transplant* 1993;12:17.

28. **Schulman LL, Anandarangam T, Leibowitz DW, et al. Four-year prospective study of pulmonary venous thrombosis after lung transplantation. *J Am Soc Echocardiogr* 2001;14(8):806–812.**

29. **Boyd SY, Sako EY, Trinkle JK, et al. Calculation of lung flow differential after single-lung transplantation: a transesophageal echocardiographic study. *Am J Cardiol* 2001;87(10):1170–1173.**

SUBJECT INDEX

Page numbers followed by *f* indicate illustrations; page numbers followed by *t* indicate tables.